P9-CKX-411

Handbook of Experimental Pharmacology

Continuation of Handbuch der experimentellen Pharmakologie

Vol. 71

Editorial Board

G. V. R. Born, London · A. Farah, Rensselaer, New York
H. Herken, Berlin · A. D. Welch, Bethesda, Maryland

Advisory Board

S. Ebashi · E. G. Erdös · V. Erspamer · U. S. von Euler · W. S. Feldberg
G. B. Koelle · M. Rocha e Silva · J. R. Vane · P. G. Waser

Interferons
and Their Applications

Contributors

J. A. Armstrong · A. Attallah · C. Baglioni · S. Baron · D. C. Burke
P. E. Came · W. A. Carter · E. De Clercq · V. G. Edy · E. C. Esber
K. H. Fantes · N. B. Finter · W. R. Fleischmann, Jr.
D. C. Gajdusek · J. A. Georgiades · C. J. Gibbs, Jr. · D. Gillespie
S. B. Greenberg · J. J. Greene · S. E. Grossberg · J. U. Gutterman
M. W. Harmon · N. O. Hill · H. E. Hopps · Y-T. Hou
P. M. Jameson · M. Krim · M. Langford · H. B. Levy
X-Y. Liu · P. I. Marcus · S. Panem · E. Pequignot · J. C. Petricciani
F. L. Riley · J. L. Sabran · A. D. Sagar · A. M. Salazar · D. S. Secher
J. J. Sedmak · P. B. Sehgal · R. A. Smith · H. Smith-Johannsen
G. J. Stanton · D. R. Strayer · D. A. Stringfellow · Y. H. Tan
J. L. Taylor · P. F. Torrence · P. O. P. Ts'o · P. K. Weck · D. A. Weigent
R. Wetzel · J. M. Zarling · K. C. Zoon

Editors

P. E. Came and W. A. Carter

Springer-Verlag
Berlin Heidelberg New York Tokyo 1984

Paul E. Came, Ph.D.
HEM Research Inc.
12280 Wilkins Avenue
Rockville, MD 20852, USA

William A. Carter, M.D.
Professor and Director, Clinical Research, Department of Oncology
Orlowitz Cancer Institute and Department of Hematology and Oncology
Hahnemann University of Health Sciences
230 North Broad Street
Philadelphia, PA 19102, USA

LIBRARY
FEB 28 1984
UNIVERSITY OF THE PACIFIC
415981
Science

With 78 Figures

ISBN 3-540-12533-7 Springer-Verlag Berlin Heidelberg New York Tokyo
ISBN 0-387-12533-7 Springer-Verlag New York Heidelberg Berlin Tokyo

Library of Congress Cataloging in Publication Data. Main entry under title: Interferons and their applications. (Handbook of experimental pharmacology; v. 71) Includes bibliographies and index. 1. Interferon – Addresses, essays, lectures. 2. Interferon – Testing – Addresses, essays, lectures. I. Armstrong, J. II. Came, P. E. (Paul E.) III. Carter, William A., 1938– . IV. Series.
QP905.H3 vol. 71 [QR187.5] 615′.1s [615′.37] 83-12436
ISBN 0-387-12533-7

This work is subject to copyright. All rights are reserved, whether the whole or part of the material is concerned, specifically those of translation, reprinting, re-use of illustrations, broadcasting, reproduction by photocopying machine or similar means, and storage in data banks. Under § 54 of the German Copyright Law where copies are made for other than private use, a fee is payable to "Verwertungsgesellschaft Wort", Munich.

© by Springer-Verlag Berlin Heidelberg 1984
Printed in Germany.

The use of registered names, trademarks, etc. in this publication does not imply, even in the absence of a specific statement, that such names are exempt from the relevant protective laws and regulations and therefore free for general use.

Product Liability: The publisher can give no guarantee for information about drug dosage and application thereof contained in this book. In every individual case the respective user must check its accuracy by consulting other pharmaceutical literature.

Typesetting, printing, and bookbinding: Brühlsche Universitätsdruckerei, Giessen
2122/3130-543210

List of Contributors

J. A. Armstrong, Department of Infectious Diseases and Microbiology, Graduate School of Public Health, A417, University of Pittsburgh, Pittsburgh, PA 15261, USA

A. Attallah, Bureau of Biologics, FDA, 8800 Rockville Pike, Bethesda, MD 20205, USA

C. Baglioni, Department of Biological Sciences, State University of New York at Albany, Albany, NY 12222, USA

S. Baron, Department of Microbiology, University of Texas Medical Branch at Galveston, Galveston, TX 77550, USA

D. C. Burke, Department of Biological Sciences, University of Warwick, Coventry CV4 7AL, Great Britain

P. E. Came, HEM Research Inc., 12280 Wilkins Avenue, Rockville, MD 20852, USA

W. A. Carter, Clinical Research, Department of Oncology, Orlowitz Cancer Institute and Department of Hematology and Oncology, Hahnemann University of Health Sciences, 230 North Broad Street, Philadelphia, PA 19102, USA

E. DeClercq, Rega Institute for Medical Research, Catholic University Leuven, Minderbroedersstraat 10, 3000 Leuven, Belgium

V. G. Edy, Flow Laboratories, Ltd., P.O. Box 17, Irvine, KA12 8NB, Scotland

E. C. Esber, Bureau of Biologics, FDA, 8000 Rockville Pike, Bethesda, MD 20205, USA

K. H. Fantes, Interferon, The Wellcome Research Laboratories, Langley Court, Beckenham, Kent BR3 3BS, Great Britain

N. B. Finter, Head, Interferon, The Wellcome Research Laboratories, Langley Court, Beckenham, Kent BR3 3BS, Great Britain

W. R. FLEISCHMANN, JR., Department of Microbiology, University of Texas Medical Branch at Galveston, Galveston, TX 77550, USA

D. C. GAJDUSEK, Laboratory of CNS Studies, NINCDS, National Institutes of Health, Building 36, Room 5B25, Bethesda, MD 20205, USA

J. A. GEORGIADES, Department of Microbiology, University of Texas Medical Branch at Galveston, Galveston, TX 77550, USA
Present address: Immuno Modulators Laboratories, Inc., 10511 Corporate Drive, Stafford, TX 77477, USA

C. J. GIBBS, JR., Laboratory of CNS Studies, NINCDS, National Institutes of Health, Building 36, Room A415, Bethesda, MD 20205, USA

D. GILLESPIE, Herbert L. Orlowitz Cancer Institute, Hahnemann Medical College, 230 North Broad Street, Philadelphia, PA 19102, USA

S. B. GREENBERG, Department of Medicine, Baylor College of Medicine, 1200 Moursund Avenue, Houston, TX 77030, USA

J. J. GREENE, Division of Biophysics, School of Hygiene and Public Health, The John Hopkins University, 615 North Wolfe Street, Baltimore, MD 21205, USA

S. E. GROSSBERG, Department of Microbiology, Medical College of Wisconsin, 8701 Watertown Plank Road, Milwaukee, WI 53226, USA

J. U. GUTTERMAN, Department of Clinical Immunology and Biological Therapy, M.D. Anderson Hospital and Tumor Institute, 6723 Bertner Drive, Houston, TX 77030, USA

M. W. HARMON, Department of Microbiology and Immunology, Baylor College of Medicine, 1200 Moursund Avenue, Houston, TX 77025, USA

N. O. HILL, President, Wadley Institutes of Molecular Medicine, P.O. Box 35988, 9000 Harry Hines Boulevard, Dallas TX 75235, USA

H. E. HOPPS, Bureau of Biologics, FDA, 8800 Rockville Pike, Bethesda, MD 20205, USA

Y-T. HOU, Institute of Virology, Chinese Academy of Medical Sciences, Beijing, China

P. M. JAMESON, Department of Microbiologie, Medical College of Wisconsin, 8701 Watertown Plank Road, Milwaukee, WI 53226, USA

M. KRIM, Head, Interferon Laboratory, Sloan-Kettering Institute for Cancer Research, 1275 York Avenue, New York, NY 10021, USA

M. Langford, Department of Microbiology, University of Texas Medical Branch at Galveston, Galveston, TX 77550, USA

H. B. Levy, National Institute of Allergy and Infectious Diseases, National Institutes of Health, Frederick Cancer Center, Bldg. 550, Frederick, MD 21701, USA

X-Y. Liu, Shanghai Institute of Biochemistry, Academia Sinica, Shanghai, China

P. I. Marcus, Microbiology Section U-44, The Biological Sciences Group, The University of Connecticut, Storrs, CT 06268, USA

S. Panem, Science Policy Fellow, The Brookings Institution, 1755 Massachusetts Avenue, N.W., Washington, DC 20036, USA

E. Pequignot, Department of Oncology, Herbert L. Orlowitz Cancer Institute, Hahnemann Medical College, 230 North Broad Street, Philadelphia, PA 19102, USA

J. C. Petricciani, Bureau of Biologics, FDA, 8800 Rockville Pike, Bethesda, MD 20205, USA

F. L. Riley, National Institute of Allergy and Infectious Diseases, National Institutes of Health, Building 5, Room B1–32, Bethesda, MD 20205, USA

J. L. Sabran, Department of Microbiology, Medical College of Wisconsin, 8701 Watertown Plank Road, Milwaukee, WI 53226, USA

A. D. Sagar, The Rockefeller University, 1230 York Avenue, New York, NY 10021, USA

A. M. Salazar, Vietnam Head Injury Study, HSHL-CI, Walter Reed Army Medical Center, Washington DC, 20307, USA

D. S. Secher, Laboratory of Molecular Biology, Medical Research Council Centre, Hills Road, Cambridge, CB2 2QH, Great Britain

J. J. Sedmak, Department of Microbiology, Medical College of Wisconsin, 8701 Watertown Plank Road, Milwaukee, WI 53226, USA

P. B. Sehgal, The Rockefeller University, 1230 York Avenue, New York, NY 10021, USA

R. A. Smith, Center for Neurologic Study, 11211 Sorrento Valley Road, San Diego, CA 91211, USA

H. Smith-Johannsen, Faculty of Medicine, Department of Medical Biochemistry, University of Calgary, Health Sciences Centre, 3330 Hospital Drive NW, Calgary, Alberta T2N 4N1, Canada

G. J. STANTON, Department of Microbiology, University of Texas Medical Branch at Galveston, Galveston, TX 77550, USA

D. R. STRAYER, Associate Professor, Institute for Cancer and Blood Diseases and Department of Hematology and Medical Oncology, Hahnemann University, 230 North Broad Street, Philadelphia, PA 19102, USA

D. A. STRINGFELLOW, Director of Preclinical Cancer Research, Bristol-Myers Company, P.O. Box 4755, Syracuse, NY 13221, USA

Y. H. TAN, Faculty of Medicine, Department of Medical Biochemistry, University of Calgary, Health Sciences Centre, 3330 Hospital Drive NW, Calgary, Alberta T2N 4N1, Canada

J. L. TAYLOR, Department of Microbiology, Medical College of Wisconsin, 8701 Watertown Plank Road, Milwaukee, WI 53226, USA

P. F. TORRENCE, National Institute of Arthritis, Metabolism, and Digestive Disease, U.S. National Institutes of Health, Bethesda, MD 20205, USA

P. O. P. TS'O, Division of Biophysics, School of Hygiene and Public Health, The John Hopkins University, 615 North Wolfe Street, Baltimore, MD 21205, USA

P. K. WECK, Immunology Section, Department of Clinical Investigation, Burroughs Wellcome Co., 3030 Cornwallis Road, Research Triangle Park, NC 27709, USA

D. A. WEIGENT, Department of Microbiology, University of Texas Medical Branch at Galveston, Galveston, TX 77550, USA

R. WETZEL, Senior Scientist, Chemical Sciences, Genentech, Inc., 460 Point San Bruno Boulevard, South San Francisco, CA 94080, USA

J. M. ZARLING, Associate Professor, Immunobiology Research Center, Department of Laboratory Medicine and Pathology, Mayo Memorial Building, University of Minnesota-Minneapolis, Box 724, Minneapolis, MN 55455, USA

K. C. ZOON, Division of Biochemistry and Biophysics, Bureau of Biologics, Food and Drug Administration, Building 29, Room 518, 8800 Rockville Pike, Bethesda, MD 20205, USA

Preface

Today, the basic mood of researchers and clinical investigators, both at the center and on the periphery of interferon studies, is optimistic regarding the future of interferons as therapeutic substances. Many also feel these polypeptides will prove invaluable probes in unraveling certain fundamental biochemical processes which control the life cycle and developmental pattern of many human cells. In contrast, only a year or two ago, this optimism had given way to an attitude almost of disenchantment as public and scientific expectations were raised steeply, then rapidly waned, as it turns out, prematurely. Both the multiple actions of interferons (a virtual cascade of biochemical reactions may be induced, as documented herein) and the high visibility of interferon research provided by the millions of dollars invested both by national health agencies and by multinational pharmaceutical companies, contributed to an upsweep in public attention to drug development probably unprecedented in this century. Virtually every oncologist, it would seem, was plagued by requests for the experimental agent, although they already had therapies of more proven value. As recently as 1980, even though interferon had achieved success against certain cancers and certain viral diseases, the variability in clinical results was seemingly ever present and little evidence emerged to suggest interferons could cure advanced diseases.

Why then the resurgence of an optimistic mood? There are almost always many elements which contribute to happiness, and this is certainly true of the broad frontier of interferon and its place in biochemical research and treatment. Still, we feel that certain descrete elements can be identified which, if you will, contribute to renewed expectations in interferons. These elements certainly include the rapid increase in basic knowledge of interferon; indeed, much of the information on the diversity of interferons has been elucidated in the last two years. Now, many of the actions of interferons can be reproduced by a set of biochemical reactions, sometimes termed the interferon "cascade", which is triggered by "mediating" substances whose expression is controlled by exposure to interferons functioning as hormonal modulators of critical cell functions. One of the main reasons for clinical variability – low purity of interferons in the various batches ised – has been addressed within the last year and largely solved. Indeed, not only can interferons be of complete biochemical purity when desired, but combinations of interferon molecules (hybrid interferons) can be produced in large yields, which often demonstrate an amplified effect much higher than that of the mixture of parent interferons. Additionally, amplifying compounds, of which modified double-stranded RNAs are the prototypes, can sometimes increase the effectiveness of interferon 50–100-fold. In addition to having their own intrinsic spectrum of biologic effects, they seem to function as catalysts of enzymes whose synthesis has been first triggered by cell exposure to the interferon polypeptide.

Thus, the optimistic mood of scientists regarding interferon seems to be well founded on a wide experimental basis. One purpose, then, of this volume is to catalog the current understanding of interferons from many different biomedical disciplines, indeed, those encompassing the whole range of topics from primary amino acid sequence to clinical application in various diseases. In so doing, we would hope to assist the growing community of laboratory researchers and students who many come to share our enthusiasm for long-term. in-depth study of the interferon systems.

PAUL E. CAME
WILLIAM A. CARTER

Contents

CHAPTER 5

Comparative Structures of Mammalian Interferons
K. C. ZOON and R. WETZEL. With 9 Figures

CHAPTER 6

Regulatory Control of Interferon Synthesis and Action
H. Smith-Johannsen, Y-T. Hou, X-Y. Liu, and Y. H. Tan
With 6 Figures

CHAPTER 7

Application of Recombinant DNA Technology to Expression of Human Interferon Genes
S. Panem

CHAPTER 8

The Molecular Mediators of Interferon Action
C. BAGLIONI. With 2 Figures

CHAPTER 9

The Cellular Effects of Interferon
J. L. TAYLOR, J. L. SABRAN, and S. E. GROSSBERG

CHAPTER 10

Interferon Induction by Viruses. P. I. MARCUS
With 8 Figures

CHAPTER 11

Interferon Induction by Nucleic Acids: Structure-Activity Relationships
P. F. TORRENCE and E. DE CLERCQ. With 4 Figures

CHAPTER 12

Production and Characterization of Human Leukocyte Interferon
N. O. Hill. With 2 Figures

CHAPTER 13

Lymphoblastoid Interferon: Production and Characterization
N. B. Finter and K. H. Fantes

CHAPTER 17

Manufacture and Safety of Interferons in Clinical Research
J. C. PETRICCIANI, E. C. ESBER, H. E. HOPPS, and A. ATTALLAH

CHAPTER 18

Nonpolynucleotide Inducers of Interferon. D. A. STRINGFELLOW
With 4 Figures

CHAPTER 19

Agents Which Modulate the Activity of Interferon
D. R. STRAYER and W. A. CARTER

CHAPTER 24

Clinical Investigation of Interferons: Status Summary and Prospects for the Future. J. U. GUTTERMAN

CHAPTER 25

Utilization of Stabilized Forms of Polynucleotides
H. B. LEVY and F. L. RILEY. With 9 Figures

CHAPTER 26

Therapeutic Applications of Double-Stranded RNAs
J. J. GREENE, P. O. P. TS'O, D. R. STRAYER, and W. A. CARTER
With 3 Figures

CHAPTER 27

Monoclonal Antibodies to Interferons
D. C. BURKE and D. S. SECHER

CHAPTER 1

Interferons and Their Applications: Past, Present, and Future

M. KRIM

A. Introduction

The interferons are powerful inducible effector molecules that can be produced by virtually all nucleated animal cells, and that can modify very basic biochemical processes in an exquisitely selective and reversible fashion. These attributes have long provided sufficient reason to lead one to believe in their importance to the proper functioning of organisms, and therefore also in their importance, ultimately, to the prevention and treatmant of disease.

The translation of such a belief into demonstrable clinical usefulness is an effort which has been possible, in the past, only on a very limited scale. Clinical trials with interferons are presently being considerably expanded to include their evaluation as therapeutic agents in several viral infections and cancers. That extensive clinical investigations can now be carried out is the fruit of over 25 years of painstaking, mostly obscure, basic research. Fundamental research must continue to be pursued vigorously because many questions remain to be answered before medicine can fully take advantage of the remarkable properties of the interferons. This chapter presents an overview of the road covered, the present exciting research achievements and clinical explorations, the course basic and clinical investigations may take in the foreseeable future, and their likely ultimate payoff.

B. Interferon Research: The Beginnings

A. ISAACS and J. LINDENMANN discovered the existence of chick interferon in 1957 through its ability to induce resistance to viral infections (ISAACS and LINDENMANN 1957). Largely for this reason, research on interferons has long been dedicated almost exclusively to the realization of their potential as medically useful antiviral agents. Such research was undertaken with high hopes, soon to be frustrated by difficulties that could not be overcome with the technologic know-how available in the 1960s. Interferons came then to be regarded by many as a curiosity, rather than a practical approach to antiviral treatment. Nevertheless, the impressively effective response of cells to interferons sustained the conviction, at least among a few, that there was here something of fundamental and perhaps momentous importance. And so a handful of laboratories persisted and set out to unravel the workings of a complicated cellular machinery at a time when molecular biology was in its infancy. Quantitative research was difficult with interferons which could be assayed only through their antiviral effect, measurable in relative units that varied from laboratory to laboratory. Particularly valuable, therefore, were those early efforts that led to the development of standard international reference preparations and so made comparisons of results possible between laboratories (FINTER 1973), and the demonstration that even in vivo, dose-related effects could be obtained reproducibly if timing and dose of interferon treatment were appropriate to kind and amount of challenge virus (FINTER 1966, 1967).

Interferon research remained hampered for a long time by difficulties in interferon production and by lack of sufficiently selective methods applicable to the purification of interferons. Prominent among the contributions to a solution of these problems was the finding that the most accessible normal human nucleated cells, the leukocytes, were capable of producing interferon (GRESSER 1961). Such cells were used thereafter in an admirable long-term effort dedicated to the development of the first dependable source of interferon preparations in substantial quantities, suitable for research on methods for their purification and for clinical studies (CANTELL et al. 1968, 1981; CANTELL and HIRVONEN 1978). The discovery that synthetic double-stranded RNAs (dsRNAs) were convenient and efficient inducers of interferon in vitro and in vivo (FIELD et al. 1967) stimulated later research, including early explorations of their clinical use (DE VITA et al. 1970).

The carefully timed use of metabolic inhibitors during interferon biosynthesis shed light on cellular control mechanisms (HELLER 1963; WAGNER and HUANG 1965; TAN et al. 1970; VILCEK and NG 1971) and resulted in a practical approach to the enhancement, or "superinduction", of interferon production by certain cells (HAVELL and VILCEK 1972). It became possible in the early 1970s realistically to plan for mass production of human interferons derived from leukocytes (CANTELL and HIRVONEN 1978; CANTELL et al. 1981), fibroblasts (HAVELL and VILCEK 1972), and established lymphoblastoid cell lines (FINTER and BRIDGEN 1977) for meaningful clinical investigations.

Concurrently, the study of cultured interferon-treated cells was revealing increasingly interesting facts. First came the discovery (paid little general attention at the time) that interferon could slow the rate of cell multiplication (PAUCKER et al. 1962). Later, it was found that interferons could affect the level of certain cellular enzymatic activities (NEBERT and FRIEDMAN 1973; GRESSER 1977b), the expression of cellular genes (GRESSER 1977b; LINDAHL et al. 1973), and immune functions, in vitro and in vivo (SVET-MOLDAVSKY et al. 1967; LINDAHL et al. 1972; DEMAEYER and DEMAEYER-GUIGNARD 1978). In recent years it was shown that interferons could modify cell structures (WANG et al. 1981) and that they were major physiologic regulators, through a positive feedback mechanism, of cells capable of killing virus-infected and tumor cells in the absence of antibody and independently of major histocompatibility antigen restriction (SANTOLI and KOPROWSKI 1979). Thus, starting a little more than a decade ago, the concept gradually emerged of the existence of an interferon system conserved through evolution – a very complex, highly regulated cellular mechanism that may have a physiologic role in both control of cell growth and function throughout the organism, and defense against viruses and aberrant cells, including, perhaps incidentally, neoplastic cells.

As soon as developments in techniques applicable to the study of biologic phenomena at the biochemical level provided the necessary tools, studies of the molecular events underlying interferon biosynthesis and actions resulted in a rich harvest of fundamental information. The translation of interferon messenger RNAs in

Xenopus oocytes and the possibility of characterizing the translation products as interferons (REYNOLDS et al. 1975) permitted the qualitative and quantitative study of these mRNAs, which heralded the application of recombinant DNA technology in interferon research, with far-reaching consequences. The finding that protein synthesis is strongly inhibited by dsRNA in extracts of interferon-treated cells (KERR et al. 1974) led to the description of two different dsRNA-activated pathways for such inhibition: a protein kinase pathway and an endonuclease pathway (SEN 1982) and to the discovery of novel, powerful inhibitors of protein synthesis, the oligoadenylates pppA(2′–5′) A_n whose synthesis is activated in interferon-treated cells (KERR and BROWN 1978). These advances are leading to an understanding of the mechanisms of interferon action at the molecular level.

As early as the 1960s, murine interferon preparations had been shown to be capable of slowing the growth, or altogether preventing the appearance, of different types of tumors in mice (GRESSER 1977a). At the time, few investigators outside the interferon field paid attention to these surprising findings. This can be attributed to others' inability to confirm them because no one could afford, or would take the considerable trouble to produce murine interferon in the quantities needed for doing so; in addition, skepticism due to an ingrained habit of thinking of interferons exclusively as antiviral agents caused the antitumor effect in the mouse to be imputed to an antiviral effect on murine tumor viruses. So, evidence obtained in Sweden in 1975 suggesting that leukocyte interferon administration may have been able to delay, or suppress, the recurrence of a highly malignant human disease, osteogenic sarcoma (STRANDER 1977), was greeted with much suspicion. And the observation, first reported in 1979 in the United States, that interferon treatment could induce the objective regression of several types of human tumors came as a major surprise (GUTTERMAN et al. 1980). This was deemed particularly remarkable because no tumor *regression* had ever been confirmed in mice; only slowed tumor growth, or delayed or suppressed tumor appearance, had been documented with animal tumors (GRESSER 1977a). The apparently greater susceptibility of human tumors to interferons should, perhaps, not have been so startling since neither the highly selected, highly malignant, transplantable murine tumor cells, nor the "spontaneous" neoplasms of inbred animal strains selected for extraordinarily high cancer incidence, are good models for rare spontaneous tumors occurring in humans. In the latter, the balance between host and tumor is far from being as inexorably skewed in favor of the tumor. Though unanticipated, interferon-induced tumor regression of human tumors was soon independently confirmed with two interferon-α (MERIGAN et al. 1979; OSSERMAN et al. 1980; BORDEN et al. 1980; PRIESTMAN 1980) and with interferon-β preparations (TREUNER et al. 1980), and the evidence became rapidly accepted as irrefutable (TYRRELL and KRIM 1981).

C. The Current Windfall in Interferon Research

Recent developments have occurred at an astonishing speed in interferon research. After being justifiably long considered one of the most complex biologic systems with which to work, in part at least because of the relatively cumbersome interferon activity assay, the interferon system turned out to be among the first to which new, highly sophisticated technologies in amino acid sequencing (Knight et al. 1980; Taira et al. 1980; Zoon et al. 1980; Okamura et al. 1980; Stein et al. 1980; Levy et al. 1980a; Levy et al. 1980b; Allen and Fantes 1980), recombinant DNA technology (Taniguchi et al. 1979, 1980; Nagata et al. 1980; Goeddel et al. 1980a, 1980b; Derynck et al. 1980), DNA sequencing and synthesis (Mantei et al. 1980; Lawn et al. 1981; Goeddel et al. 1981; Houghton et al. 1981; Degrave et al. 1981; Ohno and Taniguchi 1981; Edge et al. 1981), and hybridoma technology (Secher and Burke 1980; Montagnier et al. 1980; Hochkeppel et al. 1981; Staehelin et al. 1981; Nyari et al. 1981) could be applied in rapid succession and with complete success.

Attempts to apply new technologies to interferon purification and production were successful largely because (since even more than politics, research is the art of the possible) there existed a highly sensitive assay for the antiviral activity of interferons (Armstrong 1971; Rubinstein et al. 1981) and therefore also for products of interferon mRNA translation in *Xenopus* oocytes (Reynolds et al. 1975; Sloma et al. 1981). Not only have cDNA sequences coding for the three major human interferon antigenic types (α, β, and γ) now been cloned and expressed repeatedly in both prokaryotic and eukaryotic cells but, seemingly overnight, the fine organization of chromosomal interferon genes and the amino acid sequences of interferon polypeptides have become known. Genes for interferons-α and -β (not interferon-γ, surprisingly) have been found to share with the genes of some histones (interestingly also believed to be involved in the control of gene expression) the peculiarity of lacking introns (Houghton et al. 1981; Weck et al. 1981).

It had previously been documented that interferons-α and -β were products of distinct genes (Cavalieri et al. 1977) and that the active components of natural human interferon-α preparations were heterogeneous (Stewart and Desmyter 1975). Recent studies have revealed a surprising multiplicity of interferon-α species (Allen and Fantes 1980) and structural genes (Goeddel et al. 1981; Streuli et al. 1980; Nagata et al. 1981) most of which apparently code for functional, unique interferon polypeptides which are all "subtypes" of the α-antigenic type, "leukocyte" interferon. The existence of certain degrees of nucleotide and amino acid homology between human and mouse interferons has already led to speculations regarding the common origin of these genes, their evolutionary history, and the age of the interferon system itself (Streuli et al. 1980), a defense system which may be older than the immune system.

In addition to opening vast new research opportunities in molecular genetics and biology, the application of the new technologies has revolutionized the prospects for the medical application of interferons because these are now becoming available through industrial companies as products of recombinant organisms, in the form of pure single molecular species and in amounts the wildest dreams could not fathom as recently as 2 years ago. Furthermore, capabilities in the production and purification of "natural" interferons have also increased considerably over recent years. Leukocyte interferon [α (Le)] (Cantell and Hirvonen 1978) fibroblast interferon [β] (Clark and Hirtenstin 1981) and lymphoblastoid interferon [α] (Ly) (Fantes et al. 1980) produced by cultured human cells can now be highly purified and are now also available as highly purified preparations in quantities sufficient for extensive clinical investigations.

D. Clinical Applications

For interferon *research*, in both the laboratory and the clinic, the "future" is, indeed, "now" (FRIEDMAN 1981). For the *application* of interferons to the treatment of human disease, this is not yet the case, and therapeutic research with interferons, particularly in the field of cancer, has barely begun.

I. Viral Infections

Experiments on the prevention or treatment of human viral infections with interferon had an early start in 1962 with controlled studies in the prevention of human vaccination "takes" (SCIENTIFIC COMMITTEE ON INTERFERON 1962) and the treatment of vaccinial keratitis (JAMES et al. 1962), which clearly established its antiviral effectiveness in humans. However, it was only very much later that several trials involving the topical application of interferon preparations to the eye or upper respiratory tract demonstrated that they could be effectively prophylactic (MERIGAN et al. 1973; JONES et al. 1976; SUNDMACHER et al. 1976, 1978c; ROMANO et al. 1980; IKIC et al. 1981; GREENBERG et al. 1982; G. M. SCOTT et al. 1982) against infections by common viruses (herpes simplex virus, adenoviruses, and rhinoviruses) of public health importance. As of today, dosage regimens and methods of administration remain to be optimized for both sites. It is, nevertheless, foreseeable that the prevention and treatment of the common cold using intranasal interferon sprays may be one of the first authorized uses of interferon-α. And although it remains to be determined what additional contributions certain procedures (SUNDMACHER et al. 1978a) and/or antiviral chemotherapies (SUNDMACHER et al. 1978b) could make to interferon treatment of viral eye infections, combination therapies including interferon will soon result in useful ophthalmologic applications.

The systemic, as contrasted with topical, administration of interferons as antiviral substances has also already provided encouraging results. The infections studied in sizeable controlled trials have been varicella in children with cancer (ARVIN et al. 1982), varicella zoster in adult cancer patients (MERIGAN et al. 1978), and chronic active hepatitis B (GREENBERG et al. 1976; KINGHAM et al. 1978; WEIMAR et al. 1980; SCULLARD et al. 1981a, 1981b, 1982). In both infections due to varicella virus, benefits to patients were clear: dissemination of lesions and potentially lethal complications were significantly reduced by interferon treatment, as was the pain of postherpetic neuralgia in herpes zoster patients. In chronic active hepatitis B, several virus markers proved variously sensitive to interferon-α treatment and, in some patients, long-term treatment at appropriately high doses resulted in certain virus markers remaining suppressed long beyond the treatment period. However, what clinical benefit chronic active hepatitis B patients can derive from optimized therapy with interferon alone, and to what extent the interferon effect is superior to that of certain antiviral drugs, or could be enhanced by combination with drugs (SCULLARD et al. 1981b) or other therapies, is not yet clear. Interestingly, liver function was found to be improved in some responding patients (SCULLARD et al. 1981a), and infectious virus could no longer be demonstrated when their blood was administered to a highly susceptible test animal, the chimpanzee (SCULLARD et al. 1982). Given the considerable public health importance of chronic hepatits B infection and its very strong association with the development to hepatocarcinoma, this work should be pursued vigorously. Any contribution interferon could make, alone or in combination with other therapies, to a reduction in the incidence of chronic active hepatitis B and/or the infectivity of hepatitis B virus carriers would be very important.

Prophylactic interferon administration has been attempted in patients who were immunosuppressed in preparation for kidney transplantation. Such patients are at a very high risk of developing one or more life-threatening viral infections during a critical period prior to and following organ transplantation. These infections contribute importantly to graft-versus-host disease, graft rejection, and patient mortality. The administration of relatively low doses of interferon-α given twice or three times per week, for a total of 4–6 weeks during the period of high risk, was significantly protective against cytomegalovirus (CMV), and to a lesser extent against other viruses (CHEESEMAN et al. 1979; MEYERS et al. 1979). The contribution interferon prophylaxis may ultimately make to bone marrow and organ transplantation through improving the survival of transplant recipients will be clearly established through further work in this potentially rewarding area.

Interferon has also been administered prior to surgical resection of the trigeminal nerve done for the purpose of controlling tic douloureux, a painful spasm of the face. This treatment effectively prevented recrudescence and shedding of herpes simplex virus which commonly occurs following this operation. However, in this trial, it could not prevent later recurrences of herpes labialis lesions (PAZIN et al. 1979).

There can be little doubt regarding the eventual usefulness of interferons in the prophylaxis and therapy of certain viral infections. This will be of particular benefit to patients prone to such infections, such as cancer patients, who are often immunocompromised because of myelosuppressive treatments, malignancy itself, or both. Uncontrollable viral infections are the immediate cause of death of a significant proportion of patients with cancer (DILWORTH and MANDELL 1975; FELDMAN et al. 1975). Should interferons not prove sufficiently effective as single agents, antiviral drugs will be used in combination with them, since the drugs' mechanisms of antiviral action are different from those of interferons, and synergistic effects are possible (LEVIN and LEARY 1981; STANWICK et al. 1981). Interferons seem to have the advantage over drugs of not inducing the appearance of resistance in viruses. Recent evidence suggests that interferon-α may have suppressed the emergence of drug-resistant strains of herpesvirus when applied to herpes-infected cultured cells together with the antiviral drug, acyclovir (HAMMER et al. 1982).

II. Cancer

Regarding the treatment of cancer with interferons, all that is known for sure, as of today, is that in some patients, with certain diseases, the administration of certain doses of interferon-α or -β has elicited objective, favorable responses, i.e., that in some cases measurable, significant regressions of macroscopic tumors have been obtained and remissions have been induced (TYRRELL and KRIM 1981). This has now been reported for natural interferon-α (Le) (GUTTERMAN et al. 1980; MERIGAN et al. 1979; OSSERMAN et al. 1980; BORDEN et al. 1980; KROWN et al. 1981; MELL-

STEDT et al. 1979), interferon-α (Ly) (PRIESTMAN 1980), interferon-β (TREUNER et al. 1980; EZAKI et al. 1982) and, in a preliminary fashion, interferon-γ (GUTTERMAN 1982), as well as *Escherichia coli*-produced interferon-α A (Roche) (HORNING et al. 1982; GUTTERMAN et al. 1982). Responding tumors have been of widely different histologic types. However, even among patients with apparently similar kind and stage of disease, responses to treatment with any interferon have varied greatly: dramatic tumor regressions or remissions have been reported in only a few of them; many have had either partial or unimpressive, minimal responses and, in some others, tumor progression could not be slowed at all. Duration of interferon-induced remissions lasted from several weeks to more than 2 years. In some cases, remission could be reinduced following a second course of interferon treatment (LOUIE 1981; GUTTERMAN 1982; H. OETTGEN 1982, personal communication). The likelihood of a response to interferon treatment in any patient remains, in general, highly unpredictable. This situation reflects not only a continuing ignorance of the mechanisms of interferons' antitumor action and therefore of the clinical parameters of importance to such a response, but probably also the fact that regimens of treatment, as used so far, have not been optimal.

The first clinical antitumor trials with interferons undertaken in the United States were planned so as to answer the question of whether any human tumor was sensitive to interferon treatment and, if so, whether this could be observed as a suppression of tumor progression or, better, a reduction in tumor size. Therefore, the first trials followed the phase II trial design, i.e., they included small groups of patients with similar, objectively measurable disease and relatively good general status. Tissue-culture-produced, leukocyte interferon was used. Mainly because of the cost of the interferon preparations, treatment consisted of daily, relatively low dose ($3–10 \times 10^6$ U/day) intramuscular injections given over a relatively short period of time (usually for 4 weeks, sometimes somewhat longer) (GUTTERMAN et al. 1980; MERIGAN et al. 1979; KROWN 1981).

Antitumor activity having been objectively recorded in several such exploratory, uncontrolled trials, although not in all of them (KROWN et al. 1980), interferons entered developmental therapeutics. Clinical trials had then to proceed, systematically, starting with phase I trials whose purpose it is to establish the toxic and pharmacologic properties of the agent under study, including maximum tolerable doses. Phase I trials may involve single high doses given at long intervals of time, short courses of lower daily doses, or the administration of a small number of rapidly escalating doses until intolerable toxicity and/or side effects require cessation of administration. Usually, no patient is entered in a phase I trial who has not exhausted all likely beneficial, applicable modalities of treatment, because the agents under evaluation are still "unproven", and because there is limited probability, under the conditions of this type of trial, that patients will benefit personally from participating. Indeed, some chemotherapeutic agents, effective under optimized conditions of administration, have not shown any therapeutic effect under phase I trial conditions. Thus, patients entered in such early trials usually have advanced, uncontrollable disease and have been heavily treated previously.

In evaluating the data available today on antitumor responses to interferon treatment, it is important to remember that the majority of patients recently enrolled in trials of interferons have been, and still are, in phase I trials. Thus, far from reflecting the true, complete antitumor potential of interferons, today's data are more likely to reflect a "least response" to interferon treatment, and this only as measured through gross tumor regression in patients with advanced cancer. The broad and intensive research effort that will allow the interferons' full antitumor therapeutic potential to be assessed (including effects on prolongation of remission, prevention of metastasis, stabilization of disease, potentiation of other forms of therapy, etc.) remains to be done.

E. Looking Ahead

The research effort now necessary must involve extensive laboratory and clinical investigations. It requires, primarily, that the multifaceted biologic response of a tumor-bearing host to the tumor, and the susceptibility of each type of malignant cell to each aspect of this response, be studied in great detail in animal models and patients.

I. Tasks for the Laboratory

Research must include the study of phenotypic changes directly induced by interferons in normal, virus-infected, and tumor cells, such as in cell structures (WANG et al. 1981; BROUTY-BOYE et al. 1981), cell surface membranes (LINDAHL et al. 1973; FRIEDMAN 1979), cellular enzymatic activities (NEBERT and FRIEDMAN 1973; GRESSER 1977b; BAGLIONI 1979), and rate of cell multiplication (PAUCKER et al. 1962; PFEFFER et al. 1979). It must clarify how any or all these changes affect the behavior and, in particular, the tumorigenicity of cells (GRESSER 1971, 1977b; BROUTY-BOYE and GRESSER 1981; HICKS et al. 1981). Research must also further address itself to the changes interferons can bring about in host cells with cytotoxic potential for virus-infected and tumor cells (SVET-MOLDAVSKY et al. 1967; DEMAEYER and DEMAEYER-GUIGNARD 1978; BLOOM 1980; SCHULTZ 1980; HERBERMAN et al. 1981; ORTALDO et al. 1981), particularly autologous cancer cells, and the true significance, for the tumor-bearing host's ability to suppress the growth and spread of the tumor, of an activation of various cytotoxic cell populations. The activation of natural killer and other cytotoxic cells may represent an important, but hitherto still poorly understood, host-mediated component of the interferons antitumor effect.

Each cloned molecular species of interferon must be studied alone and also in combination with others. Although pure molecular species of interferon (αA, α_2) have been found to have in vivo properties, including antitumor properties, very similar to those of the natural interferon mixtures produced by human cells (HORNING et al. 1982; GUTTERMAN et al. 1982; SMOLIN et al. 1982), each subtype differs from others in structure and may also differ in the kind of activities it can exert (WECK et al. 1981), particularly, perhaps, in its affinity for, and activity on, different types of cells (STREULI et al. 1981). Structure–function studies remain largely to be done which may allow the selection of particularly effective types or subtypes of interferons for particular clinical situations, and/or the construction of molecules with properties superior to those of the natural interferon polypeptides.

The properties of interferons-γ (which have, so far, not been available in a state of purity) remain entirely to be explored in vitro and in vivo. This work is urgent since this true lymphokine is clearly distinct from interferons-α and -β in several respects such as amino acid sequence, antigenicity, and biologic activity. Highly impure preparations (rich in other lymphokines in addition to containing interferon-γ) have been more powerful growth suppressors (RUBIN and GUPTA 1980; BLALOCK et al. 1980) and antitumor agents in animals (CRANE et al. 1978) than interferons-α and -β. Whether this reflects a property of the interferons-γ themselves is a question, among many others, that needs an urgent answer.

Since clinical trials cannot be carried out with each and every known molecular species of interferon, in vitro correlates of in vivo interferon effects need to be discovered. Rapid in vitro tests with predictive value for various in vivo responses must be developed. The use of tumor cells derived from biopsy material and growing as discrete colonies in semisolid media (tumor stem cell clonogenic assay) shows some promise for testing the sensitivity of tumor cells to interferons (SALMON et al. 1981), but this assay system is likely to measure mainly direct effects on tumor cells, and not host-mediated effects. Assessment of the latter in vitro may require complex cocultivation schemes involving one or more subsets of effector and other cells derived from tumor-bearing hosts, the target cells being freshly derived from autologous tumors. There also remains to be developed an in vitro assay predictive of the ability of interferon molecules to elicit, sometimes, formation of specific antibody in patients (VALLBRACHT et al. 1981; J. GUTTERMAN 1981, personal communication). Whether such occurrences represent a form of autoimmunity or an immune response to molecules which have lost their native conformation, remains to be established. Though relatively rare, such cases cause justifiable worry.

II. Challenges for Clinical Investigators

Clinicals trials with various interferons will continue at an accelerating pace, spurred by competitiveness among the industrial interferon producers who have begun sponsoring them. Standard early trials will provide information on interferon-induced side effects and highest tolerable doses (phase I), and will screen various neoplastic diseases for relative sensitivity to the antitumor effect of interferons (phase II). As for phase III trials – designed to arrive at an optimum regimen of treatment for each kind and stage of disease – they will require much additional information to be derived from the laboratory, and they will last through the present decade and beyond.

Predictably, phase II and III trials with interferons will raise some difficult questions. Neither the maximum tolerable dose, nor the most prolonged continuous treatment, may be most effective with physiologic, biologically active agents, since biologic systems have feedback mechanisms, and interferon action may be self-limiting. There is evidence suggesting that tolerance to daily interferon administration could develop. This seems apparent for certain interferon-induced effects in vitro (GUPTA et al. 1981) and side effects in vivo (GUTTERMAN et al. 1980; LOUIE et al. 1981; KROWN 1981). For example, weekly or monthly short courses of treatment with high doses may prove more effective than daily doses given over long periods of time.

Physiologic substances do not have gross toxicity, but interferons do elicit significant side effects, which are unpleasant to patients. However, if these side effects are integral manifestations of a desirable biologic response, their control through medication could be counterproductive. Interferon-induced fever and chills are an example. On the one hand, elevated temperatures have been reported to potentiate several biologic effects of interferons in vitro (HERON and BERG 1978); if so, fever may be beneficial. On the other hand, interferon-induced fever may result from induction of prostaglandins (YARON et al. 1977) which appears to occur also in vivo since interferon-induced fever is controllable by indomethacin (SCOTT et al. 1981). The role of prostaglandins in human cancer remains to be clarified (GOODWIN 1981), but at least some of them may be part, or activators, of a feedback mechanism which shuts off the response of cells to interferons (DROLLER et al. 1978; BRUNDA et al. 1980; KOREN et al. 1981). If the latter is true in vivo, prostaglandin synthesis (and fever) may best be suppressed by the administration of inhibitors of prostaglandin synthesis. In an animal tumor system, indomethacin alone has been reported capable of suppressing tumor growth (JENKIN and SUNDHAREDAS 1981).

Following the administration of cytotoxic drugs, leukopenia reflects bone marrow depression and, as such, is alarming. Leukopenia following interferon administration may only partly be due to a reduced rate of cell multiplication in the bone marrow: its extent does not always correlate with the degree of thrombocytopenia, it is rapidly reversible upon cessation of treatment, and interferon-treated patients do not display an increased susceptibility to infections. In interferon-treated animals, changes in white blood cell distribution patterns in the organism, which can be mistaken for true leukopenia, have been observed (GRESSER et al. 1981). Furthermore, some clinicians believe that the extent of leukopenia observed in cancer patients during interferon treatment may correlate with response to treatment (GUTTERMAN et al. 1980). Thus, with regard to the side effects of interferons, clinical thinking (and standard protocols) may have to be revised in order to take into account the properties of these particular biologic response modifiers.

The selection of patients for phase II and III trials with interferons raises the question of the validity of data obtained in patients whose immune defense mechanisms have been compromised to various extents by prior cytotoxic treatments. Although such previous treatments apparently do not preclude a response (MERIGAN et al. 1979; BORDEN et al. 1980; GUTTERMAN et al. 1980; OSSERMAN et al. 1980; PRIESTMAN 1980; TREUNER et al. 1980; KROWN 1981; EZAKI et al. 1982; GUTTERMAN 1982; GUTTERMAN et al. 1982; HORNING et al. 1982; H. OETTGEN 1982, personal communication), it may well hinder it. Because interferons are immunomodulators and act at least in part through host-mediated mechanisms, the integrity of natural defense systems must be beneficial, if not essential, to a good response to interferon treatment in humans, as has clearly been shown in animals (GRESSER 1977a). Therefore, very early treatment with interferon in otherwise untreated patients would generally seem desirable. However, for ethical reasons, it may long remain impossible, in most cases, not to use first a proven, but perhaps immunosuppressive therapy.

The need for controls raises the same problem. Also for ethical reasons, the use of true placebo preparations in experimental cancer therapy is generally impossible nowadays. Therefore, phase II and III trials with interferons, as with all new drugs, will require their being tested first as adjuvants, so that patients serving as controls can receive treatment. Certain drugs currently used in cancer therapy have inhibitory effects on cellular metabolic processes that are required for a response to interferon. For the sake of a fair assessment of interferons in cancer therapy, careful attention will have to be paid to the mechanisms of action of the drugs selected to be given prior to, or in combination with them.

The study of in vivo interactions between chemotherapeutic drugs (or other therapies) and interferons is also important because it may lead to synergistic combination therapies. In laboratory animals, the use of certain cytoreductive (CHIRIGOS and PEARSON 1973; BEKESI et al. 1976; SLATER et al. 1981) or immunostimulating (CERUTTI et al. 1979) drugs preceding interferon treatment has produced antitumor responses which suggest not only lack of antagonistic effects, but the possibility of synergistic ones. The mechanisms of such synergisms remain unknown and deserve through study.

On the other hand, interferon treatment may inhibit, or enhance, the therapeutic and/or toxic effects of cell-cycle-specific drugs (R. L. STOLFI et al. 1982) and/or, through depressing the hepatic cytochrome P-450-linked monooxygenase system, have profound effects on the toxicity and therapeutic properties of many drugs (SINGH and RENTON 1981; SONNENFELD et al. 1982). Since cancer chemotherapeutic drugs may have a narrow margin of safety, such effects of interferons must be carefully investigated. The therapeutic properties of interferon-γ preparations must not only be tested with this interferon given alone, but in combination with preparations of interferons-α and -β. Probably because interferons-α/β and -γ bind to different receptors (BRANCA and BAGLIONI 1981), potentiation of their effects has been observed in vitro and in the mouse when they are used in combination (FLEISCHMAN et al. 1980).

Administration of interferons by systemic routes is now generally used in antitumor trials because the control of inoperable primary or metastatic lesions is a continuing, overriding need in cancer therapy. This need has also motivated the development and wide use of systemic chemotherapies. However, systemic administration may not always be the optimal route for interferons. Delivery of high interferon concentrations at the tumor site through intraarterial perfusion (HAWKINS et al. 1982) or direct infiltration of solid tumor masses (SAWADA et al. 1979; NAGAI and ARAI 1980; ISHIHARA and HAYASAKA 1980; PADOVAN 1981) may have distinct advantages in certain situations. Such routes of administration have shown promise and must be explored further.

F. Future Prospects

It has often been pointed out that no single overnight "breakthrough" is to be expected in the treatment of cancer. It is abundantly clear that this will hold true also for therapies making use of interferons. Although it is foreseeable, on the basis of evidence already at hand, that interferon treatment may have broad-spectrum efficacy in terms of the variety of sites where it can be effective and the histologic types of tumors susceptible to it, certain diseases will certainly yield sooner than others. For juvenile laryngeal papilloma and various forms of warts (as well as a variety of benign and premalignant tumors of viral etiology), response to interferon-α as single therapy has already been the rule rather than the exception (HAGLUND et al. 1981; UYENO and OHTSU 1980; BLANCHET-BARDON et al. 1981).

Interferon may therefore emerge as the treatment of choice for such diseases. This has started happening in Sweden, where juvenile laryngeal papilloma is now routinely treated with biweekly intramuscular injections of interferon-α produced in a local laboratory from human white blood cells, rather than through repeated surgery (H. STRANDER 1981, personal communication). Should, as a result of presently ongoing studies (K. CLARK 1982, personal communication; GUTTERMAN 1982, personal communication), this come to be considered desirable in the United States as well, this rare disease could easily be controlled with interferon-α produced, for example, by the New York Blood Center alone (K. WOODS 1982, personal communication). The treatment would cost far less in both money and human suffering than repeated surgical procedures.

Certain types of true neoplasms which have responded to interferon treatment in ongoing phase I and II trials are also emerging as being relatively sensitive to interferon-α therapy, such as nodular poorly differentiated or mixed lymphoma (MERIGAN et al. 1979; KROWN 1981; LOUIE et al. 1981; EZAKI et al. 1982; GUTTERMAN et al. 1982; HORNING et al. 1982; H. OETTGEN 1982, personal communication), and certain forms of malignant myeloma (perhaps only those involving secretion of IgA and Bence Jones protein, as opposed to IgG) (H. STRANDER 1981, personal communication). In those particular diseases, response rates to interferon-α treatment may be, now, in phase I and II trials, within the range of those obtained with established chemotherapeutic regimens (H. STRANDER 1981, personal communication). If and when interferon administration should become acknowledged as a superior from of therapy for any kind of malignancy, it will become possible to treat certain patients early in their disease, when "tumor load" is small and immune defense mechanisms apparently intact, conditions under which the stimulation of a vigorous host response may still be possible. Only then, it must be stressed, will it also be possible to start evaluating the true therapeutic potential of interferons as biologic response modifiers, when used alone, against certain forms of cancer.

Although it cannot be stated today with any degree of certainty that interferons will ever be sufficiently effective in the treatment of any cancer when used as primary, single therapy, it seems already possible to predict a significant role for one or more interferons in adjuvant therapy. They could effectively help host defense mechanisms "mop up" residual tumor cells and micrometastases which now escape surgery or cytoreductive modalities of treatment. The major shortcoming of current treatments, even when several modalities are given in combination or sequentially, is their still frequent failure to eliminate all neoplastic cells, and therefore their failure to protect patients from residual, often drug- and/or radiation-resistant cells, whose outgrowth is the cause of local and/or metastatic recurrences. Current cytoreductive treatment modalities and interferons appear to have completely different mechanisms of action. Interferon administration may: (a) restrain the tumor cells' malignant behavior; (b) slow tumor cell growth rate, and so reduce opportunities for genetic variation and the emergence of resistant cell clones; (c) stimulate cytotoxic cells to kill target tumor cells even though the latter may have developed resistance to drugs or radiation. Through all these effects, interferons may be able to contribute significantly to cancer cure rates achievable with current treatments.

The future availability of inexpensive and relatively nontoxic interferons in abundant amounts will also permit to contemplate experiments in secondary cancer prevention. In the mouse, interferon treatment has been quite effective in delaying or altogether suppressing the appearance of carcinogen-, radiation-, and virus-induced tumors (GRESSER 1977a). In humans, genetic or environmental conditions predisposing to cancer are known, in which prevention could be tried. Certain high-risk or premalignant states are readily identifiable in certain situations (BEKESI et al. 1982). Prospective studies involving interferon administration to several hundred such cases will not be out of the realm of possibility within the foreseeable future. Interferon-induced suppression of virus shedding by carriers of herpesvirus type II and hepatitis virus B, would, in all likelihood, in itself result in the prevention of many cases of cancer.

As for the role, in all this work, of human cell-produced, "natural" interferons (as opposed to cloned ones), a plea is made here as has been made by others (DUNNICK et al. 1981) for their continuing laboratory and clinical use for comparison purposes, and therefore also a plea for the survival of the laboratories producing them. The "natural" interferons can now be extensively purified and they remain, for the time being, competitive with cloned materials in terms of production cost. They may always remain research reagents, but they are essential to investigations of the physiologic role of the interferon system in health and disease and, perhaps, for the selection of effective "cocktails" of different single, clones interferon subtypes for optimal therapeutic use.

G. Possible Socioethical Problems

Looking, beyond the scientific and medical, to the sociological consequences of developments in applications of interferons to medicine, it is predictable that these will confront society with certain serious issues, as have other rapid advances in techniques with life-saving potential, such as, for example, renal dialysis. For a certain time to come, the public will experience a new "scarcity era" with respect to interferons. This is, of course, at odds with public expectations. The new scarcity will be due to an unavailability of interferons to patients who are not involved in clinical trials, imposed by regulations applying to the use of any experimental drug. It will not, as in the past, be a scarcity primarily due to limitations in production capabilities. In the foreseeable future, interferons will be available only to clinical investigators (as opposed to practicing physicians and patients), and then only for very specific research purposes. ("Compassionate" use of regulated agents in individual cases is authorized by the U.S. Food and Drug Administration, but it must be applied for and reported on, which, for all practical purposes, excludes its application to more than a handful of special cases.) Ethical, legal, and economic issues will be raised by the conflict inherent in the strictly limited availability of interferon preparations (for the sole purpose of accumulating data needed by investigators, producing companies, and regulatory agencies), while the public at large, and probably many physicians, will perceive them as having sufficient potential in the treatment of life-threatening diseases to warrant their immediate availability to terminally ill patients on the basis of equity and justice.

An American Cancer Society's press release in 1978, one that merely announced the award of a large grant for the purchase of interferon preparations destined for clinical trials, elicited on outpouring of urgent, pathetic requests for interferon. If, as is likely, a certain percentage of good – even if temporary – responses are obtained in serious malignant or viral diseases over the next few years, no matter how small that percentage may be, the clamor will rise again. When it comes from patients who have exhausted all available modalities of treatment, how will physicians, in a society that claims to be just and humane, be able, in good conscience, to justify not providing an essentially available material?

The problem will, paradoxically, be less acute if response rates to interferons become rapidly and clearly superior to those obtained with other available therapies. In the face of compelling evidence and public pressure, it is conceivable that regulatory agencies would waive certain requirements, at least selectively, and that governments would purchase interferon preparations and provide cancer centers with them, much as they often do today for costly experimental cancer drugs, so that virtually all patients who may benefit from the treatment may be able to receive it. But, much more likely, response rates will be low to start with and will improve only progressively. The public demand will not lessen if the odds of deriving true benefit from interferon treatment may be only one in five, and if that benefit may only be temporary. For terminally ill persons, one chance in five to liver longer are very attractive odds. Commercial companies and nonprofit laboratories (such as blood centers) involved in interferon production will not be able to offer their products to the tune of several thousand dollars' worth per patient requesting them. On the other hand, patients will not be able to buy interferon legally, and treating physicians will not be able to administer it freely, as long as it is not approved for general use. The danger that an illegal market will develop is real, in fact an "interferon black market" already exists on a small scale. It will grow, fed by the money of the desperate, and supplied with interferon preparations of doubtful quality. How wisely to deal with such a contingency is a matter which promptly requires more discussion (ANONYMOUS 1980).

H. Conclusion

Much basic and clinical research work remains to be done before interferons can be used effectively and predictably. Particularly with regard to the treatment of human cancer, the present decade will certainly go by before their effectiveness – whatever it might turn out to be – will have been thoroughly explored and optimized. However, in the course of this decade, the use of various interferons is likely gradually to develop into a new modality of treatment comprising several forms of single, adjuvant, and combination therapies, each tailored for the treatment of one or a few diseases from among a broad variety of acute and chronic viral infections, benign tumors, and malignancies. The evidence at hand today justifies the prediction that, eventually, these new forms of treatment will enter medical practice and bring significant benefit to many patients.

References

Allen G, Fantes KH (1980) A family of structural genes for human lymphoblastoid (leukocyte-type) interferon. Nature 287:408–411

Anonymous (1980) What not to say about interferon. Nature 285:603–604

Armstrong J (1971) Semi-micro, dye-binding assay for rabbit interferon. Appl Microbiol 21:723–725

Arvin AM, Kushner JH, Feldman Bachner RL, Hammond D, Merigan TC (1982) Human leukocyte interferon for the treatment of varicella in children with cancer. N Engl J Med 306:761–765

Baglioni C (1979) Interferon-induced enzymatic activities and their role in the antiviral state. Cell 17:255–264

Bekesi JG, Roboz JP, Zimmerman E, Holland JF (1976) Treatment of spontaneous leukemia in AKR mice with chemotherapy, immunotherapy or interferon. Cancer Res 36:631–636

Bekesi JG, Roboz JP, Fishbein E, Selikoff IJ (1982) Immune dysfunctions due to xenobiotics. Cancer Detect Prev 5:85

Blalock IE, Georgiades JA, Langford MP, Johnson HM (1980) Purified human immune interferon has more potent anticellular activity than fibroblast or leukocyte interferon. Cell Immunol. 49:390–394

Blanchet-Bardon C, Puissant A, Lutzner M, Orth G, Nutini MT, Guesry P (1981) Interferon treatment of skin cancer in patients with epidermodysplasia verruciformis. Lancet I:274

Bloom BR (1980) Interferons and the immune system. Nature 284:593–595

Borden E, Dao T, Holland J, Gutterman J, Merigan TC (1980) Interferon in recurrent breast carcinoma: Preliminary report of the American Cancer Society clinical trials program. Proc Am Assoc Cancer Res 21:abstract 750

Branca AA, Baglioni C (1981) Evidence that types I and II interferons have different receptors. Nature 294:768–770

Brouty-Boye D, Gresser I (1981) Reversibility of the transformed and neoplastic phenotype. I. Progressive reversion of the phenotype of X-ray-transformed C3H/10T ½ cells under prolonged treatment with interferon. Int J Cancer 28(2):165–174

Brouty-Boye D, Cheng YSE, Chen LB (1981) Association of phenotypic reversion of transformed cells induced by interferon with morphological and biochemical changes in the cytoskeleton. Cancer Res 41:4174–4784

Brunda MF, Herberman RB, Holden HT (1980) Inhibition of murine natural killer cell activity by prostaglandins. J Immunol 124:2628–2687

Cantell K, Hirvonen S (1978) Large-scale production of human leukocyte interferon containing 10^8 units per ml. J Gen Virol 39:541–544

Cantell K, Strander H, Hadhazy GY, Nevanlinna HR (1968) How much interferon can be prepared in human leukocyte suspensions? In: Rita G (ed) The Interferons. Academic, New York, p 223–232

Cantell K, Hirvonen S, Kauppinen HL, Myllyla G (1981) Production of interferon in human leukocytes from normal donors with the use of Sendai virus. In: Pestka S (ed) Interferons, part A. Academic, New York, pp 29–38

Cavalieri RL, Havell EA, Vilcek J, Pestka S (1977) Synthesis of human interferon by Xenopus laevis oocytes: two structual genes for interferon in human cells. Proc Natl Acad Sci USA 74:3287–3291

Cerutti I, Chany C, Schlumberger JF (1979) Isoprinosine increases the antitumor action of interferon. Int J Immunopharmacol 1:59–63

Cheeseman SH, Rubin RH, Stewart JA, Tolkoff-Rubin NE, Cosimi AB, Cantell K, Gilbert J, Winkle S, Herrin JT, Black PH, Russell PS, Hirsch MS (1979) Controlled clinical trials of prophylactic human leukocyte interferon in renal transplantation. N Engl J Med 300:1345–1349

Chirigos M, Pearson JW (1973) Cure of murine leukemia with drug and interferon treatment. J Natl Cancer Inst 51:1367–1368

Clark JM, Hirtenstin MD (1981) High yield cultured human fibroblasts on microcarriers: A first step in production of fibroblast-derived interferon (human beta interferon). J Interferon Res 1:391–400

Crane JL Jr, Glasgow LA, Kern ER, Youngner JS (1978) Inhibition of murine osteogenic sarcomas by treatment with type I or type II interferon. J Nat Cancer Inst 61:871–874

Degrave W, Derynck R, Tavernier J, Haegeman G, Fiers W (1981) Nucleotide sequence of the chromosomal gene for human fibroblast (2_1) interferon and of the flanking regions. Gene 14:137–143

DeMaeyer E, DeMaeyer-Guignard J (1978) Interferons and the immune system. In: Doria G, Eshkol A (eds) Immune system, vol 27. Academic, London, pp 213–226

Derynck R, Remant E, Saman E, Stanssens P, DeClercq E, Content J, Fiers W (1980) Expression of human fibroblast interferon gene in Escherichia coli. Nature 287:193–197

De Vita V, Canellas G, Carbone P, Baron S, Levy H, Gralnick H (1970) Clinical trials with the interferon inducer polyinosinic-cytidylic acid. Proc Am Assoc Cancer Res 11:21–30

Dilworth JA, Mandell GL (1975) Infections in patients with cancer. Semin Oncol 2:349–359

Droller MJ, Schneider MU, Perlmann P (1978) A possible role of prostaglandins in the inhibition of natural and antibody-dependent cell mediated cytotoxicity. Cell Immunol 39:165

Dunnick J, Merigan TC, Galasso G (1981) NIAID News: Report on a workshop on DNA recombinant technology in interferon cloning. J Inf Dis 143:297–300

Edge MD, Greene AR, Heathcliffe GR, Meacock PA, Schuh W, Scanlon DB, Atkinson TC, Newton CR, Markham AF (1981) Total synthesis of a human leukocyte interferon gene. Nature 292:756–761

Ezaki K, Ogawa M, Okabe K, Abe K, Inoue K, Horikoshi N, Inagaki J (1982) Clinical and immunological studies of human fibroblast interferon. Cancer Chemother Pharmacol 8:47–55

Fantes KH, Burman CJ, Ball GD, Johnston MD, Finter NB (1980) Production, purification and properties of human lymphoblastoid interferon. In: DeWeck AL, Kristensen F, Landy M (eds) Biochemical characterization of lymphokines. Academic, New York, pp 343–357

Feldman S, Hughes WT, Daniel CB (1975) Varicella in children with cancer: seventy seven cases. J Pediatr 56:388–397

Field AK, Tytell AA, Lampson GP, Hilleman MR (1967) Inducers of interferon and host resistance. II. Multistranded synthetic polynucleotide complexes. Proc Natl Acad Sci USA 58:1004–1010

Finter NB (1966) Interferon as an antiviral agent in vivo: quantitative and temporal aspects of the protection of mice against Semliki Forest virus. Br J Exp Pathol 47:361–371

Finter NB (1967) Interferon in mice: protection against small doses of virus. J Gen Virol 1:395–397

Finter NB (1973) The assay and standardization of interferon and interferon inducers. In: Finter NB (ed) Interferons and interferon inducers. Elsevier, Amsterdam, pp 135–170

Finter NB, Bridgen D (1977) Large scale production of human interferons and their possible uses in medicine. Trends Biochem Sci 3:76–80

Fleischman WR Jr, Kleyn KM, Baron S (1980) Potentiation of antitumor effect of virus-induced interferon by mouse immune interferon preparations. J Natl Cancer Inst 65:963–966

Friedman RM (1979) Interferons: Interactions with cell surfaces. In: Gresser I (ed) Interferon 1979, vol 1. Academic, London, pp 53–75

Friedman RM (1981) Interferons, a primer. Academic, New York

Goeddel DV, Shepard HM, Yelverton E, Leung D, Crea R, Sloma A, and Pestka S (1980a) Synthesis of human fibroblast interferon by E. coli. Nucleic Acids Res 8:4057–4074

Goeddel DV, Yelverton E, Ullrich A, Heymeker HL, Miozzari G, Holmes W, Seeburg TD, Dull T, May L, Stebbing N, Crea R, Maeda S, McCandliss R, Sloma A, Tabor JM, Gross M, Familletti P, Pestka S (1980b) Human leukocyte interferon produced by E. coli is biologically active. Nature 287:411–416

Goeddel DV, Leung DW, Dull TJ, Gross M, Lawn RM, McCandliss R, Seeburg PH, Ullrich A, Yelverton E, Gray PW (1981) The structure of eight distinct cloned human leukocyte interferon cDNAs. Nature 290:20–26

Goodwin JS (1981) Prostaglandin E and cancer growth: Potential for immunotherapy with prostaglandin synthetase inhibitors. In: Hersch EM, Chirigos MA, Mastrangelo MJ (eds) Augmenting agents in cancer therapy. Raven, New York, pp 393–415

Greenberg HB, Pollard RB, Lutwick LI, Gregory PB, Robinson WS, Merigan TC (1976) Effect of human leukocyte interferon on hepatitis B virus infection in patients with chronic active hepatitis. N Engl J Med 295:517–522

Greenberg SB, Hamison MW, Gueh RB, Johnson PE, Wilson SZ, Bloom K, Quarles S (1982) Prophylactic effect of low doses of human leukocyte interferon against infection with Rhinovirus. J Inf Dis 145:542–566

Gresser I (1961) Production of interferon by suspensions of human leukocytes. Proc Soc Exp Biol Med 108:799–803

Gresser I (1977a) Antitumor effects of interferon. In: Becker F (ed) Cancer A comprehensive treatise, vol 5, Chemotherapy. Plenum, New York, pp 521–571

Gresser I (1977b) On the varied biologic effects of interferon. Cell Immunol 34:406–415

Gresser I, Thomas MT, Brouty-Boye D (1971) Effect of interferon treatment of L1210 cells in vitro on tumour and colony formation. Nature 231:20–21

Gresser I, Guy-Graud D, Maury C, Maunoury M-T (1981) Interferon induces peripheral lymphadenopathy in mice. J Immunol 127:1569–1575

Gupta SL, Rubin BY, Holmes SL (1981) Regulation of interferon action in human fibroblasts: Transient induction of specific proteins and amplification of the antiviral response by Actinomycin D. Virology 111:331–340

Gutterman JN (1982) Presentation at UCLA symposium on molecular and cell biology, Squaw Valley, 10–12 March

Gutterman JN, Blumenschein GR, Alexanian R, Yap HY, Buzdar AV, Cabanillas F, Hortobagyi GN, Distefano A, Hersch EM, Rasmussen SL, Harmon M, Kramer M, Pestka S (1980) Leukocyte interferon induced tumor regression in human metastatic breast cancer, multiple myeloma and malignant lymphoma. Ann Intern Med 93:399–406

Gutterman JN, Fein S, Quesada J, Horning S, Levine JL, Alexanian R, Bernhardt L, Kramer M, Speigel H, Colburn W, Trown P, Merigan TC, Dziewanowska Z (1982) Recombinant human leukocyte interferon (IFLrA): a clinical study of pharmacokinetics, single dose tolerance and biologic effects in cancer patients. Ann Intern Med 96:549–556

Haglund S, Lundquist PG, Cantell K, Strander H (1981) Interferon therapy in juvenile laryngeal papillomatosis. Arch Otolaryngol 107:327–332

Hammer SM, Kaplan JC, Lowe BR, Hirsch MS (1982) Alpha interferon and acyclovir treatment of herpes simplex virus in lymphoid cell cultures. Antimicrob Agents Chemother 21:634–640

Havell EA, Vilcek J (1972) Production of high titered interferon in cultures of human diploid cells. Antimicrob Agents Chemother 2:476–484

Hawkins MJ, Borden EC, Cantell K, Wirtanen GW, Sielaff KM, McBain JA, Fox RW, Smith-Zaremba KM (1982) Phase I evaluation of human interferon α following intraarterial, intratumor infusion pharmacokinetic and immunologic analysis. Merigan TC, Friedman RM (eds) Interferons. UCLA symposia on molecular and cellular biology, Vol 25. Academic, New York, pp 407–420

Heller E (1963) Enhancement of Chikungunya virus replication and inhibition of interferon production by actinomycin D. Virology 21:652–656

Herberman RB, Ortaldo JR, Rubinstein M, Pestka S (1981) Augmentation of natural and antibody-dependent cell-mediated cytotoxicity by pure human leukocyte interferon. J Clin Immunol 1:149–153

Heron I, Berg K (1978) The actions of interferon are potentiated at elevated temperature. Nature 274:508–510

Hicks NJ, Morris AG, Burke DC (1981) Partial reversion of the transformed phenotype of murine sarcoma virus-transformed cells in the presence of interferon: a possible mechanism for the anti-tumor effect of interferon. J Cell Sci 49:225–236

Hochkeppel HK, Menge U, Collins J (1981) Monoclonal antibodies against human fibroblast interferon. Eur J Biochem 118:437–442

Horning SJ, Levine JF, Miller RA, Rosenberg SA, Merigan TC (1982) Clinical and immunological effects of recombinant leukocyte A interferon in eight patients with advanced cancer. J Am Med Assoc 247:1718–1722

Houghton M, Jackson IJ, Porter AG, Doel SM, Catlin GH, Barber C, Caray NH (1981) The absence of introns within a human fibroblast interferon gene. Nucleic Acids Res 9:247–266

Ikic D, Trayer D, Cupak K, Petricevic I, Prazio M, Soldo I, Jusic D, Smerdel S, and Soos E (1981) The clinical use of human leukocyte interferon in viral infections. Int J Clin Pharm Ther Toxicol 19:498–505

Isaacs A, Lindenmann J (1957) Virus interference: I. The interferon. Proc R Soc Lond B147:258–267

Ishihara K, Hayasaka K (1980) Treatment of malignant melanoma by intratumoral administration of human fibroblast interferon (HFIF). In: Conference on clinical potentials of interferons in viral diseases and malignant tumors, Jpn Med Res Found, Tokyo, 2–4 December

James BR, Galbraith JEK, Al-Hussaini MK (1962) Vaccinial keratitis treated with interferon. Lancet 2:875–879

Jenkin B, Sundharedas G (1981) Tumor growth inhibition by indomethacyn in mice. Abstr of the 10th annual meeting midwest autumn immunology conference, University of Minnesota, October

Jones BR, Costa DJ, Falcon MG, Cantell K (1976) Topical therapy of ulcerative herpetic keratitis with human interferon. Lancet II:128

Kerr IM, Brown RE (1978) ppA2′p5′A2′p5′A: An inhibitor of protein synthesis synthesized with an enzyme fraction from interferon-treated cells. Proc Natl Acad Sci USA 75:256–260

Kerr IM, Brown RE, Ball LA (1974) Increased sensitivity of cell-free protein synthesis to double-stranded RNA after interferon treatment. Nature 250:57–59

Kingham JG, Ganguly NK, Shaari ZD, Mendelson R, McGuire MJ, Holgate SJ, Cartwright T, Scott GM, Richards BM, Wright R (1978) Treatment of HBsAg-positive chronic active hepatitis with human fibroblast interferon. Gut 19:91–94

Knight E Jr, Hunkapiller MW, Korant BD, Hardy RWF, Hood LE (1980) Human fibroblast interferon: Amino acid analysis and amino terminal amino acid sequence. Science 207:525–526

Koren HS, Anderson SJ, Fischer DG, Copeland CS, Jensen PJ (1981) Regulation of human natural killing. I. The role of monocytes, interferon and prostaglandins. J Immunol 127:2007–2013

Krown SE (1981) Prospects for the treatment of cancer with interferon. In: Burchenal JH, Oettgen HF (eds) Cancer, achievements, challenges and prospects for the 1980s, vol 1. Grune and Stratton, New York, pp 367–379

Krown SE, Stoopler MB, Cunningham-Rundles S, Oettgen HF (1980) Phase II trial of human leukocyte interferon (IF) in non-small-cell lung cancer (NSCLC). Proc Amer Assoc Cancer Res 21:179

Krown SE, Burk M, Kirkwood JM, Kerr D, Nordlund JJ, Morton DL, Oettgen HF (1981) Human leukocyte interferon (HuLeIF) in malignant melanoma (MM): Preliminary report of the American Cancer Society clinical trials. Proc Amer Assoc Cancer Res 22:158

Lawn RM, Gross M, Houck CM, Franke AE, Gray PV, Goeddel DV (1981) DNA sequence of a major human leukocyte interferon gene. Proc Natl Acad Sci USA 78:5435–5439

Levin MJ, Leary PL (1981) Inhibition of human herpes viruses by combinations of acyclovir and human leukocyte interferon. Infect Immun 32:995–999

Levy WP, Rubinstein M, Shively J, DelValle U, Lai CY, Maschera J, Brink L, Gerber L, Stein S, Pestka S (1980a) Amino acid sequence of human leukocyte interferon. Proc Natl Acad Sci USA 78:6186–6190

Levy WP, Shively J, Rubinstein M, DelValle U, Pestka S (1980b) Amino-terminal amino acid sequence of human leukocyte interferon. Proc Natl Acad Sci USA 77:5102–5104

Lindahl P, Leary P, Gresser I (1972) Enhancement by interferon of the specific cytotoxicity by sensitized lymphocytes. Proc Natl Acad Sci USA 69:721–725

Lindahl P, Leary P, Gresser I (1973) Enhancement by interferon of the expression of surface antigens on murine leukemia L 1210 cells. Proc Natl Acad Sci USA 70:2785–2788

Louie AC, Gallagher JG, Sikora K, Levy R, Rosenberg SA, Merigan TC (1981) Follow-up observations on the effect of human leukocyte interferon in non-Hodgkins lymphoma. Blood 58:712–718

Mantei N, Schwarzstein M, Streuli M, Panem S, Nagata S, Weissmann C (1980) The nucleotide sequence for a cloned human leukocyte interferon cDNA. Gene 10:1–10

Mellstedt H, Bjorkholm M, Johansson B, Ahre A, Holm G, Strander H (1979) Interferon therapy in myelomatosis. Lancet I:245–247

Merigan TC, Reed SE, Hall TS, Tyrrell DA (1973) Inhibition of respiratory virus infection by locally applied interferon. Lancet I:563–567

Merigan TC, Rand KH, Pollard RB, Abdallah PS, Jordan GW, Fried RP (1978) Human leukocyte interferon for the treatment of herpes zoster in patients with cancer. N Engl J Med 298:981–987

Merigan TC, Sikora K, Breeden JH, Levy R, Rosenberg SA (1979) Preliminary observations on the effect of human leukocyte interferon in non-Hodgkin's lymphoma. N Engl J Med 299:1449–1453

Meyers JD, McGuffin RW, Neimann PE, Singer JW, Thomas ED (1979) Toxicity and efficacy of human leukocyte interferon for treatment of cytomegalovirus pneumonia after marrow transplantation. J Infect Dis 141:555–562

Montagnier L, Laurent AG, Gruest J (1980) Isolation of a cellular hybrid secreting an antibody specific for human leukocyte interferon. Compt Rend Acad Sci D291:893–896

Nagai M, Arai T (1980) Interferon therapy on malignant brain tumors. In: Conf Clin Potentials of Interferons in Viral Diseases and Malignant Tumors. Jpn Med Res Found. Tokyo, 2–4 December

Nagata S, Taira H, Hall A, Johnsrud L, Streuli M, Ecsodi J, Boll W, Cantell K, Weissmann C (1980) Synthesis in E. coli of a polypeptide with human leukocyte interferon activity. Nature 284:316–320

Nagata S, Brack C, Henco K, Schambock A, Weissmann C (1981) Partial mapping of ten genes of the human interferon α family. J Interferon Res 1:333–336

Nebert DW, Friedman RM (1973) Stimulation of aryl hydrocarbon hydroxylase induction in cell cultures by interferon. J Virol 11:193–197

Nyari LJ, Tan YH, Erlich HA (1981) Production and characterization of monoclonal antibodies to human fibroblast (β) interferon. In: DeMaeyer E, Galasso G, Schellekens H (eds) The biology of the interferon system. Elsevier, Amsterdam, pp 67–71

Ohno S, Taniguchi T (1981) Structure of a chromosomal gene for human interferon β. Proc Natl Acad Sci USA 78:5305–5309

Okamura H, Berthold W, Hood L, Hunkapiller M, Inoue M, Smith-Johannsen H, Tan YH (1980) Human fibroblastoid interferon: Immunoabsorbent column chromatography and N-terminal amino acid sequence. Biochemistry 19:3831–3835

Ortaldo JR, Timonen T, Mantovani A, Pestka S (1981) The effect of interferon on natural immunity. In: DeMaeyer E, Galasso G, Schellekens H (eds) The biology of the interferon system. Elsevier, Amsterdam, pp 241–244

Osserman EF, Sherman WH, Alexanian R, Gutterman JV, Humphrey RL (1980) Preliminary results of the American Cancer Society sponsored trial of human leukocyte interferon in multiple myeloma. Proc Am Assoc Cancer Res 21:Abstract 643

Padovan I, Broderec I, Ikic D, Kuezevic M, Soos E (1981) Effect of interferon therapy of skin and head and neck tumors. J Cancer Res Clin Oncol 100:295–310

Paucker K, Cantell K, Henle W (1962) Quantitative studies on viral interference in suspended L-cells. III. Effect of interfering viruses and interferon on the growth rate of cells. Virology 17:324–334

Pazin GJ, Armstrong JA, Lem MT, Tarr GC, Jannetta PJ, Ho M (1979) Prevention of reactivated herpes simplex infection by human leukocyte interferon. N Engl J Med 301:225–229

Pfeffer LM, Murphy JS, Tamm I (1979) Interferon effects on the growth and division of human fibroblasts. Exp Cell Res 121:111–120

Priestman TJ (1980) Initial evaluation of human lymphoblastoid interferon in patients with advanced malignant disease. Lancet I:113–118

Reynolds FH Jr, Premkumar E, Pitha PM (1975) Interferon activity produced by translation of human interferon messenger RNA in cell-free ribosomal systems and in Xenopus oocytes. Proc Natl Acad Sci USA 72:4881–4887

Romano A, Revel M, Gurari-Rotman D, Blumenthal M, Stein R (1980) Use of human fibroblast-derived (β) interferon in the treatment of epidemic adenovirus keratoconjunctivitis. J Interferon Res 1:95–100

Rubin BY, Gupta SL (1980) Differential efficacies of human type I and type II interferons as antiviral and antiproliferative agents. Proc Natl Acad Sci USA 77:5928–5932

Rubinstein S, Familletti PC, Pestka S (1981) Convenient assay for interferons. J Virol 37:755–758

Salmon SE, Young L, Stebbing L (1981) Antitumor activity of natural and cloned human interferons (IF) in the human tumor stem cell assay (HTSCA). Proc American Assoc Cancer Res, abstract no 1794

Santoli D, Koprowski H (1979) Mechanism of activation of human natural killer cells against tumor and virus-infected cells. Immunol Rev 44:125–163

Sawada T, Fujita T, Kusunoki T, Imanishi J, Kishida T (1979) Preliminary report on the clinical use of human leukocyte interferon in neuroblastoma. Cancer Treat Rep 63:2111–2113

Schultz RM (1980) Macrophage activation by interferon. In: Pick E (ed) Lymphokine reports, vol 1. Academic, New York, pp 63–97

Scientific Committee on Interferon (1962) Effect of interferon on vaccination in volunteers. Lancet I:873

Scott GM, Secher DS, Flowers D, Bate J, Cantell K, Tyrrell DAJ (1981) Toxicity of interferon. Br Med J 282:1345–1348

Scott, GM, Phillpotts RJ, Wallace J, Secher DS, Cantell K, Tyrell DAJ (1982) Purified interferon as protection against rhinovirus infection. Brit Med J 284:1822–1825

Scott GM, Phillpotts RJ, Wallace J, Gauci CL, Tyrrell DAJ, Greiner J (1982) Prevention of rhinovirus colds by human interferon Alpha-2 from *Escherichia coli*. Lancet II: 186–188

Scullard GH, Andres LL, Greenberg HB, Smith JL, Sawhney VK, Neal EA, Mahal AS, Popper H, Merigan TC, Robinson WS, Gregory PB (1981 a) Antiviral treatment of chronic hepatitis B virus infection: improvement in liver disease with interferon and adenine arabinoside. Hepatology 1:228–232

Scullard GH, Pollard RB, Smith JL, Sacks SL, Gregory PB, Robinson WS, Merigan TC (1981 b) Antiviral treatment of chronic hepatitis B virus infection. I. Changes in viral markers with interferon combined with adenine arabinoside. J. Infect Dis 143:772–783

Scullard GH, Greenberg AB, Smith JL, Gregory PB, Merigan TC, Robinson WS (1982) Antiviral treatment of chronic hepatitis B virus infection: infectious virus cannot be detected in patient serum after permanent responses to treatment. Hepatology 2:39–49

Secher DS, Burke DC (1980) A monoclonal antibody for large-scale purification of human leukocyte interferon. Nature 285:446–450

Sen GC (1982) Mechanism of interferon action: progress towards its understanding. Prog Nucleic Acid Res Mol Biol 27:105–156

Singh G, Renton KW (1981) Interferon-mediated depression of cytochrome P-450-dependent drug biotransformation. Mol Pharmacol 20:681–684

Slater LM, Wetzel MW, Cesario T (1981) Combined interferon-antimetabolite therapy of murine L1210 leukemia. Cancer 48:5–9

Sloma A, McCandliss R, Pestka S (1981) Translation of human interferon mRNA in Xenopus laevis oocytes. Methods Enzymol 79:68–71

Smolin G, Stebbing N, Friedlaender M, Friedlaender R, Okumoto (1982) Natural and cloned human leukocyte interferon in herpes virus infections of rabbit eyes. Arch Ophthalmol 100:481–483

Sonnenfeld G, Smith P, Nerland DE (1982) Interferons and drug metabolism. In: Merigan TC, Friedman RM (eds) Interferon. UCLA symposium on molecular and cellular biology, vol 25. Academic, New York, pp 329–340

Staehelin T, Durrer B, Schmidt J, Takacs B, Stocker J, Miggiano V, Stahli C, Rubinstein M, Levy WP, Hershberg R, Pestka S (1981) Production of hybridomas secreting monoclonal antibodies to the human leukocyte interferons. Proc Natl Acad Sci USA 78:1848–1852

Stanwick TL, Schinazi RF, Campbell DE, Nahmias AJ (1981) Combined antiviral effect of interferon and acyclovir on herpes simplex virus types 1 and 2. Antimicrob Agents Chemother 19:672–674

Stein S, Kenny C, Friesen HJ, Shively J, DelValle U, Pestka S (1980) Aminoterminal amino acid sequence of human fibroblast interferon. Proc Natl Acad Sci USA 77:5716–5719

Stewart WE II, Desmyter J (1975) Molecular heterogeneity of human leukocyte interferon: two populations differing in molecular weights, requirements for renaturation and cross-species antiviral activity. Virology 67:68–78

Stolfi RL, Martin DS, Sawyer, RC, Spiegelman S (1983) Modulation of 5-Fluorouracil-induced toxicity in mice with interferon or with the interferon inducer, polyinosinic-polycytidylic acid. Cancer Res 43:561–566

Strander H (1977) Interferons: Anti-neoplastic drugs? Blut 35:277–288

Streuli M, Nagata S, Weissmann C (1980) At least three human type α interferons: Structure of α_2. Science 209:1343–1347

Streuli M, Hall A, Boll W, Stewart WE II, Nagata S, Weissmann C (1981) Target cell specificity of 2 species of human interferon-α produced in Escherichia coli and of hybrid molecules derived from them. Proc Natl Acad Sci USA 78:2848–2852

Sundmacher A, Neumann-Haefelin D, Cantell K (1976) Successful treatment of dendritic keratitis with human leukocyte interferon. Albrecht Von Graefes Arch Klin Exp Ophthalmol 201:39–45

Sundmacher R, Cantell K, Hang P, Neumann-Haefelin D (1978a) Role of debridement and interferon in the treatment of dendritic keratitis. Albrecht Von Graefes Arch Klin Exp Ophthalmol 207:77–82

Sundmacher R, Cantell K, Neumann-Haefelin D (1978b) Combination therapy of dendritic keratitis with trifluoro thymidine and interferon. Lancet II:687

Sundmacher R, Cantell K, Skoda R, Hallermann C, Neumann-Haefelin D (1978c) Human leukocyte and fibroblast interferon in a combination therapy of dendritic keratitis. Albrecht Von Graefes Arch Klin Exp Ophthalmol 208:229–233

Svet-Moldavsky GJ, Chernyakhovskaya J, Yu I (1967) Interferon and the interaction of allogeneic normal and immune lymphocytes with L-cells. Nature 215:1299–1300

Taira H, Broeze RJ, Jayaram BM, Lengyel P, Hunkapiller MW, Hood LE (1980) Mouse interferons: Aminoterminal amino acid sequences of various interferon species. Science 207:528–530

Tan YH, Armstrong JA, Ke JH, Ho M (1970) Regulation of cellular interferon production: Enhancement by antimetabolites. Proc Natl Acad Sci USA 67:464–471

Taniguchi T, Sakai M, Fujii-Kuriyama Y, Muramatsu M, Kobayashi S, Sudo T (1979) Construction and identification of a bacterial plasmid containing the human fibroblast interferon gene sequence. Proc Jpn Acad 55:464–468

Taniguchi T, Buarente L, Roberts TM, Kimelman D, Donhan J III, Ptashne M (1980) Expression of the human fibroblast interferon gene in Escherichia coli. Proc Natl Acad Sci USA 77:5230–5233

Treuner J, Niethammer D, Dannecker G, Hagmann R, Neef V, Hofschneider RH (1980) Successful treatment of nasopharyngeal carcinoma with interferon. Lancet I:817–818

Tyrrell DA, Krim M (1981) Interferon. In: Hadden J, Chedid L, Mullen P, Spreafico F (eds) Advances in immunopharmacology. Pergamon, Oxford, pp 469–476

Uyeno K, Ohtsu A (1980) Interferon treatment of viral warts and some skin diseases. In: Conference on clinical potentials of interferons in viral diseases and malignant tumors, Jpn Med Res Found, Tokyo, 2–4 December

Vallbracht A, Treuner J, Flehmig B, Joester K-E, Niethammer D (1981) Interferon neutralizing antibodies in a patient treated with human fibroblast interferon. Nature 289:496–497

Vilcek J, Ng MH (1971) Post-transcriptional control of interferon synthesis. J Virol 7:588–594

Wagner RR, Huang AS (1965) Reversible inhibition of protein synthesis by puromycin. Evidence of interferon specific mRNA. Proc Natl Acad Sci USA 54:1112–1118

Wang E, Pfeffer LM, Tamm I (1981) Interferon increases the abundance of submembranous microfilaments in HeLa-S3 cells in suspension culture. Proc Natl Acad Sci USA 78:6281–6285

Weck PK, Apperson S, May L, Stebbing N (1981) Comparison of the antiviral activities of various cloned human interferon-α subtypes in mammalian cell cultures. J Gen Virol 57:233–237

Weimar W, Heijtink RA, Ten Kate FJP, Schulms W, Masurel N, Schellekens H (1980) Double blind study of leukocyte interferon administration in chronic HBsAg-positive hepatitis. Lancet I:336–338

Yaron M, Yaron I, Gurari-Rotman D, Revel M, Lindner HR, Zor U (1977) Stimulation of prostaglandin E production in cultured human fibroblasts by poly I · C and human interferon. Nature 267:457–459

Zoon KC, Smith ME, Bridgen PJ, Anfinsen CB, Hunkapiller MW, Hood LE (1980) Amino terminal sequence of the major component of human lymphoblastoid interferon. Science 207:527–528

CHAPTER 2

Assay of Interferons

S. E. GROSSBERG, P. M. JAMESON, and J. J. SEDMAK

A. Introduction

The definition of interferon (IFN) as a cellular protein capable of making cultured cells resistant to virus infection depends upon a biologic assay. The purpose of the assay is to determine biologic activity, or potency, in ways comparable to what has been done with antibiotics, vitamins, or hormones. The components of the IFN bioassay include suitable cultured cells, a virus that will replicate in these cells to provide a given effect or product, and the means to measure this. The attributes of an ideal assay are precision, reproducibility, objectivity, sensitivity, efficiency, rapidity, and economy of time, effort, and supplies.

In this context, there are two aspects of the assay which influence the observed precision: (1) the measurement of the viral manifestation or product; and (2) the determination of potency of replicate samples of IFN. Precision is evaluated by the degree of reproducibility, to wit, the demonstration that similar values can be obtained sequentially on different days in measurements of the same material. We shall avoid the term "accuracy" since it refers to the degree to which results approach the "true" value, which may be indeterminate. As discussed in Sect. C, unitage is relative, and the determination of how much IFN, is in a sample depends primarily upon the ultimate sensitivity of the assay. Assay "sensitivity" is the ability of the assay to determine some proportion of the IFN actually present. The term "titer" expresses, as in other microbiologic assays, the potency of a sample in terms of the highest dilution of the original material that manifests an endpoint. "Endpoint" can be defined as the arbitrarily selected point at which a given effect is achieved, in this case, a significant reduction in virus growth or effect. A "unit" can be defined either as the point to which a sample can be diluted to obtain and endpoint, or in proportionate terms relative to a standard having an assigned degree of potency (as discussed in Sect. C.III); the preferred expression of IFN unitage is one which relates it to an international reference preparation, if one exists. A titer is then expressed as a concentration of IFN, e.g., international units (IU) per milliliter of sample.

There are a number of variables in the assay, the most significant of which are the biologic fluctuations in cultured cells as they are propagated, the effects of biologic constituents of medium (especially serum), the conditions that influence the interaction of virus and cell, and the factors that influence the growth of both virus and cells. Inapparent contamination with mycoplasma or extraneous viruses certainly may alter assay results. Due consideration must be given to pH optima for IFN effect and viral growth as well as cell maintenance. In general, increasing the number of replicate cultures treated with a dilution of IFN increases reproducibility.

There are several factors in the selection of an assay that in part may depend upon the taste or background of the investigator. Conventional wisdom would suggest that an endpoint that must be determined by objective means, e.g., a spectrophotometer or enumeration of foci, would be preferred to a subjective one, such as visual appreciation of cytopathic effect (CPE), or that an assay that generates several data points to determine more precisely the slope of a curve would be preferred to one that does not. A compromise may often have to be made among different factors to select the most desirable assay for particular needs.

This chapter attempts to delineate the major types of IFN bioassays employed and the kinds of data they generate. It further addresses the approach to analyzing such data and how potency can appropriately be expressed in IU. Problems in standardization and derivation of standards are also addressed. Finally, the development of immunoassays and the problems they pose in relation to determining potency are discussed.

B. Bioassays

The various kinds of IFN assays have been extensively reviewed (FINTER 1973, 1977; GROSSBERG et al. 1974; GREEN 1977; OIE 1977; STEWART 1979), and detailed descriptions of a number of assays have been recently published in *Methods in Enzymology*, Vol. 78. We shall build upon earlier reviews in discussing the different kinds of IFN assays, especially more recently reported methods.

I. Cytopathic Effect Inhibition Assay

Currently, the most popular assays for IFN are variations of a method first described by HO and ENDERS (1959). These assays depend upon using a virus that causes extensive damage to the cultured cells (approaching 100%). The potency of an IFN preparation is then determined by its ability to prevent virus-induced CPE. The CPE can be assessed either subjectively or objectively.

1. Subjective Endpoints

An estimate of CPE is scored, usually by microscopic observation of each infected culture. Discontinuous scores usually cover the range 0 and integers from 1 to 4, corresponding to an intact monolayer, and 25%, 50%, 75%, or 100% destruction of the indicator cells. The titer of the interferon is usually taken as the reciprocal of the dilution of IFN which will allow only 50% destruction of cells. Although this kind of assay has been used with a wide variety of viruses, the most commonly used challenge viruses are vesicular stomatitis virus (VSV) and encephalomyocarditis virus (EMCV) because of their wide host range. These CPE inhibition assays have been used for most, if not all, species of IFNs (SELLERS and FITZPATRICK 1962; FANTES et al. 1964; WHEELOCK and SIBLEY 1965; KONO and HO 1965; BUCKNALL 1967; TILLES and FINLAND 1968; FINTER 1969, 1973; BILLIAU and BUCKLER 1970; BUCKNALL 1970; DAHL and DEGRE 1972; DAHL 1973; AHL and RUMP 1976; LVOV-

SKY and LEVY 1976; VIEHAUSER 1977; FERREIRA et al. 1979; STEWART 1979; FAMILETTI et al. 1981; RUBINSTEIN et al. 1981). CPE inhibition assays can be completed in 16 h if virus and IFN are added simultaneously, but the assay is 30-fold less sensitive than if IFN addition precedes virus challenge by 6 h or more (FAMILETTI et al. 1981). The time at which the CPE is observed is critical since IFN effect, i.e., the difference in CPE from the controls, can be gradually overcome, even within hours. Generally, infection is established with relatively low virus multiplicities, say 0.1–0.01 infectious particles per cell, requiring several cycles of virus replication to achieve significant CPE. The data generated are usually not satisfactory for constructing dose–response curves, since the IFN dilution interval is very small between full protection and complete CPE, making for very steep curves that do not permit comparisons of different slopes observed in other assays with different IFNs.

2. Objective CPE Inhibition Assays

The subjective element of viral CPE can be eliminated by measuring spectrophotometrically the amount of vital dye, such as neutral red, that is taken up by cells (FINTER 1969; PIDOT 1971; MCMANUS 1976; BORDEN and LEONHARDT 1977; DUVALL et al. 1980; WEIL et al. 1980; IMANISHI et al. 1981; JOHNSTON et al. 1981) or the binding of a dye such as crystal violet (gentian violet) (ARMSTRONG 1971, 1981). These dye uptake methods usually involve extracting the dye from the IFN-treated cells; IMANISHI et al. (1981) have reported a method in which the dye taken up by the cells can be measured without extraction.

Both the subjective and objective CPE inhibition assays can be done in microtiter plates so that large numbers of samples can be assayed simultaneously. However, microscopic recording of CPE can be tedious. DUVALL et al. (1980) have expedited the reading and recording of samples by using a spectrophotometer equipped with a sample programmer, a rapid sampler, and a thermal printer. EPSTEIN et al. (1981) quantitatively assessed IFN protection in a microtiter system by reading the absorbance due to eluted crystal violet dye at 550 nm with a Titertek Multiskan (Flow Laboratories, McLean, Virginia). The optical density of 96 samples can be automatically read and printed out within 1 min.

II. Plaque Reduction Assays

WAGNER (1961) first reported the use of a plaque reduction assay for chicken IFN. Generally, after cells are treated between 6 h and overnight with IFN, cultures are inoculated with a dilution of virus that will give a sufficiently large number of countable plaques to interpret the inhibitory effect of the IFN. After infection, the cells are overlaid with a solid or semisolid medium until plaques develop (1–3 days); the plaques can then be enumerated after adding a second solid overlay with a vital dye, such as neutral red, or the original semisolid overlay can be removed, and the remaining cells washed and then stained with crystal violet. The most commonly used challenge virus for plaque reduction assays has been VSV (WAGNER 1961; MERIGAN 1971; ROSSI et al. 1980). FERREIRA et al. (1979) found VSV, Sindbis virus, and poliovirus to be equally susceptible to human IFN in monkey Vero cells. FERREIRA et al. (1979), also found the plaque reduction assays to be more sensitive and reproducible than CPE assays with the three viruses mentioned.

Although plaque reduction assays are relatively precise and reproducible (OIE 1977), they are laborious, time consuming, and expensive. Further, they fail to take into account the IFN effect observable as reducing the size of plaques as well as the number. Like the CPE assays, the time of reading the assay is critical since "breakthrough", or appearance of previously unobservable plaques, does occur, reducing the difference from the controls. Sometimes, unintended variation of the plaque numbers results in too few or too many (uncountable) plaques to derive a valid IFN titer.

To overcome some of the difficulties associated with doing plaque reduction assays, CAMPBELL et al. (1975) devised a microplaque reduction assay for mouse and human IFNs, which gives titers comparable to those obtained with a macroplaque system. Although the microplaque assay requires less sample, less time, fewer cells, and is much less expensive than macroplaque assays for IFN, foci must be counted in a microscope (LANGFORD et al. 1981). GREEN et al. (1980) reported a rapid, quantitative, semiautomated microplaque reduction assay for human IFN. Semiautomated equipment was used for dilution and distribution of IFN samples onto cell monolayers. Although this assay can be completed 30 h from time of addition of IFN, it still requires visual counting of plaques.

III. Virus Yield Reduction Assays

In virus yield reduction assays, the ability of IFN to reduce the yield of infectious virus, viral hemagglutinin (HA), viral enzymes, or viral nucleic acid is measured. These assays generally use high multiplicities of challenge virus and determine the extent of inhibition of the viral parameter after a single cycle of viral growth.

1. Reduction in Infectious Virus Yield

These bioassays are based upon titration of infectious virus produced by IFN-treated cells and measured by plaque or CPE assay (FOURNIER et al. 1969; STEWART and LOCKART 1970; GALLAGHER and KHOOBYARIAN 1971; ITO and MONTAGNIER 1970; WEIGENT et al. 1981). These assays are laborious and expensive and thus are not widely employed, although because of their relative precision, as well as other attributes, they have been recommended for use in determining potency of international standards (GROSSBERG 1979; see Sect. B.V).

2. Hemagglutinin Yield Reduction

During their studies on viral interference which resulted in the discovery of IFN, ISAACS and LINDENMANN (1957) used the inhibition of influenza virus HA production to quantitate IFN. OIE et al. (1972) developed methods to measure IFN with the GD VII strain of mouse encephalomyelitis virus in mouse cells and Sindbis virus in human, chicken, and mouse cells. An improved method using Sindbis virus has recently been described by STANTON et al. (1981), in which the sensitivity of virus detection is increased by extraction of HA using Tween 80 and ether. Unextracted arbovirus HA can now be measured directly by using trypsin-treated human O erythrocytes (SEDMAK et al. 1983). An HA yield reduction method using EMCV has been applied to measurement of IFN in human, monkey, cow, pig, rabbit, cat, hamster, dog, and mouse cells (JAMESON et al. 1977; JAMESON and GROSSBERG 1981). EMCV HA yield is determined with human O erythrocytes. HA yield reduction assays are practical, sensitive, rapid, objective, reproducible, require no sophisticated instruments, and have been adapted to microtiter methods (STANTON et al. 1981; JAMESON and GROSSBERG 1981). The yield of EMCV HA is directly proportional to the amount of plaque-forming units (PFU) of virus produced, with about 10^6 PFU = 1 HA unit. In these assays, 1 U IFN is taken as the dilution that reduces HA yield by 70% (0.5 $\log_{10}$).

3. Inhibition of Retrovirus Reverse Transcriptase

Generally, to demonstrate an IFN-induced antiviral state, cells are treated with IFN prior to infection with a challenge virus. However, ABOUD et al. (1976) were able to circumvent the need for a challenge virus by measuring the inhibition of virus production in mouse NIH/3T3 cells chronically infected with the Moloney strain of murine leukemia virus. They measured virus production after exposure of cells to IFN by quantitating viral reverse transcriptase activity in the medium (incorporation of thymidine methytriphosphate ^{3}H into acid-insoluble material). This assay is reported to be simple, rapid, accurate, reproducible, and as sensitive as the VSV plaque reduction assay. SALZBERG et al. (1979) extended this assay to human IFNs by measuring reverse transcriptase activity in cells chronically infected with a feline retrovirus.

4. Neuraminidase Yield Reduction

The reduction in yield of influenza A virus neuraminidase is a sensitive and reproducible bioassay for various species of IFN (SEDMAK and GROSSBERG 1973 a; SEDMAK et al. 1975; SEDMAK and GROSSBERG 1981). A recombinant influenza virus X7(F1), of antigenic composition HON2, is used as challenge because of its wide host range and its ability to produce large amounts of neuraminidase. In some cultured cells, e.g., the human cells tested, the viral replication cycle of X7(F1) is incomplete, with the production of HA and neuraminidase, but no infectious virus. Various neuraminidase substrates can be used, but a synthetic substrate, methoxyphenylneuraminic acid, has greatly simplified the assay (SEDMAK and GROSSBERG 1973 b). One advantage of an enzyme bioassay for IFN is that if virus-infected cells produce low levels of enzyme, the yield of product from the neuraminidase substrate can be amplified by prolonging the incubation of enzyme with substrate until an acceptable quantity of reaction product is obtained for the virus-infected control cells not treated with IFN. A 30% inhibition endpoint was selected because it fell at the midpoint of the linear portion of the dose–response curve.

5. Inhibition of Viral RNA Synthesis

Several methods of assaying IFN based on inhibition of viral nucleic acid synthesis ($INAS_{50}$ method) have been reported. ALLEN and GIRON (1970) and GIRON (1981) measured incorporation of uridine ^{3}H into MM virus-infected cells in the presence of actinomycin D, which inhibits DNA-dependent RNA synthesis, but allows picornavirus RNA synthesis to proceed. At 6 h after infection, acid-insoluble radioactivity was determined. The endpoint is the dilution that inhibits incorporation by 50%. This method is reported to be three times more sensitive than a plaque reduction assay with VSV. VASSEF et al. (1973) employed reovirus as the challenge virus and measured incorporation of uridine ^{3}H into double-stranded RNA accumulated in infected cells. ISHITSUKA et al. (1977) measured incorporation of uridine ^{3}H into released VSV particles.

Several modifications have been reported for these kinds of assay in order to reduce handling and cost (MILLER et al. 1970; MCWILLIAMS et al. 1971; KOBLET et al. 1972; ATKINS et al. 1974; SUZUKI et al. 1974, 1981; RICHMOND et al. 1980). Even these modified assays still require considerable labor to wash and dry samples before they can be counted with a liquid scintillation counter.

IV. Other Assays

1. Hemadsorption Inhibition Assay

Hemadsorption is the adherence of erythrocytes to cells that are infected with either orthomyxoviruses or paramyxoviruses. FINTER (1964) was the first to use quantitative hemadsorption assay for IFN. IFN-treated cells were infected with Sendai virus. After 22–24 h, a suspension of erythrocytes was added to the infected cells for the erythrocytes to bind to cell membranes containing viral HA. The unbound red cells were washed away and the attached red cells lysed in water. The hemoglobin liberated from the lysed erythrocytes was then quantitated with a spectrophotometer. In this assay, 1 U IFN reduced extracted hemoglobin by 50%.

A hemadsorption inhibition assay for IFN that entails enumeration of hemadsorbing virus-infected cells has also been reported (HAHON and BOOTH 1974; HAHON et al. 1975; HAHON 1981). Cell monolayers on coverslips were treated with IFN and then challenged with Sendai virus; 22 h after viral infection, guinea pig erythrocytes were added to the coverslips and the hemadsorbing cells enumerated by microscopic examination. The endpoint for this assay is that dilution of IFN which depresses the number of hemadsorbing cells by 50%. Although this assay is simple, the microscopic enumeration of hemadsorbing cells is very time consuming when large numbers of IFN samples are assayed. A modification of the method uses ^{51}Cr-labeled erythrocytes to quantitate hemadsorption (EMODI et al. 1975).

2. Immunofluorescent Cell-Counting Assay

This assay combines histochemical and immunologic procedures to detect a specific viral antigen in cells. Antibody against a virus is coupled with a dye that fluoresces when excited by ultraviolet (UV) irradiation. BOXACA and PAUCKER (1967) and SAKAGUCHI et al. (1982) used an immunofluorescence assay to quantitate L-cells infected with VSV. The endpoint is the IFN dilution that reduces the number of infected cells by 50%. HAHON and associates applied this assay to human IFNs (KOZIKOWSKI and HAHON 1969; HAHON et al. 1975; HAHON 1981). Such assays have not been widely used, perhaps because antiserum has to be prepared against the challenge virus and the antibody conjugated to a dye such as fluorescein isothiocyanate. Additionally, a UV microscope is required to enumerate virus-infected cells. Immunofluorescent cell-counting assays for IFN are comparable in sensitivity to hemadsorption assays (HAHON 1981), and both kinds of assays generate dose–response curves which are parallel to each other with a given IFN.

3. Reduction of DNA Synthesis

EIFE et al. (1981) described a so-called unified assay for comparing the antiviral (AV) and antiproliferative (AP) effects of IFN, based on the reduction in DNA synthesis in IFN-treated, VSV-infected cells. The cells were treated with IFN for 24 h and then infected with VSV; 24 h after VSV infection, thymidine ^{3}H (TdR) was added to the cells for 3 h. The IFN dilution allowing TdR ^{3}H incorporation two standard derivations above untreated VSV-infected controls was considered as the AV titer inasmuch as, in the absence of IFN, the VSV would have killed the cells, thereby permitting only low levels of TdR ^{3}H incorporation. The IFN dilution allowing maximal TdR ^{3}H incorporation was considered as the AP titer since higher concentrations of IFN inhibited the replication of cells. As the authors indicate, this assay is not intended for routine use in comparing IFN potencies of large numbers of IFN samples, but might serve to compare AP : AV ratios of selected IFN preparations.

4. Other Assays of Limited Use

STEWART (1979) briefly discusses an agar diffusion method (PORTERFIELD 1959), pH indicator assays (PAUCKER 1965), cytochemical assays (SUELTENFUSS and POLLARD 1963), Epstein–Barr virus-expression assays (ADAMS et al. 1975), and various nonantiviral assays of several different types (see Chap. 9).

V. A Reference Bioassay

In 1978 at an international workshop held in Woodstock, Illinois, a reference bioassay was proposed to be used in collaborative studies on IFN standards (GROSSBERG et al. 1979). The reference assay recommended was an infectivity yield reduction assay with EMCV. This virus has a wide host range and low pathogenicity for humans. It is also stable, easily grown and assayed, and accepted for use worldwide. The cells recommended at that time were the human diploid fibroblast BUD-8 cell strain for assay of human IFN, L-cells for mouse IFN, and the RK-13 cell line for rabbit IFN; however, for human IFN a stable cell line that is sensitive to all three types of IFN, e.g., the A549 human lung carcinoma cells, may be more convenient than a cell strain.

The proposed assay consists of treating cultured cells with IFN for 16 h and then challenging the cells with EMCV at a multiplicity of infection of 3–5; after 7–8 h, or more conveniently overnight incubation, the infected cells are frozen. To determine virus yields, the frozen cells are thawed and tenfold dilutions of disrupted cells and supernatant fluids are added to several replicate cultures of cells per dilution of virus. After 36–72 h, virus yield is calculated for the sample and control by counting the cultures showing CPE and calculating a median tissue culture infectious dose ($TCID_{50}$). The IFN titer is taken as the reciprocal of the IFN dilution, determined from dose–response curves, that produces a 0.5 $\log_{10}$ reduction in virus yield.

C. Data Analysis, Unitage, and Standardization

I. Dose–Response Curves

To determine a unit of antiviral activity of IFN, an arbitrarily established decrease in some parameter of viral replication, or endpoint, is selected. Some assays establish this endpoint at the 50% level, that is, where the dilution of IFN reduces the virus activity to one-half that observed in untreated control cultures; other assays take the endpoint at the 0.5 $\log_{10}$ reduction level, or about one-third the amount observed in the untreated control cultures. An endpoint should fall reproducibly within the rectilinear portion of the dose-response curve. Calculations of endpoints by linear regression analysis of data or by interpolation assume, for the points used in the calculation, that a linear correlation exists between the dose and response. The IFN potency, or titer, is then expressed as the reciprocal of the dilution, thereby denoting the number of units per milliliter in the original sample. The volume of the IFN dilution (amount of IFN) added to the cells does not appear to be as important as the concentration of IFN in determining the effects on the cells. Potency is commonly reported as a concentration, namely U/ml, and as specific activity, i.e., U per milligram protein.

1. Construction of Graphical Representations

The graph is usually a log–log or semilogarithmic representation of the data, with the IFN dilution expressed as a logarithm or plotted on a logarithmic scale. The viral parameter may be expressed as a percentage, either plotted on an arithmetic or probit scale, or as $\log_{10}$ or $\log_2$ plotted on an arithmetic scale. For calculation of linear regression it is often convenient to use the natural logarithm, ln, of the IFN dilution and ln, $\log_{10}$, or $\log_2$ of the virus parameter. The resulting curve (extended by sufficient data points) is sigmoidal, with the estimation of endpoint made to fall within the rectilinear portion of the curve.

a) Cytopathic Effect Reduction

The endpoint of the IFN effect in the CPE reduction assay most frequently is obtained either by direct observation of the stained monolayers or by microscopic visualization of the IFN dilution corresponding to 50% destruction (ARMSTRONG 1981; FAMILLETTI et al. 1981). Because CPE appears and changes so abruptly as the IFN is diluted, it is difficult to construct satisfactory dose–response curves. More objective quantitation can be obtained by the dye uptake method of measuring surviving cells, using a photometric measurement with either crystal violet (ARMSTRONG 1981) or neutral red (JOHNSTON et al. 1981). The sigmoidal curves obtained in such assays have a very limited rectilinear portion that may encompass only two points of a 0.3 or 0.2 $\log_{10}$ dilution series usually used for this particular type of assay (JOHNSTON et al. 1981). Either very small dilution intervals such as 0.2 $\log_{10}$ should be employed, or a "point-slope" method used to calculate endpoints from the one or two points within the rectilinear portion of the curve. The latter calculation requires that all samples have dose–response curves with identical slopes; however, IFN samples of diverse sources or samples composed of multiple subtypes of IFN may not give curves with the same slope.

b) Infectious Focus Assays

Most of the assays depending upon the inhibition of the number of virus-induced foci employ the 50% endpoint for graphical analysis or mathematical interpolation. These techniques include the plaque reduction method (WAGNER 1961; LANGFORD 1981), hemadsorption and fluorescence detection of infected cells (HAHON 1981), as well as of cell transformation or "focus" formation by retroviruses (FITZGERALD 1969). Generally, the 50% reduction endpoint is made to relate to the dilution of IFN by either a semilogarithmic or probit plot of the percentage response versus the logarithm of the IFN dilution. A noticeable change in the shape of the dose–response curve results from the mathematical transformation from percentage to probit (JORDAN 1972), but this does not appear to affect the resulting estimation of IFN potency corresponding to the 50% endpoint. The recommendation for the use of a 73% reduction rather than 50% reduction as the endpoint is based upon statistical grounds to provide a more precise determination of endpoint, but gives a lower value for the titer (JORDAN 1972).

c) Yield Reduction Assays

The yield of virus or viral components (HA, neuraminidase, viral RNA, reverse transcriptase) is typically plotted as a logarithmic transformation on an arithmetic scale (WEIGENT et al. 1981; STANTON et al. 1981; JAMESON and GROSSBERG 1981), or as percentage of the control response, using the 50% endpoint (SALZBERG et al. 1979; GIRON 1981; SEDMAK and GROSSBERG 1981; SUZUKI et al. 1981), whereas the IFN dilution is usually plotted on a $\log_{10}$ scale. In one case (STANTON et al. 1981), the endpoint selected was a 0.5 $\log_5$ reduction in yield of viral HA; this represents slightly less than one-half the yield obtained in the untreated control cultures, whereas most assays of this type use the 0.5 $\log_{10}$ endpoint.

2. Factors Affecting Slope and Assay Results

There are many variables of the bioassay system which may alter the dose–response relationships, thereby increasing or decreasing the apparent potency of an IFN preparation. Such variables include the presence of contaminating biologically active antiviral substances, duration of exposure to IFN, culture conditions, virus dose, virus sensitivity, as well as cell sensitivity (GROSSBERG et al. 1974; FINTER 1977, 1981; BUCKLER 1977; OIE 1977; GROSSBERG et al. 1979; STEWART 1979). One difficulty in the comparative evolution of assay system is that the variables of different assays are usually not tested within a given laboratory. If a common assay technique is used with the same challenge virus, it can be demonstrated that cells can vary independently in their sensitivity to different types of IFN (P. JAMESON and J. J. SEDMAK, unpublished work). The type of IFN influences the slope of the dose–response curves in different cells; illustrative curves are shown in Fig. 1 for a typical IFN titration in A549 cell cultures.

II. Determination of Variability of Assay Results

The factors contributing to variability of results are generally attributable to biologic variation in cell behavior and therefore cannot be so easily defined. Standard-

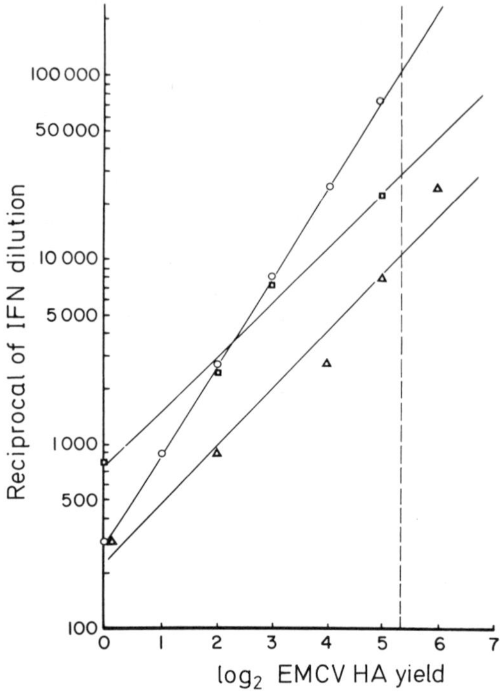

Fig. 1. Linear regression dose–response curves of three types of human IFN in the encephalomyocarditis virus (EMCV) hemagglutinin (HA) yield reduction assay with the A549 human lung carcinoma cell line. Representative curves for samples of HuIFN-α (*circles*), HuIFN-β (*triangles*), and HuIFN-γ (*squares*) were selected from a series of 8–16 repeated titrations of a given type of IFN; the slope of the curve selected approximates that of the mean for the group of titrations of each sample. The slope is calculated as the quotient of the change in the $\log_2$ reciprocal of the IFN dilution divided by the change in $\log_2$ reciprocal of the HA yield of EMCV. The mean slope values obtained for the three types of interferon are 1.60 for HuIFN-α ($N=10$), 1.08 for HuIFN-β ($N=8$), and 0.95 for HuIFN-γ ($N=16$). The endpoint is represented by the *vertical broken line* (at the EMCV HA yield of 5.34 in this titration) which indicates the intercept of the 0.5 $\log_{10}$ reduction in virus HA yield, or 1.66 $\log_2$ below the HA yield in untreated infected cells, from which the observed IFN titer is derived

izing materials and procedures relating to the use of cells and viruses within a laboratory can be helpful: control of quality of virus lots, serum used in cell cultures, and water for medium, as well as freedom of all materials from microbial contamination. Increasing the number of replicates should reduce the degree of variability. In titrating two or more samples repeatedly the variation between assays done on different days is generally greater than, but can be similar to, that observed within an assay. It is necessary therefore to base precise comparisons of titers of two samples upon more than four assays.

III. Standards

Because of the variation in results within and between titrations of a given type of assay, between different types of assays, and among different laboratories performing similar or different assays, it is necessary to compare results of IFN titrations by means of an accepted IFN preparation designated as a standard. This reagent, in the form of an international standard, (or, if none is available, a national standard) is used to calibrate the sensitivity of a given assay method relative to the assigned value of the standard, and to establish a geometric mean titer of a laboratory IFN preparation for subsequent use as an internal reference for monitoring the reproducibility of the assay results between titrations. The laboratory preparation should be of the same type of IFN and if possible have the same characteristics as the international standard, and they must give parallel dose–response curves.

1. Calibration of Assay

Simultaneous titrations of a laboratory standard and the international reference standard should be done five or more times. The ratio of the assigned value to the observed potency (geometric mean titer) of the international standard describes the relative sensitivity of the assay and establishes the conversion factor by which the observed activities in samples can be reported in international units (IU). The unitage (IU) of the laboratory standard is then calculated by multiplying the observed potency by the conversion factor. Unitage should be expressed in IU if there is available an international reference preparation designated by the World Health Organization.

2. Use of Laboratory and International Standards

After the laboratory standard has been properly calibrated by reference to the international standard as described in Sect. C.III.1, it must be used in every titration not only as a monitor of assay reproducibility, but as a reference for the conversion of observed units of activity to IU, accomplished in the same manner as for the laboratory standard itself. However, it is essential that the conversion of units be made only for IFN preparations that are of the same species and type (α, β, γ) as the reference reagent itself. It is not yet clear whether the multiple subtypes of HuIFN-α give parallel dose–response curves to each other or to the natural leukocyte product. There are instances in the literature in which the HuIFN-α reference reagent has been used as a standard for the presentation of titers of HuIFN-γ in IU, an unfortunate misuse of the α standard since the dose–response curves of the two IFN types are not parallel (see Fig. 1; GROSSBERG and GALASSO 1981; GROSSBERG 1981).

D. Interferon Standards

The reference standards for calibration of assays are IFN preparations the potency of which has been assigned a unitage, or content of IFN per container, on the basis of results of repeated titrations in several laboratories and, if appropriate, relating it to previously available IFN standards with designated titers. There are several categories of standards: local (or laboratory standard), national (e.g., U.S. National Institutes of Health or British Medical Research Council working reference reagents), and international standards (approved by the World Health Organization) (GROSSBERG et al. 1979). Information about available standards is listed in Table 1.

I. Derivation

The current standards have been prepared as a single large batch after little or no purification and characterized as an IFN of a given type. An effective stabilizing agent, generally inert protein, has been added to the IFN and a buffer system selected to provide optimal pH during the handling, freeze-drying, storage, and subsequent reconstitution of the IFN to prevent loss of activity. A uniform volume of the IFN preparation usually containing more than 1,000 U is then dispensed into each ampoule under aseptic conditions. The IFN is freeze-dried to provide optimal stability during prolonged storage and shipping at ambient temperatures to various laboratories (GROSSBERG et al. 1979; JAMESON et al. 1979; FINTER 1977; GALASSO 1969).

After the freeze-dried IFN has been characterized as having an adequate amount of antiviral activity with typical physicochemical properties, sufficient stability, and freedom from undesirable biologic contaminants, it is then submitted to many laboratories for a collaborative calibration of the antiviral activity. From the results of the collaborative titration of the IFN, with reference to previously established standards, if available, a unitage is assigned to the preparation which reflects the geometric mean activity obtained in the various laboratories. The assigned titer must also reflect the proportional relationship between the the activity of a new standard and the unitage of the existing standard. Since the titers of identical samples titrated in different laboratories by several methods can vary widely, statistical analysis of their logarithmically transformed values more nearly approaches a normal distribution than does an arithmetic distribution. Therefore, geometric mean titers have been used to report the results of collaborative titrations of standards we have produced for the U.S. National Institutes of Health.

II. Quality

The need for assessment of the quality of various properties of a given standard depend upon the purpose of the reagent and its anticipated applications. The purity of IFN (content of biologic activity relative to total protein) may not be important for a standard which is intended for use only as a biologically active reference reagent as long as it does not contain extraneous substances which could degrade or inactivate the IFN or interfere with the assay systems being calibrated. Current standards have not been evaluated, and therefore no values assigned, for their effect on cell growth or immunologic tests, such as enhancement of natural killer cell activity. Purity or high specific activity might become a primary requisite for a standard intended for use as a reference in an assay that does not depend upon measurement of biologic activity. For example, immunoassay methods would require standards in which the immunologically identifiable IFN molecules could be shown to be related to biologic activity. Therefore, it is important that standards be used only for the purpose for which they were intended and with appreciation of their limitations.

III. Stability and Its Prediction

A standard preparation is useful only if it either retains full activity during storage or its long-term degradation rate can be predicted. Freeze-drying of IFN has been selected as the stabilization method of choice since it causes virtually no loss of activity and does not require additives which might interfere with assay procedures. Methods have been devised for the evaluation of stability using modifications of accelerated storage tests originally developed for estimation of shelf life for pharmaceutical products (JAMESON et al. 1979). Short-term thermal tests extending up to 1 year in duration are used to test the stability of a standard and to predict the long-term stability at various storage temperatures. Confirmation of the validity of the predicted stability is done by periodically measuring the activity of samples stored at temperatures between −20° and +56 °C for several years. To date, four different standards have been tested for 5–10 years. Although all four were inactivated at 56 °C, about 50% of the activity was retained at 37 °C, as expected from predicted stabilities. All have maintained 100% of their activity at 20°, 4°, and −20 °C relative to samples held at −70 °C.

IV. Use and Limitations of Standards

Available standards have been prepared and tested for use as reference reagents only for the determination of sensitivity of assays for antiviral effects and calibration of laboratory standards for such assays. Their use as reference reagents for tests of anticellular (nonantiviral) activities, or physicochemical properties, or radioimmunoassay methods is not justified on the basis of available information. The international standards are valuable because they permit more meaningful comparison of IFN potencies among laboratories that employ either similar or different assay procedures. The major limitation on the use of a standard is the unavoidable variability of bioassay systems, a fact which originally dictated the need for such standards. The calibration of activity by means of a standard does not imply an accurate determination of the number of IFN units present in the sample; it provides a relative value to form a reference point or basis for comparison. An assay method which measures 20,000 U/ml in a standard having an assigned value of 20,000 is not a perfect assay, but rather has a relative sensitivity of 1 vis-à-vis another assay which measures 5,000 U which would have 0.25 times the sensitivity; while yet another which measures 80,000 U would be considered to have 4 times the sensitivity. The use of a reference assay (see Sect. B.IV.4.) with defined components may decrease the variation observed among laboratories participating in collaborative attempts to fix the value of an international standard.

V. Sources of Standards

The national and international standards can be obtained from the Director, National Institute for Biological Standards and Control, Holly Hill, London NW3 6RB, England, or the Research Resources Branch, National Institute for Allergy and Infectious Disease, National Institutes of Health, Bethesda, Maryland 20205, United States, upon request to the appropriate agency, as indicated in Table 1 (GROSSBERG et al. 1979; GROSSBERG 1981).

Table 1. Characteristics of international reference preparations and other freeze-dried interferon standards available from the U.S. National Instituts of Health (NIH) and the British Medical Research Council (MRC)

Agency	Catalog number	Animal species and predominant IFN type cell	Inducer	Inactivation or removal of inducer	Titer assigned ($\log_{10}$)	Predicted stability (years to lose 1,000 U)	
						At 20 °C	At 4 °C
NIH	G002-904-511 [a]	Mouse α and β (L929)	Newcastle disease virus	$HClO_4$	12,000 (4.1)	5.5	110
NIH	G023-901-527 [b]	Human α (leukocyte)	Sendai virus	pH 2	20,000 (4.3)	1.4	28.8
NIH	G019-902-528 [a]	Rabbit (kidney)	Bluetongue virus	pH 3.5	10,000 (4.0)	1.0	6.3
NIH	G023-902-527 [a]	Human β (fibroblast)	Poly(I)·poly(C)	Washing	10,000 (4.0)	> 1.5	> 29
NIH	Gg23-901-530	Human γ (lymphocyte)	Staphylococcal enterotoxin A	Porous glass chromatography	4,000 (3.6)	(In progress)	
NIH	Gg02-901-533	Mouse γ (splenocyte)	Lentil lectin of *Lens culinaris*	(In progress)	(To be done)	(To be done)	
MRC	Standard B [a] 69/19	Human α (leukocyte)	Sendai virus	pH 2	5,000 (3.7)	> 1.5	> 29
MRC	Standard B [a] 67/18	Chicken (allantois in ovo)	Influenza virus (B/Eng)	Centrifugation, pH 2	80 (1.9)		

[a] International reference preparation
[b] Designated by WHO as international working reference preparation

E. Radioimmunoassays

Unlike the IFN bioassays described thus far, the measurement of IFN antigen in a mixture of proteins and other antigens does not involve cell culture methods. Like other immunoassays, such methods require either pure IFN or antibody to pure IFN without contaminating antibodies to other antigens; either the IFN or the specific anti-IFN antibody must be labeled in some appropriate way. Calibration of antigenic content with units of activity remains a major problem. A summary of the polyclonal antibodies available from the U.S. National Institutes of Health (GROSSBERG and GALASSO 1981) is given in Table 2.

SECHER (1981) has described an immunoradiometric assay for HuIFN-α utilizing ^{125}I-labeled monoclonal antibody to IFN-α. This assay uses a crude sheep anti-IFN-α antibody of known potency bound to a solid-phase polystyrene support to which an IFN preparation is added for 4 h at 4 °C. The amount of IFN bound to the solid support can be calculated from the amount of ^{125}I-labeled NK2 monoclonal antibody to IFN bound to the solid phase support following a 16-h incubation at 4 °C; thus, the quality of the sheep antiserum bound to the support is not a critical factor of the assay. In sensitivity this assay can measure IFN reliably at concentrations greater than or equal to 50 IU/ml. Its reproducibility appears to be better than bioassays since it had a standard error of about 10% for independent assays on the same sample. The expense of the assay largely depends on the cost of the antibodies. The immunoassay lends itself to automation, and hundreds of samples can be assayed within 24 h. One serious potential problem with using this monoclonal immunoglobulin is that only the IFN-α species that have the NK2 antigenic site will be detected, but it has yet to be demonstrated how many of the approximately 14 species of HuIFN-α have the NK2 antigenic site. Further, this assay assumes that the sheep antibody attached to the solid support does not hinder the attachment of the ^{125}I-labeled antibody to the NK2 antigenic site.

INOUE and TAN (1981) have developed an assay for HuIFN-β employing ^{125}I-labeled purified polyclonal anti-HuIFN-β immunoglobulin in which HuIFN-β preparations are incubated for 1.5 h with rabbit anti-IFN-β immunoglobulin immobilized on Sepharose 4B beads. The resultant IFN-β–antibody complex is then incubated with purified ^{125}I-labeled rabbit anti-HuIFN-β immunoglobulin, after which the solid-phase complex is washed, and the amount of ^{125}I present in the complex determined. This assay can detect as little as 5 IU/ml IFN-β and the entire assay is completed in 5 h. The titers obtained by this method were highly correlated with a dye uptake antiviral assay for IFN. The coefficient of variability of this radioimmunoassay was only 1.1% at 500 IU/ml and 9.4% at 5 IU/ml whereas the antiviral assay could not distinguish a twofold difference in IFN titers. This assay requires highly purified radiolabeled antibody prepared against highly purified IFN; these reagents are currently expensive and hard to obtain.

The other type of radioimmunoassay reported for IFN relies upon radiolabeled nearly pure IFN. DAUBAS and MOGENSEN (1982) described a competitive inhibition assay for human leukocyte IFN. IFN-α is incubated with purified rabbit anti-HuIFN-α immunoglobulin for 1 h at 20 °C and then ^{125}I-IFN-α (highly purified) is added, and the mixture incubated overnight at 20 °C after which *Staphylococcus aureus* containing protein A is added to bind to the Fc portion of the rabbit anti-

Table 2. Antisera to interferons available from the U.S. National Institutes of Health (NIAID)

NIH antiserum or control antiserum	Production of antigen	Catalog number	Neutralizing titer[a]
Anti-human fibroblast IFN, sheep	Diploid cell; poly(I) · poly(C) purified on controlled pore glass (CPG) to 10^6 U per milligram protein	G028-501-568	12,000 vs 8–10 U IFN
Control anti-human fibroblast IFN, sheep	Void material from CPG column	G029-501-568	< 50 vs 8–10 U IFN[b]
Anti-human leukocyte IFN, sheep	Buffy coat; Sendai virus purified on Sepharose 4B to 10^4 U per milligram protein	G026-502-568	750,000 vs 8–10 U IFN[c]
Control anti-human leukocyte IFN, sheep	Void material from Sepharose 4B column	G027-501-568	< 50 vs 8–10 U human IFN
Anti-human lymphoblastoid (Namalwa) IFN, bovine	Namalwa; Sendai virus, partially purified	G030-501-553	40,000 vs Namalwa[d]
Control anti-human lymphoblastoid (Namalwa) IFN control, bovine	(unstated)	G031-501-553	< 25 vs Namalwa IFN[e]
Anti-mouse L-cell IFN, sheep	L929 NDV purified to 10^6 U per milligram protein	G024-501-568	300,000 vs 8–10 U IFN[f]
Control anti-mouse L-cell IFN, sheep	Void material from Sepharose 4B column	G025-501-568	< 50 vs 8–10 U mouse IFN

[a] These titers are those stated in the NIH reference reagent notes describing each preparation
[b] May be cytotoxic at $\leqq 1:100$ dilutions
[c] 2,000 titer vs 8–10 U human fibroblast IFN
[d] 40,000 titer vs primary leukocyte IFN; 10,000 titer vs fibroblast IFN
[e] < 25 titer vs leukocyte IFN; < 25 titer vs fibroblast IFN
[f] Low levels of antibody to human leukocyte IFN

IFN IgG complexed with the HuIFN-α. The immune complexes bound to the *S. aureus* are washed, centrifuged, and the amount of ^{125}I in the complex is determined. The specificity of the assay depends solely on the purity of the labeled IFN. Electrophoretic profiles indicate that their IFN-α preparation had one minor low molecular weight protein contaminant which did not interfere with the assay since it was not detectable in the immune complexes. The lower limit of sensitivity of this assay is 10 IU/ml with a standard error of 5.5% compared with 54.5% for a bioassay. This technique may offer a greater probability of recognizing more HuIFN-α species than do assays using monoclonal antibody.

Immunoassays for IFNs offer advantages over bioassays in terms of rapidity and reproducibility. However, immunoassays can only be as specific as the purity of the labeled immunoglobulin or IFN. Further, it is assumed that labeling with ^{125}I has no effect on the interaction of IFN and immunoglobulin. Because of their advantages immunoassays may replace bioassays for IFN in the next decade, provided that there is an acceptable correspondence between the antigenic content of preparations, including clinical samples, and biologic potency. Enzyme-linked and fluorescence-labeled immunoassays should obviate the stability problems which characterize the use of radiolabeled reagents (EAKINS 1981).

F. Summary

The increasing clinical use of IFN and the expanding quantity of experimental work reported require the proper reporting of IFN research results in ways that permit their comparison with the results of others. The varieties of bioassays of IFN with different attributes (some desirable, some undesirable) make it possible to select one or more bioassays most applicable to the particular needs of the researcher or agency, provided that the correct use is made of available international reference preparations of IFN. The proper use of such standards will permit the expression of results in IU. In this chapter, considerable attention has been paid to the use of such international reference preparations and laboratory standards for the calibration of assays and how results should be expressed. Greater attention should be paid, for example, to the necessity for parallelism between the dose–response curves of the international standards and the laboratory standard as well as the unknown samples being tested for potency. A reference bioassay is described that was recommended for use in the assignment of potency to international or national research IFN standard preparations. The recent description of some few radioimmunoassays and the availability of high quality polyclonal as well as monoclonal antibodies should make it possible in the future to utilize immunoassays, provided that there is an acceptable correspondance between biologic potency and the antigenic content of preparations, including those of clinical origin.

Acknowledgments. This work was supported by NIH awards NO1-AI02658 and NO1-AI12671.

References

Aboud M, Weiss O, Salzberg S (1976) Rapid quantitation of interferon with chronically oncornavirus-producing cells. Infect Immun 13:1626–1632

Adams A, Strander H, Cantell K (1975) Sensitivity of the Epstein-Barr virus transformed human lymphoid cell lines to interferon. J Gen Virol 28:207–217

Ahl R, Rump A (1976) Assay of bovine interferons in cultures of porcine cell line IB-RS-2. Infect Immun 14:603–610
Allen PT, Giron DJ (1970) Rapid sensitive assay for interferons based on inhibition of MM virus nucleic acid synthesis. Appl Microbiol 20:317–322
Armstrong JA (1971) Semi-micro, dye-binding assay for rabbit interferon. Appl Microbiol 21:723–725
Armstrong JA (1981) Cytopathic effect inhibition assay for interferon: microculture plate assay. Methods Enzymol 78:381–387
Atkins GJ, Johnston MD, Westmacott LM, Burke DC (1974) Induction of interferon in chick cells by temperature-sensitive mutants of Sindbis virus. J Gen Virol 25:381–390
Billiau A, Buckler CE (1970) Production and assay of rat interferon. Symp Ser Immunobiol Stand 14:37–40
Borden EC, Leonhardt PH (1977) A quantitative semimicro, semiatomated colorimetric assay for interferon. J Lab Clin Med 89:1036–1042
Boxaca M, Paucker K (1967) Neutralization of different murine interferons by antibody. J Immunol 98:1130–1135
Buckler CE (1977) Interferon assays: general considerations. Tex Rep Biol Med 35:150–153
Bucknall RA (1967) Species specificity of interferons: a misnomer? Nature 216:1022–1023
Bucknall RA (1970) The assay of human interferon. Symp Ser Immunobiol Stand 14:97–100
Campbell JB, Grunberger T, Kochman MA, White SL (1975) A microplaque reduction assay for human and mouse interferon. Can J Microbiol 21:1247–1253
Dahl H (1973) A micro assay for mouse and human interferon. II. Dose-response in different cell-virus systems. Acta Pathol Microbiol Scand [B] 81:359–364
Dahl H, Degre M (1972) A microassay for mouse and human interferon. Acta Pathol Microbiol Scand [B] 80:863–867
Daubas P, Mogensen E (1982) A radioimmuno-assay of human leukocyte interferon using protein-A containing Staphylococcus aureus. J Immunol Methods 48:1–12
Duvall J, Khan A, Hill NO, Ground M, Muntz D, Lanius R (1980) A computer assisted micro-dye uptake human interferon assay. In: Khan A, Hill NO, Dorn GL (eds) Interferon: properties and clinical uses. Leland Fikes Foundation, Dallas, P 529
Eakins R (1981) Merits and disadvantages of different labels and methods of immunoassay. In: Voller A, Bartlett A, Bidwell D (eds) Immunoassays for the 80s. University Park Press, Baltimore, P 5
Eife R, Hahn T, DeTavera M, Schertel F, Holtmann H, Eife G, Levin S (1981) A comparison of the antiproliferative and antiviral activities of alpha-, beta-, and gamma-interferons: description of a unified assay for comparing both effects simultaneously. J Immunol Methods 47:339–347
Emodi G, Just M, Hernandez R, Hirt HR (1975) Circulating interferon in man after administration of exogenous human leukocyte interferon. J Natl Cancer Inst 54:1045–1048
Epstein LB, McManus NH, Hebert SJ, Woods-Hellman J, Oliver DG (1981) Microtiter assay for antiviral effects of human and murine interferon utilizing a vertical light path photometer for quantitation. In: Adams DO, Edelso PJ, Koren HS (eds) Methods for studying mononuclear phagocytes. Academic, New York, p 619
Familletti PC, Rubinstein S, Pestka S (1981) A convenient and rapid cytopathic effect inhibition assay for interferon. Methods Enzymol 78:387–394
Fantes K, O'Neill CF, Mason PJ (1964) Purification of chick interferon. Biochem J 91:20–24
Ferreira PCP, Peixoto MLP, Silva MAV, Golgher RR (1979) Assay of human interferon in Vero cells by several methods. J Clin Microbiol 9:471–475
Finter NB (1964) Quantitative haemadsorption: a new assay technique. I. Assay of interferon. Virology 24:589–597
Finter NB (1969) Dye uptake methods for assessing viral cytopathogenicity and their applications to interferon assays. J Gen Virol 5:419–427
Finter NB (1973) The assay and standardization of interferon inducers. In: Finter NB (ed) Interferons and interferon inducers. North-Holland, Amsterdam, p 135
Finter NB (1977) The precision and comparative sensitivity of interferon assays. Tex Rep Biol Med 35:161–166

Finter NB (1981) Standardization of assay of interferons. Methods Enzymol 78:14–22
Fitzgerald GR (1969) The effect of interferon on focus formation and yield of murine sarcoma virus in vitro. Proc Soc Exp Biol Med 130:960–965
Fournier F, Rousset S, Chang C (1969) Investigations on a tissue antagonist of interferon (TAI). Proc Soc Exp Biol Med 132:943–950
Galasso GJ (ed) (1969) Standards for interferon. Symp Ser Immunobiol Standard 14:271–295
Gallagher JG, Khoobyarian N (1971) Sensitivity of adenovirus types 1, 3, 4, 5, 8, 11, and 18 to human interferon. Proc Soc Exp Biol Med 136:920–924
Giron DJ (1981) Assay of interferon by measurement of reduction of MM virus RNA synthesis. Methods Enzymol 78:399–402
Green JA (1977) Rapid assay of interferon. Tex Rep Biol Med 35:167–172
Green JA, Yeh T-J, Overall JC Jr (1980) Rapid, quantitative, semiautomated assay for virus-induced and immune human interferons. J Clin Microbiol 12:433–438
Grossberg SE (ed) (1979) Interferon standards: a memorandum. J Biol Standard 7:383–396
Grossberg SE (1981) On reporting interferon research. Ann Intern Med 95:115–116
Grossberg SE, Galasso GJ (1981) Problems in standardization: an interferon standards committee report. In: DeMaeyer E, Galasso GJ, Schellekens H (eds) The biology of the interferon system. Elsevier/North-Holland, Amsterdam, pp 19–22
Grossberg SE, Jameson P, Sedmak JJ (1974) Interferon bioassay methods and the development of standard procedures; a critique and analysis of current observations. In: Waymouth C (ed) The production and use of interferon for the prevention of human virus infections. Tissue Culture Association, Rockville, p 26
Hahon N (1981) Hemadsorption and fluorescence determinations for assay of virus-yield reduction by interferon. Methods Enzymol 78:373–381
Hahon N, Booth JA (1974) Hemadsorption cell-counting assay of interferon. Arch Ges Virusforsch 44:160–163
Hahon N, Booth JA, Eckert HL (1975) Interferon assessment by the immunofluorescent, immunoperoxidase and hemadsorption cell-counting techniques. Arch Virol 48:239–243
Ho M, Enders JF (1959) An inhibitor of viral activity appearing in infected cell cultures. Proc Natl Acad Sci USA 45:385–389
Imanishi J, Hoshino S, Hoshino A, Oku T, Kita M, Kishida T (1981) New simple dye-uptake assay for interferon. Biken J 24:103–108
Inoue M, Tan YH (1981) Radioimmunoassay for human beta interferon. Infect Immun 33:763–768
Isaacs A, Lindenmann J (1957) Virus interference. I. The interferon. Proc R Soc Lond B147:258–267
Ishitsuka H, Nomura Y, Takano K (1977) A simple and efficient microassay method for titration of interferon. Microbiol Immunol 21:583–591
Ito Y, Montagnier L (1970) Heterogeneity of the sensitivity of vesicular stomatitis virus to interferons. Infect Immun 18:13–27
Jameson P, Grossberg SE (1981) Virus yield-reduction assays for interferon: picornavirus hemagglutination measurements. Methods Enzymol 78:357–368
Jameson P, Dixon MA, Grossberg SE (1977) A sensitive interferon assay for many species of cells: encephalomyocarditis virus hemagglutinin yield-reduction. Proc Soc Exp Biol Med 155:173–178
Jameson P, Greiff D, Grossberg SE (1979) Thermal stability of freeze-dried mammalian interferons. Analysis of freeze-drying conditions and accelerated storage tests for murine interferon. Cryobiology 16:301–314
Johnston MD, Finter NB, Young PA (1981) Dye uptake method for assay of interferon activity. Methods Enzymol 78:394–399
Jordan GW (1972) Basis for the probit analysis of an interferon plaque reduction assay. J Gen Virol 14:49–61
Koblet H, Kohler V, Wyler R (1972) Optimization of the interferon assay using inhibition of Semliki Forest virus-ribonucleic acid synthesis. Appl Microbiol 24:323–327
Kono Y, Ho M (1965) The role of the reticuloendothelial system in interferon formation in the rabbit. Virology 25:162–166

Kozikowski EH, Hahon N (1969) Quantitative assay of interferon by the immunofluorescent cell-counting technique. J Gen Virol 4:441–443

Langford MP, Weigent DA, Stanton GJ, Baron S (1981) Virus plaque-reduction assay for interferon: micro-plaque and regular macroplaque reduction assays. Methods Enzymol 78:339–346

Lvovsky E, Levy HB (1976) Interferon assay of high sensitivity. Proc Soc Exp Biol Med 153:511–513

McManus NH (1976) Microtiter assay for interferon: microspectrophotometric quantitation of cytopathic effect. Appl Environ Microbiol 31:35–38

McWilliams M, Finkelstein MS, Allen PT, Giron DJ (1971) Assay of chick interferons by the inhibition of viral ribonucleic acid synthesis. Appl Microbiol 21:959–961

Merigan TC (1971) A plaque inhibition assay for human interferon employing human neonate skin fibroblast monolayers and bovine vesicular stomatitis virus. In: Bloom BR, Glade PR (eds) In vitro methods in cell mediated immunity. Academic, New York, p 489

Miller PA, Lindsay HL, Cormier M, Mayberry BR, Trown PW (1970) Rapid semiautomated procedures for assaying antiviral activity. Ann NY Acad Sci 173:151–159

Oie HK (1977) Conventional assay systems. Tex Rep Biol Med 35:154–160

Oie HK, Buckler CE, Uhlendorf CP, Hill DA, Baron S (1972) Improved assays for a variety of interferons. Proc Soc Exp Biol Med 140:1178–1181

Paucker K (1965) The serologic specificity of interferon. J Immunol 94:371–378

Pidot ALR (1971) Dye uptake assay: An efficient and sensitive method for human interferon titration. Appl Microbiol 22:671–677

Porterfield JS (1959) A simple plaque inhibition test for antiviral agents: application to assay of interferon. Lancet 2:326–327

Richmond JY, Polatnick J, Knudsen RC (1980) Microassay for interferon, using [3H]uridine, microculture plates, and a multiple automated sample harvester. Appl Environ Microbiol 39:823–827

Rossi CR, Kiesel GK, Hoff EJ (1980) Factors affecting the assay of bovine type I interferon on bovine embryonic lung cells. Am J Vet Res 41:552–556

Rubinstein S, Familletti PC, Pestka S (1981) Convenient assay for interferons. J Virol 37:755–758

Sakaguchi AY, Stevenson D, Gordon I (1982) Species specificity of interferon action: a functioning homospecific nucleus is required for induction of antiviral activity in heterokaryons. Virology 116:441–453

Salzberg S, Heller A, Aboud M, Gurari-Rotman D, Revel M (1979) Effect of interferon on human cells releasing oncornaviruses: an assay for human interferon. Virology 93:209–214

Secher DS (1981) Immunoradiometric assay of human leukocyte interferon using monoclonal antibody. Nature 290:501–503

Sedmak JJ, Grossberg SE (1973a) Interferon bioassay: reduction in yield of myxovirus neuraminidases. J Gen Virol 21:1–7

Sedmak JJ, Grossberg SE (1973b) Comparative enzyme kinetics of influenzae neuraminidases with the synthetic substrate methoxyphenylneuraminic acid. Virology 56:658–661

Sedmak JJ, Grossberg SE (1981) Virus yield-reduction assays for interferon with the influenza virus neuraminidase assay. Methods Enzymol 78:369–373

Sedmak JJ, Dixon M, Schoenherr C, Sabran JL, Grossberg SE (1983) Interferon and antibody titrations using haemagglutinating Togaviridae and trypsinized human erythrocytes. J Virol Meth 6:99–105

Sedmak JJ, Grossberg SE, Jameson P (1975) The neuraminidase yield-reduction bioassay of human and other interferons. Proc Soc Exp Biol Med 149:433–438

Sellers RF, Fitzpatrick M (1962) An assay of interferon produced in Rhesus monkey and calf kidney tissue cultures using bovine enterovirus M6 as challenge. Br J Exp Path 43:674–683

Stanton GJ, Langford MP, Dianzani F (1981) Virus yield-reduction assay for interferon by titration of Sindbis virus hemagglutinin. Methods Enzymol 78:351–357

Stewart WE II (1979) Interferon assays. In: Stewart WE II (ed) The interferon system. Springer, Berlin Heidelberg New York, p 13
Stewart WE II, Lockart RZ Jr (1970) Relative antiviral resistance induced in homologous and heterologous cells by cross-reacting interferons. J Virol 6:795–799
Sueltenfuss EA, Pollard M (1963) Cytochemical assay of interferon produced by duck hepatitis virus. Science 139:595–596
Suzuki J, Akaboshi T, Kobayashi S (1974) A rapid and simple method for assaying interferon. Jpn J Microbiol 18:449–456
Suzuki J, Iizuka M, Kobayashi S (1981) Assay of interferon by reduction of viral RNA synthesis: a convenient assay for tracer experiments with monolayer cultures. Methods Enzymol 78:403–409
Tilles JG, Finland M (1968) Microassay for human and chick cell interferons. Applied Microbiol 16:1706–1708
Vassef A, Beaud G, Paucker K, Lengyel P (1973) Interferon assay based on the inhibition of double-stranded reovirus RNA accumulation in mouse L-cells. J Gen Virol 19:81–87
Viehauser G (1977) Simple procedure for large-scale assays for chick interferon. Appl Environ Microbiol 33:740–752
Wagner RR (1961) Biological studies of interferon. I. Suppression of cellular infection with eastern equine encephalomyelitis virus. Virology 13:323–337
Weigent DA, Stanton GJ, Langford MP, Lloyd RE, Baron S (1981) Virus yield-reduction assay for interferon by titration of infectious virus. Methods Enzymol 78:346–351
Weil J, Epstein LB, Epstein CJ (1980) Synthesis of interferon-induced polypeptides in normal and chromosome 21-aneuploid human fibroblasts: relationship to relative sensitivities in antiviral assays. J Interferon Res 1:111–124
Wheelock EF, Sibley WA (1965) Circulating virus interferon and antibody after vaccination with 17-D strain of yellow-fever virus. N Engl J Med 273:194–198

CHAPTER 3

Evolution of Interferon Genes

D. GILLESPIE, E. PEQUIGNOT, and W. A. CARTER

A. Introduction

Interferon genes are particularly interesting from an evolutionary viewpoint because they are multiple gene families from which are emerging data relevant to several levels of biologic organization: DNA structure, protein function, varied and complex biologic processes. Presently, we recognize three interferon gene families: α, β, and γ – leukocyte, fibroblast, and immune interferon, respectively. Interferons-α and -β have been examined at the DNA level; interferon-γ has not. DNA studies suggest that human interferon-α is coded by at least ten genes (NAGATA et al. 1980; GOEDDEL et al. 1981). DNA studies suggest that interferon-β is coded by only one gene (TAVERNIER et al. 1981; HOUGHTON et al. 1981; LAWN et al. 1981a), but less direct evidence indicates the existence of more than one human interferon-β gene (SAGAR et al. 1981). Therefore, while interferon genes are multiple gene families, the number of genes is not the same for the different types of interferon and may differ for the same type from different mammals. The latter conclusion would of course imply that recent alterations have taken place in the interferon gene families.

Some insight into the evolution of interferon gene families can be gained by comparing the nucleotide sequence of several of the human interferon-α genes. The published sequences derive primarily from cloned copies of interferon-α mRNA, but these serve also as chromosomal gene sequences since the chromosomal interferon-α and -β genes apparently possess no intervening sequences (LAWN et al. 1981b; TAVERNIER et al. 1981). Like other genes, the interferon gene elements which are transcribed into mRNA consist of a 5′ noncoding region, a coding region, and a 3′ noncoding region. The available sequence data include very little information relative to the 5′ noncoding region; therefore, we cannot consider evolution of this element. However, conclusions can be drawn concerning the evolution of the coding and 3′ noncoding elements as described in Sects. B–D.

B. Coding Region Nucleotide Sequence

The human interferon-α coding region consists of some 567 nucleotides which presumably code for polypeptides about 189 amino acids long. Of eight human interferon-α genes sequenced by GOEDELL et al. (1981) (see also NAGATA et al. 1980), six have coding regions of equal length. Of the remaining two, interferon-αA has one code word deleted (for amino acid 66), while the interferon-αE has an extra nucleotide at position 187. Though the interferon-αB coding region has the char-

```
        00                   20                   40                   60                   80                  100
β       |ATGaCCaacAagTgTctccTcCaaATtGCtCTcCTGtTGtgCttCTcCActaCAgctcttTCcaTGaGCTacaActTGCtTggattCCtacaaagaaGcA
αA      *ATGGCCTTGACCTTTGCTTTACTGgTGGCCCTcCTGGTGCTCAGCTGCAAGTCAAGCTGCTCTgTGGGCTGTGATCTGCCTCAaACCCACAGCCTGGGTA
αB      *ATGGCCTTGACtTTTTaTTTAaTGgTGGCCCTaGTGGTGCTCAGCTACAAGTCAtTCaGCTCTCTGGGCTGTGATCTGCCTCAGACtCACAGCCTGGGTA
αC      *ATGGCCcTGTCCTTTTCTTTACTtATGGCCgTGCTGGTGCTCAGCTACAAaTCcATCTGtTCTCTGGGCTGTGATCTGCCTCAGACCCACAGCCTcGGTA
αD      *ATGGCCTcGCCCTTTGCTTTACTGATGGtCCTGGTGGTGCTCAGCTGCAAGTCAAGCTGCTCTCTGGGCTGTGATCTcCCTgAGACCCACAGCCTGGaTA
αE      *                                                           ctgcCTCTGGGCTGTGATCTGCCTCAGgCCCACAGCgTGGGTA
αF      *ATGGCCcTGTCCTTTTCTTTACTGATGGCCgTGCTGGTGCTCAGCTACAAaTCcATCTGtTCTCTGGGCTGTGATCTGCCTCAGACCCACAGCCTGGGTA
αG      *
αH      *ATGGCaTTGCCCTTTGCTTTAaTGATGGCCCTGGTGGTGCTCAGCTGCAAGTCAAGCTGCTCTCTGGGCTGTaATCTGtCTCAaACCCACAGCCTGaaTA
PROG    *ATGGCCTTGXCCTTTXCTTTACTGATGGCCCTGXTGGTGCTCAGCTXCAAGTCAAXCTGCTCTCTGGGCTGTGATCTGCCTCAGACCCACAGCCTGGGTA

        100                  120                  140                  160                  180                  200
β       |gCAatttcagTgtcagaagCTcctgtggcaattGAatgggaggCtTgaaTatTGCCTcAAGGACAGgatgaACTTTGacaTcCCtgAGGAGattaagcA
αA      *gCAGGAGGaCCTTGATgCTCCTGGCACAgATGAGGAaAATCTCTCtTTTCTCCTGCtTGAAGGACAGACATGACTTTGGATTTCCCCAGGAGGAGTTT
αB      *ACAGGAGGGCCTTGATACTCCTGGCACAAATGcGAAGAATCTCTCCTTTCTCCTGCCTGAAGGACAGACATGACTTTGaATTcCCCCAGGAGGAGTTTGA
αC      *AtAGGAGGGCCTTGATACTCCTGGgACAAATGgGAAGAATCTCTCCTTTCTCCTGCCTGAAGGACAGACATGAtTTccGAaTcCCCCAGGAGGAGTTTGA
αD      *ACAGGAGGaCCTTGATgCTCCTGGCACAAATGAGcAGAATCTCTCCTTcCTCCTGtCTGAtGGACAGACATGACTTTGGATTTCCCCAGGAGGAGTTTGA
αE      *ACAGGAGGGCCTTcATACTCCTGaCACAAATGAGGAGAATCTCTCCTTTtTCtTaCCTGAAGGACAGACATGACTTTGatTTTCCaCAtcAGGtGTTTcA
αF      *AtAGGAGGGCCTTGATACTCCTGGCACAAATGgGAAGAATCTCTCCTTTCTCCTGCCTGAAGGACAGACATGACTTTGGATTcCCCCAaGAGGAGTTTGA
αG      *                                                                   CATGACTTTGGATTTCCtCAGGAGGAGTTTGA
αH      *ACAGGAGGaCtTTGATgCTCaTGGCACAAATGAGGAGAATCTCTCCTTTCTCCTGCCTGAAGGACAGACATGACTTTGaATTTCCCCAGGAGGAaTTTGA
PROG    *ACAGGAGGGCCTTGATACTCCTGGCACAAATGAGGAGAATCTCTCCTTTCTCCTGCCTGAAGGACAGACATGACTTTGGATTTCCCCAGGAGGAGTTTGA

        200                  220                  240                  260                  280                  300
β       |gctgcAgCAGTTCCAGAAGGaggAcGCCgcaTtgacCaTCtATGAGATGcTCCAGaAcAtCTTtgcTaTtTTCAGacaAgAttcaTCtagcaCTGgcTGG
αA      * GGCAACCAGTTCCAaAAGGCTgAAaCCATCcCTGTCCTCCATGAGATGATCCAGCAGAtCTTCAATCTCTTCAGCACAAAGGACTCATCTGCTGCTTGG
αB      *TGatAAaCAGTTCCAGAAGGCTCAAGCCATCTCTGTCCTCCATGAGATGATCCAGCAGACCTTCAAcCTCTTCAGCACAAAGGACTCATCTGCTGCTTtG
αC      *TGGCAACCAGTTCCAGAAGGCTCAAGCCATCTCTGTCCTCCATGAGATGATCCAGCAGACCTTCAATCTCTTCAGCACAgAGGACTCATCTGCTGCTTGG
αD      *TGGCAACCAGTTCCAGAAGGCTCcAGCCATCTCTGTCCTCCATGAGcTGATCCAGCAGAtCTTCAAcCTCTTtAcCACAAAaGAtTCATCTGCTGCTTGG
αE      *TGGCAACCAcTTCCAGAAGGtTCAAGCtATCTtccTttTCCATGAGATGATgCAGCAGACCTTCAAcCTCTTCAGCACAAAGGACTCATCTGaTaCTTGG
αF      *TGGCAACCAGTTCCAGAAGGCTCAAGCCATCTCTGTCCTCCATGAGATGATCCAGCAGACCTTCAATCTCTTCAGCACAAAGGACTCATCTGCTaCTTGG
αG      *TGGCAACCAGTTCCAGAAGGCTCAAGCCATCTCTGTCCTCCATGAGATGATCCAGCAGACCTTCAATCTCTTCAGCACAAAGGACTCATCTGCTaCTTGG
αH      *TGGCAACCAGTTCCAGAAaGCTCAAGCCATCTCTGTCCTCCATGAGATGATgCAGCAGACCTTCAATCTCTTCAGCACAAAGaACTCATCTGCTGCTTGG
PROG    *TGGCAACCAGTTCCAGAAGGCTCAAGCCATCTCTGTCCTCCATGAGATGATCCAGCAGACCTTCAATCTCTTCAGCACAAAGGACTCATCTGCTGCTTGG

        300                  320                  340                  360                  380                  400
β       |aATGAGACtaTtgTtGAgAAccTCctggCTaAtgTcTAtCAtCAGaTaAAccAtCTGaAgaCagtccTGgaAsAaaAacTgGaGaaaGAAGAtttcaCCa
αA      *GATGAGACCCTCCTAGACAAATTCTACACTGAACTcTACCAGCAGCTGAATGACCTGGAAGCCTGTGTGATACAGGgGGTgGGGGTGacAGAGACTCCCC
αB      *GATGAGACCCTtCTAGAtgAATTCTACAtcGAACTTgACCAGCAGCTGAATGACCTGGAAGtCctgtgtgatCAGGAaGTgGGGGTGatAGAGtCTCCCC
αC      *GAacAGAgCCTCCTAGAaAAATTtTcCACTGAACTTTACCAGCAaCTGAATGACCTGGAAGCaTGTGTGATACAGGAGGTTGGGGTGGAAGAGACTCCCC
αD      *GATGAGgaCCTCCTAGACAAATTCTgCACcGAACTcTACCAGCAGCTGAATGACtTGGAAGCCTGTGTGATgCAGGAGGagaGGGTGGgAGAaACTCCCC
αE      *GATGAGACCCTttTAGACAAATcCTACACTGAACTTTACCAGCAGCTGAATGACCTGGAAGCCTGTGTGATgtAGaAGGTTGGaGTGGAAGAGACTCCCC
αF      *GAacAGAgCCTCCTAGAaAAATTtTcCACTGAACTTaACCAGCAGCTGAATGACaTGGAAGCCTGcGTGATACAGGAGGTTGGGGTGGAAGAGACTCCCC
αG      *GATGAGACaCTtCTAGACAAATTCTACACTGAACTTTACCAGCAGCTGAATGACCTGGAAGCCTGTaTGATgCAGGAGGTTGGaGTGGAAGAcACTCCtC
αH      *GATGAGACCCTCCTAGAaAAATTCTACAtTGAACTTTtCCAGCAaaTGAATGACCTGGAAGCCTGTGTGATACAGGAGGTTGGGGTGGAAGAGACTCCCC
PROG    *GATGAGACCCTCCTAGACAAATTCTACACTGAACTTTACCAGCAGCTGAATGACCTGGAAGCCTGTGTGATACAGGAGGTTGGGGTGGAAGAGACTCCCC

        400                  420                  440                  460                  480                  500
β       |gGggaAAacTcatgagCAgtCTGcaceTGAaaAsATAtTatgggAGgATtctgCaTTAcCTGAagGccAAGgAgTACAGtCacTGTGCCTGGaccaTaGT
αA      *TGATGAAgGAGGACTCCATtCTGGCTGTGAGGAAATACTTCCAAAGAATCACTCTcTATCTGAaAGAGAAGAAATACAGCCCTTGTGCCTGGGAGGTTGT
αB      *TGATGtAcGAGGACTCCATCCTGGCTGTGAGGAAATACTTCCAAAGAATCACTCTaTATCTGACAGAGAAGAAATACAGCtCTTGTGCCTGGGAGGTTGT
αC      *TGATGAATGAGGACTCCATCCTGGCTGTGAGGAAATACTTCCAAAGAATCACTCTTTATCTaAtAGAGAgGAAATACAGCCCTTGTGCCTGGGAGGTTGT
αD      *TGATGAATGTGGACTCCATCtTGGCTGTGAaGAAATACTTCCgAAGAATCACTCTcTATCTGACAGAGAAGAAATACAGCCCTTGTGCCTGGGAGGTTGT
αE      *TGAgGAATGTGGACTCCATCCTGGCTGTGAGaAAATACTTtCAAAGAATCACTCTTTATCTGACAaAGAAGAAgTAtAGCCCTTGTtCCTGGGAGGcTGT
αF      *TGATGAATGTGGACTCCATCtTGGCTGTGAaGAAATACTTCCAAAGAATCACTCTTTATCTGACAGAGAAGAAATACAGCCCTTGTGCtTGGGAGGTTGT
αG      *TGATGAATGTGGACTCtATCCTGaCTGTGAGaAAATACTTtCAAAGAATCACcCTcTATCTGACAGAGAAGAAATACAGCCCTTGTGCaTGGGAGGTTGT
αH      *TGATGAATGAGGACTCCATCCTGGCTGTGAaGAAATACTTCCAAAGAATCACTCTTTATCTGAtgGAGAAGAAATACAGCCCTTGTGCCTGGGAGGTTGT
PROG    *TGATGAATGXGGACTCCATCCTGGCTGTGAGGAAATACTTCCAAAGAATCACTCTTTATCTGACAGAGAAGAAATACAGCCCTTGTGCCTGGGAGGTTGT

        500                  520                  540                  560
β       |CAGAGtgGAAATCcTaAGgaaCTTtTacTTccttAacAgacTtacAGgttaccTccGaAactgaagATct
αA      *CAGAGCAGAAATCATGAGATCtTTtTCTTTgTCAACAAACTTGCAAGAAAGtTTAAGaAGtAAGGAATGA
αB      *CAGAGCAGAAATCATGAGATCCTTCTCTTTATCAAtcAACTTGCAAaAAAGATTgAaGAGtAAGGAATGA
αC      *CAGAGCAGAAATCATGAGATCCcTCTCgTTtTCAACAAACTTGCAAaAAAGATTAAGGAGGAAGGAtTGA
αD      *CAGAGCAGAAATCATGAGATCCcTCTCTTTATCAACAAACTTGCAAGAAAGATTAAGGAGGAAGGAATaA
αE      *CAGAGCAGAAATCATGAGATCCTTCTCTTTATgAACgAACTTGCAgGAAAGATTAAGGAGGAAGGAATGA
αF      *CAGAGCAGAAATCATGAGATCCTTCTCTTTATCAAaAAttTTtCAAGAAAGATTAAGGAGGAAGGAATGA
αG      *CAGAGCAGAAATCATGAGATCCTTCTCTTTATCAgCAAACTTGCAAGAAAGATTAAGGAGGAAGGAATGA
αH      *CAGAGCAGAAATCATGAGATCCTTCTCTTTtTCAACAAACTTGCAAaAAAGATTAAGGAGGAAGGAtTGA
PROG    *CAGAGCAGAAATCATGAGATCCTTCTCTTTATCAACAAACTTGCAAGAAAGATTAAGGAGGAAGGAATGA
```

Fig. 1. Interferon-α nucleotide sequences. The sequences of GOEDELL et al. (1981) are reproduced. The 3′ noncoding regions have been realigned for maximum homology. The sequence of the putative progenitor sequence is included. *Capital letters* indicate nucleotides in common with the progenitor sequence. *Lowercase letters* indicate nucleotides different from the progenitor sequence. The nucleotide sequences of insertions 1–12 are specified in Fig. 6

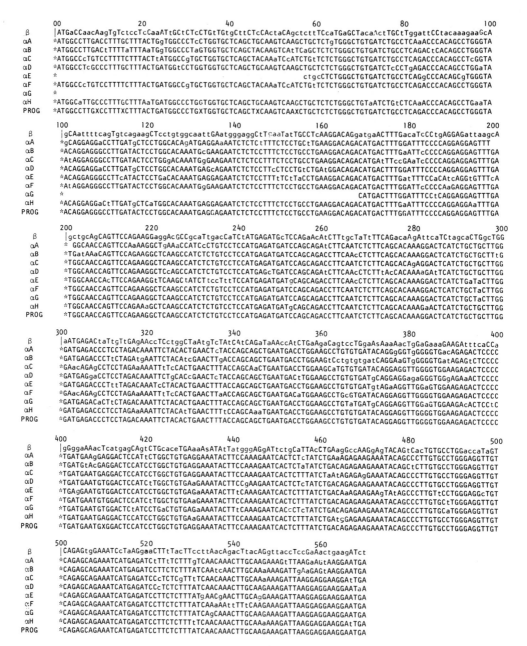

```
        00                  20                  40                  60                  80                  100
        |                   |                   |                   |                   |                   |
αA      *AAACTGGTTCAACATGGAAATGA-TTtTCATTGAtTcgTAtgCCAGCTCACctTTTtATGA  TCTGCCATTTCAAAGACTCATGTTTCTGCTATgACCA
αB      *gAcCTGGTaCAACAcGGAAATGA-TTCTCATaGACTAATACAgCAGtctACACTTTgAcaAGTTgTGCtcTTTCAAAGACcCtTCTTTCTGCcAaAACCA
αC      *AAACTGGTTCAACATGGcAATGA-TcCTgATTGACTAATACAttATCTCACACTTTCATGAGTTCTtCCATTTCAAAGACTCA     CTtCTATAACCA
αD      *tAtCTGGTcCAACATGaAAAcaA-TTCTtATTGACTcATACACCAGgTCACgCTTTCATGAaTTCTGtCATTTCAAAGACTCtCAcccCTGCTATAACtA
αE      *AAACTGGTTCAACATGGAAATGAlaTtTCcaTGAtTAATACAtCATCTCACACaTTCATGAaTTCTGCCATTTC        tCATTTtTGCTATAtCCA
αF      *AAcC GtTTCAACATGGAAATGA-TctgtATTGACTAATACACCAGtcCACACTTctATGAcTTCTGCCATTTCAAAGACTCA  TTTCTcCTATAACCA
αG      *AAACTGGTTCAACATcGAAATGA-TTCTCATTGACTAgTACACCATtTCACACTTct TGAGTTCTGCCgTTTCAAAtAtTaA  TTTCTGCTATAtCCA
αH      *AAACTGGTTCAtCATGGAAATGA-TTCTCATTGACTAATACAtCATCTCACACTTTCAT . TTCTtCCATTTCAAAGACTCA  cTTC   TATAACCA
PROG    *AAACTGGTTCAACATGGAAATGA-TTCTCATTGACTAATACACCAXCTCACACTTTCATGAGTTCTGCCATTTCAAAGACTCAXXTTTCTGCTATAACCA

        100                 120                 140                 160                 180                 200
        |
αA      *TGACAcGAtTTaAAT2CAAAtgTTTt3cAtTGTaTTCAGc  TcTTAA                               GGCACTAGTCCcTTACAGAgGACCATGCT
αB      *TGctATGAaTTGAAT-CAAAtgTgTC-AAgTGTTTTCAGGAGTGTTAAGCAACATCcTGTTcAGCTGTAtgGGCACTAGTCCcTTACAGATGACCATGCT
αC      *cGAgcG   TTGAAT-CAAAATTTTC-AAATGTTTTCAGcAGTGTaAAGAAGtgTCGTGTaTACCTGTGCAGGCACTAGTCCTTTACAGATGACCATtCT
αD      *TG                                                                                             ACCATGCT
αE      *TGACATGAGTTGAAT-CAAAATTTTa-AAATGTTTTCAGGAaTGTTAAGCAGCATCATGTTcAGCTGTACAGGCACTAGTtCcTTACgGATGAtCATGCT
αF      *ccgCATGAGTTGAAT-CAAAATTTTC-AgATcTTTTCAGGAGTGTaAgGAAACATCATGTTTACCTGTGCAGGCACTAGTCCTTTACAGATGACCATGCT
αG      *TGACtTGAGTTGAAT-CAAAATTTTC-AAAcG TTTCAcacGTGTTAAGCAACA CtTcTTTAGCTccACAGGgACaAaatCTTTACAGATGAtCATGCc
αH      *ccACA  AGTTGAAT-CAAAATTTcC-AAATGTTTTCAGGAGTGTTAAGAAGCATCGTGTTTACCTGTGCAGGCACTAGTCCTTTACAGATGACCATtCT
PROG    *TGACATGAGTTGAAT-CAAAATTTTC-AAATGTTTTCAGGAGTGTTAAGXAXCATCXTGTTTAXCTGTXCAGGCACTAGTCCTTTACAGATGACCATGCT

        200                 220                 240                 260                 280                 300
        |
αA      *GActGATCcA-TT ATCTATTT5ATTTtA7T-ATTTATTT-AACTATTTATAAaAc  AAcTTATTTT--TGTTCATaTtAcgTCATGTGcACCTTTgC
αB      *GATGGATCTA-TTCATCTATTT-ATTTAAA-T-cTTTATTT9AACTAcTataggGAcTTAAATTAgTTT--TGTTCATaTtATATtATGTGaACtTTTAC
αC      *GATGtcTCTg-TTCATCT TTT-gTTTAAA-T-ATTTATTT-AAtTATTTtTAAaATTTA                   TGTAATATCATGaGTcgCTTTAC
αD      *GATaaA CTg4TTTATCTA      TTTAAA-T-ATTTATTT-AACTATTcATAAGATTTAAATTATTTT--TGTTCATaTAAcqTCATGTGcACCTTTAC
αE      *GATGGATCTg-TTTATCTATTT-gTcTAAA-T-AaTTATTT-AACTATTTATAAtATTTAAAaTcTTcT--T TTCATGTA   TCATGTaT  tTTTAC
αF      *GATaGATCTA-aTTATCTATcT-ATTgAAA-T-ATTTATTT        ATTTATtAGATTTAAATTATTTT--TGTcCATGTAATATtATGTGTACtTTTAC
αG      *aATctATCTA-TT   CTATcT6ATTTAAA-T-ATTTATTT        ATTTATAAGATTTAAATTATTTT10TGTTCAgGTAATATtA catccaCcTTAC
αH      *GATGtcTCct-TTCATCTATTT-ATTTAAA-T8ATTTATTT-AACTATTTtTAttATTTAAATTATTTT--Tt   ATGTAATATCATGaGTACCTTTAC
PROG    *GATGGATCTA-TTXATCTATTT-ATTTAAA-T-ATTTATTT-AACTATTTATAAGATTTAAATTATTTT--TGTTCATGTAATATCATGTGTACCTTTAC

        300                 320                 340                 360                 380                 400
        |
αA      *AcaGTGGTTAATGTAAtAAAA--TATGTTC--TTTgTATTTgGT(end)
αB      *ATTGTGaaTtgTGTAACAAAA11cATGTTC--TT ATATTTAtT        atTTTgCCaTgTTtATTAAATTTTTACTATGAAAAAATTCTT TATTT
αC      *ATTGTGGTTAATGTAACAAtA--TATGTTC--TTcATATTTAGcCAATATATTAATTTCCTTTTTCATTAAATTTTTACTATAC(end)
αD      *AcTGTGGTTAgTGTAAtAAAA--cATGTTC--cTTATATTTAcTC(end)
αE      *tTTGTGGTTAATaTAACAAcA--cATGTTC--TTTATATTTAGTCAATATATTACTTTgCTTTTTCATTAAATTTTTACTATGG(end)
αF      *ATTGTGtT    aTAtCAAAA--TATGTTa12cTaATATTTAGTCAATATATTATTTT CTTTTT ATTAAATTTTTACTATTAAAA CTTCTTATATTA
αG      *tTTGTGGcTAATaTAAtAAAA--TATGTTC--TTTATgTTTtGTC(end)
αH      *ATTGTGGTTAATGTAACAAA --TATGTTC--TTcATATTTAGcCAATATATTAATTTCCTTTTTCATTAAATTTTTACTAT(end)
PROG    *ATTGTGGTTAATGTAACAAAA--TATGTTC--TTTATATTTAGTC(end)

        400                 420                 440                 460

αA      *
αB      *ATTCTTTAAAATT      GAA CTCCAA CCCATGAATTGTGCAAACTGATTAAAGAATGGATGGT(end)
αC      *
αD      *
αE      *
αF      *TTTGGTTATTCTTTAATAAAGAAATTCCAAGCCC(end)
αG      *
αH      *
PROG    *
```

Fig. 1

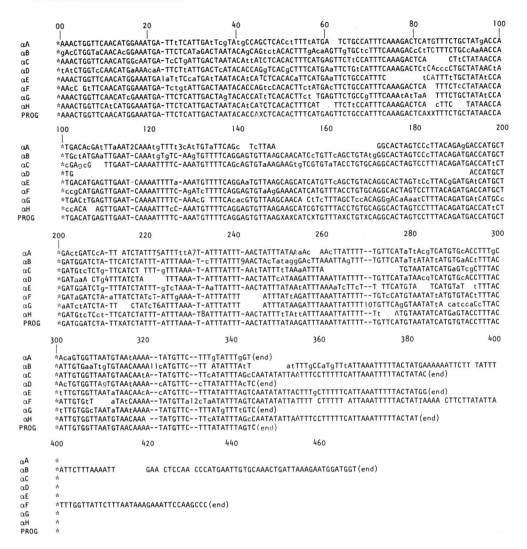

acteristic 567 nucleotides, there appears to have been an insertion of a T residue at position 363 followed by a deletion of the A residue at position 373 (GOEDDEL et al. 1981). The eight human interferon-α genes which have been characterized are closely interrelated in the nucleotide sequence. Therefore, they probably descended from a common progenitor sequence. The descent of the existing interferon genes from this progenitor sequence is recent enough that the sequence of the progenitor gene can be deduced from the most common nucleotide at each position of the eight present-day sequences (Fig. 1). Comparison of each of the present-day sequences to the progenitor gene and to the interferon-β gene reveals that six of the eight genes have mutated at approximately equivalent rates and more or less uniformly throughout the length of the coding region (Fig. 2). Interferon-αE has ex-

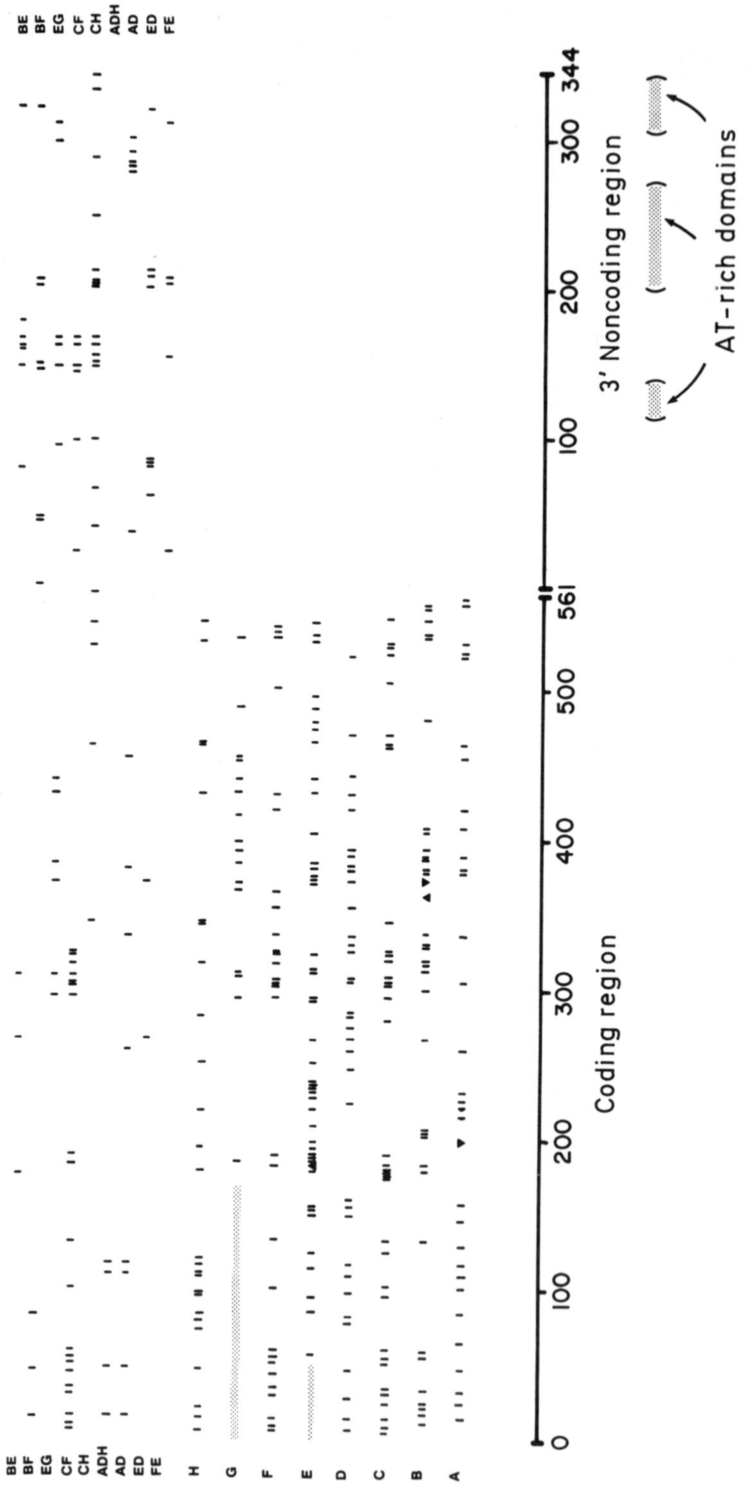

Fig. 2. Position of mutations in interferon-α genes. Mutations are indicated by *short, vertical lines. Letters* on the ordinate denote interferon genes. *Pairs of letters* indicate two genes and the corresponding mutations refer to coincident mutations involving those two genes. *Upward triangles,* insertions; *downward triangles,* deletions

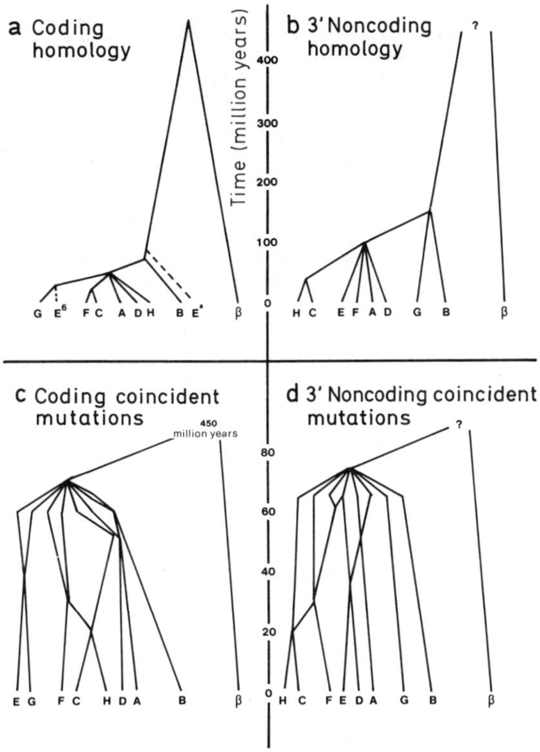

Fig. 3a–d. Evolutionary tree of interferon genes. See text for explanation

hibited the highest mutation rate, consistent with the idea that it is not functionally active due to the insertion mutation of position 187 (GOEDDEL et al. 1981). A large share of the extra mutations in the interferon-αE gene are near the insertion site. Interferon-αB has also mutated significantly faster than the average. This gene, too, has had an insertion mutation.

A simple model for human interferon-α and -β gene evolution (Fig. 3a) is that about 450 million years ago an ancestral gene was duplicated, one copy destined to become a progenitor of the interferon-α gene family and the other destined to become the interferon-β gene or a progenitor of the interferon-β gene family (TANIGUCHI et al. 1980). This scheme requires that, on the average, the interferon-β gene will be more closely related to the interferon-α progenitor gene (ca. 450+400 million years divergent) than to any individual present-day interferon-α gene (ca. 450+450 million years divergent). This expectation was fulfilled as well as can be expected (Fig. 4). The analysis was only marginally useful, however, since the amplification of the interferon-α genes was apparently recent, compared with the time of the α–β split. A more telling argument involved comparing those positions where present-day interferon-α gene differs from the progenitor gene and asking in which direction most of the changes lead to a sequence more closely like the interferon-β gene sequence. Considering the interferon-αD gene of the present, of 36 positions

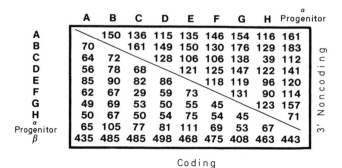

	A	B	C	D	E	F	G	H	α Progenitor
A		150	136	115	135	146	154	116	161
B	70		161	149	150	130	176	129	183
C	64	72		128	106	106	138	39	112
D	56	78	68		121	125	147	122	141
E	85	90	82	86		118	119	96	120
F	62	67	29	59	73		131	90	114
G	49	69	53	50	55	45		123	157
H	50	67	50	54	75	54	45		71
α Progenitor	65	105	77	81	111	69	53	67	
β	435	485	485	498	468	475	408	463	443

3' Noncoding (above diagonal); Coding (below diagonal)

Fig. 4. Divergence of interferon genes. The numbers indicate millions of years since any given pair of interferon genes possessed a common ancestor. The calculations relied on the Markov chain approach developed by GILLESPIE et al. (1980) for satellite DNA

where interferon-αD and the putative interferon-α progenitor gene are different, 22 cases found the progenitor nucleotide the same as that in interferon-β; in only 5 cases is the interferon-αD nucleotide the same as that found in interferon-β. Thus, the general picture in Fig. 3 is likely to be correct.

If interferon genes mutated at a rate of 0.1% per million years, an unproven assumption but an average mutation rate for single-copy DNA, and if they diverged from the progenitor simultaneously, this divergence would have occured some 50–75 million years ago (Figs. 3 and 4). The separation of this progenitor from the related interferon-β gene was considerably earlier, having apparently occurred 400–500 million years ago. We cannot say whether the interferon-α progenitor gene was maintained as a single-copy sequence from then until its recent amplification, but this is the simplest assumption. The notion that the present-day interferon-α genes simultaneously separated from the progenitor gene predicts that, within statistical limits, pairs of interferon-α genes will exhibit sequence differences consistent with a divergence 50–75 million years ago. In fact, a Markov chain analysis suggests that this is not so (Fig. 4). Interferons-αC and -αF are more closely related than expected, as are interferons-αA, -αD, and -αH. Interferon-αE is distantly related to all interferons except interferon-αG.

Either: (1) these variations are statistically insignificant; (2) the separate interferon-α genes descended independently from the progenitor, but at different times in evolution; or (3) they descended simultaneously from the progenitor gene, but have not evolved randomly or independently. As mentioned earlier, all the genes, except αB and αE, have evolved at about the same rate over the last 50 million years (Fig. 4).

There is evidence from the coding sequences that the interferon-α genes interacted with one another during evolution. In several instances two or more genes differ from the rest at the same position in exactly the same way. For example, at position 303 genes αC and αF carry an A residue while the remaining six genes have a T residue at this site. By deduction, the progenitor gene had a T residue at position 303 and both genes αC and αF mutated to an A residue at that position. Given the number of mutations which have occurred since the origination of the inter-

	A	B	C	D	E	F	G	H
A		**8**	2	**6**	3	1	3	0
B	5		3	3	**7**	5	5	3
C	1	4		1	1	**6**	2	**16**
D	**8**	3	0		**8**	4	1	1
E	0	3	0	2		5	**6**	3
F	1	3	**18**	2	1		**7**	5
G	1	1	1	2	**6**	1		2
H	5	5	5	**8**	2	1	0	

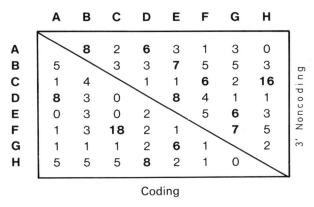

3' Noncoding

Coding

Fig. 5. Coincident mutations in interferon-α genes. The numbers indicate the number of coincident mutations shared by a given pair of interferon-α genes

feron-α gene family and assuming all mutations are equally likely, the chance of independent mutations of two genes at the same position to the same nucleotide is low, less than 1 in 500[1] Moreover genes αC and αF exhibit this phenomenon repeatedly – at positions 7, 10, 16, 31, 47, 51, 54, 60, 102, 133, 183, 303, 304, 308, 318, 324, 326, 464, 531, 547, and 567 – a total of 21 positions (Fig. 5). One interpretation of this fact is that the interferon genes occasionally "correct" their sequence by recombining with other interferon genes. Correction by unequal crossover would change interferon gene number if recombination were extragenic and would additionally produce a hybrid gene if the recombination event were intragenic. In the case of interferon genes αC and αF, described earlier, coincident mutations were found more or less uniformly throughout the coding sequence and in the 3′ noncoding sequence (Fig. 2). If this reflects an extragenic crossover, it probably occurred some 30 million years ago, since αC and αF possess only 24 differences from each other. Interferons-αC and -αH, in contrast, show coincident mutations only in the 3′ portion of the coding sequence, suggesting correction by an intragenic recombination event. This hypothesis is supported by the existence of coincident mutations in the 3′ noncoding regions of the αC and αH genes (Fig. 2). This exchange was probably earlier than the αC–αF exchange since αC and αH show more differences from each other. The αC and αH genes are probably linked on chromosome 9 (LAWN et al. 1981 b).

A striking example of coincident mutations is the αA–αDαH trio, exhibiting four coincident mutations at the 5′ end of the coding sequence. The prediction that these three interferon genes will exhibit coincident mutations in the 5′ noncoding sequence cannot be tested until more sequence data are available. Evolutionarily, we view this three-way correction as a pair of two-member recombinations closely spaced in time. Aside from the αA–αD–αH trio, there are 14 other cases of triple

1 Selection mechanisms favoring certain types of mutations (e.g., transition mutations or mutations not changing code words) will produce coincident mutations. This probably accounts for the "background" of 1–3 coincident mutations per pair of genes. The correction argument derives from pairs of genes displaying an unusually high number of coincident mutations

coincident mutations involving different trios of interferon genes. These probably arose from selection for specific nucleotides at those positions.

It is apparent that the interferon-α genes have exchanged sequences among themselves. No evidence suggests that exchanges have taken place between interferon-α and interferon-β. If the exchanges among interferon-α genes were occasional, then the conclusion that they derived recently and approximately simultaneously from a common progenitor gene follows well. If the human interferon-α genes originated as recently as 50–75 million years ago by amplification of a progenitor gene which was itself maintained as a single-copy gene for the preceding 400 million years (as depicted in Fig. 3a), then interferon-α genes from an animal having an ancestor in common with humans longer than 50–75 million years ago (e.g., mice) will be more closely related in sequence to the putative human progenitor gene than to most present-day interferon-α genes.

If, however, genetic exchanges among interferon-α genes have been frequent, then divergence from the progenitor gene would have been earlier than we calculate. Also, formation of the multiple present-day genes in that case need not have been simultaneous. Finally, the sequence of the progenitor gene would not be deducible from present-day sequences. Frequent recombination would have served to "homogenize" the interferon genes, producing a set of sequences which are more closely interrelated than would be predicted on the basis of independent accumulation of mutations in each gene. This evolutionary mechanism has been proposed for satellite and other repeated DNAs to explain how these families of DNA sequences can remain as closely interrelated members within the genome of a species while allowing the family from one species to diverge from the homologous family in a second species. Were it true that exchanges among interferon-α genes have been frequent, great differences in interferon-α gene organization among humans, apes, and monkeys will be expected and polymorphisms of interferon gene organization and number between infrequently breeding groups within the human population will probably be common. Though some domains of the interferon polypeptide may have been more evolutionarily conserved than others (TANIGUCHI et al. 1980), no parts of the interferon-β gene bear unexpected homology to any parts of any interferon-α gene; thus, the interferon-β gene has apparently not recently exchanged sequences with any known interferon-α gene.

C. 3′ Noncoding Region Nucleotide Sequence

The 3′ noncoding regions of human interferon-α genes are related to one another (Fig. 1) and were apparently generated from a common ancestor at about the same time as the coding regions were generated (Fig. 3b). However, during subsequent evolution, the 3′ noncoding regions have experienced many more multisite alterations and there has been less of a tendency to preserve the linear extent of the 3′ noncoding region. The 3′ noncoding region of the eight sequenced interferon-α genes can be aligned for maximum homology and a putative progenitor sequence can be written for it (Fig. 1), as was done for the coding region. The deduced alignment was similar, but not identical to that presented by GOEDDEL et al. (1981). The 40 insertion or deletion mutations are each considered to be a single change from the progenitor gene.

INSERTIONS

1. **TGGAAACC**
2. **CTTTTCA**
3. **TAGG AGTA TCAA TCAA** cA
4. **TgAxA**
5. ATTT **AAAT** ATTT
6. ATTT **ATTT ATCT ATCT GTCT GTCT TCTA TCTA ATCT** ATTT
7. ATTT **TTAA AATAT** ATTT
8. ATTT AAAT **ATTT** ATTT
9. ATTT **AAGT** AACT ATTT
10. ATTT **TAAA CTTA TGTT** TG
11. **A**c**ATG**
12. **AA**

DELETIONS

13. AC**TG**GT
14. C**AT**G
15. **CATG**
16. TGA**GT**
17. **CAAAG ACTCA** TG/CA
18. CA TG/CA **TTT**C TG
19. CA TG/CA
20. **TGC**
21. CA TG **AC delete 86 TG** AC CA
22. CA**TG**
23. CA **T GAG**TTG
24. TG**T**
25. **AG** TG
26. **G** t **AACATCCTGTTTAGCTGTACA**
27. CA **T**
28. **T**
29. ATT t
30. ATT t **AT**
31. **A**TTT ATTT
32. **ATTT** ATTT
33. ATTT **AACT** ATTT
34. A**TTT**
35. ATTTA **AATT ATTT TTGT TCA** TG
36. TG **TTC**ATG
37. **ATA**
38. **TG**
39. **AC**
40. **TAAT**

Fig. 6. Insertions and deletions in the 3′ noncoding region of interferon-α genes. *Boldface letters* indicate nucleotides added or deleted, relative to the deduced progenitor sequence. *Lightface letters* indicate boundary nucleotides. *Underlining* indicates TG or CA dinucleotide. *Small letters* indicate boundary nucleotide not in progenitor sequence, but in mutated gene

There have been 12 insertions and 28 deletions during evolution of the progenitor interferon-α gene to the eight characterized, present-day genes (Fig. 6). The multisite mutations range from 1 to 90 nucleotides in length. In the progenitor gene sequence they are generally flanked by the nucleotides ATTT, TG, or AC. The tetramer ATTT and variants of it comprise a substantial portion of the 3′ noncoding sequence (Fig. 1 and see Sect. D). This simple sequence is capable of aligning out of register with homologs to create insertions and deletions by unequal crossover. The dimer TG and its invert AC have been noticed at the end of some transposable elements. However, in the 3′ noncoding region of interferon-α, it is not often found cleanly at the deletion or insertion boundary. Moreover, while in some TG and AC clusters multisite mutations are found frequently (e.g., see 3′ noncoding positions 99–112 and 276–289), in other clusters multisite mutations are not frequent (e.g., positions 10–51 and 303–317). Nevertheless, the boundaries of multisite mutations in the 3′ noncoding regions carry a few favored sequences and it is reasonable to suppose that their proximity is a facet of the origin of these mutations. Also, it is clear that insertions and deletions have contributed significantly to the evolution of the 3′ noncoding region, unlike the case of the coding regions which have evolved primarily by single-site substitutions.

The 3′ noncoding region of the interferon-α genes is not demonstrably related in nucleotide sequence to the 3′ noncoding region of the interferon-β gene. As in the case of the coding regions, the noncoding regions of the interferon-α genes display coincident mutations, suggesting that genetic exchanges have occurred between nonhomologous gene pairs (Figs. 2 and 3 d). However, the genetic exchanges evidenced by coincident mutations in the 3′ noncoding regions do not often involve the same gene pairs or multiples which display coincident mutations in the coding region. Therefore, there must be a crossover "hot spot" near the boundary between the coding region and the 3′ noncoding region and, consequently, the two regions have corrected independently of each other, for the most part. Considering each multisite mutation to be a single event and assuming the same time of amplification of both the 3′ noncoding regions and the coding regions from a progenitor gene, the 3′ noncoding region has accumulated mutations at roughly twice the rate of the coding region. This is considerably less than predicted for a freely mutating DNA. Presumably, there are functional or structural constraints preventing accelerated evolution of the 3′ noncoding region.

D. Structural Evolution of the 3′ Noncoding Region

The overall linear extent of the 3′ noncoding region has not been preserved during evolution. Some of this is undoubtedly due to large blocks of simplesequence, "AT-rich" clusters, especially at positions 206–270 and 346–end. The simple "ATTT"-based, AT-rich cluster in positions 206–270 provides a suitable sequence mileu for unequal crossover. Interestingly, a majority of 3′ noncoding sequences in other genes exhibit regions based on an approximately repeating, simple sequence. Have any spatial relationship been conserved during evolution of the 3′ noncoding region of the interferon genes? Three sequence boundaries are recognizable: (1) the coding–noncoding junction; (2) the signal for polyadenylation (AATAAAA or AATTAAA); and (3) the noncoding region–poly (A) junction.

In the genes of interferon-β and interferons-αA, -αD, and αG, the signal for polyadenylation is AATAAAA and in each case it is located 19–20 nucleotides from the poly(A) tract. These are properties common to other structural genes. The linear distance between the signal for polyadenylation and the coding–noncoding boundary has not been preserved however, being 312, 223, and 346 nucleotides, re-

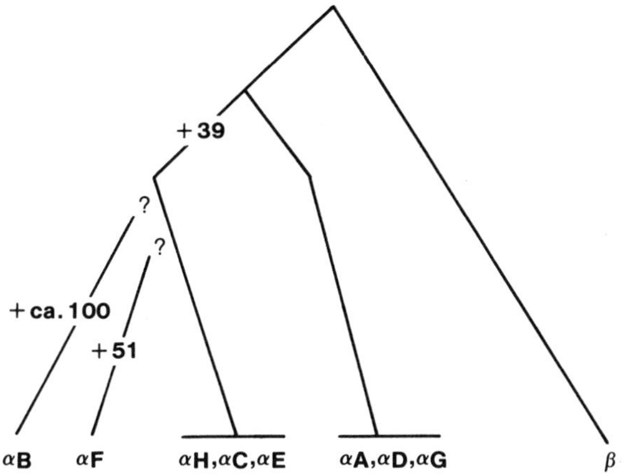

Fig. 7. Evolutionary tree of interferon gene 3′ additions. Numbers indicate number of nucleotides added. A corresponding subtraction model was not considered because the sequence downstream of the interferon-αD gene is not clearly detectably related to nucleotides 345–385 in genes αB, αC, αE, αF, or αH

spectively, in interferon genes αA, αD, and αG (Table 1). This distance in the progenitor gene was 315 nucleotides. In the remaining interferon-α genes the AATAAAA sequence reads AACAAAA and long ATC-rich sequences of varying lengths have apparently been added onto the noncoding region (Fig. 1). Except for the gene for interferon-αF, the added bases carry ATTAAA, a variant signal for polyadenylation, 10–14 nucleotides from the poly(A) tract. In the additions to the interferons-αB and -αF, a third polyadenylation signal was added – in αB it is an ATTAAA 11 bases from the poly(A) tract and in αF it is AATAAA 14 nucleotides from the poly(A) region. The sequence downstream from the end of gene αD is not detectably related to nucleotides 345–385 of genes αB, αC, αE, αF, or αH. The chromosomal gene for interferon-β possesses a second polyadenylation signal some 200 nucleotides downstream from the first. The alternative use of two polyadenylation signals might help explain the two forms of interferon-β mRNA in certain induced cells (Sagar et al. 1981).

The simple evolutionary flow for the 3′ noncoding region which satisfies these length differences and is also consistent with sequence comparisons is contained in Fig. 7. The noncoding regions of genes αC, αE, αH, αF, and αB reflect the addition of a common 39 nucleotides AT-rich sequence to the "original" interferon-α noncoding terminus exemplified by the genes of interferons-αA, -αD, and -αG. Interferon genes αC, αE, and αH remained at this length. Additional tracts were added to interferons-αB and -αF to form the present genes.

This evolutionary picture of terminal noncoding tracts does not coincide with the branch points derived from homology and coincident mutation data on the body of the 3′ noncoding region or the coding region. If the 3′ terminal tracts are not cloning artifacts then the evolution of the interferon-α gene family involved a larger number of important exchanges than we recognized earlier or the coding, 3′ noncoding and 3′ terminal regions evolved independently. Regardless of the tim-

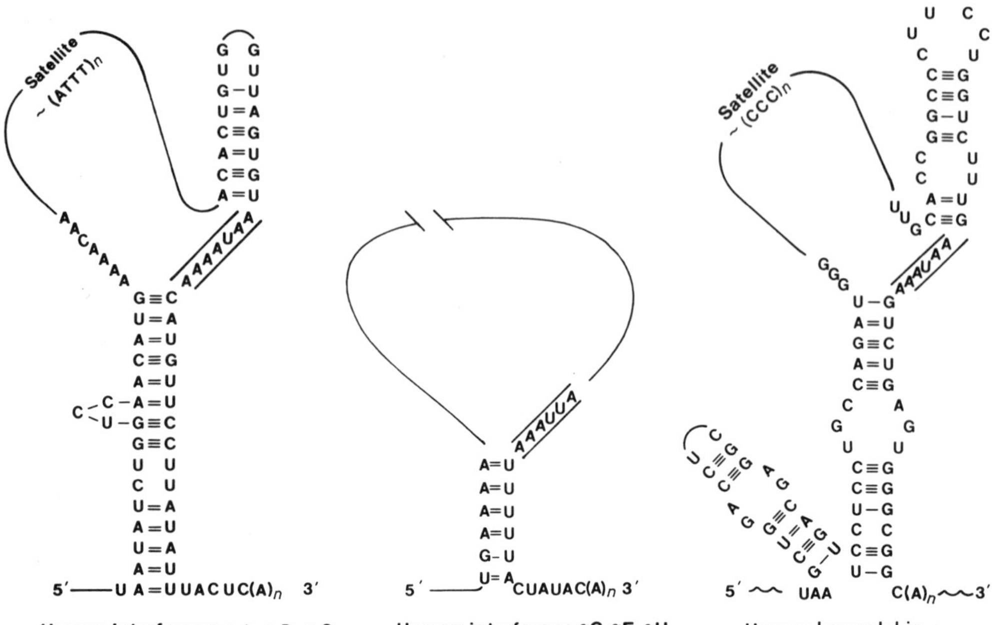

Fig. 8. Possible secondary structures of 3′ noncoding regions. See text for explanation

ing of the evolution of the 3′ terminus of the interferon gene family, it is generally true that when the 3′ end of the genes was changed, a new polyadenylation signal was added and the poly(A) tract was changed.

However, the linear distances may be irrelevant. For some of the interferon genes it is possible to draw molecules with secondary structures that position all three elements close to one another. Such a structure is drawn for the 3′ noncoding region of the interferon-αD gene in Fig. 8. Similar structures can be written for the interferon-α genes αA, αC, αE, αG, and αH and for the genes for the α chain of human hemoglobin, human preproinsulin, and bovine growth hormone, but not as yet for the interferon-β gene or for the interferon-αB or -αF genes. The contribution of secondary structure constraints to the evolution of the interferon genes is not known.

E. Coding Region Amino Acid Sequence

The evolution of the coding region of the interferon genes must be constrained by the functional contribution of individual amino acids to the three-dimensional structure and thereby to the biologic activity of the interferon molecule. The amino acid sequence of interferons-α and -β can be predicted from the genes' nucleotide sequence (Fig. 9a). Moreover, the interferon-αA protein has been sequenced and the position of its two disulfide bonds has been determined (WETZEL et al. 1981). The sequence of interferon-αA is reproduced in Fig. 9b, along with an analogous representation for interferon-β in Fig. 9c. One disulfide bridge in interferon-β is missing because both Cys residues have been mutated (WETZEL et al. 1981).

Fig. 9a

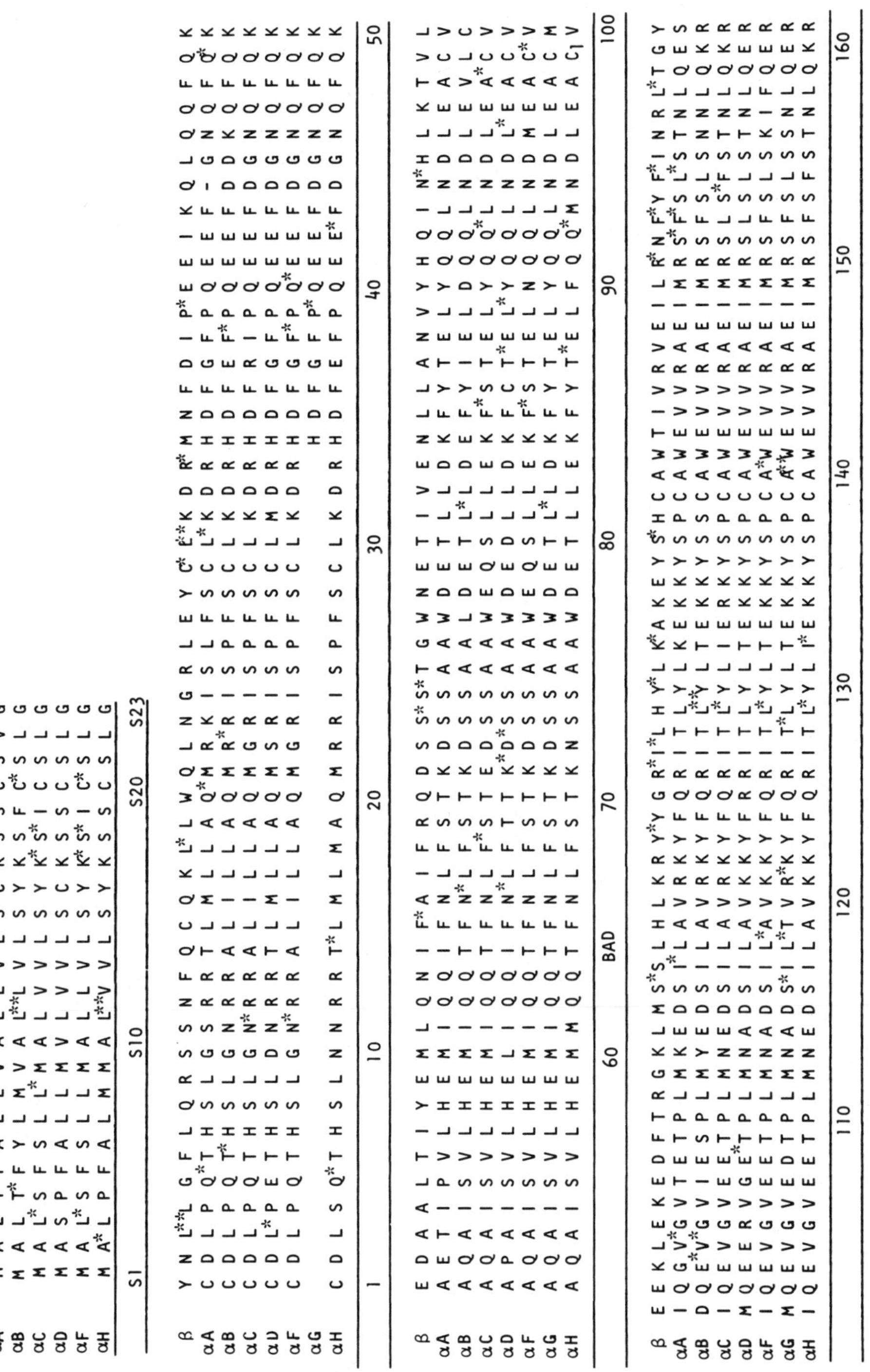

Fig. 9a–c. Amino acid sequences of interferons-α and -β. See text for explanation. Ala = A, Arg = R, Asn = N, Asp = D, Cys = C, Gln = Q, Glu = E, Gly = G, His = H, Ile = I, Leu = L, Lys = K, Met = M, Phe = F, Pro = P, Ser = S, Thr = T, Trp = W, Tyr = Y, Val = V. Nomenclature is that of IUPAC-IUB Commission on Biochemical Nomenclature (1968)

Fig. 9b

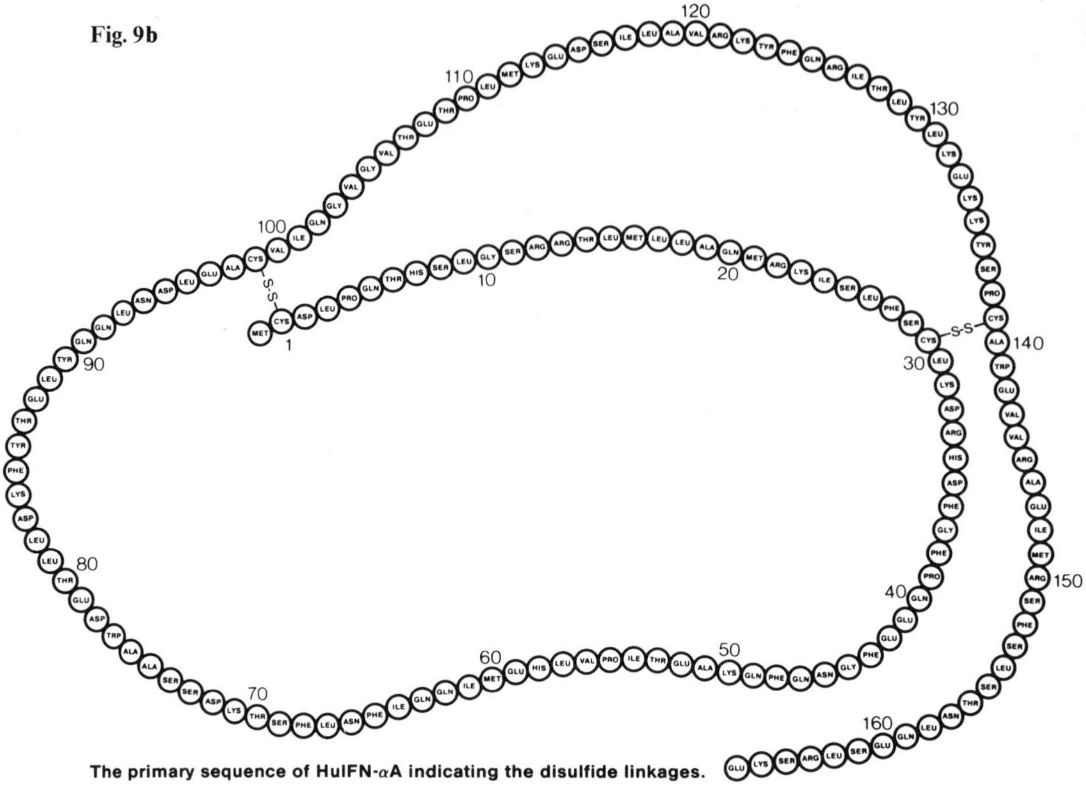

The primary sequence of HuIFN-αA indicating the disulfide linkages.

Fig. 9c

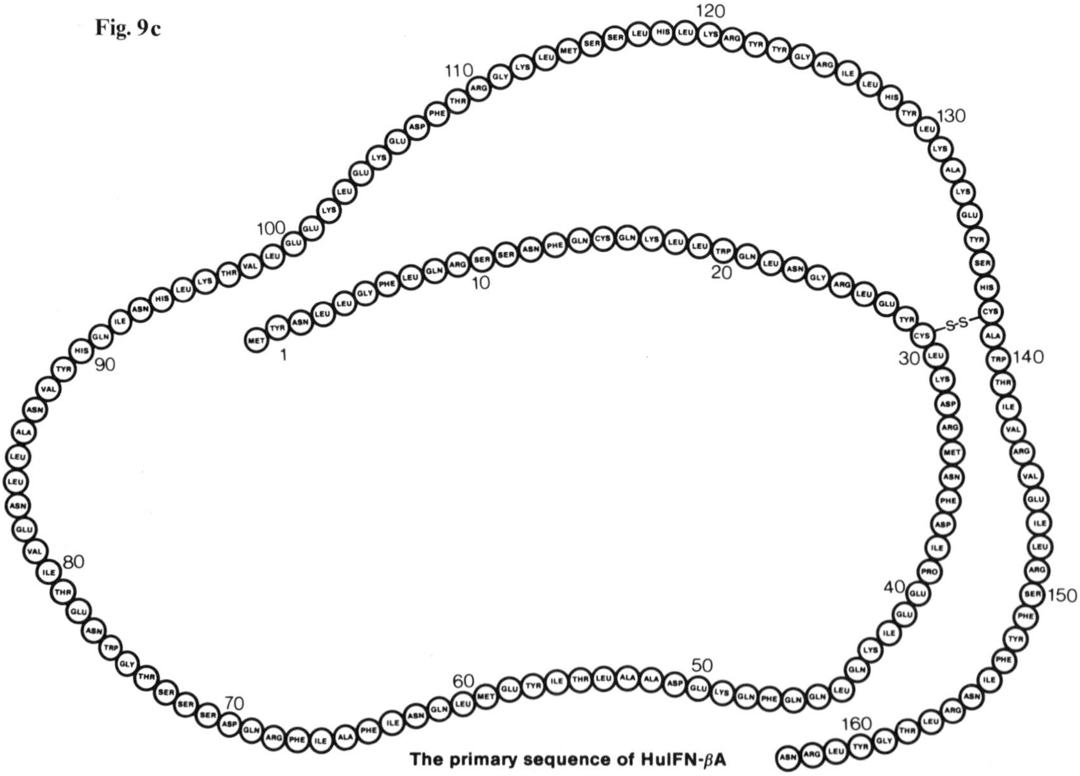

The primary sequence of HuIFN-βA

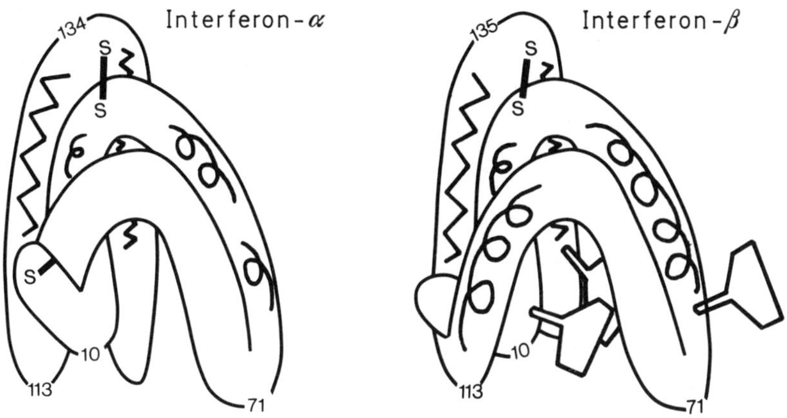

Fig. 10. Possible three-dimensional structure of interferons-α, and -β. Positions of reverse turns, α-helices, and β-sheets were predicted according to CHOU and FASMAN (1978). Features are emphasized which are common to both interferon types and which have been conserved among species of interferon-α. *Loops* indicate α-helical regions. *Zigzags* indicate β-sheet regions

As TANIGUCHI et al. (1980) point out, after comparing interferon-α and -β, certain regions of the interferon polypeptide have apparently been conserved. Similarly, conserved regions can be seen when comparing the amino acid sequences of seven of the interferon-α proteins (interferon-αE is excluded from this evaluation). In particular, the region around the disulfide bond (Cys-29–Cys-139) has been conserved. This corresponds to amino acids 23–36 and 121–151. The region of amino acids 45–95 is moderately conserved while the regions 1–20 and 95–115 show the least conservation.

A start toward predicting the three-dimensional structure of interferon can be made by determining regions which are probably involved in reverse turns, α-helices, and β-sheets (CHOU and FASMAN 1978). Individual amino acids have a propensity to be involved in, or excluded from, such structures and these probabilities have been quantitated. Such an analysis of the interferon-α and -β polypeptides leads us to propose the general structure schematized in Fig. 10. It should be realized that certain aspects of the structure will be subject to alteration in the future but, as developed in the following paragraphs, some aspects have a very high probability of being correct.

Eight regions of interferon-β and six in interferon-α are possible reverse turn regions; five are common to both interferon-β and -α (Fig. 11). Two of the five are near one another, so probably only one is actually used. The region of amino acids 71–74 has a very high P_t, 1.3, and is poor in amino acids which favor an α-helix or β-sheet [2]. Moreover, all seven interferon-α sequences retained the 71–74 reverse turn. Thus, the chance that amino acids 71–74 participate in a reverse turn is high. This reverse turn can have the effect of bringing the area around amino acids 80–90 in proximity to the disulfide bridge that interferon-α and -β have in common (Fig.

2 P_t, P_α, and P_β are the probabilities of reverse turns, α-helices, and β-sheets as defined by CHOU and FASMAN (1978)

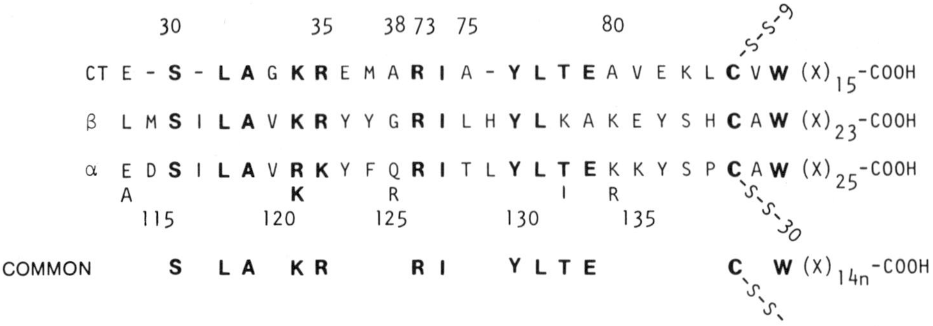

Fig. 11. Homology between cholera toxin, subunit B, and interferon. CT = cholera toxin; β = interferon-β; α = interferon-α, common = identical amino acids among CT, β, and α. Numbers indicate position in the protein

10). Similarly, the reverse turns of amino acids 10–13 and 134–137 have acceptably high P_t values and low P_α and P_β values and are also conserved among the seven interferon-α sequences and the one interferon-β sequence. The reverse turns around amino acid 110 are present in interferon-β and most species of interferon-α.

The conservation of reverse turn amino acids in the interferons is remarkable. For example, all four amino acids found in position 10 strongly favor reverse turns. In other positions (11, 72, 73, 74, 115, 116, 137) amino acids strongly favoring reverse turns have been conserved, either by preserving one amino acid or by substituting one reverse turn favorer for another. In only one position (114) have reverse turn breakers been introduced into the sequence (in interferons-αD, -αF, and -αG). Thus, the conservation of the four reverse turns in the sequence of eight interferons, one only distantly related to the remainder, strongly supports the existence of these turns and argues for their importance in interferon function.

Two good regions of α-helicity can be identified in interferon-β. These extend from amino acids 40 to 70 and from 90 to 109. These regions have P_α values of over 1.2 and are not involved in reverse turns or β-sheets. The helical regions possess hydrophobic amino acids every 3–4 amino acids. In interferon-β there is Ile-42, Leu-45, Phe-48, Ala-54, Tyr-58, Leu-61, Phe-65, Phe-68 in the 40–70 α-helix region. Presuming that these eight hydrophobic residues are buried, seven hydrophobic residues remain to contribute to surface hydrophobicity of the interferon molecule (Phe-43, Ala-53, Leu-55, Ile-57, Ile-64, Ala-66, Ile-67). The general feature of hydrophobic resides spaced 3–4 amino acids apart also characterized the α-helix at positions 90–104 of interferon-β and has been conserved in interferons-α.

There are no entirely satisfactory β-sheet candidate regions in the interferon molecules. The regions 118–131 and 140–155 have P_β values of 1.08 and 1.21, respectively, in interferon-β and 1.19 and 1.04, respectively, in interferon-αA. In the representation of Fig. 10 the putative β-sheet regions are in a position to interact with one another and with α-helical areas of the interferon protein.

Interferon-β carries glycosyl residues, probably three, judging from the molecular weight difference between glycosylated and deglycosylated molecules (CARTER 1979). For illustrative purposes these were placed in Fig. 10 at asparagine residues in positions 12, 63, and 156. These are also regions of decreased hydrophobicity in interferon-α. The position of hydrophyllic carbohydrates can profoundly alter the shape of the hydrophobic interferon protein and thereby could alter function. Interferon-β, for example, displays considerably more species specificity than the natural mixture of interferons-α. Until the carbohydrate moieties on interferon-β are located, however, their contribution to function and their role in interferon evolution will remain obscure.

F. Concluding Remarks

It would be desirable to end a chapter on interferon evolution with a discussion of the evolution of interferon function. Unfortunately, little can be said in this regard. In order for interferon to exert its biologic effects it must first be recognized by the target cell surfaces, at least in part through a receptor coded in humans by a gene on chromosome 21. The specificity and strenght of this interaction will depend upon interferon's amino acid sequence and will provide an element of evolutionary selection. Interferons-αA and -β bind the same sites on the cell surface (A. BRANCA and C. BAGLIONI, personal communications) so one might expect homologous amino acid sequences in the cell binding region of interferons-α and -β. However interferon-β from a variety of animals binds cells with considerably more avidity for the homologous species than is exhibited by the "natural" mixture of interferons-α, and possibly binds homologous cells with a higher affinity constant (see GILLESPIE and CARTER 1982). Moreover, STREULI et al. (1981) have shown that target cell specificity of interferons-α can be modified by altering either the COOH terminal or the NH_2 terminal amino acid sequence of the protein. Thus, the binding determinants on the interferon molecule are likely to be complex and difficult to evaluate evolutionarily.

FRIEDMAN and KOHN (1976) identified a ganglioside receptor whose binding to interferon is blocked by cholera toxin. It is known that it is the B subunit of cholera toxin which binds cells. DUFFY and LAI (1979) found that modification of Arg-35 by cyclohexanedione abolished the ability of the B subunit of cholera toxin to bind to the cell membrane. There is little homology of amino acid sequence between the B subunit of cholera toxin (LAI 1977) and interferon-α or -β. The region of closest homology is shown in Fig. 11. This homologous region contains the Arg-35 residue of cholera toxin and the amino acids immediately to its NH_2 side, Ser-Leu-Ala-Lys-Arg. There is no homology of the next 35 amino acids toward the COOH terminus, but cholera toxin residues 73–87 show homology to interferon residues 126–141. Thus, a continuous stretch of about 25 amino acid residues in the interferon polypeptide is homologous to two cholera toxin domains interrupted by an unrelated polypeptide sequence. As in cholera toxin, the homologous arginine residue is part of a basic dipeptide. Unlike cholera toxin, however, the interferon basic dipeptide is in a highly hydrophobic environment. There is no asparagine residue in the immediate linear vicinity of the basic dipeptide in interferon-β.

We surmise that the basic dipeptide at residues 121–122 of interferon participates in binding to the cell surface. We note that the most target cell-specific form of human interferon yet characterized, interferon-β, has a Lys-Arg dipeptide at residues 121–122 while the least specific, interferon-α_1 of STREULI et al. (1981), which is equivalent to interferon αD of GOEDDEL et al. (1981), has a Lys-Lys dipeptide in that position. Interferon-αA, which is intermediate in specificity, has an Arg-Lys dipeptide in positions 121–122. Possibly the presence and position of an arginine residue in this area of the interferon protein dictates the target cell specificity by determining binding to the cell membrane.

Once bound to the cell, interferon exerts a variety of effects on macromolecular synthesis and often an cellular morphology itself. Apparently, very few interferon molecules are required to elicit these changes in function and structure. As detailed elsewhere in this book, interferon prevents the multiplication of many viruses, inhibits cell growth, prevents lymphoblastogenesis, reverses neoplastic phenotypes, and stimulates or prevents differentiation. Where it has been studied, interferon-β and all species of interferon-α elicit each of the various biologic responses, although these studies have been largely confined to examinations of inhibition of virus multiplication and cell growth. It is possible that the various interferons will differ in their antitumor activity or their ability to modify cellular differentiation programs.

The question of interferon function is directly related to the question of why there are multiple interferon genes. If all interferon proteins have the same function, why is more than one gene necessary? Either: (1) multiple genes are required for reasons of dosage; (2) interferon genes are selfish; (3) interferon is functionally imperfect and new, more functional members are being duplicated and modified; or (4) the individual interferon genes do not have identical functions.

It is conceivable that a few cells produce massive quantities of interferon in order to compensate for an inefficient induction mechanism. Even so, until there is reason to believe differently, we consider the gene dosage idea to be unlikely. Similarly, the idea that the interferon-α genes are multiple because they possess an innate propensity to multiply seems unreasonable. There is no evidential basis for rejecting the hypothesis that the interferon-α genes carry DNA duplication or recombination sequences which favored the amplification pictured in Fig. 3 and are present for no reason of evolutionary fitness or physiologic advantage. The present-day genes would then be viewed as a tolerated genetic load. Indeed, the presence of the interferon-αE gene, presumably inactive because of a frame-shift insertion in the evolutionary past, indicates that unnecessary interferon genes can be tolerated.

Nevertheless, we prefer the view that, while the multiplication of the human interferon-α genes does reflects some structural feature of them, the presence of this structural feature is evolutionarily advantageous. It is conceivable that the advantage of multiplicity is the presence of protein variants to test, modify, and select for enhanced function, i.e., that present-day interferons are functionally imperfect. However, this thought implies that there is an inverse relationship between functional adequacy of proteins and the number of genes that code for them, a relationship as yet without expermental precedent.

Therefore, we favor the possibility that the different interferon genes code for interferon proteins which have somewhat different functions. If amplification of the human interferon-α gene family occurred as recently as depicted in Fig. 3, i.e., after the primate lineage split from rodents, carnivores, ungulates, etc., then these genes may be involved in a process which distinguishes one phylogenetic group from another, e.g., in implementing programs of development or differentiation.

From this idea it follows that interferon genes and developmental programs coevolve, implying a level of information transfer in "tailoring" interferon molecules that is beyond our present knowledge, but perhaps not beyond our experimental grasp over the foreseeable future.

References

Carter WA (1979) Mechanisms of cross-species activity of mammalian interferons. Pharm Ther 7:245–252

Chou PY, Fasman GD (1978) Empirical predictions of protein conformation. Ann Rev Biochem 47:251–276

Duffy LK, Lai CY (1979) Involvement of arginine residues in the binding site of cholera toxin subunit B. Biochem Biophys Res Comm 91:1005–1010

Friedman RM, Kohn LD (1976) Cholera toxin inhibits interferon action. Biochem Biophys Res Comm 70:1078–1087

Gillespie D, Carter WA (1982) Species specificity of interferon. Texas Rep Biol Med 41:37–42

Gillespie D, Pequignot E, Strayer D (1980) An ancestral amplification of DNA in primates. Gene 12:103–111

Goeddel DV, Leung DW, Dull TJ, Gross M, Lawn RM, McCandliss R, Seeburg PH, Ullrich A, Yelverton E, Gray PW (1981) The structure of eight distinct cloned human leukocyte interferon cDNAs. Nature 290:20–26

Houghton M, Jackson IJ, Porter AG, Doel SM, Catlin GH, Barber C, Carey NH (1981) The absence of introns within a human fibroblast interferon gene. Nucleic Acids Res 9:247

IUPAC-IUB Commission on Biochemical Nomenklature (1968) A one-letter notation for amino acid sequences. Eur J Biochem 5:151

Lai CY (1977) Determination of the primary structure of cholera toxin B subunit. J Biol Chem 252:7249–7256

Lawn RM, Adelman J, Franke AE, Houck CM, Gross M, Najarian R, Goeddel DV (1981 a) Human fibroblast interferon gene lacks introns. Nucleic Acids Res 9:1045

Lawn RM, Adelman J, Dull TJ, Gross M, Goeddel D, Ullrich A (1981 b) DNA sequence of two closely linked human leukocyte interferon genes. Science 212:1159–1162

Nagata S, Mantei N, Weissman C (1980) The structure of one of the eight or more distinct chromosomal genes for human interferon-α. Nature 287:401–408

Sagar AD, Pickering LA, Sussman-Berger P, Stewart WE, Sehgal PB (1981) Heterogeneity of interferon mRNA species from Sendai Virusinduced human lymphoblastoid (Namalva) cells and Newcastle disease virusinduced murine fibroblastoid (L) cells. Nucleic Acids Res 9:149–160

Streuli M, Hall A, Boll W, Stewart W, Nagata S, Weissman C (1981) Target cell specificity of two species of human interferon produced from Escherichia coli and of two hybrid molecules from them. Proc Natl Acad Sci USA 78:2848–2852

Taniguchi T, Mantei N, Schwarzstein M, Nagata S, Muramatsu M, Weissman C (1980) Human leukocyte and fibroblast interferons are structurally related. Nature 285:547–549

Tavernier J, Derynck R, Fiers W (1981) Evidence for a unique human fibroblast interferon (IFN β_1) chromosomal gene, devoid of intervening sequences. Nucleic Acids Res 9:461–471

Wetzel R, Perry LJ, Estell DA, Lin N, Levine HL, Slinker B, Fields F, Ross MJ, Shively J (1981) Properties of human alphainterferon purified from E. coli extracts. J Interferon Res 1:381–390

CHAPTER 4

Comparative Analysis of Interferon Structural Genes

P. B. SEHGAL and A. D. SAGAR

A. Introduction

Interferons (IFNs) are a family of inducible proteins which exert potent biologic effects on target cells. These proteins render animal cells resistant to infection by a wide spectrum of viruses, inhibit cell proliferation and exert immunomodulatory effects on a variety of target cells (SEHGAL et al. 1982). IFNs can be induced in a large number of different animal species (STEWART 1979) and usually exert their effects on cells of homologous species. However, certain IFNs are also active on cells of heterologous species (STEWART 1979).

Human and murine IFNs are presently classified into α (leukocyte), β (fibroblast), and γ (immune) subtypes based primarily on their antigenic relationships. Thus, antisera raised against IFN-α, -β, or -γ do not cross-react with IFNs of a different type. However, antisera raised against human IFN-α do cross-react with certain species of murine IFN-α (STEWART and HAVELL 1980). This relationship between the IFN proteins also extends to the structure of the respective IFN genes. Thus human IFN-α cDNA sequences do not cross-hybridize human IFN-β or -γ-genes, but do cross-hybridize murine IFN-α genes (OWERBACH et al. 1981).

Recent advances in the characterization of IFN mRNA species, the molecular cloning of some of the corresponding cDNA molecules, and the elucidation of the structure of some of the human IFN genes have provided remarkable insights into the structural and evolutionary relationships that exist in this complex multigene family that codes for proteins which exert potent antiviral, anticellular, and immunomodulatory effects on animal cells. Some of the human IFN genes are closely related (cross-hybridize), others only distantly related (do not cross-hybridize); some are located in tandem on the same chromosome in the human genome, others are widely dispersed; some of the genes are coordinately expressed while others are expressed in a grossly noncoordinate manner. The structural and functional complexity of the human IFN gene family suggests that the induction of specific IFNs may represent finely tuned responses by different cells or tissues to particular physiologic or pathologic stimuli. The recent elucidation of the precise structural relationships between some of the human IFN genes represents a major advance in understanding the complex functions of this gene family.

B. Molecular Cloning of Some Human IFN-α cDNA and Chromosomal Genes

NAGATA and his colleagues (NAGATA et al. 1980a; STREULI et al. 1980) have described the molecular cloning of two distinct IFN-α cDNA species derived from

12 *S* polyadenylated RNA extracted from Sendai virus-induced human peripheral blood leukocytes. These two cDNA species, designated IFN-α_1 and IFN-α_2, were then used to screen a human DNA gene bank. This led to the isolation of at least ten distinct human IFN-α genes which cross-hybridize an α_1 cDNA probe (NAGATA et al. 1980 b, 1981). Similarly, GOEDDEL and his colleagues isolated an IFN-α cDNA clone derived from 12 *S* polyadenylated RNA extracted from Sendai virus-induced human myeloblastoid cells (KG-1) (GOEDDEL et al. 1980 a). This cDNA clone (LeIF A) [1] was then used as a DNA hybridization probe to isolate at least eight distinct, but cross-hybridizing cDNA clones from their 12 *S* mRNA library in pBR322 (GOEDDEL et al. 1980 a, 1981). These investigators have also used these cDNA clones to screen a human DNA gene bank and have isolated up to 12 distinct, but cross-hybridizing IFN-α genes (LAWN et al. 1981 a, b). This set of cross-hybridizing human IFN-α genes and their derived mRNAs and proteins has been designated IFN-α_S in order to distinguish it from a second set of human IFN-α_L mRNAs which do not appear to cross-hybridize IFN-α_S-specific DNA probes (SAGAR et al. 1981; SEHGAL et al. 1981 a, b).

C. Molecular Cloning of a Human IFN-β cDNA and Its Chromosomal Gene

TANIGUCHI and his colleagues (TANIGUCHI et al. 1979, 1980 a, b) were the first to report the molecular cloning of a single species of IFN-β cDNA derived from 12 *S* polyadenylated RNA extracted from poly(I)·poly(C)-induced diploid human fibroblasts. This species of cDNA is designated IFN-β_1 in order to distinguish it from other IFN-β mRNAs which do not appear to cross-hybridize an IFN-β_1 cDNA probe (SEHGAL and SAGAR 1980; WEISSENBACH et al. 1980; SAGAR et al. 1981, 1982). Numerous other investigators have also cloned and characterized IFN-β_1 cDNA (GOEDDEL et al. 1980 b; DERYNCK et al. 1980 a, b). Several investigators have screened human DNA gene banks using IFN-β_1 cDNA probes and have isolated and characterized a single gene corresponding to IFN-β_1 (HOUGHTON et al. 1981; TAVERNIER et al. 1981; DEGRAVE et al. 1981; LAWN et al. 1981 c; OHNO and TANIGUCHI 1981; GROSS et al. 1981).

D. Comparative Structure of Some IFN-α and -β mRNAs and Proteins Deduced from cDNA Clones

The IFN-α cDNA clones described in Sect. B correspond to a group of cross-hybridizing mRNA species of length between 0.7 and 1.4 kilobases (SEHGAL et al. 1981 a, b). This set of IFN-α mRNAs is collectively designated IFN-α_S. A second set of IFN-α_L mRNAs which corresponds to mRNA species of length between 1.6 and 3 kilobases (peak activity 1.8 kilobases) has not yet been cloned (SEHGAL et

1 IFN nomenclature is in a state of flux at the present time, with different laboratories using different designations. In the case of the human α system, LeIF A and LeIF D (GOEDDEL et al. 1981) are equivalent to HuIFN-α_2 and HuIFN-α_1 respectively (NAGATA et al. 1980 a; STREULI et al. 1980)

al. 1981 a, b). The IFN-β_1 cDNA described in Sect. C corresponds to an mRNA species of length approximately 0.9 kilobases (SEHGAL and SAGAR 1980). Although a total of five distinct human IFN-β mRNA species have been described recently (SEHGAL and SAGAR 1980; SAGAR et al. 1981, 1982) four of these have not yet been cloned. Thus, the discussion in Sect. D and E is restricted to the human IFN-α_S set and to the IFN-β_1 gene.

I. The Coding Regions

A detailed characterization of the 8–10 distinct IFN-α cDNA clones available at the present time has revealed that most of these would code for proteins which consist of 166 amino acids, except for IFN-α_2, which would code for a protein containing 165 amino acids (Fig. 1). There is approximately 80% homology in the amino acid sequences of the mature proteins, but 85%–95% homology in the DNA sequence in the coding region. Two domains, amino acids 28–80 and 115–150 are highly conserved in all of these IFN-α proteins. These regions may represent the biologically active sites on these proteins. Studies on the activity of hybrid interferons derived from fused cloned IFN cDNA (STREULI et al. 1981) where codons for the NH_2 terminal amino acids 63 or 92 of IFN-α_1 are fused with codons for the remainder of the COOH terminal amino acids of IFN-α_2 and vice versa suggest that species-specific IFN activity segregates with the NH_2 terminal portion of the IFN molecule. These data suggest that the region 28–80 may contain the site which binds to the cell surface receptor. It has been suggested that the second region (amino acids 115–150) may have a role in modulating this binding or may contain a site responsible for some other biologic function (STREULI et al. 1981).

IFN-β_1 cDNA also codes for a mature protein of 166 amino acids (TANIGUCHI et al. 1980 a, c). IFN-β_1 is only 29% homologous with IFN-α_1 at the protein level, but is ~45% homologous in the DNA sequence of the coding region (TANIGUCHI et al. 1980 c). The two conserved domains in codons 28–80 and 115–150 observed in IFN-α_1 and -α_2 proteins are also conserved in IFN-β_1. However, the degree of nucleotide sequence conservation is not sufficient for cross-hybridization of IFN-β_1 RNA or DNA with IFN-α_1 DNA probes, even under relaxed hybridization conditions. Furthermore, the degree of amino acid sequence conservation is not sufficient for cross-reaction between antisera raised against IFN-α or -β and the heterologous interferons.

The IFN-protein sequences deduced from the cDNA clones indicate marked conservation of cysteine at positions 1, 29, 98 or 99, and 138 or 139 in the IFN-α proteins and the presence of cysteine residues at positions 31 and 141 in IFN-β_1 (Fig. 1; STREULI et al. 1980; GOEDDEL et al. 1981; WETZEL 1981). In the IFN-α proteins, Cys-1 is bonded to Cys-98 or -99 and Cys-29 to Cys-138 or -139 by disulfide bridges (WETZEL 1981). Similarly, IFN-β_1 may contain Cys-31 bonded to Cys-141.

The natural IFN-α proteins characterized to date are devoid of carbohydrate moieties (RUBINSTEIN et al. 1981; ALLEN and FANTES 1980) whereas IFN-β_1 has been shown to be a glycoprotein (KNIGHT 1976; TAN et al. 1979). Attachment of carbohydrate through *N*-glycosidic linkage is known to occur on the asparagine in the triplets Asn-X-Ser or Asn-X-Thr and the presence of this sequence is a necessary, but not a sufficient condition for glycosylation (NEUBERGER 1972). IFN-β_1

```
                                            10                  20
Mouse IFN-C               A D L P Q T Y N L G N K G A L K V L A Q
                                                                                      30                  40
HuIFN-α1                  C D L P E T H S L D N R R T L M L L A Q M - S R I S P S S C L M D R H D F G F P Q E
HuIFN-α2                  C D L P Q T H S L G S R R T L M L L A Q M - R R I S L F S C L K D R H D F G F P Q E
Lymphoblastoid IFN        S D L P Q T H S L G N R R A L I L L A Q M - G R I S L F S C L K D R
                                      10                  20                      30                  40
HuIFN-β1            M S Y N L L G F L Q R S S N F Q C Q K L L W Q L N G R - - L E Y C L K D R M N F D I P E E
Mouse IFN-A         I N Y K Q L Q L Q E R T N I R K ? Q E L L E Q L

All                           L                           L L   Q       R           C L   D R     F     P   E

                                          50                  60                  70                  80
HuIFN-α1                  E F D G N Q F Q K A P A I S V L H E L I Q Q I F N L F T T K D S S A A W D E D L L D
                                            50                  60                  70                  80
HuIFN-α2                  E F - G N Q F Q K A E T I P V L H E M I Q Q I F N L F S T K D S S A A W D E T L L D
                                      50                  60                  70                  80
HuIFN-β1                  I K Q L Q Q F Q K E D A A L T I Y E M L Q N I F A I F R Q D S S S T G W N E T I V E

All                                 Q F Q K                 E     Q   I F     F         S S     W   E

                                      90                  100                 110                 120
HuIFN-α1                  K F C T E L Y Q Q L N D L E A C V M Q E E R V G E T P L M N A D S I L A V K K Y F R
                                        90                  100                 110                 120
HuIFN-α2                  K F Y T E L Y Q Q L N D L E A C V I Q G V G V T E T P L M K E D S I L A V R K Y F Q
                                90                    100                 110                 120
HuIFN-β1                  N L L A N V Y H Q I N H L K T V L E E K L E K E D F T R G K L M S S L H L K R Y Y G

All                                   Y   Q   N   L                                       S   L         Y

                                  130                 140                 150                 160
HuIFN-α1                  R I T L Y L T E K K Y S P C A W E V V R A E I M R S L S L S T N L Q E R L R R K E
                                    130                 140                 150                 160
HuIFN-α2                  R I T L Y L K E K K Y S P C A W E V V R A E I M R S F S L S T N L Q E S L R S K E
                              130                 140                 150                 160
HuIFN-β1                  R I L H Y L K A K E Y S H C A W T I V R V E I L R N F Y F I N R L T G Y L R N

All                       R I     Y L     K   Y S   C A W     V R   E I   R               L       L R   K
```

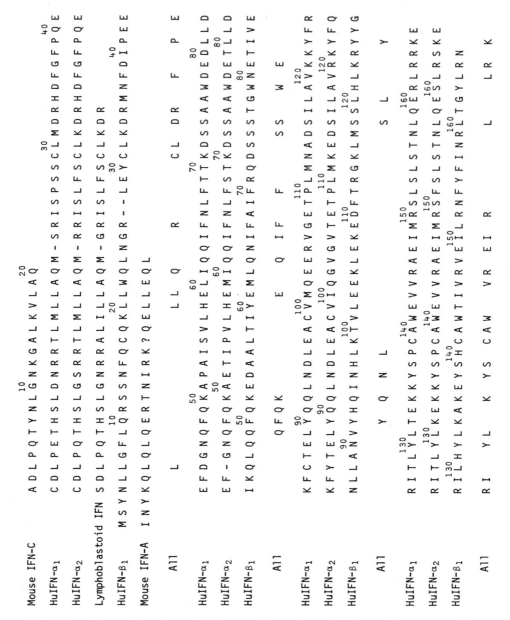

Fig. 1. The coding region of some IFN genes. Comparison of amino acid sequences of human IFN-α_1 and -α_2, deduced from the cDNA sequence (Mantei et al. 1980), with human lymphoblastoid IFN, deduced from amino acid analyses, murine IFN-A and -C, deduced from NH_2 terminal amino acid analyses (Taira et al. 1980), and human fibroblast IFN-β_1 from the cDNA sequence (Taniguchi et al. 1980a). The amino acids are written according to the one-letter notation as recommended by the IUPAC-IUB Commission on Biochemical Nomenclature (Dayoff 1978). A-alanine; C-cysteine; D-aspartic acid; E-glutamic acid; F-phenylalanine; G-glycine; H-histidine; I-isoleucine; K-lysine; M-methionine; N-asparagine; P-proline; Q-glutamine; R-arginine; S-serine, T-threonine; V-valine; W-tryptophan; Y-tyrosine. A *question mark* indicates a sequence not yet identified. *Dashes* have been introduced to obtain maximum homology. Mouse IFN-C corresponds to IFN-α and mouse IFN-A corresponds to IFN-β. Streuli et al. (1980)

contains such an asparagine at position 80 of the amino acid sequence while none of the IFN-α protein sequences deduced to date indicates the presence of this amino acid triplet.

A number of cDNA molecules which have unusual features in their coding regions have been cloned:

1. The IFN-α cDNA designated "LeIFN E" (GOEDDEL et al. 1981) contains one nucleotide more than the other IFN-α cDNAs at position 187, corresponding to amino acid 40. Subsequent to this translation termination condons are encountered in all three phases. Thus "LeIFN E" cDNA appears to represent a pseudogene that is transcribed and expressed at a low level in virus-induced myeloblastoid cells.

2. Two IFN-α cDNA clones designated "LeIFN H" and "LeIFN H_1" are virtually identical except for a single nucleotide deletion in H_1 (at nucleotide 545, C) which is followed six nucleotides later by a correcting insertion (after nucleotide 551, G), thus restoring the original reading frame. These two clones probably represent allelic genes (GOEDDEL et al. 1981).

3. An IFN-β_1 cDNA has been isolated in which the deduced protein sequence includes the change of Cys-141 to Tyr-141. The protein expressed in *Escherichia coli* corresponding to this unusual cDNA displays no antiviral activity, does not compete with anti-IFN-β immunoglobulin, and does not bind to cell membranes (SHEPARD et al. 1981). Thus, it appears that Cys-141 may play an important role in the biologic activity of IFN-β_1.

While many of the conclusions about these IFN-α and -β_1 proteins deduced from the nucleotide sequences of the cDNA clones have been confirmed by direct analyses of the mature proteins (KNIGHT et al. 1980; TANIGUCHI et al. 1980a, c; MAEDA et al. 1980; ALLEN and FANTES 1980), a recent report (LEVY et al. 1981) suggests that three particular species of mature IFN-α proteins derived from virus-induced human leukocyte cell cultures (the cells were obtained from patients with chronic myelogenous leukemia) lack the ten COOH terminal amino acids predicted by the DNA sequence.

II. The Signal Peptides

IFNs are secretory proteins. Thus, each of the IFN cDNA clones that has been characterized reveals the presence of a hydrophobic signal peptide 21–23 amino acids long (TANIGUCHI et al. 1980a, c; MANTEI et al. 1980a; GOEDDEL et al. 1980a, b). There is a greater degree of variability in the signal sequence than in the coding regions. The six IFN-α signal peptides that have been deduced consist of 23 amino acids, are approximately 70% homologous to each other with 11 (43%) of the amino acids completely conserved. On the other hand the 21 amino acid IFN-β_1 signal peptide is markedly different from the IFN-α signal peptides (~60% divergence in nucleotide sequence) (TANIGUCHI et al. 1980c; STREULI et al. 1980).

III. The Noncoding Regions

The 5′ noncoding region in the IFN-α and β_1 mRNAs is approximately 65–75 nucleotides long (HOUGHTON et al. 1981; NAGATA et al. 1980b; LAWN et al. 1981b).

	(e)	(d)	(c)	(b)	(a)	Corresponding designation
	−125	−80	−59	−30	−1	
1	TGAAAACCCATG	G–AAAGTA	TTTGGAA	TATTTAA	CA	IFN-α_2
2	TCTACACCCATG	GAAAAAAA	TTCAGAA	TATTTAA	CA	
3	CTTAAACACATG	G–AAAGTA	TTTAGAA	TATTTAA	CA	
4	TTTAAACACATG	G–AAAGTA	TTTAGAA	TATTTAA	CA	
5	TTTAAACACATG	G–AAAGTA	TTTAGAA	TATTTAA	CA	
6	TCTAAAATCATG	G–AAAGTG	TTAAGAA	TATTTAA	CA	IFN-α_1
7	TCTATACCCATG	G–AAAGTA	TTCTGAA	TATTTAA	CA	
	−114	−72	−57	−31	−1	
8	TACTAAAATG	GAAAGTGG	CTCTGAA	TATAAA	CA	IFN-β_1

Fig. 2a–e. The 5′ flanking region of some IFN genes. Comparison of homologous nucleotide sequences, upstream from the transcription initiation site of several human IFN-α genes and the IFN-β_1 gene. These sequences could conceivably play a role in gene regulation. **a** transcription initiation site; **b** Goldberg–Hogness box; **c** and **e** presumably involved in induction; **d** CCAAT box thought to be involved in RNA polymerase II binding. Sequences 1–7 taken from LAWN et al. (1981 b); 8 from DEGRAVE et al. (1981)

There is marked (~75%) sequence homology in the 5′ noncoding regions of seven of the IFN-α genes sequenced so far. On the other hand the 5′ noncoding region of IFN-β_1 has a much lower degree of homology with the IFN-α sequences. The 3′ noncoding regions of IFN-α and -β_1 mRNAs are highly variable. The length of the 3′ noncoding region can vary from 203 (IFN-β_1) to approximately 506 (LeIF A (+175)) nucleotides preceding the poly(A). There is approximately 50% homology in the nucleotide sequence in this region among the IFN-α mRNAs. Thus, DNA restriction fragments corresponding to this region can be used as hybridization probes for the individual IFN-α mRNA species (STREULI et al. 1980; GOEDDEL et al. 1981). There is only 30% homology between the nucleotide sequence in this region in IFN-β_1 mRNA and IFN-α_1 and -α_2 mRNAs (STREULI et al. 1980).

The hexanucleotide, AAUAAA precedes the site of polyadenylation in many eukaryotic cellular mRNAs by 15–25 nucleotides (PROUDFOOT 1976). IFN-β_1 mRNA contains the AAUAAA sequence 20 nucleotides internal to the poly(A) site. One-half of the IFN-α cDNAs sequenced contain the corresponding AATAAA sequence approximately 15–20 nucleotides from the poly(A) site (LeIFN A, D, F, and G; GOEDDEL et al. 1981) while several others (LeIFN B, C, E, and H; GOEDDEL et al. 1981) contain the related sequence ATTAAA. LeIFN B contains the ATTAAA approximately 400 nucleotides from the end of the coding region, but is not polyadenylated until after a second ATTAAA sequence is reached approximately 485 nucleotides into the 3′ noncoding region (GOEDDEL et al. 1981). Whereas LeIF A or IFN-α_2 is usually polyadenylated approximately 330 nucleotides from the end of the coding region and contains the AAUAAA sequence 20 nucleotides proximal to this poly(A) site (GOEDDEL et al. 1981), a variant cDNA [LeIFN A (+175)] has been cloned which represents an mRNA species in which polyadenylation did not occur at this site, but at a location 175 nucleotides further downstream (LAWN et al. 1981 b). A second AATAAA hexanucleotide precedes the 3′ end of this extended cDNA clone (LAWN et al. 1981 b).

The length of the 3′ poly(A) tails present in IFN-α mRNA species has not been investigated. The length of the 3′ poly(A) in cytoplasmic IFN-β_1 mRNA has been estimated to be approximately 100 nucleotides and that of IFN-β_2 mRNA to be approximately 200 nucleotides (SOREQ et al. 1981). Since the group of IFN-α_S genes and the IFN-β_1 gene are known to be devoid of introns (Sect. E) it is intriguing to determine whether newly synthesized mRNAs derived from these genes have shorter poly(A) than newly synthesized mRNA molecules derived from most other cellular split genes (150–250 nucleotides). mRNAs derived from mammalian histone genes, which also lack introns, are devoid of 3′ poly(A). The degree of variability in the 3′ noncoding sequence suggests that this region may not be particularly crucial to the translational function of IFN mRNAs. Indeed, deletion of the poly(A) and large (100–200 nucleotides) segments of the 3′ noncoding sequence internal to the poly(A) does not affect the translational function of IFN-β_1 and -β_2 mRNAs in *Xenopus laevis* oocytes (SOREQ et al. 1981).

E. Comparative Structure of Some IFN-α and -β_1 Chromosomal Genes

A set of up to 12 distinct, but cross-hybridizing genes and pseudogenes has been isolated by screening human DNA gene banks (e.g., in lambda phage charon 4A) using IFN-α cDNA probes (NAGATA et al. 1980b, 1981; LAWN et al. 1981 a, b). In contrast, a single IFN-β_1 gene has been isolated in this manner (HOUGHTON et al. 1981; OHNO and TANIGUCHI 1981; TAVERNIER et al. 1981; LAWN et al. 1981 c; GROSS et al. 1981). These chromosomal genes and their flanking 5′ and 3′ regions have been extensively characterized.

All of the cloned chromosomal IFN-α and -β_1 genes lack introns. The chromosomal DNA sequence is completely colinear with the nucleotide sequence of IFN-α and -β_1 mRNA species. The absence of intervening sequences in these IFN-α and -β_1 genes is unusual in that eukaryotic genes (except the histones) contain "redundant" noncoding DNA (introns) interspersed within the coding regions (exons) (HAMER and LEDER 1979). The DNA sequence in the introns frequently diverges much more rapidly than in the exons of related genes (HEILIG et al. 1980). Several of the cross-hybridizing and closely related IFN-α genes are also closely linked in tandem and contain inverted repeats in the flanking regions, suggestive of a gene duplication mechanism in the evolution of these IFN-α genes (NAGATA et al. 1981; LAWN et al. 1981 a, b).

Figure 2 presents a comparison of the nucleotide sequences in the 5′ noncoding and the 5′ flanking region in several IFN-α genes and in the IFN-β_1 gene. The 5′ flanking region immediately upstream from an mRNA sequence is thought to play an important role in the regulation of gene expression. Specific sequence homologies are present in the 5′ flanking region of eukaryotic structural genes. These regions could represent loci where RNA polymerase II binds to the DNA to initiate transcription or where other inducers of regulatory molecules could bind to activate or repress the transcriptional acitivity of genes. Figure 2 reveals regions of distinct homology between the IFN genes, several of which are also seen in other eukaryotic genes and may thus be important in the regulation and expression of these genes.

a. There is a transcription initiation/capping site CA* approximately 70 nucleotides upstream from the translation initiation codon ATG.

b. A sequence TATTTAA approximately 31 nucleotides upstream from the presumed cap site is common to all the IFN-α genes. A similar sequence TATAAA 30 nucleotides upstream from the cap site is seen in the IFN-β_1 gene. This sequence is thought to play an important role in positioning the initiation of transcription and is generally found at a similar distance from the transcriptional start sites of eukaryotic genes (GOLDBERG 1979; GROSVELD et al. 1981; BAKER et al. 1981).

c. The sequence GAAAGT$^{A}_{G}$ is present at position −77 in the IFN-α genes and at −72 in the IFN-β_1 genes. This region presumably serves as a controlling or recognition region for transcription by RNA polymerase II (BENOIST et al. 1980; WASYLYK et al. 1980).

d. The sequence CTCTGAA (−57 to −51 in IFN-β_1) in present at about the same distance in chicken ovalbumin (BENOIST et al. 1980) and conalbumin (COCHET et al. 1979), and in modified form in the IFN-α genes.

e. Further upstream, the sequence TACTAAAATG is observed in IFN-β_1 and to some degree in the IFN-α genes. A similar sequence also occurs at a considerable distance (−125 to −140 nucleotides) from the cap site in human insulin, chicken ovalbumin, and chicken conalbumin genes (BENOIST et al. 1980; COCHET et al. 1979; BELL et al. 1980). Homologies indicated in e and c may be common to inducible proteins.

f. Small direct repeats are present several hundred (300) nucleotides upstream from some of the IFN-α genes and the IFN-β_1 gene in addition to a palindromic sequence in positions −280 to −240 (LAWN et al. 1981 a, b; GROSS et al. 1981).

These homologies in 5′ flanking sequence suggest not only that these genes may have evolved from a common ancestor, but that these regions may also have an important function in the expression of IFN genes. Multiple polyadenylation signals (AATAAA or ATTAAA) are seen in the 3′ flanking region of several IFN-α genes. It is clear that the same gene can give rise to mRNA species which utilize different poly(A) sites (GOEDDEL et al. 1981; LAWN et al. 1981 b).

F. Other Human IFN-α and -β Genes

Recent evidence suggests the existence of a second set of human IFN-α mRNAs which code for IFNs which are serologically of the α type but which do not cross-hybridize IFN-α_1-related cDNA probes, even under relaxed hybridization conditions (SAGAR et al. 1981; SEHGAL et al. 1981 a, b). This set of unusual mRNA species of length 1.6–3 kilobases (designated IFN-α_L) can be resolved from the conventional IFN-α mRNAs of length 0.7–1.4 kilobases (designated IFN-α_S) by electrophoresis of RNA through agarose–CH_3HgOH gels.

Similarly, electrophoresis of RNA through agarose–CH_3HgOH gels has led to the recognition of five distinct IFN-β mRNAs designated IFN-β_1 through IFN-β_5

(of lengths 0.9, 1.3, 1.8, 0.7, 0.9 kilobases, respectively) (SEHGAL and SAGAR 1980; SEHGAL et al. 1981 a; SAGAR et al. 1981, 1982). Even though these mRNAs code for IFNs which are serologically of the β type, their nucleic acids do not appear to cross-hybridize (SEHGAL and SAGAR 1980; WEISSENBACH et al. 1980; SAGAR et al. 1982). The molecular cloning of IFN-β_2 cDNA has been recently reported (WEISSENBACH et al. 1980). Thus, the IFN-α and -β gene family is even more complex than has been described in Sects. D and E. There appears to be even greater variability in IFN structural genes than had been anticipated.

G. Chromosomal Localization

Several of the IFN-α_S genes are closely linked and are arranged in tandem in chromosomal DNA (NAGATA et al. 1981; LAWN et al. 1981 a). Although most of these genes have been localized to human chromosome 9 (OWERBACH et al. 1981), it is unclear whether all of these are present on chromosome 9. The IFN-β_1 gene has also been localized to human chromosome 9 (MEAGER et al. 1979; OWERBACH et al. 1981). Nevertheless, the IFN-β_1 gene is not closely linked to the IFN-α_S genes since large (35–40 kilobases) segments of chromosomal DNA containing IFN-β_1 have been found to lack IFN-α sequences (GROSS et al. 1981).

The chromosomal localization of IFN-α_L genes (SEHGAL et al. 1981a, b) is not known. It has been clearly shown that the other human IFN-β genes are widely dispersed in the human genome (TAN et al. 1974; SLATE and RUDDLE 1979, 1980; SAGAR et al. 1982). The available data are consistent with the localization of IFN-β_2 to human chromosome 5, and IFN-β_3 and -β_5 to chromosome 2 (SAGAR et al. 1982). In addition, there may exist another IFN-β on a chromosome other than 2, 5, or 9 (SAGAR et al. 1982). Although IFN-β_1 is a gene without introns, there is suggestive evidence that IFN-β_2 may be a gene with introns (SEHGAL and TAMM 1980; M. REVEL 1980, personal communication).

Several of the IFN-α_S genes localized to chromosome 9 are expressed in a coordinate manner (GOEDDEL et al. 1980 a, 1981). The IFN-β_1 gene which is also localized to chromosome 9 can be expressed independently of these α genes following poly(I)·poly(C) induction of diploid human fibroblasts (TANIGUCHI et al. 1979; 1980 a, b) as well as coordinately with the IFN-α genes following virus induction of human myeloblastoid cells (GOEDDEL et al. 1980 b). Furthermore, the various IFN-β genes can be expressed in a grossly noncoordinate manner in poly(I)·poly(C)-induced diploid human fibroblasts (SEHGAL and SAGAR 1980; SAGAR et al. 1982).

The expression of IFN-α_S genes can be inhibited and that of IFN-α_L genes enhanced when human peripheral blood leukocytes are induced with Sendai virus in the presence of 5,6-dichloro-1-β-D-ribofuranosylbenzimidazole (SEHGAL et al. 1981 b). It is likely that this variability in the expression of human IFN genes reflects the complex structural relationships between them. Insights into these phenomena may have to await the molecular cloning and characterization of the recently discovered human α and β genes. Similarly, human IFN-γ genes await detailed characterization.

H. IFN Structural Genes in Other Species

IFNs are expressed in a wide range of animal species (STEWART 1979). The murine IFN genes are likely to be as complex as the human IFN genes. Murine IFN-α, -β, and -γ have been clearly recognized (YAMAMOTO and KAWADE 1980; OSBORNE et al. 1979). The NH_2 terminal amino acid sequence of a species of murine IFN-α reveals good homology with a species of human IFN-α and that of murine IFN-β reveals some homology with human IFN-β_1 (Fig. 1; TAIRA et al. 1980). Antisera to human IFN-α cross-react with a species of murine IFN-α (STEWART and HAVELL 1980; HAVELL and CARTER 1981). DNA probes derived from human IFN-α genes appear to cross-hybridize with analogous sequences in the murine genome (OWERBACH et al. 1981). While the known human IFN-α proteins lack carbohydrate moieties and human IFN-β_1 contains carbohydrate, both murine IFN-α and -β proteins are glycoproteins (HAVELL and CARTER 1981). Appropriate differences (e.g., Asn-X-Ser or Asn-X-Thr sequences) between the structure of human IFN-α and murine IFN-α genes can be anticipated. It is likely that there will be rapid progress in the elucidation of the structure of not only the murine IFN genes, but of those in a wide variety of animal species.

J. Conclusions

IFNs represent a highly complex multigene family which consists of numerous closely related as well as several distantly related genes. Some of the genes which are closely related are present in a cluster on chromosome 9 (IFN-α_S genes) whereas several of the genes which are more distantly related are dispersed in the human genome (IFN-β genes). Although recent advances in the characterization of some human IFN genes have provided fascinating insights into some of the structural relationship that exist in this gene family, several of the newly recognized IFN genes still remain to be characterized. It is likely that even more exciting insights lie ahead.

Acknowledgments. We thank Dr. IGOR TAMM for numerous helpful discussions. Research in the authors' laboratory is supported by Grant AI-16262 from the NIAID. P. B. S. is the recipient of a Junior Faculty Research Award from the American Cancer Society and A. D. S. is supported by an NIH Institutionl predoctoral fellowship.

References

Allen G, Fantes KH (1980) A family of structural genes for human lymphoblastoid (leucocyte-type) interferon. Nature 287:408–411

Baker CC, Herisse J, Courtois G, Galibert F, Ziff E (1979) Messenger RNA for the Ad 2 DNA binding protein: DNA sequences encoding the first leader and heterogeneity at the mRNA 5′ end. Cell 18:569–580

Bell GI, Pictet RL, Rutter WJ, Cordell B, Tischer E, Goodman HM (1980) Sequence of the human insulin gene. Nature 284:26–32

Benoist C, O'Hare K, Breathnach R, Chambon P (1980) The ovalbumin genese-quence of putative control regions. Nucleic Acids Res 8:127–142

Cochet M, Gannon F, Hen R, Maroteaux L, Perrin F, Chambon P (1979) Organization and sequence studies of the 17 piece chicken conalbumin gene. Nature 282:567–574

Dayoff MO (1978) Atlas of protein sequence and structure, vol 5, suppl 3. National Biomedical Research Foundation, Washington, DC
Degrave W, Derynck R, Tavernier J, Haegeman G, Fiers W (1981) Nucleotide sequence of the chromosomal gene for human fibroblast (β_1) interferon and of the flanking regions. Gene 14:137–143
Derynck R, Content J, DeClercq E, Volckaert G, Tavernier J, Devos R, Fiers W (1980a) Isolation and structure of a human fibroblast interferon gene. Nature 285:542–546
Derynck R, Remaut E, Saman E, Stanssens P, DeClercq E, Content J, Fiers W (1980b) Expression of human fibroblast interferon gene in Escherichia coli. Nature 287:193–197
Goeddel DV, Yelverton E, Ullrich A, Heyneker HL, Miozzari G, Holmes W, Seeburg PH, Dull T, May L, Stebbing N, Crea R, Maeda S, McCandliss R, Sloma A, Tabor JM, Gross M, Familletti PC, Pestka S (1980a) Human leucocyte interferon produced by E. coli is biologically active. Nature 287:411–416
Goeddel DV, Shepard HM, Yelverton E, Leung D, Crea R, Sloma A, Pestka S (1980b) Synthesis of human fibroblast interferon by E. coli. Nucleic Acids Res 8:4057–4074
Goeddel DV, Leung DW, Dull TJ, Gross M, Lawn RM, McCandliss R, Seeburg PH, Ullrich A, Yelverton E, Gray P (1981) The structure of eight distinct cloned human leucocyte interferon cDNAs. Nature 290:20–26
Goldberg M (1979) Ph. D. Thesis, Stanford University
Gross G, Mayr U, Bruns W, Grosveld F, Dahl HHM, Collins J (1981) The structure of a thirty-six kilobase region of the human chromosome including the fibroblast interferon gene IFN β. Nucleic Acids Res 9:2495–2507
Grosveld CC, Shewmaker CK, Jat P, Flavell RA (1981) Localization of DNA sequences necessary for transcription of the rabbit β globin gene in vitro. Cell 25:215–226
Hamer DH, Leder P (1979) Splicing and the formation of stable RNA. Cell 18:1299–1302
Havell EA, Carter WA (1981) Effects of tunicamycin on the physical properties and antiviral activities of murine L cell interferon. Virology 108:80–86
Heilig R, Perrin F, Cannon F, Mandel JL, Chambon P (1980) The ovalbumin gene family: structure of the X gene and evolution of duplicated split genes. Cell 20:625–637
Houghton M, Jackson IJ, Porter AG, Doel SM, Catlin GH, Barber C, Carey NH (1981) The absence of introns within a human fibroblast interferon gene. Nucleic Acids Res 9:247–266
Knight E Jr (1976) Interferon: Purification and initial characterization from human diploid cells. Proc Natl Acad Sci USA 73:520–523
Knight E Jr, Hunkapiller MW, Korant BD, Hardy RWF, Hood LE (1980) Human fibroblast interferon: amino acid analysis and amino terminal amino acid sequence. Science 207:525–526
Lawn RM, Adelman J, Dull TJ, Gross M, Goeddel D, Ullrich A (1981a) DNA sequence of two closely linked human leucocyte interferon genes. Science 212:1159–1162
Lawn RM, Gross M, Houck CM, Franke AE, Gray PV, Goeddel DV (1981b) DNA sequence of a major human leucocyte interferon gene. Proc Natl Acad Sci USA 78:5435–5439
Lawn RM, Adelman J, Franke AE, Houck CM, Gross M, Najarian R, Goeddel DV (1981c) Human fibroblast interferon gene lacks introns. Nucleic Acids Res 9:1045–1052
Levy WP, Rubinstein M, Shively J, Delvalle U, Lai CY, Moschera J, Brink L, Gerber L, Stein S, Pestka S (1981) Amino acid sequence of a human leucocyte interferon. Proc Natl Acad Sci USA 78:6186–6190
Maeda S, McCandliss R, Gross M, Sloma A, Familletti PC, Tabor JM, Evinger M, Levy WP, Pestka S (1980) Construction and identification of bacterial plasmids containing nucleotide sequence for human leukocyte interferon. Proc Natl Acad Sci USA 77:7010–7013
Mantei N, Schwarzstein M, Streuli M, Panem S, Nagata S, Weissman C (1980) The nucleotide sequence of a cloned human leucocyte interferon cDNA. Gene 10:1–10
Meager A, Graves M, Burke DC, Swallow DM (1979) Involvement of a gene on chromosome 9 in human fibroblast interferon production. Nature 280:493–495

Nagata S, Taira H, Hall A, Johnsrud L, Streuli M, Escodi J, Boll W, Cantell K, Weissmann C (1980a) Synthesis in E. coli of a polypeptide with human leucocyte interferon activity. Nature 284:316–320
Nagata S, Mantei N, Weissmann C (1980b) The structure of one of the eight or more distinct chromosomal genes for human interferon-α. Nature 287:401–408
Nagata S, Brack C, Henco K, Schamböck A, Weissmann C (1981) Partial mapping of ten genes of the human interferon-α family. J Interferon Res 1:333–336
Neuberger A, Gottschalk A, Marshall RD, Spiro RG (1972) In: Gottschalk A (ed) The glycoproteins: their composition, structure and function. Elsevier, Amsterdam, p 450
Ohno S, Taniguchi T (1981) Structure of a chromosomal gene for human interferon β. Proc Natl Acad Sci USA 78:5305–5309
Osborne LC, Georgiades JA, Johnson HM (1979) Large scale production and partial purification of mouse immune interferon. Infect Immun 23:80–86
Owerbach D, Rutter WJ, Shows TB, Gray P, Goeddel DV, Lawn RM (1981) Leukocyte and fibroblast genes are located on human chromosome 9. Proc Natl Acad Sci USA 78:3123–3127
Proudfoot NJ, Brownlee GG (1976) 3′ Noncoding region sequences in eukaryotic messenger RNA. Nature 263:211–214
Rubinstein M, Levy WP, Moschera JA, Lal GY, Hershberg RD, Bartlett RT, Pestka S (1981) Human leucocyte interferon: isolation and characterization of several molecular forms. Arch Biochem Biophys 210:307–318
Sagar AD, Pickering LA, Sussman-Berger P, Stewart WE II, Sehgal PB (1981) Heterogeneity of interferon mRNA species from Sendai virus-induced human lumphoblastoid (Namalva) cells and Newcastle disease virus-induced murine fibroblast (L) cells. Nucleic Acids Res 9:149–159
Sagar AD, Sehgal PB, Slate DL, Ruddle FH (1982) Multiple human β interferon genes. J Exp Med 156:744–755
Sehgal PB, Sagar AD (1980) Heterogeneity of poly(I) · poly(C)-induced human fibroblast interferon mRNA species. Nature 287:95–97
Sehgal PB, Tamm I (1980) The transcription unit for poly(I) · poly(C)-induced human fibroblast interferon messenger RNA. Virology 102:245–249
Sehgal PB, Sagar AD, Braude IA, Smith D (1981a) Heterogeneity of human α and β interferon mRNA species. In: DeMaeyer E, Schellekens H (eds) The biology of the interferon system, North-Holland/Elsevier, Amsterdam, p 43
Sehgal PB, Sagar AD, Braude IA (1981b) Further heterogeneity of human α interferon mRNA species. Science 214:803–805
Sehgal PB, Pfeffer LM, Tamm I (1982) Interferon and its inducers. In: Came PE, Caliguiri LA (eds) Chemotherapy of viral infections. Hdbk Exp Pharm 61:205–311 Springer Berlin, Heidelberg, New York
Shepard M, Leung D, Stebbing N, Goeddel DV (1981) Synthesis in E. coli of a naturally occurring mutant fibroblast interferon. Abstr of the 5th international congress of virology, Strasbourg, p 89
Slate DL, Ruddle FH (1979) Fibroblast interferon in man is coded by two loci on separate chromosomes. Cell 16:171–180
Slate DL, Ruddle FH (1980) Somatic cell genetic analysis of interferon production and response. Ann NY Acad Sci 350:174–178
Soreq H, Sagar AD, Sehgal PB (1981) Translational activity and functional stability of human fibroblast β_1 and β_2 interferon mRNAs lacking 3′-terminal RNA sequences. Proc Natl Acad Sci USA 78:1741–1745
Stewart WE II (ed) (1979) The interferon system. Springer Berlin Heidelberg New York
Stewart WE II, Havell EA (1980) Characterization of a subspecies of mouse interferon cross-reactive on human cells and antigenically related to human leukocyte interferon. Virology 101:315–318
Streuli M, Nagata S, Weissmann C (1980) At least three human type α interferons: Structure of α2. Science 209:1343–1347

Streuli M, Hall A, Boll W, Stewart WE II, Nagata S, Weissmann C (1981) Target cell specificity of two species of human interferon-α produced in Escherichia coli and of hybrid molecules derived from them. Proc Natl Acad Sci USA 78:2848–2852

Taira H, Broeze RJ, Jayaram BM, Lengyel P, Hunkapillar MW, Hood LE (1980) Mouse interferons: Amino terminal amino acid sequences of various species. Science 207:528–529

Tan YH (1974) The somatic cell genetics of human interferon: Assignment of human interferon loci to chromosomes 2 and 5. Proc Natl Acad Sci USA 71:2251–2255

Tan YH, Barakat F, Berthold W, Smith-Johannsen H, Tan C (1979) The isolation and amino acid/sugar composition of human fibroblastoid interferon. J Biol Chem 254:8067–8073

Taniguchi T, Sakai M, Fujii-Kuriyama Y, Muramatsu M, Kobayashi S, Sudo T (1979) Construction and identification of a bacterial plasmid containing the human fibroblast interferon gene sequence. Proc Jpn Acad Ser B 55:464–469

Taniguchi T, Ohno S, Fujii-Kuriyama Y, Muramatsu M (1980a) The nucleotide sequence of human fibroblast interferon cDNA. Gene 10:11–15

Taniguchi T, Guarente L, Roberts TM, Kimelman D, Douhan J, Ptashne M (1980b) Expression of the human fibroblast interferon gene in Escherichia coli. Proc Natl Acad Sci USA 77:5230–5233

Taniguchi T, Mantei N, Schwarstein M, Shigekazu N, Muramatsu M, Weissmann C (1980c) Human leucocyte and fibroblast interferons are structurally related. Nature 285:547–549

Tavernier J, Derynck R, Fiers W (1981) Evidence for a unique human fibroblast interferon (IFN β_1) chromosomal gene, devoid of intervening sequences. Nucleic Acids Res 9:461–471

Wasylyk B, Derbyshire R, Guy A, Molko D, Roget A, Tedule R, Chambon P (1980) Specific in vitro transcription of conalbumin gene is drastically decreased by single-point mutations in T-A-T-A box homology sequence. Proc Natl Acad Sci USA 77:7024–7028

Weissenbach J, Chernajovsky Y, Zeevi M, Shulman L, Soreq H, Nir U, Wallach D, Perricaudet M, Tiollais P, Revel M (1980) Two interferon mRNAs in human fibroblasts: In vitro translation and Escherichia coli cloning studies. Proc Natl Acad Sci USA 77:7152–7156

Wetzel R (1981) Assignment of the disulphide bonds of leucocyte interferon. Nature 289:606–607

Yamamoto Y, Kawade Y (1980) Antigenicity of mouse interferons: Distinct antigenicity of the two L cell interferon species. Virology 103:80–88

CHAPTER 5

Comparative Structures of Mammalian Interferons

K. C. ZOON and R. WETZEL

A. Introduction

Our knowledge of the structure of mammalian interferons has been limited in the past, predominantly because only minute quantities were available for structureal studies. Advances in amino acid analysis and sequence determination of picomolar quantities of protein have permitted the acquisition of composition and partial sequence data for several native human and mouse interferons. However, the majority of information on the structure of interferon has been the direct result of recombinant DNA (rDNA) technology. Not only has this application of genetic engineering provided amino acid sequence data for a number of human interferons, but has also allowed the isolation of sufficient quantities of human interferon for other structural studies, e.g., disulfide bond analysis and circular dichroism spectroscopy. Studies aimed at determining the composition and structure of the carbohydrate moiety of interferon are, of course, dependent upon the availability of naturally derived material, and thus have been more limited.

B. Purification and Characterization of Native Interferons

I. Human Interferons-α

1. Purification

A summary of the major procedures developed for the purification of native human interferons-α (HuIFN-α)[1] was reported recently (ZOON 1981). Some of the most powerful steps include immunoabsorbant affinity chromatography using either monoclonal or polyclonal antibodies, sodium dodecylsulfate polyacrylamide gel electrophoresis (SDS PAGE), and high pressure liquid chromatography (HPLC). Multiple species of native HuIFN-α have been isolated from virus-induced cultures of buffy coat (ZOON et al. 1982a; BERG and HERON 1980), Namalwa (ZOON et al. 1979; ALLEN and FANTES 1980), chronic myelogenous leukemia (RUBINSTEIN et al. 1981), and KG-1 (D. HOBBS 1981, personal communication) cells.

---

1 We have attempted to use current recommended nomenclature (leukocyte = α, fibroblast = β, immune = γ) as much as possible in this review. The following exceptions will be found, however: cloned interferon genes or their products derived from the work of GOEDDEL et al. (1981) are referred to as either IFN-αA, B, C, etc., or LeIF-A, B, C, etc.; single subtype interferons originally purified at the protein level (RUBINSTEIN et al. 1981) are designated as α, β, γ based on their high pressure liquid chromatography retention times; in this case, the use of Greek letters in both systems of nomenclature is accommodated by placing the designations of RUBINSTEIN et al. in parentheses. For instance, IFN-α(Le_1 β_1) is purified subtype β_1 of human interferon-α

Table 1. Amino acid compositions of several native human interferons

Amino acid	HuIFN-$\alpha(\alpha_1)$[a,b]	HuIFN-$\alpha(\beta_1)$[a,b]	HuIFN-$\alpha(\gamma_2)$[c,d]	HuIFN-α (Ly, 18,500 daltons)[d,e]	HuIFN-β[d,f]
Asx	14.9	12.5	14.4	14.9	18.9
Thr	8.3	9.7	10.4	8.0	6.8
Ser	9.9	11.2	8.4	10.7	10.5
Glx	21.9	22.6	27.2	27.3	27.0
Pro	6.6	5.7	5.2	9.0	2.7
Gly	5.5	5.4	5.4	10.7	7.8
Ala	9.1	8.0	8.8	11.0	10.0
Val	8.0	6.5	7.6	7.7	6.0
Met	3.9	5.3	4.2	4.0	2.9
Ile	8.0	7.0	8.7	6.9	9.0
Leu	19.4	19.9	21.8	17.8	20.4
Tyr	4.3	4.8	5.2	3.8	7.5
Phe	7.4	9.5	9.7	7.1	9.4
His	3.3	3.1	3.6	4.4	4.9
Lys	11.4	9.7	10.9	10.4	11.6
Arg	6.7	8.8	9.3	9.6	10.9
Cys	4.2	3.4	3.2	1.8	1.7

[a] Levy et al. (1981)
[b] Based on 155 amino acid residues total (including 2 tryptophan residues)
[c] Rubinstein et al. (1981)
[d] Based on 166 amino acid residues total
[e] Zoon et al. (1981)
[f] Knight et al. (1980)

2. Characterization

Purified native HuIFN-α have an apparent molecular weight range of 16,000–23,000 (Rubinstein et al. 1981). The amino acid compositions of these interferons show a great deal of similarity. Several examples are shown in Table 1. These HuIFN-α exhibit extensive amino acid sequence homology among themselves (Fig. 1) as well as to those derived from DNA technology (see Fig. 3).

It is noteworthy that three major species of HuIFN-α: HuIFN-$\alpha(\alpha_1)$, HuIFN-$\alpha(\alpha_2)$, and HuIFN-$\alpha(\beta_1)$, isolated from chronic myelogeneous leukemia cells appear to lack the ten COOH terminal amino acids predicted from cDNA sequences of a number of HuIFN-α (see Fig. 3) as well as the sequences of several native HuIFN-α (Fig. 1) (Levy et al. 1981). No alterations in the specific activity of these abbreviated interferons have been observed (Levy et al. 1981). In addition, the amino acid sequences of HuIFN-$\alpha(\alpha_2)$ and HuIFN-$\alpha(\beta_1)$ appear to be virtually identical to the sequence of one of the major rDNA-derived interferons, HuIFN-αA, or HuIFN-α_2. Interestingly, the multiple species of native HuIFN-α show a range of antiviral activity titers on a number of animal cell lines and, in addition, they exhibit different ratios of cell growth inhibition to antiviral activity (Evinger et al. 1981). Similar properties are observed for the rDNA-derived HuIFN-α (see Table 3).

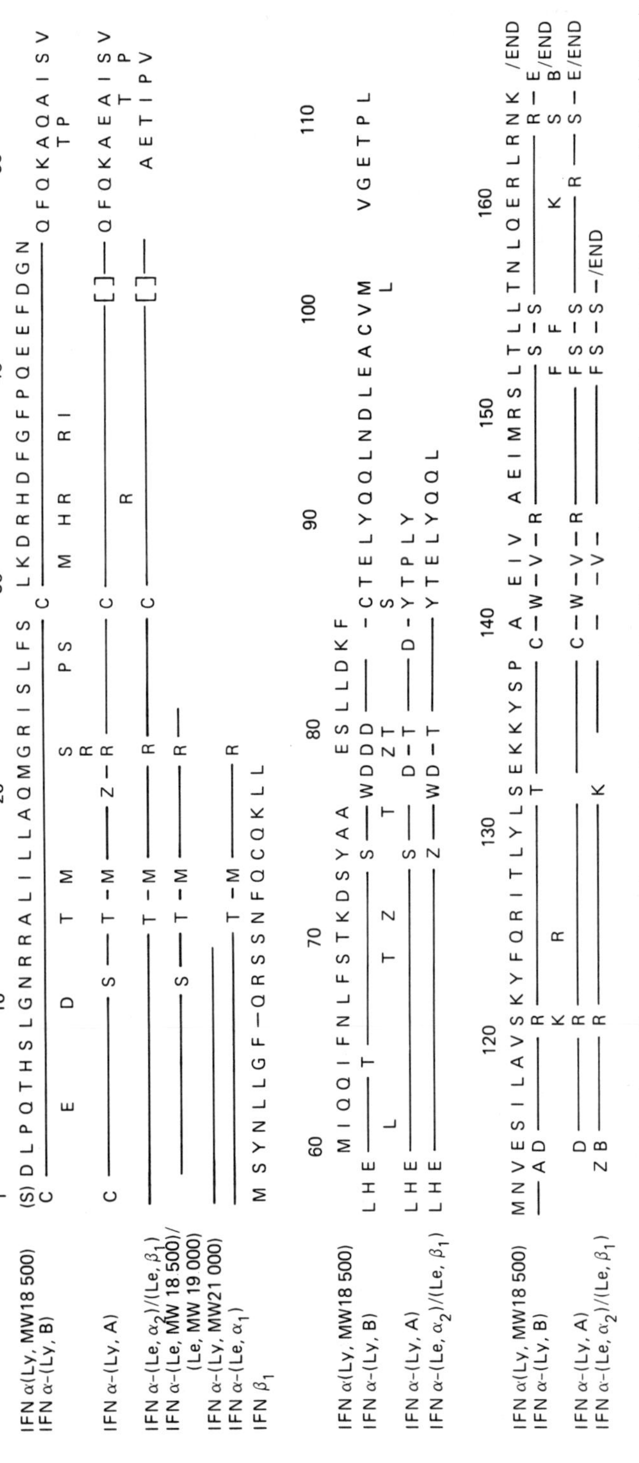

Fig. 1. Comparison of the partial amino acid sequences of several native human interferons. *Lines* indicate identity to IFN-α (Ly, 18,500 daltons). *Brackets* at position 44 indicate a deletion. *Blanks*-indicate sequence not identified or uncertain

Table 2. Amino acid composition of interferons from mouse Ehrlich ascites tumor cells (Cabrer et al. 1979)

	MuIFN-β (35,000 daltons) (residues/100 amino acids)	MuIFN-α (20,000 daltons) (residues/18,000 daltons)
Asx	9.3	14.2
Thr	7.7	9.4
Ser	4.8	9.2
Glx	16.4	23.9
Pro	2.8	5.7
Gly	3.9	6.3
Ala	5.3	9.8
Val	4.7	7.0
Met	3.5	4.2
Ile	4.4	5.2
Leu	11.7	16.7
Tyr	4.6	4.8
Phe	4.6	5.9
His	1.3	4.0
Lys	7.8	16.0
Arg	7.2	9.6
GLCN[a]	8.0	8.1
Cys	N.D.[b]	4.0

[a] GLCN = glucosamine
[b] N.D. = not determined

II. Human Interferon-β

1. Purification

Several purification schemes have been successfully developed to isolate human interferon-β (HuIFN-β) (Stewart 1981). Particularly noteworthy is the one-step purification procedure employing Blue Sepharose chromatography (Knight and Fahey 1981). At present only one species of biologically active HuIFN-β has been identified.

2. Characterization

Native HuIFN-β has an apparent molecular weight of 20,000. The amino acid composition is similar to that observed for the family of HuIFN-α (Table 1) and mouse interferons (Table 2). The partial amino acid sequence data obtained from microsequencing studies of the native protein (or proteins) is shown in Fig. 1 (Knight et al. 1980; E. Knight 1981, personal communication). This sequence is identical to that predicted from the nucleotide sequence of the HuIFN-β cDNA, excluding the signal peptide (see Fig. 4). Of the first 21 NH_2 terminal amino acids, only 1 residue at position 9 corresponds to that residue in the NH_2 terminal sequences of the native HuIFN-α.

```
                          1       5         10        15        20      24

MuIFN-β (MW 35 000)       I N Y K Q L Q L Q E R T N I R K ? Q E L L E Q L
        (MW 26 000)

MuIFN-α (MW 20 000)       A D L P Q T Y N L G N K G A L K V L A Q
```

Fig. 2. NH_2 terminal amino acid sequences of MuIFN-α and MuIFN-β

III. Human Interferon-γ

The purification of native human interferon-γ (HuIFN-γ) has been recently described (Yip et al. 1981). Two species with apparent molecular weights of 20,000 and 25,000 were detected by SDS PAGE (Yip et al. 1982). In contrast, with gel filtration, HuIFN-γ has an apparent molecular weight between 40,000 and 70,000. These studies suggest that native HuIFN-γ may be an aggregate. Currently, neither amino acid composition nor sequence data is available for native HuIFN-γ.

IV. Mouse Interferons

Three mouse interferons, one MuIFN-α and two MuIFN-β, have been purified to homogeneity (DeMaeyer-Guignard et al. 1978; Iwakura et al. 1978; Kawakita et al. 1978). In contrast to MuIFN-α and MuIFN-β, no homogeneous species of MuIFN-γ has been obtained. The amino acid compositions of MuIFN-β (molecular weight 35,000), MuIFN-β (molecular weight 26,000), and MuIFN-α (molecular weight 20,000) are shown in Table 2. Again a similarity is apparent among the MuIFN and between the MuIFN and the HuIFN-α and -β. Partial amino acid sequence data for MuIFN-α and both types of MuIFN-β are shown in Fig. 2 (Taira et al. 1980).

V. Comparison of Amino Acid Sequences of Human and Mouse Interferons

A comparison of the NH_2 terminal amino acid sequences of MuIFN-α and MuIFN-β to those of HuIFN-α and HuIFN-β clearly shows homology. Of the first 20 NH_2 terminal amino acids of native and rDNA-derived HuIFN-α, 8–13 are identical to those of MuIFN-α. Of the first 24 NH_2 terminal amino acid residues of HuIFN-β, 8 are identical to those of both forms of MuIFN-β.

C. Purification and Characterization of rDNA-Derived Interferons

I. Human Interferons-α

The DNA sequences of 13 distinct HuIFN-α cDNA clones indicate that these multiple HuIFN-α genes represent a family of homologous proteins. The primary

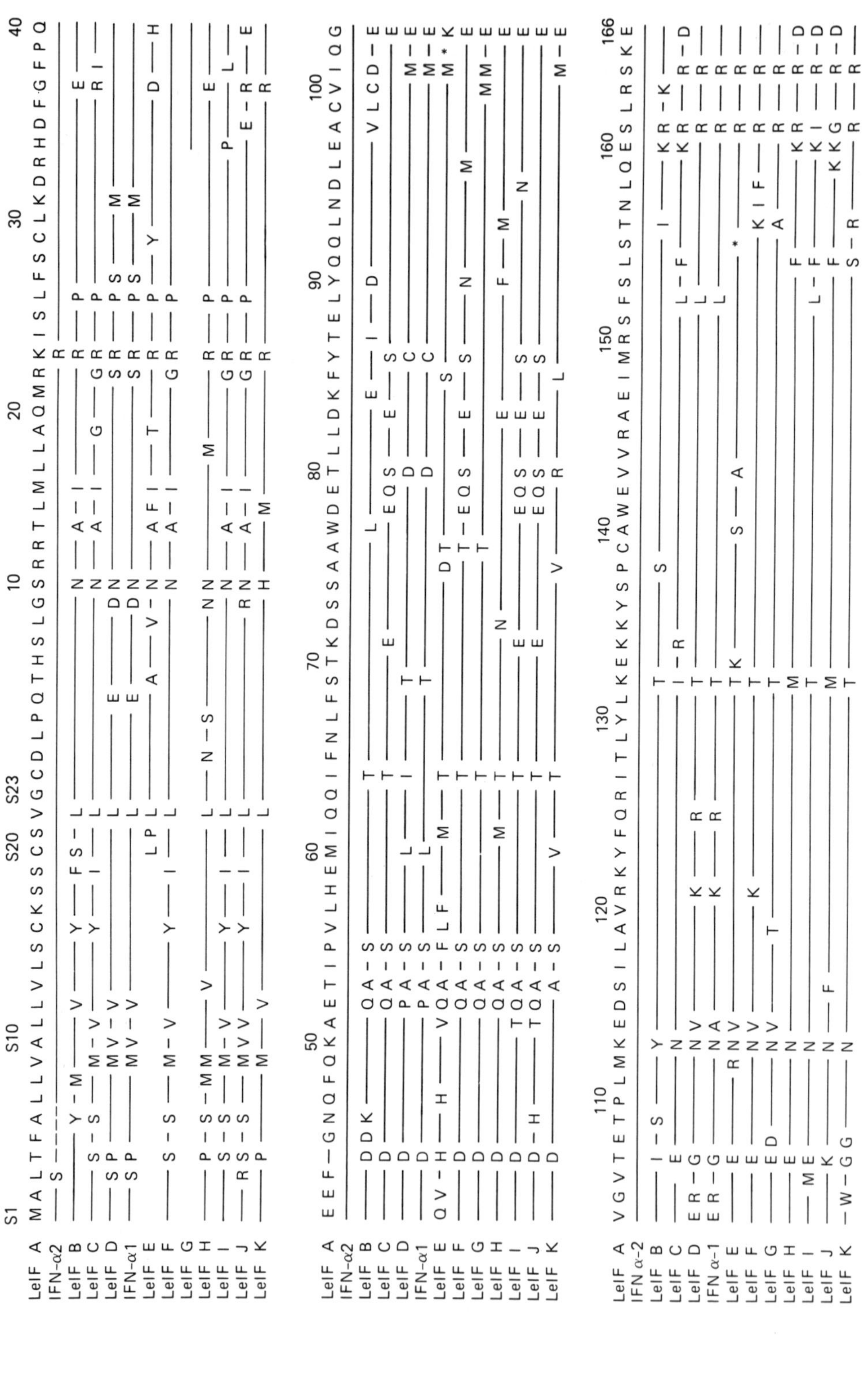

Fig. 3. Comparison of the protein sequences of 13 HuIFN-α deduced from nucleotide sequences. *Lines* indicate identity to HuIFN-αA (LeIF A). *Dash* for LeIF A indicates a deletion. *Asterisk* indicates inphase termination codons. S1 etc. denote signal peptide amino acid residues

amino acid sequences deduced from the DNA sequences of the clones are shown in Fig. 3 (GOEDDEL et al. 1981; STREULI et al. 1980). Each species consists of a 23 amino acid residue signal peptide and a 165 (or 166) amino acid residue mature HuIFN-α protein, except for subtype E which appears to be a pseudogene copy (GOEDDEL et al. 1981). Greater than or equal to 73% homology is observed for the mature HuIFN-α amino acid sequences. Disregarding subtype E, approximately 60% of the amino acids are identical in all sequences (GOEDDEL et al. 1981). Many of the amino acid changes can be attributed to single nucleotide alterations. The predicted cysteine residues at positions 1, 29, 99 (or 100), and 139 of the mature HuIFN-α are highly conserved. HuIFN-αA and HuIFN-α_2 differ by only one amino acid (Fig. 3). A single amino acid substitution was also observed for HuIFN-αD and HuIFN-α_1 (Fig. 3). The signal peptide amino acid sequences show >65% homology with 11 out of 23 positions identical. These signal peptides, which are not found in isolated interferons, are presumably involved in cellular secretion, during which they are proteolytically removed. Some interferon genes have been expressed in yeast as well (HITZEMAN et al. 1982). Genes coding for preinterferon, when expressed in yeast, secrete correctly processed interferon into the growth medium (HITZEMAN et al., to be published).

Many of the native interferon structural genes have been engineered for expression in bacteria (for review, see WETZEL and GOEDDEL, to be published). *Escherichia coli*-derived HuIFN-αA has been purified to homogeneity using monoclonal antibody chromatography as the major purification step (STAEHELIN et al. 1981). The specific activity of the purified molecule is $1–3 \times 10^8$ U/per milligram protein (STAEHELIN et al. 1981; WETZEL et al. 1981) which is in the same range of specific activities observed for native human interferons. The apparent molecular weight of purified subtype A is approximately 19,500 (STAEHELIN et al. 1981; WETZEL et al. 1981), again within the range observed for native human interferons. The amino acid composition (STAEHELIN et al. 1981; WETZEL et al. 1981) of this species is similar to those published for native human and mouse interferons-α and -β (Tables 1 and 2). The amino acid sequence of *E. coli*-derived HuIFN-αA is identical to that predicted by the nucleotide sequence of the gene for the mature protein (Fig. 3). This was determined by sequence analysis of the molecule's NH_2 terminus (WETZEL et al. 1981) and of tryptic fragments collected from HPLC (KOHR and WETZEL, to be published). HPLC analysis of trypsin digests also allowed characterization of the disulfide bond arrangements in subtypes A (WETZEL 1981) and D (R. WETZEL 1982, unpublished work). Depending on fermentation conditions and on the strain of bacteria used, variable amounts of NH_2 terminal methionine are observed. The rDNA-derived HuIFN-α like the native HuIFN-α exhibit a spectrum of antiviral activities on a variety of cell lines (STREULI et al. 1981; WECK et al. 1981a). In addition, genetically engineered hybrid HuIFN-α (see Sect. III.3) have antiviral properties distinct from the parent molecules (STREULI et al. 1981; WECK et al. 1981b).

II. Human Interferons-β

In contrast to the multigene family of HuIFN-α, only a single HuIFN-β gene has been found (DERYNCK et al. 1980; OHNO and TANIGUCHI 1981). The amino acid se-

```
S1            S10           S20 1              10             20             30             40
M T N K C L L Q I A L L L C F S T T A L S M S Y N L L G F L Q R S S N F Q C Q K L L W Q L N G R L E Y C L K D R M N F D I

                50             60             70             80             90             100
P E E I K Q L Q Q F Q K E D A A L T I Y E M L Q N I F A I F R Q D S S S T G W N E T I V E N L L A N V Y H Q I N H L K T V L E

              110            120            130            140            150            160
E K L E K E D F T R G K L M S S L H L K R Y Y G R I L H Y L K A K E Y S H C A W T I V R V E I L R N F Y F I N R L T G Y L R N
```

Fig. 4. Protein sequence of HuIFN-β deduced from nucleotide sequence. S1 etc. indicate signal peptide amino acid residues

quence deduced from the HuIFN-β gene sequence is shown in Fig. 4. This sequence predicts, like the HuIFN-α cDNA sequences, a signal peptide (21 residues instead of the 23 residues observed for HuIFN-α) and 166 amino acid mature HuIFN-β polypeptide. The signal peptide is absent from native HuIFN-β as was observed for native HuIFN-α. The 30 amino acids nearest the NH_2 terminus of mature IFN-β expressed in *E. coli* have been determined and are as expected from the gene sequence (HARKINS et al., to be published). The NH_2 terminal initiator methionine of HuIFN-β is about 80% removed by *E. coli*, giving a molecule one amino acid shorter than that isolated from fibroblast cell culture. No effect on interferon activity of this difference has been observed.

III. Human Interferons-γ

Sequence analysis of the cloned cDNA coding for HuIFN-γ (GRAY et al. 1982) allows some insight into the structure of the protein molecule. This clone was identified as interferon-γ by the ability of derived DNA to command expression in mouse cells of an antiviral activity that could be neutralized by authentic anti-γ antibodies, but not by anti-α or anti-β antibodies. In addition, other properties of the protein, predicted from the gene sequence, are consistent with those observed during purification of lymphocyte-derived interferon-γ (see Sect. B.III). The amino acid sequence predicted for this molecule is shown in Fig. 5. The first 20 amino acids are probably a signal peptide for protein secretion, similar to sequences found in HuIFN-α and HuIFN-β genes. The mature protein coded on the gene is 146 amino acids long, approximately 20 amino acids shorter than HuIFN-α and HuIFN-β. Several groups have reported detection of limited homologies between HuIFN-γ and HuIFN-α or HuIFN-β (GRAY et al. 1982; GRAY and GOEDDEL 1982; EPSTEIN 1982; DEGRADO et al. 1982). The molecular weight, 17, 110, of the molecule predicted by the DNA sequence is smaller than that reported for the activity derived from induced lymphocyte culture (LANGFORD et al. 1979; DELEY et al. 1980; YIP et al. 1981). This may be due to glycosylation and/or a dimeric native structure. There are two potential *N*-glycosylation sites in the predicted sequence, at amino acid 28 and 100.

One striking feature of the amino acid sequence is the basicity of the molecule. There are 27 basic amino acids (Arg+Lys) and only 19 acidic residues (Asp+Glu). Some of the excess positive charge may be neutralized in the glycosylated form by sialic acid, but the glycosylated, lymphocyte-derived form is basic as well, with a pI of about 8.7 (YIP et al. 1981). Eight of the basic residues occur in two clusters of four each (amino acids 89–92 and 131–134), similar to one of the cleavage sites in the corticotropin–β-lipotropin precursor (NAKANISHI et al. 1979).

Assuming the signal peptide is processed as expected (GRAY et al. 1982), the mature HuIFN-γ molecule has only two cysteine residues, at positions 1 and 3. There are no proteins known which contain a disulfide bond between cysteines separated by only one amino acid (RICHARDSON 1981). In addition, the activity of naturally derived HuIFN-γ is not sensitive to reducing agents tested (YIP et al. 1981). While the actual thiol structure of the unusual NH_2 terminal end of HuIFN-γ remains uncharacterized, there are clearly no disulfides in HuIFN-γ analogous

S1 S10 1 10 20 30
MKYTSYILAFQLCIVLGSLGCYCQDPYVKEAENLKKYFNAGHSDVADNGTLFLGIL

40 50 60 70 80 90
KNWKEESDRKIMQSQIVSFYFKLFKNFKDDQSIQKSVETIKEDMNVKFFNSNKKKR

100 110 120 130 140
DDFEKLTNYSVTDLNVQRKAIHELIQVMAELSPAAKTGKRKRSQMLFRGRRASQ

Fig. 5. Protein sequence of HuIFN-γ deduced from nucleotide sequence. S 1 etc. denote signal peptide amino acid residues. Gray et al. (1982)

to those found in HuIFN-α and presumed in HuIFN-β (Sect. D.I). Like interferons-α and -β, HuIFN-γ contains a large number of aromatic residues: ten phenylalanine, five tyrosine, and one tryptophan. A high α-helix content is expected based on structural prediction calculations (Sect. E).

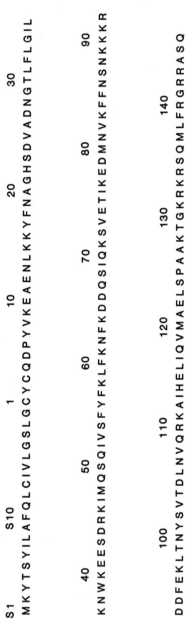

D. Protein Structure and Interferon Activity

Until recently, structure–function studies on interferon suffered from: (a) the relatively low amount of protein available; (b) the lack of purity of most preparations; and (c) the heterogeneity of the preparations with respect to molecules possessing interferon activity. Recent work under these restrictions has centered on following extracted interferon activity by SDS PAGE. Limited proteolysis experiments (OTTO et al. 1980; BRAUDE et al. 1979, 1981 a) show that the apparent molecular weight of gel-extracted activity can be reduced when interferon preparations are exposed to some proteinases.

The availability of relatively large amounts of single subtypes of HuIFN-α (WETZEL et al. 1981; STAEHELIN et al. 1981) as well as HuIFN-β (HARKINS et al., to be published) has recently made possible structure–function studies on single molecular species (WETZEL et al. 1982). The following section includes preliminary results from some of the studies, as well as results taken from structure–function studies pursued at the DNA level.

I. Disulfide Bonds

There are four or five cysteines in the HuIFN-α, three in HuIFN-β, and two in HuIFN-γ. None of the naturally derived interferons, however, has been characterized for disulfide arrangements. It is known that while HuIFN-α (MOGENSEN and CANTELL 1974) and HuIFN-β (SHEPARD et al. 1981) antiviral activity is sensitive to reducing agents, HuIFN-γ is insensitive (YIP et al. 1981).

Among the HuIFN-α, all cloned genes so far isolated contain conserved cysteines at positions 1, 29, 99, and 139 (numbering based on 166 amino acid length), which suggests two conserved disulfide bonds. Two disulfide bonds, between Cys-1 and Cys-98, and between Cys-29 and Cys-138, were characterized in HuIFN-αA synthesized in *E. coli* (WETZEL 1981; WETZEL et al. 1981). A similar arrangement is likely in HuIFN-αD (R. WETZEL 1982, unpublished work).

A chemical derivative of IFN-αA containing only the Cys-29–Cys-138 bond was found to possess full in vitro antiviral activity (WETZEL et al. 1982; MOREHEAD et al., to be published). The lack of importance of the Cys-1–Cys-99 bond is also implied in the results of STREULI et al. (1980), who obtained active interferon from *E. coli* transformed with a plasmid containing an incomplete HuIFN-α_2 gene inserted into the β-lactamase gene of pBR322. If, as seems likely, their gene product is not a hybrid β-lactamase–interferon molecule, then it must arise from reinitiation of protein synthesis at the first interferon AUG in the "polycistronic" mRNA. Because the cDNA is incomplete at the 5′ end of the HuIFN-α gene, the first AUG occurs at amino acid 16 of the HuIFN-α molecule, and the isolated protein product thus can begin no earlier than Met-16. Thus, at least in HuIFN-α_2, the Cys-1–Cys-98 (or 99) disulfide as well as amino acids 1–15 seem to be nonessential or antiviral activity.

Previous work on crude IFN-α (MERIGAN et al. 1965; MOGENSON and CANTELL 1974) or cloned *E. coli* material (STEWART et al. 1980) has revealed differing responses of IFN-α to reducing agent. Antiviral activity is either reversibly or irreversibly destroyed, depending on conditions and the IFN preparation used. Reduction of IFN-αA under native conditions inactivates the molecule and produces, depending upon reducing agent, varying amounts of disulfide-linked oligomers (WETZEL, to be published). Such thermally denatured preparations can be reactivated by a denaturation/renaturation cycle (using guanidine hydrochloride, urea, or sodium dococylsulfate) followed by thiol–disulfide interchange or air oxidation.

This behavior of IFN-αA has been further studied using an *S*-sulfonate derivative of IFN-αA (WETZEL et al. 1982; MOREHEAD et al., to be published). While this inactive disulfide-free derivative retains immunochemical relatedness to IFN-αA as well as the ability to regain antiviral activity after thiol–disulfide interchange, both these properties are lost after incubation of the derivative at 37 °C under native conditions. This denaturation was shown to be driven by a conformational change to a monomeric from of lower free energy. Exposure of this form to denaturants, followed by dialysis, regenerates the "proactive" conformation. This suggests that the inability of IFN-αA to survive reduction is due to the fact the the initial conformation of reduced IFN-αA decays at 37 °C (the minimum temperature for complete reduction) to a form which is incapable, under native conditions, of recovering an active or proactive conformation. The 29–138 disulfide, which is required for antiviral activity, is thus also important in maintaining IFN-αA in a critical conformation. In its absence, IFN-αA is subject to irreversible thermal denaturation (WETZEL, to be published).

II. Physical Studies

1. rDNA-Derived Interferons

a) Human Interferons-α

Preliminary investigation of HuIFN-αA by circular dichroism and ultraviolet spectroscopy indicates that the molecule is a typical globular protein with a densely packed, hydrophobic core. One can measure an α-helix content at neutral pH ranging from 45% to 70% (BEWLEY et al. 1982; M. BOUBLIK and H. KUNG 1982, personal communication), while no major β-sheet structure is apparent. Raman spectroscopy of IFN-αA gave these approximate values: α-helix, 49%; disordered helix, 25%; extended β-sheet, 8%; turns, 10% (R. WETZEL and R. WILLIAMS 1982, unpublished results). At least one of the molecule's tryptophans is tightly held in an asymmetric environment. This interaction, as well as about 50% of the α-helix, is reversibly lost on titration of the molecule to pH 2 (BEWLEY et al. 1982).

Ultracentrifugation studies on IFN-αA show a concentration-dependent aggregation in the neutral range, with sedimentation coefficients consistent with a dimeric or trimeric structure. The molecule behaves as a monomer at pH 2 and at lower concentrations (SHIRE 1982). A major conformational change at low pH can also be detected when IFN-αA is studied by pH titration. The change occurs around pH 3 and is entirely reversible. Several residues (Lys or Tyr) were found to ionize at abnormally low pH (SHIRE 1982).

b) Human Interferon-β

Circular dichroism studies on HuIFN-β purified from *E. coli* show it to contain about 55% α-helix (M. BOUBLIK and H. KUNG 1982, personal communication), consistent with structure predictions (Fig. 7).

2. Interferon Fragments

COOH terminal fragments of HuIFN-α_1 containing residues 121–166 and 111–166 have been chemically synthesized using solid-phase synthesis techniques (ARNHEITER et al. 1981; SMITH et al. 1981). These fragments do not exhibit antiviral activity nor do they compete with radiolabeled native HuIFN-α for its binding site on bovine kidney cells (ZOON et al. 1982b). However, they are antigenically cross-reactive with HuIFN-α_1 and exhibit secondary structure as observed by circular dichroism studies. Fragment 111–166 yielded values of 24% α-helix and 36% β-sheet (ARNHEITER et al. 1981). The fragment 121–166 exhibited an α-helix content consistent with the predicted α-helix content of HuIFN-α average (SMITH et al. 1981). Trypsin and cyanogen bromide fragments of IFN-αA, individually or in mixtures, had no detectable antiviral or receptor binding activities (WETZEL et al. 1982).

III. Effect of Sequence Changes on Activity

1. NH_2 Terminal Variations

The first 15 amino acids of IFN-α_2 are probably not essential for antiviral activity (see Sect. D.I).

2. COOH Terminal Variations

Some of the COOH terminal amino acids of the cDNA-predicted interferon-α amino acid sequence are not essential for antiviral activity. LEVY et al. (1981) have characterized by microsequencing of tryptic fragments several active interferons-α isolated from cell culture and were unable to locate the ten amino acids nearest the COOH terminus of these molecules. An interferon isolated from limited proteolysis of HuIFN-αA, which lacks the 13 amino acids nearest the COOH terminus, has full in vitro antiviral activity (WETZEL et al. 1982). In addition , a short HuIFN-αA has been made by introducing an early stop codon in the cloned gene after position 154. The gene product synthesized in *E. coli* exhibits 30% of the specific activity of the full length subtype (FRANKE et al., to be published).

3. cDNA-Encoded Analogs

At least 14 subtypes of interferon-α have been cloned, leading to structure–function information derived from comparisons of specific activities with amino acid sequences in the different proteins (STREULI et al. 1980; YELVERTON et al. 1981; WECK et al. 1981a). In addition, these cloned genes can in some bases be used to generate artifical subtypes, by making hybrid genes that encode new sequence variants. This can be done by in vitro recombination of gene fragments generated by cleavage at

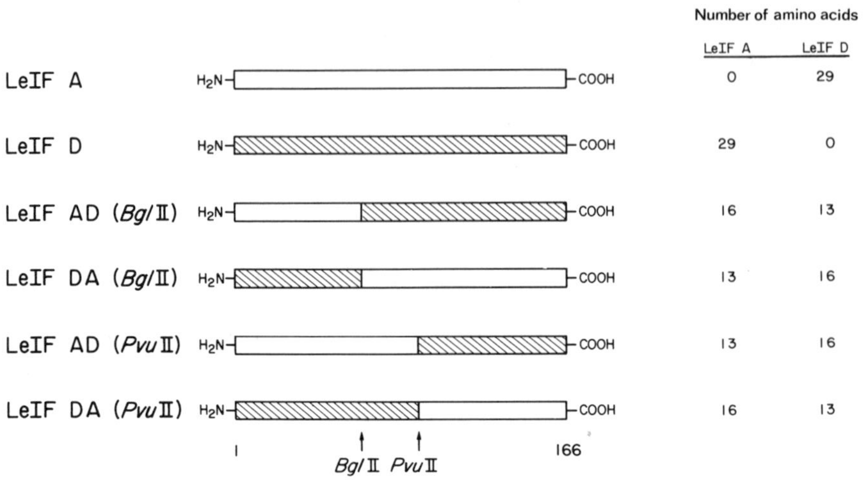

Fig. 6. Design of hybrid interferons-α produced by expression of cloned cDNAs derived from in vitro recombination of naturally derived cDNA WECK et al. (1981 b)

Table 3. Relative specific activities of interferons

LeIF	STREULI et al. (1981)			WECK et al (1981 b)		
	MDBK	WISH	L 929	MDBK	WISH	L 929
A	100	100	3	100	100	6
D	131	14	100	74	15	100
AD (*Bgl*)	54	28	667	97	190	100,000
AD (*Pvu*)	46	144	333	47	280	4,000
DA (*Bgl*)	46	< 1	< 2	110	< 1	20
DA (*Pvu*)	46	< 1	< 1	110	< 2	100

a DNA restriction site common to two subtype genes. Using cloned cDNA for HuIFN-αA (α_2) and D (α_1), STREULI et al. (1981) and WECK et al. (1981 b) reported the construction of AD and DA hybrids and specific activity comparisons in a number of cell lines.

Figure 6 (WECK et al. 1981 b) shows the nature of these constructions at the *Bgl*II site (amino acid 61 of IFN-αA) and the *Pvu* site (amino acid 91 of IFN-αA). Despite the facts that the interferons produced in one study (STREULI et al. 1981) were synthesized at the ribosome as 21 amino acid NH_2 terminal extensions of the native interferons produced in the other study (WECK et al. 1981 b), and that the two groups used different techniques to compensate for possible differential stability in vivo of interferon analogs, the data produced are quite similar. Table 3 shows data from each group in which the analogs as well as the parent molecules were assayed in vitro on different cell lines.

Although some dramatic effects were observed on interferon activity on different cell lines, the data cannot be rationalized with respect to any simple structure–function model. Activity seems to be associated with one end of the molecule in one series and with the other end in another series (STREULI et al. 1981). STREULI et al. (1981) propose a model in which both ends of the molecule are involved in binding to receptor components capable of differentially responding to these NH_2 and COOH termini.

Hybrid experiments like these are valuable initial forays into interferon structure–function studies, and, aided by other physical or biochemical studies on the purified proteins, may yet provide real clues to the way the interferon molecule functions. In addition, some hybrid interferons may prove to be of clinical use. Nonetheless, it appears that higher resolution methods of analog generation, such as transpositions of shorter gene fragments, and ultimately site-specific mutagenesis, are more likely to elucidate interferon structure–function relationships. One such analog has already been made. By constructing a gene containing a Cys to Tyr mutation at position 141 of HuIFN-β, SHEPARD et al. (1981) demonstrated the importance of cysteine at this position. The lack of antiviral activity of this interferon analog may be due to its loss of ability to form a disulfide bond.

IV. Carbohydrate Content

1. Native Human Interferons-α

Studies designed to elucidate whether native HuIFN-α are in fact glycoproteins have yielded conflicting results (GROB and CHADHA 1979; BOSE et al. 1976; ALLEN and FANTES 1980). Recent amino acid composition and sequence studies of native and rDNA-derived HuIFN-α suggest HuIFN-α are not glycosylated. Amino acid analyses of native HuIFN-α do not show the presence of amino sugars (ALLEN and FANTES 1980). Amino acid sequence data of these interferons show the absence of an Asn-X-Ser(Thr) sequence, which is required for the glycosylation of asparagine residues. These observations do not omit the possibility of an *O*-glycosidic carbohydrate–peptide linkage. While it is controversial as to whether native HuIFN-α are glycosylated, it appears that the carbohydrate portion of the molecule is not necessary for biologic activity, since: (a) treatment of HuIFN-α with a glycosidase mixture from *Streptococcus pneumoniae* does not result in the loss of biologic activity (BOSE et al. 1976); and (b) rDNA-derived *E. coli* HuIFN-α lacking carbohydrate have similar specific activities to native HuIFN-α.

2. Native Human Interferons-β

In contrast to HuIFN-α, HuIFN-β appears to be a glycoprotein. Amino acid analysis of native HuIFN-β indicates the presence of the amino sugars galactosamine and mannosamine (TAN et al. 1979), and amino acid sequence data obtained from rDNA-derived HuIFN-β shows a potential *N*-glycosidic linkage site at the asparagine in position 80 (see Fig. 4). It is important to note that the biologic specific activity of rDNA-derived HuIFN-β is similar to that of native HuIFN-β, thus again indicating the carbohydrate moiety is not essential for eliciting the activities of HuIFN-β. In addition, treatment of homogeneous native HuIFN-β with a glycosidase mixture results in an apparent molecular weight change of approximately 5,000 as observed by SDS PAGE (KNIGHT and FAHEY 1982). These studies suggest native HuIFN-β is a glycoprotein and that the carbohydrate portion is not essential for expression of its biologic activity.

3. Native Human Interferons-γ

Although HuIFN-γ has been purified to apparent homogeneity, no amino acid or amino sugar composition is available. The amino acid sequence deduced from the nucleotide sequence of the HuIFN-γ cDNA clone shows two potential *N*-glycosidic linkage points at asparagine residues 28 and 100 (see Fig. 5). In addition, chromatographic and inhibitor studies indicate HuIFN-γ are glycoproteins. They exhibit lectin specificity, i.e., they bind to concanavalin A (con A)–Sepharose and are eluted with α-methylmannopyranoside (Mizrahi 1978). Species of HuIFN-γ produced in the presence of tunicamycin, an inhibitor of the synthesis of *N*-acetylglucosaminylpyrophosphorylpolyisoprenol, do not bind to con A-Sepharose, but still exhibit antiviral activity (Mizrahi 1978).

4. Native Mouse Interferons

Many if not all MuIFNs (α, β, and γ) appear to be glycoproteins. Purified MuIFN-α and MuIFN-β stain with periodate Schiff's Reagent on SDS gels, indicating the presence of carbohydrate (DeMaeyer-Guignard et al. 1978). Two interferon species with apparent molecular weights of 15,000 and 18,000 are produced by NDV-induced mouse C243 cells in the presence of tunicamycin in lieu of the 24,000 daltons (MuIFN-α) and 35,000 daltons (MuIFN-β) species produced in the absence of the inhibitor (Raj and Pitha 1981). Experiments on con A-Sepharose binding suggest that MuIFN-α, MuIFN-β (Besancon and Bourgeade 1974), and MuIFN-γ (E. Havell 1982, personal communication) possess carbohydrate moieties. Changes in the isoelectric point of MuIFN-γ following neuramidinase treatment also support its glycoprotein nature (E. Havell 1982, personal communication). Amino acid analyses of MuIFN-α and MuIFN-β show the presence of the amino sugar, glucosamine (Table 2).

E. Structure Prediction

The predicted secondary structures for interferons shown in Figs. 7, 8 (Wetzel et al. 1982), and 9 (R. Wetzel 1982, unpublished work) were calculated by the method of Garnier et al. (1978). Predictions by this method benefit in principle from the availability of a series of homologous protein sequences. Since it is based upon eight cDNA-predicted IFN-α amino acid sequences, the average IFN-α structure in Fig. 7 is thus expected to be significantly more reliable (5%–10%) than predictions of any individual interferon-α. Secondary structure calculations using the Chou-Fasman (1974) method for HuIFN-β_1 and HuIFN-αD have been published (Hayes 1980).

All the interferons are predicted to be highly helical (50%–70%) by either method. Available experimental data (Sect. D.II) for HuIFN-α and HuIFN-β is in agreement with these calculations. While overall helical contents were confirmed by experiment, the calculations are limited in their ability to locate elements of structure precisely. Other predictive or experimental methods must be used to refine the calculations.

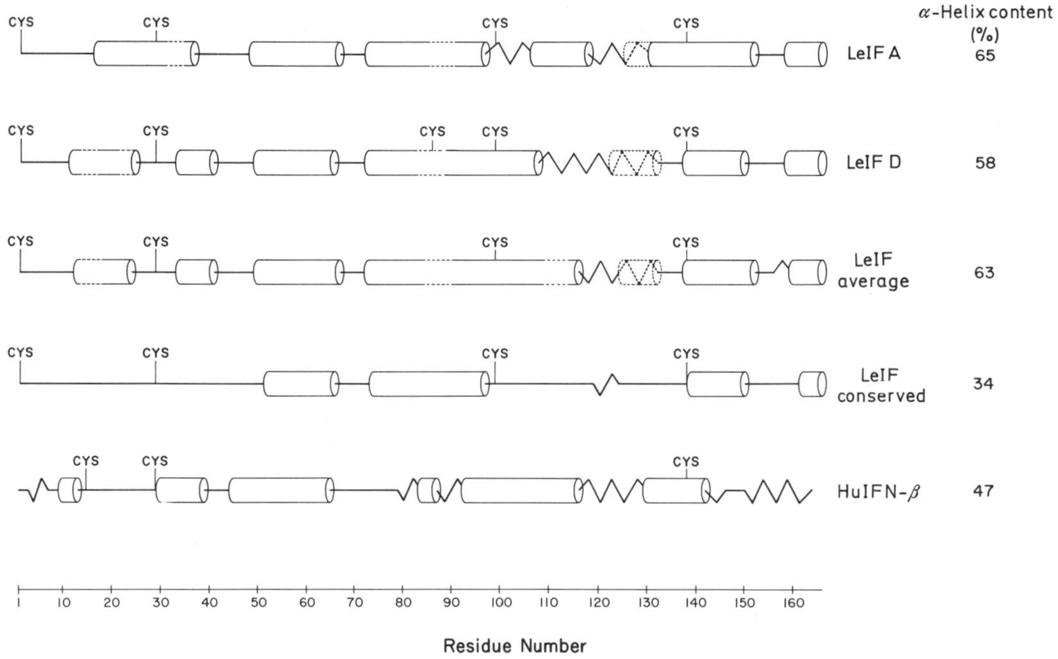

Fig. 7. Secondary structure predictions for HuIFN-α and HuIFN-β applying the algorithm of GARNIER et al. (1978) to amino acid sequences predicted from sequences of cloned cDNA. Residues were scored for their relative tendencies to exist in four possible states (α-helix, extended chain, reverse turn, and coil) based on values for each amino acid obtained by examination of 26 protein crystal structures. Only α-helix (*barrels*) and extended chain (β-sheet, *zigzags*) are shown since they are predicted most accurately. Stretches equally likely to be in α-helix or extended chain are shown with these structures *dotted and superimposed.* Regions with moderate helical potential which might be strengthened by adjoining helical regions are shown as *dotted connections* between helices

Figure 7 shows that HuIFN-αA and HuIFN-αD, differing in amino acid sequence, are predicted to have some structural homology, but also some differences. The "average" structure shown is a best guess at HuIFN-α secondary structure, which is assumed to be constant throughout the subtypes. The "conserved" HuIFN-α structure shows the strongest predicted structural elements, which are consistently predicted in all subtypes. One method of further refining the average prediction is to use a different algorithm to predict folding. Figure 8 shows a hydrophilicity profile for IFN-αA. These calculated affinities of polypeptide segments for an aqueous environment should be highest (most negative free energy) at solvent-exposed regions such as β-turns. The four reverse turns predicted by the algorithm of GARNIER et al. (1978) are supported by their coincidence with maxima in the hydrophilicity curve. Predicted regions of flexible, solvent-exposed polypeptide can also be tested experimentally by limited proteolysis experiments. The arrows of Fig. 8 indicate points on the polypeptide chain cleaved by limited digestion with a variety of endoproteases. Cleavages at positions 7, 28, and 152 support the predictions, while cleavages at positions 103, 109, and 117 cast doubt on a strong α-helical character in this region of IFN-αA.

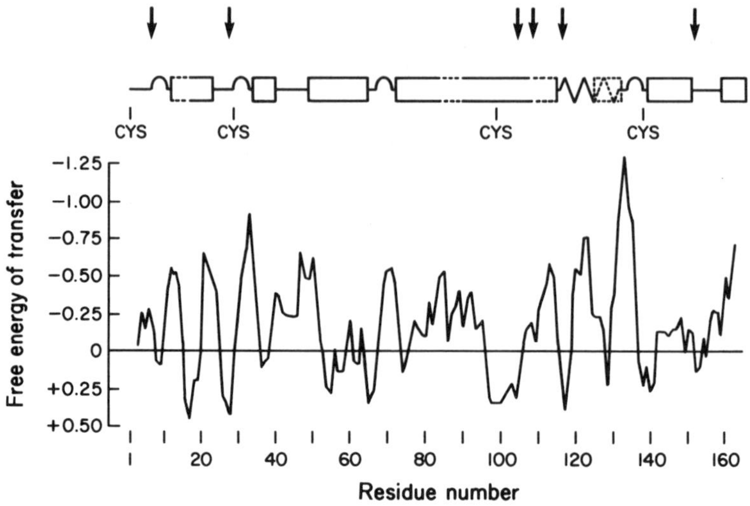

Fig. 8. Tests of the predicted average IFN-α structure. The average IFN-α structure from Fig. 7 is redrawn, including the four strongly predicted reverse turns, shown as loops. The hydrophilicity profile was computed using as a data base the free energies of transfer for the 20 amino acids determined by Janin (1979) from static accessibility tests on amino acids in 22 protein crystal structures. In jumps of one amino acid, average free energies along the primary sequence of IFN-αA were calculated for a moving window of five amino acids, and the values plotted with respect to the central amino acid. The Janin (1979) values were chosen based on their agreement with experimentally determined hydration potentials for amino acid side chains (Wolfenden 1981). The *arrows* on the top of the figure indicate loci along the primary sequence which suffered initial nicks by a variety of endoproteases under limiting conditions. W. Kohr and R. Wetzel (1981, unpublished work); Wetzel et al. (1982)

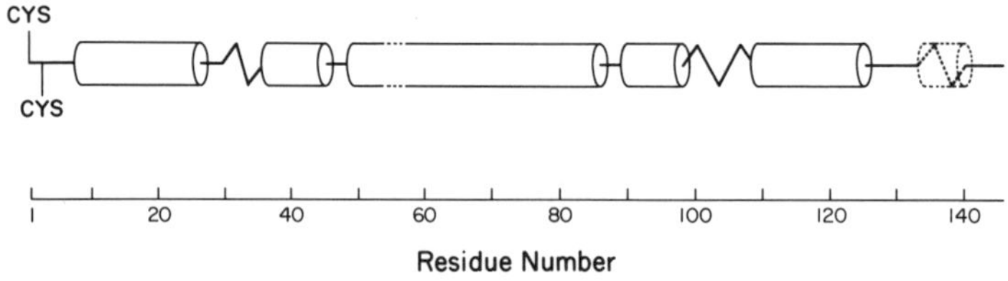

Fig. 9. Secondary structure prediction for HuIFN-γ by the algorithm of Garnier et al. (1978). See Fig. 7

Except for overall helix content, the HuIFN-β structure prediction very little resembles that for HuIFN-α (Fig. 7). This may be due in part to an error in the algorithm, to some real difference between interferon-α and -β structure, or may be a true prediction of a structural difference that is compensated in the real molecule by glycosylation. The potential *N*-glycosylation site of HuIFN-β at residue 80 is in fact in an area of the molecule which is predicted to have different structure from HuIFN-α. HuIFN-γ also predicted to contain over 50% α-helix (Fig. 9). While the prediction for IFN-α has had some experimental support (Sect. II.1.b), the predicted structures for IFN-β and IFN-γ have not been further tested.

Using the helical wheel analysis of SHIFFER and EDMUNDSON (1967), DEGRADO et al. (1982) have built a convincing case for significant *structural* homology between interferons-α, -β, and -γ in a presumed α-helix in the middle portion of their primary sequences. They interpreted their results as evidence for divergent evolution of interferons-α, -β, and -γ from a common precursor.

References

Allen G, Fantes KH (1980) A family of structural genes for human lymphoblastoid (leukocyte-type) interferon. Nature 287:408–411

Arnheiter H, Thomas RM, Leist T, Fountoulakis M, Gutte B (1981) Physico-chemical and antigenic properties of synthetic fragments of human leukocyte interferon. Nature 294:278–280

Berg K, Heron I (1980) The complete purification of human leukocyte interferon. Scand J Immunol 11:489–502

Besancon F, Bourgeade M (1974) Affinity of murine and human interferon for concanavalin A. J. Immunol 113:1061–1063

Bewley TA, Levine HL, Wetzel R (1982) Structural features of human leukocyte A as determined by circular dichroism spectroscopy. Int J Pept Protein Res 20:93–96

Bose S, Gurari-Rotman D, Ruegg UT, Corley L, Anfinsen CB (1976) Apparent dispensability of the carbohydrate moiety of human interferon for antiviral activity. J Biol Chem 251:1659–1662

Braude IA, Lin LS, Stewart WE (1979) Differential inactivation of homologous and heterologous antiviral activity of human leukocyte interferon by a proteolytic enzyme. Biochem Biophys Res Comm 89:612–619

Braude IA, Lin LS, Stewart WE (1981 a) Isolation of a biologically active fragment of human alpha interferon. J Interferon Res 1:245–252

Braude IA, Lin LS, Stewart WE (1981 b) Size characteristics of human leukocyte interferon under reducing and nonreducing conditions. Biochem J 193:947–951

Cabrer B, Taira H, Broeze RT, Kempe TD, Williams K, Slattery E, Konigsberg WH, Lengyel P (1979) Structural characteristics of interferons from mouse. Ehrlich ascites tumor cells. J Biol Chem 254:3681–3684

Chou PY, Fasman GD (1974) Prediction of protein conformation. Biochemistry 13:222–245

DeGrado WF, Wasserman ZR, Chowdhry V (1982) Sequence and structural homologies among type I and type II interferons. Nature 300:379–381

De Ley M, Van Damme J, Claeys H, Weening H, Heine JW, Billiau A, Vermylen C, De Somer P (1980) Interferon induced in human leukocytes by mitogens: production, partial purification and characterization. Eur J Immunol 10:877–883

DeMaeyer-Guignard J, Tovey MG, Gresser I, DeMaeyer E (1978) Purification of mouse interferon by sequential affinity chromatography on poly(U)- and antibody-agarose columns. Nature 271:622–625

Derynck R, Content J, DeClercq E, Volckaert G, Tavernier J, Devos R, Fiers W (1980) Isolation and structure of a human fibroblast interferon gene. Nature 285:542–546

Epstein LB (1982) Interferon-gamma: success, structure, and speculation. Nature 295:453–454

Evinger M, Rubinstein M, Pestka S (1981) Antiproliferative and antiviral activities of human leukocyte interferons. Arch Biochem Biophys 210:319–329

Franke AE, Shepard HM, Houck CM, Leung DW, Goeddel DV, Lawn RM (to be published) Carboxy terminal region of hybrid interferons affects antiviral specificity

Garnier J, Osguthorpe DJ, Robson B (1978) Analysis of the accuracy and implications of simple methods for prediciting the secondary structure of globular proteins. J Mol Biol 120:97–120

Goeddel DV, Leung DW, Dull TJ, Gross M, Lawn RM, McCandliss R, Seeburg PH, Ullrich A, Yelverton E, Gray PW (1981) The structure of eight distinct cloned human leukocyte interferon cDNAs. Nature 290:20–26
Gray PW, Goeddel DV (1982) Structure of the human immune interferon gene. Nature 298:859–863
Gray PW, Leung DW, Pennica D, Yelverton E, Najarian R, Simonsen CC, Derynck R, Sherwood PJ, Wallace DM, Berger SL, Levinson AD, Goeddel DV (1982) Expression of human immune interferon cDNA in E. coli and monkey cells. Nature 295:503–508
Grob PM, Chadha KC (1979) Separation of human leukocyte interferon components by concanavalin A-agarose affinity chromatography and their characterization. Biochemistry 18:5782–5786
Harkins RN, Weck PK, Apperson S, Haas P, Agarwal B (to be published) Structural and biological properties of purified bacteria derived human fibroblast interferon.
Hayes TG (1980) Chou-Faman analyses of the secondary structure of F and Le interferons. Biochem Biophys Res Commun 95:872–879
Hitzeman RA, Hagie FE, Levine HL, Goeddel DV, Ammerer G, Hall BD (1981) Expression of a human gene for interferon in yeast. Nature 293:717–722
Hitzeman RA, Leung DW, Perry LJ, Kohr WJ, Levine HL, Goeddel DV (to be published) Secretion of human interferons by yeast
Iwakura J, Yonehara S, Kawade Y (1978) Purification of mouse L cell interferon. J Biol Chem 253:5074–5079
Janin J (1979) Surface and inside volumes in globular proteins. Nature 277:491–492
Kawakita M, Cabrer B, Taira H, Rebello M, Slattery E, Weideli H, Lengyel P (1978) Purification of interferon from mouse Ehrlich ascites tumor cells. J Biol Chem 253:598–602
Knight E Jr, Fahey D (1981) Human fibroblast interferon: an improved purification. J Biol Chem 256:3609–3612
Knight E Jr, Fahey D (1982) Human interferon-β: effects of deglycosylation. J Interferon Res 2:421–429
Knight E Jr, Hunkapiller MW, Korant BD, Hardy RWF, Hood LE (1980) Human fibroblast interferon: amino acid analysis and amino terminal amino acid sequences. Science 207:525–526
Kohr W, Wetzel R (to be published) Amino acid sequence of E. coli-produced human alpha interferon subtype A by characterization of the HPLC/tryptic map.
Langford MP, Georgiades JA, Stanton GJ, Dianzani F, Johnson HM (1979) Large-scale production and physicochemical characterization of human immune interferon. Infect Immun 26:36–41
Levy WP, Rubinstein M, Shively J, Del Valle U, Lai CY, Moschera J, Brink L, Gerber L, Stern S, Pestka S (1981). Amino acid sequence of a human leukocyte interferon. Proc Natl Acad Sci USA 78:6186–6190
Merigan TC, Winget CA, Dixon CB (1965) Purification and characterization of vertebrate interferons. J Mol Biol 13:679–681
Mizrahi A, O'Malley JA, Carter WA, Takatsuki A, Tamura G, Sulkowski E (1978) Glycosylation of interferon: effects of tunicamycin on human immune interferon. J Biol Chem 253:7612–7615
Mogensen KE, Cantell K (1974) Human leukocyte interferon: a role for disulfide bonds. J Gen Virol 22:95–103
Morehead H, Johnston P, Wetzel R (to be published) The role of the disulfide bonds of human alpha interferon. I. Contribution to antiviral avtivity
Nakanishi S, Inoue A, Kita T, Nakamura M, Chang ACY, Cohen SN, Numa S (1979) Nucleotide sequences of cloned cDNA for bovine corticotropin-β-lipotropin prescursor. Nature 278:423–427
Ohno S, Taniguchi T (1981) Structure of a chromosomal gene for human interferon β. Proc Natl Acad Sci USA 78:5305–5309
Otto MJ, Sedmak JJ, Grossberg SE (1980) Enzymatic modifications of human fibroblast and leukocyte interferons. J Virol 35:390–399
Raj NBK, Pitha PM (1981) Interferon heterogeneity resulting from differences in glycosylation. J Interferon Res 1:595–600

Richardson JS (1981) The anatomy and taxonomy of protein structure. Adv Protein Chem 34:168–330

Rubinstein M, Levy WP, Moschera JA, Lai CY, Hershberg RD, Bartlett RT, Pestka S (1981) Human leukocyte interferon: isolation and characterization of several molecular forms. Arch Biochem Biophys 210:307–318

Shepard HM, Leung D, Stebbing N, Goeddel DV (1981) A single amino acid change in human fibroblast interferon (IFN-β1) abolishes antiviral activity. Nature 294:563–565

Shiffer M, Edmundson AB (1967) Use of helical wheels to represent the structures of proteins and to identify segments with helical potential. Biophys J 7:121–135

Shire S (1982) pH dependent behavior of purified biosynthetic human leukocyte interferon A (LIF-A). Biophys J 37:384a

Smith ME, Komoriya A, Anfinsen CB (1981) Chemical synthesis and properties of fragments of human leukocyte interferon. In: DeMaeyer E, Galasso G, Schellekens H (eds) The biology of the interferon system. Elsevier/North Holland, Amsterdam, pp 39–42

Staehelin T, Hobbs DS, Kung H, Lai CY, Pestka S (1981) Purification and characterization of recombinant leukocyte interferon (IFLra) with monoclonal antibodies. J Biol Chem 256:9750–9754

Stewart WE II (ed) (1981) The interferon-system. Springer, Berlin Heidelberg New York, pp 168–171

Stewart WE II, Sarkar FH, Taira H, Hall A, Nagata S, Weissman C (1980) Comparison of several biological and physicochemical properties of human leukocyte interferons produced by human leukocytes and by E. coli. Gene 11:181–186

Streuli M, Nagata S, Weissman C (1980) At least three human type α interferons: structure of α2. Science 209:1343–1347

Streuli M, Hall A, Boll W, Stewart WE II, Nagata S, Weissman C (1981) Target cell specificity of two species of human interferon-α produced in Escherichia coli and of hybrid molecules derived from them. Proc Natl Acad Sci USA 78:2848–2852

Taira H, Broeze RJ, Jayaram GM, Lengyel P, Hunkapiller MW, Hood LE (1980) Mouse interferons: amino terminal amino acid sequences of various species. Science 207:528–530

Tan YH, Barakat F, Berthold W, Smith-Johannsen H, Tan C (1979) The isolation and amino acid/sugar composition of human fibroblastoid interferon. J Biol Chem 254:8067–8073

Weck PK, Apperson S, May L, Stebbing N (1981 a) Comparison of the antiviral activities of various cloned human-α subtypes in mammalian cell cultures. J Gen Virol 57:233–237

Weck PK, Apperson S, Stebbing N, Gray PW, Leung D, Shepard HM, Goeddel DV (1981 b) Antiviral activities of hybrids of two major human leukocyte interferons. Nucleic Acids Res 9:6153–6166

Wetzel R (1981) Assignment of the disulfide bonds of leukocyte interferon. Nature 289:606–607

Wetzel R (to be published) The role of the disulfide bonds of human alpha interferon. II. Contribution to conformational stability

Wetzel R, Goeddel DV (1983) Synthesis of polypeptides by recombinant DNA methods. In: Gross E, Meienhofer J (eds) The peptides: analysis, synthesis, biology. Academic, New York (in press)

Wetzel R, Perry LJ, Estell DA, Lin N, Levine HL, Slinker B, Fields F, Ross MJ, Shively J (1981) Properties of a human alpha-interferon purified from E. coli extracts. J Interferon Res 1:381–390

Wetzel R, Levine HL, Estell DA, Shire S, Finer-Moore J, Stroud R, Bewley TA (1982) Structure-function studies on human alpha interferon. In: Merigan T, Friedman R, Fox CF (eds) Chemistry and biology of interferons: relationship to therapeutics. UCLA symposia 25. Academic, New York, pp 365–376

Wolfenden R, Andersson L, Cullis PM, Southgate CCB (1981) Affinities of amino acid side chains for solvent water. Biochemistry 20:849–855

Yelverton E, Leung DW, Weck PK, Gray PW, Goeddel DV (1981) Bacterial synthesis of a novel human leukocyte interferon. Nucleic Acids Res 9:731–741

Yip YK, Pang RHL, Urban C, Vilcek J (1981) Partial purification and characterization of human-γ (immune) interferon. Proc Natl Acad Sci USA 78:1601–1605
Yip YK, Barrowclough BS, Urban C, Vilcek J (1982) Molecular weight of human gamma interferon is similar to that of other human interferons. Science 215:411–413
Zoon K (1981) Purification, sequencing, and properties of human lymphoblastoid and leukocyte interferon. In: DeMaeyer E, Galasso G, Schellekens H (eds) The biology of the interferon system. Elsevier/North Holland, Amsterdam, pp 47–55
Zoon KC, Smith ME, Bridgen PJ, ZurNedden D, Anfinsen CB (1979) Purification and partial characterization of human lymphoblastoid interferon. Proc Natl Acad Sci USA 76:5601–5605
Zoon KC, Miller D, ZurNedden D, Hunkapiller M (1982a) Human leukocyte interferon: purification and amino terminal amino acid sequence of two components. J Interferon Res 2:253–260
Zoon KC, ZurNedden D, Arnheiter H (1982b) Specific binding of human alpha interferon to a high affinity cell surface binding site on bovine kidney cells. J Biol Chem 257:4695–4697

CHAPTER 6

Regulatory Control of Interferon Synthesis and Action

H. SMITH-JOHANNSEN, Y-T. HOU, X-Y. LIU, and Y-H. TAN

A. Regulatory Control of IFN Synthesis

I. Introduction

The induction of interferon (IFN) consists of a series of cellular events resulting in the transcription and translation of the IFN genes followed by events leading to the curtailment of these activities. After induction, cells remain refractory for several hours before they can be stimulated for IFN synthesis again. Much could be learned of mammalian gene regulation from the mechanism or mechanisms by which IFN genes are stimulated and regulated. This chapter reviews the evidence regarding the number and nature of human IFN genes and the progress toward understanding the regulation of their expression.

II. Human IFN Genes

1. A Multigene Family

Several lines of evidence indicate that both IFN-α and IFN-β are families consisting of a number of genes. Molecular cloning studies have revealed the existence of at least 15 gene-like sequences for IFN-α, including 5 pseudogenes (NAGATA et al. 1980; BRACK et al. 1981; GOEDDEL et al. 1981). None of the IFN-α genes so far examined contains introns (NAGATA et al. 1980; LAWN et al. 1981 a, b). Based on restriction mapping, sequencing, and R-loop and heteroduplex analyses, BRACK et al. (1981) conclude that nine of the IFN-α genes are nonallelic and one is allelic. The data also indicate that some of the genes are clustered in linkage groups. One linkage group is 36 kilobases long and consists of three genes interspersed with three pseudogenes. A second group is 25 kilobases long and contains one gene and one pseudogene. The presence of extensive homologies in the flanking sequences of some of these genes, in particular the 35 kilobase linkage group, led BRACK et al. to speculate that these flanking regions may play a role in the regulation of the expression of these IFN-α genes.

When human leukocytes are induced to produce IFN by Sendai virus, a heterogeneous mixture of IFN-α mRNAs can be detected in the cytoplasmic extracts (SEHGAL et al. 1981). These mRNAs can be resolved into two size classes. The major population (IFN-α_S) corresponds to a size range of 0.8–1.4 kilobases and a minor population (IFN-α_L) corresponds to a size range of 1.6–3.5 kilobases. The induction of the IFN-α_S mRNAs is preferentially inhibited by treatment of the induced leukocytes with 5,6-dichloro-1-D-ribofuranosylbenzimidazole (DRB). In contrast, synthesis of IFN-α_L mRNAs appears to be increased in the presence of

DRB. When translated in oocytes, the IFN-α_S mRNA yields a molecular species which is more active on bovine cells than is the product of IFN-α_L mRNA. This suggests that the two forms of IFN-α are biologically different, even though they are neutralizable by IFN-α antibodies.

To date, one gene for IFN-β has been detected by molecular cloning techniques. As in the case of IFN-α, the genomic DNA coding for IFN-β contains no introns (DERYNCK et al. 1980; GROSS et al. 1981; HOUGHTON et al. 1981; LAWN et al. 1981c; OHNO and TANIGUCHI 1981). Analysis of the DNA sequences flanking the IFN-β gene has revealed sites possibly involved in regulation. For example, GROSS et al. (1981) isolated a 36 kilobases region of human DNA containing the IFN-β gene. In the upstream region, they found a Goldberg–Hogness box and a series of short repeated sequences which may serve as transcription signals. DEGRAVE et al. (1981) reported that a significant homology exists between the upstream flanking sequences of IFN-α and IFN-β genes. They speculate that this homology may reflect similarities in the induction and control of the IFN-α and IFN-β genes. Gene transfer studies have been carried out in a number of laboratories in an effort to elucidate further the regulatory sequences governing IFN expression (HAUSER et al. 1981, 1982; CANAANI and BERG 1982; GHEYSEN and FIERS 1982; OHNO and TANIGUCHI 1982; REYES et al. 1982; ZINN et al. 1982). These studies, which have all involved the IFN-β gene and nonhuman mammalian cells, indicate that the regulatory sequences influencing the inducibility of IFN-β are localized to a region proximal to the structural gene, presumably at the 5′ end. The precise nature and location of these sequences, however, remain obscure.

Although recombinant DNA techniques have indicated the presense of a single IFN-β gene (TAVERNIER et al. 1981), other studies have revealed the possibility that more than one IFN-β gene may exist. SEHGAL (1981) was able to detect at least four different types of IFN-β mRNA in induced human fibroblasts ranging from 0.7 to 1.8 kilobases. The extracted mRNAs were purified on methylmercury gels and translated in *Xenopus* oocytes. The resulting antiviral activities were neutralized by monoclonal antibodies (NYARI et al. 1982) as well as polyclonal antibodies to pure human IFN-β. IFN-β_1 is the 20,000 daltons glycoprotein which has been partially sequenced (KNIGHT et al. 1980; OKAMURA et al. 1980; STEIN et al. 1980) and whose mRNA is 0.8 kilobases long. Preliminary immunologic characterization of IFN-β_2 indicates that one antiviral unit corresponds to 0.1–0.25 U IFN-β_1 by radioimmunoassay (INOUE and TAN 1981; P. B. SEHGAL and Y. H. TAN, unpublished work). Little is known of the proteins corresponding to IFN-β_3 and IFN-β_4 except that the sizes of their mRNAs are 1.8 and 0.7 kilobases, respectively. When human fibroblast cells are stimulated to produce IFN, the major species identified is IFN-β_1. However, normal human fibroblasts can also produce some IFN-β_2 (P. B. SEHGAL and Y. H. TAN, unpublished work), but the precise conditions responsible for preferential synthesis of IFN-β_2 remain unknown. Furthermore, it is not known whether the IFN-β_3 mRNA and the IFN-β_4 mRNA are even translated in fibroblasts.

At this time, the discrepancy between the results of TAVERNIER et al. (1981) who do not detect more than one IFN-β sequence in the human genome and the data from mRNA studies (SEHGAL et al. 1981; SEHGAL 1981) is difficult to explain. If additional IFN-β sequences do exist, but do not cross-hybridize with IFN-β_1

Table 1. Human IFN-β gene chromosomal assignment

Type of human IFN gene	Chromosomal assignment
β_1	9
β_2	5
β_3	2
β_4	?
β_5	2

cDNA, then it is puzzling why antibodies to IFN-β_1 can cross-react with the corresponding IFN-β subspecies. Hopefully, this contradiction will be resolved with careful investigation.

2. Location of IFN Genes

Until recently, much controversy surrounded the chromosomal assignment of IFN structural genes. Previous evidence was based on somatic cell genetics. For example, TAN et al. (1974a) found that human chromosomes 2 and 5 were involved in human IFN-β production in human/mouse cell hybrids. Other studies suggested that chromosome 5 alone was responsible for human IFN-β production (MORGAN and FAIK 1977; TAN et al. 1977). SLATE and RUDDLE (1979) also obtained evidence for IFN-β loci on chromosomes 2 and 5. In contrast, MEAGER et al. (1979) reported data for a single IFN-β locus chromosome 9. Finally, CHANY et al. (1981) has proposed that chromosomes 9 and 13 contain IFN genes.

These apparently conflicting results would be resolved if IFN-β were multigenic with loci on more than one chromosome. Although the evidence awaits confirmation, SAGAR et al. (1982) report that the presence of the various IFN-βmRNA species previously described (SEHGAL 1981) does correlate with the presence of certain human chromosomes in human/mouse cell hybrids: chromosomes 2, 5, and 9 (see Table 1).

All of the assignments by somatic cell genetics so far have been for human IFN-β, even when the parental human cell line used in the fusion was capable of producing IFN-α. The loss of other differentiated phenotypes has been previously observed in hybrids derived from two differentiated parent cells (DARLINGTON et al. 1974). However, no satisfactory explanation is currently available to account for this loss of expression of certain phenotypes, including synthesis of IFN-α. More recently, evidence based on nucleic acid hybridization studies with DNA for somatic cell hybrids indicates that a set of IFN-α genes, as well as an IFN-β gene, is located on chromosome 9 (OWERBACH et al. 1981).

Until very recently, nothing was known of the nature, number, or location of IFN-γ gene (or genes). Now GRAY et al. (1982) have described the cloning of IFN-γ cDNA into *Escherichia coli* pBR322. In hybridization experiments with restricted human DNA, no evidence was found for more than one IFN-γ gene in contrast to the multigene family for IFN-α. In addition, the results indicated that the IFN-γ gene contains at least one intron and is thus structurally distinct from the IFN-α

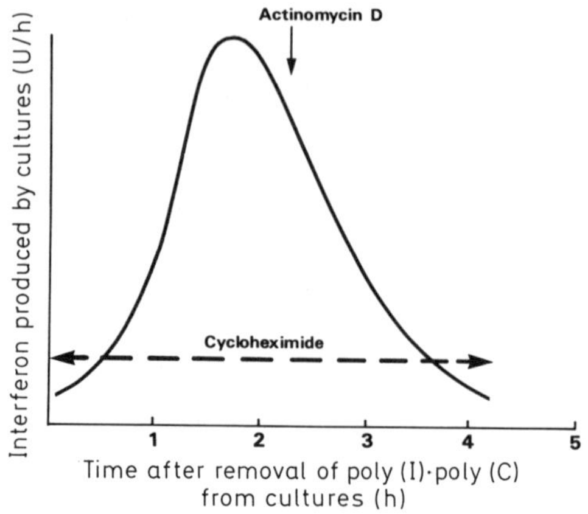

Fig. 1. Possible regulatory mechanisms controlling IFN production

and IFN-β genes. The location of the DNA sequences coding for IFN-γ is still unknown, but with the availability of IFN-γ cDNA as a probe this information should soon be forthcoming.

III. Regulation of IFN Synthesis

1. Superinduction

As a rule, normal cells do not synthesize IFN in the absence of inducer. Some exceptions to the rule have been reported. For example, PICKERING et al. (1980) have described human lymphoblastoid cell lines which produce IFN spontaneously. WEISSENBACH et al. (1981) obtained evidence for the release of IFN by Friend cells at confluency. However, in general, the expression of IFN genes appears to be under stringent control. When cloned IFN-β cDNA is used as a sensitive probe for detecting the corresponding mRNAs, no IFN-β mRNA sequences can be found in uninduced human fibroblasts (RAJ and PITHA 1981; HU et al. 1982).

The mechanism by which induction of IFN is initiated remains unknown. Many different agents are capable of inducing IFN, including all major classes of viruses, bacterial endotoxins, double-stranded RNA (dsRNA), and mitogens (see STEWART 1979). Since there is no common structural feature among all these IFN inducers, it is likely that they may instead share an ability to alter cellular metabolism in such a way as to trigger IFN synthesis. In this regard, it is interesting that reversible inhibitors of macromolecular synthesis such as cycloheximide or DRB alone can induce IFN synthesis (TAN and BERTHOLD 1977; DIANZANI et al. 1981; E.A. HAVELL 1981, personal communication). This suggests that the IFN gene is normally blocked by a labile repressor and depletion of this repressor allows transcription to occur (Fig. 1).

TAN (1981) has observed that IFN can induce its own synthesis in the absence of antimetabolites or conventional inducers. When cells were incubated with 1,000 U/ml human IFN-α for 8 h, they subsequently produced 200 U/ml antiviral activity. This activity could be neutralized by rabbit antibody to pure IFN-β, but not

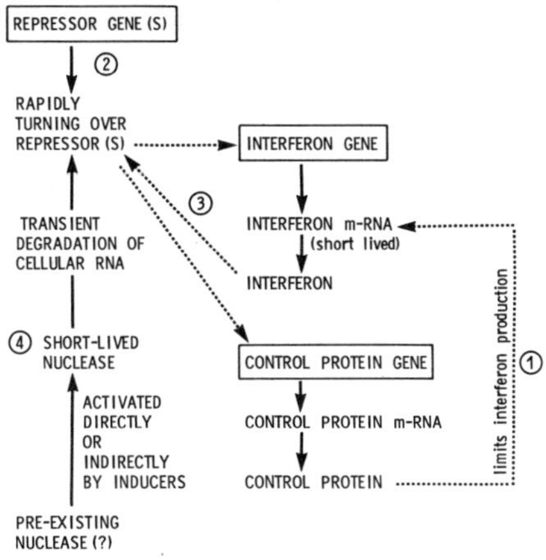

Fig. 2. Kinetics of poly(I) · poly(C)-induced IFN synthesis

by antiserum to IFN-α. The possibility that the human IFN-α preparation may have contained residual Sendai virus which induced the IFN in the cells is unlikely since the IFN-α was an NIH standard certified to be virus free. Alternatively, this observation could be explained by a depletion of labile repressor caused by the inhibitory action of IFN on macromolecular synthesis. Similarly, the well-known priming effect of IFN might also be related to diminution of repressor.

As seen in Fig. 2, the kinetics of IFN-β production are a "one-shot" affair. Fibroblasts synthesize IFN rapidly within hours of exposure to inducer, but this synthesis lasts for only a short time. This phenomenon implies the existence of an inherent mechanism which limits IFN production as soon as the cells are stimulated to make IFN. By treating induced cells with a sequential combination of cycloheximide and actinomycin D, one can apparently interfere with this mechanism and greatly enhance the synthesis of IFN. Such a superinduction procedure was first reported for rabbit kidney cells by Ho and associates (Armstrong 1970; Tan et al. 1970, 1971) and was confirmed by Vilček and Ng 971). When applied to human fibroblast cultures, superinduction increased the yield of IFN-β 20–100-fold (Ho et al. 1972, 1973; Billiau et al. 1973; Havell and Vilček 1974).

The kinetics of IFN production and the phenomenon of superinduction are consistent with the possibility that a regulatory gene is cotranscribed with the IFN gene. The product of the regulatory gene would then be involved in shutting off IFN synthesis (Fig. 1). The refractory period following IFN production during which cells cannot be restimulated to synthesize IFN may thus represent the turnover of such a regulatory protein. However, the existence of the regulatory gene, as well as that of the labile repressor described previously, is still a hypothesis.

With the recent availability of cloned IFN cDNA with which to detect IFN mRNAS, the induction of IFN and its regulation can be explored in greater detail. Using IFN-β cDNA as a probe, Hu et al. (1982) demonstrated that, in poly(I) · poly(C)-induced fibroblasts, newly transcribed IFN-β mRNA appears in the cytoplasm in the polyadenylated form and is converted to the nonpolyadenylated form by 4 h postinduction, suggesting that the newly synthesized IFN-β mRNA is rapidly deadenylated. After priming and/or superinduction, the level of polyadenylated IFN-β mRNA is not only increased, but maintained for at least another 7 h. In a similar study, RAJ and PITHA (1981) estimated the half-life of IFN-β mRNA to be 30 min and that this is extended under conditions of superinduction. These investigators point out that ongoing protein synthesis is required for degradation of the IFN-β mRNA, suggesting that the delay in decay of the IFN-β mRNA can account for enhanced yields of IFN after superinduction. However, they also concede that their results cannot rule out an increased rate of transcription as contributing to the greater accumulation of IFN-β mRNA in the presence of inhibitors.

Another approach to further understanding of the regulation of IFN synthesis is to study the expression of IFN genes after transfer to a heterologous system. HAUSER et al. (1981) have reported that mouse LTk^- $Aprt^-$ cells transformed with herpes TK gene and pCos IFN-β produce human IFN-β constitutively. This observation could be interpreted as indicating that the putative labile murine IFN gene repressor does not recognize the corresponding human IFN-β gene which then becomes accessible for transcription. Under the conditions of this experiment, one might not predict that a postulated murine regulatory protein would be elaborated in the absence of inducer. Nevertheless, constitutive production of human IFN-β in mouse cells might be sustained even so since evidence suggests that posttranscriptional control of IFN synthesis is species specific (GREEN et al. (1980).

The synthesis of IFN-α and IFN-γ is apparently subject to control mechanisms different from that governing IFN-β production since neither IFN-α nor IFN-γ synthesis is enhanced by exposing induced cells to inhibitors of macromolecular synthesis (NG et al. 1981). Alternatively, the mechanisms regulating the synthesis of IFN0b and IFN-α/-γ may be similar, but the response of fibroblasts and lymphoid cells to antimetabolites may differ. With the availability of cDNA probes, it should be possible to test the validity of the scheme presented in Fig. 1 and to define the mechanism or mechanisms which control the synthesis of IFN-α, -β, and -γ.

2. Cellular RNA Metabolism During Induction

When C-10 cells are induced with poly(I)·poly(C), cycloheximide, and actinomycin D, unique changes in cellular RNA metabolism ensue (HUANG and TAN, to be published). Although the rate of total RNA synthesis in induced and noninduced cells is similar, the recoverable poly(A)-containing mRNA fraction is less in the induced cultures than in the controls (Table 2). This effect is transient and the amount of poly(A) mRNA is restored to normal levels as soon as the inducers are removed from the cultures. It is uncertain if this reduction of mRNA is due to inhibition of its synthesis exclusively or also to degradation. Possibly, when cells are induced by dsRNA, a case very similar to viral challenge, the cells respond by degrading viral as well as newly synthesized cellular RNA (perhaps through a short-lived nuclease) as a first step in antiviral defense. The degradation of labile mRNA in a cell could affect the concentration of proteins with high turnover rates like the postulated IFN repressor (Fig. 1), allowing the IFN gene to be transcribed.

Table 2. The effect of interferon induction on cellular RNA

Treatment	Total RNA	Poly(A) RNA [a]	Total RNA	Poly(A) RNA [a]
	($cpm \times 10^{-6}$)		(mg)	
Control (^{3}H)	12.4	0.76 (6.1)	352	19.2 (5.4)
Induced (^{3}H)	15.7	0.052 (0.3)	316	4.8 (1.5)
Superinduced (^{3}H)	11.1	0.056 (0.5)	243	3.0 (1.2)
Control (^{3}H)	30	0.56 (1.8)		
Superinduced (^{32}P)	4	0.02 (0.5)		
Control (^{3}H)	15.5	0.20 (1.3)		
Induced (^{32}P)	1.7	0.01 (0.5)		
Cells recovered from superinduction (^{3}H)	12.9	1.2 (9.3)		
Cells recovered from superinduction (^{32}P)	1.0	0.3 (3.0)		

[a] Figures in brackets indicate percentages

IV. Virus-Resistant Cell Mutants

There is evidence to suggest that IFN genetic expression may be related to the cells' ability to support viral replication. HOFFMAN et al. (1968) reported that cultured cells from golden hamsters (*Mesocricetus auratus*), which are highly susceptible to many virus infections, were also more susceptible to lytic infection with viruses, including the influenza virus and group B togaviruses, which multiply poorly in most other cell cultures. The unusual susceptibility of the hamster and cricetine cells to viruses may be related to defects in their IFN mechanism, for attempts at induction either in the whole animal or in cell cultures with different inducers generally failed to demonstrate IFN (CARVER et al. 1968; TAYLOR-PAPADIMITRIOU and STOKER 1971). GROSSBERG et al. (1975) reported detectable IFN only in 4 of 17 experiments in the intact hamster and 1 out of 21 experiments in cricetine cell cultures, using different viral inducers as well as poly(I) · poly(C).

Vero cells, a line of African green monkey kidney cells, are suitable for the replication of many viruses. DESMYTER et al. (1968) demonstrated that these cells failed to produce IFN when infected with viruses, although they were sensitive to IFN: The virus-sensitive diploid cell strains, WI-38 and MRC-5, have been shown to be low IFN producers. Comparing the sensitivity to viruses with the IFN-inducing ability of six human diploid cell strains, WU et al. (1979) demonstrated that high IFN-inducing cell strains were accompanied by a decrease of sensitivity to vesicular stomatitis virus (VSV) replication.

BURKE (1978) described pluripotential embryonal carcinoma (EC) cells failing to produce IFN after treatment with a variety of inducers and being concurrently insensitive to IFN action. Several differentiated lines derived from the EC cells, however, produced IFN and were sensitive to it. Apparently, differentiation of EC cells in vitro was accompanied by the development of IFN inducibility and sensitivity. The EC cells had been shown to be sensitive to infection with encephalomyocarditis virus (EMCV), Sindbis virus, VSV, and vaccinia virus. Furthermore, Semliki Forest virus, which is known to be IFN sensitive, grew better in cell lines that could not produce IFN than in those that could, possibly because of the lack of an active IFN system. On the other hand, several groups have shown that EC cells were resistant to Simian virus 40 (SV40), polyomavirus, and ecotropic C-type viruses (PERIES et al. 1977; TEICH et al. 1977), but these viruses replicated in differentiated EC cell lines. The failure to activate genes responsible for the IFN system and the failure of tumor virus multiplication suggest that in both cases, the genome is masked in some way.

It is of particular interest to select cell lines containing mutations in the regulating genes for IFN in order to understand the mechanism of IFN genetic expression and its relationship to antiviral activities. MORGAN et al. (1973) described a method for the isolation of virus-resistant mutants of mammalian cells in culture. Actively growing monolayers of a mouse embryo fibroblast line (3T6) at 50% confluence were incubated for 24 h at 37 °C with *N*-methyl-*N'*-nitronitrosoguanidine at 8 µg/ml. The surviving cells were allowed to grow out in fresh medium for several days. Confluent cell monolayers were infected with *ts* mutant of Sindbis virus which was allowed to proceed through one cycle of replication at the permissive temperature. When the cells were transferred to the nonpermissive temperature, further cycles of virus replication were prevented and noninfected cells allowed to grow out. Repetition of this procedure over several months resulted in the isolation of a virus-resistant cell line by micropipet cloning. This line of mutant cells was resistant to VSV, Mengo virus, and Semliki Forest virus as well as Sindbis virus, and did not shed infectious Sindbis virus. No viral genetic information was detected in the mutant cell line that could rescue other *ts* mutant Sindbis viruses and no alteration in either virus adsorption of penetration was found.

COLBY et al. (1975) and JARVIS and COLBY (1978) described the isolation of a virus-resistant mutant of murine 3T6 cells, designated 3T6-V^rB2. This mutant cell displayed a high degree of resistance to infection by members of the togavirus, rhabdovirus, and picornavirus groups. They suggested that 3T6-V^rB2 cells behaved phenotypically as cells engaged in the semiconstitutive synthesis of small, but detectable amounts of IFN as demonstrated as follows:

First, though no detectable amount of IFN was demonstrated by conventional methods in mutant cell cultures in the absence of induction, the untreated cultures of 3T6-V^rB2 produced VSV, Mengo virus, and Sindbis virus in titers similar to those produced by 3T6 cells that had been pretreated with approximately 100 IU/ml IFN.

Second, IFN-induced intracellular enzymatic activities, namely, the dsRNA-dependent phosphorylation of a protein, and the dsRNA-dependent production of a low molecular weight inhibitor of protein synthesis, were detected in extracts prepared from 3T6-V^rB2 cultures which had not been pretreated with IFN.

Third, upon cocultivation of 3T6-V^rB2 cells with IFN-sensitive mouse cells, L929, an antiviral state was induced in the latter cells as measured by a reduction of virus yield following infection. This effect was noticeable at a ratio as small as 10% 3T6-V^rB2 to 90% L929, but was maximal when the mixed cultures contained equal numbers of the two cell types. In this case, there was a 33-fold increase in

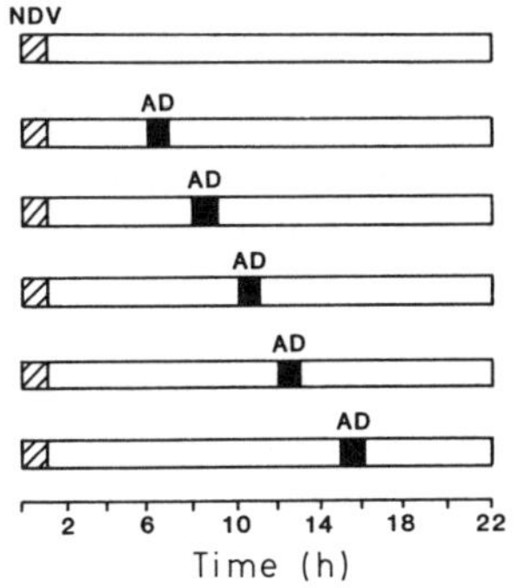

L929B (log₄ U/0.5 ml)	LVR-2 (log₄ U/0.5 ml)	LVR-2 / L929B
8.50	7.00	0.125*
4.00	4.50	
4.43	6.00	8.8*
5.33	5.50	
6.00	5.50	
8.00	7.00	0.25*

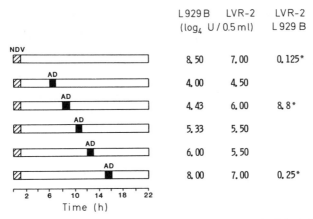

Fig. 3. Kinetics of synthesis of IFN mRNA in LVR-2 cells induced with NDV. AD, actinomycin D, 2 μg/ml at 37 °C for 1 h. Each number represents the mean from three samples. *Asterisks* indicate percentage of the geometric mean of IFN titer in LVR-2 against that in L929B

viral resistance over what would be expected. It was found that a diffusible molecule was inducing an antiviral response in L929 cells.

Fourth, in the presence of mouse IFN antiserum, the ability of the mutant cells to induce an antiviral state in IFN-sensitive mouse cells upon cocultivation was eliminated. Additionally, growing mutant cells in the presence of IFN antiserum caused a reversion to the virus-resistant phenotype.

Hou et al. (1981) reported the selection of three virus-resistant L-cell mutants (LVR-1, -2, -5) by a mutagenesis selection method similar to that described by Morgan et al. (1973). These cell mutants were highly resistant to infection by VSV, Sindbis, and vaccinia viruses, and retained their phenotype unchanged during 50 passages. VSV was adsorbed onto antiviral mutant cells more quickly than onto parent cells, suggesting that the antiviral character of mutant cells was not due to cell membrane changes resulting in refractoriness to virus adsorption. Spontaneous IFN production was not detected in repeatedly frozen and thawed suspensions of 4×10^6 mutant cells. Cytopathic effect was not observed in chick embryo cell cultures challenged with suspensions prepared from concentrated mutant cells (LVR-1, 5) after 1 week incubation at 33° and 37 °C.

These mutant cell lines were found to show marked changes in their IFN induction system. For example, the final IFN yield of antiviral cell mutant (LVR-2) after induction with Newcastle disease virus (NDV) was definitely lower as compared with that of parent cells. In contrast, the amount of IFN induced in LVR-1 and LVR-2 cells with poly(I)·poly(C) alone, poly(I)·poly(C)–DEAE-dextran complex, or poly(I)·poly(C) with cycloheximide and actinomycin D was higher than that induced in parent cells. Studies on the kinetics of IFN induction with NDV in different cell sublines indicated that the IFN response of antiviral cell lines was more rapid than that of parent cells. As illustrated in Fig. 3, the IFN yield obtained in LVR-2 cell cultures treated with actinomycin D 8 h after induction was 8.8 times higher than that obtained in its parent cells. However, at 15 h, the IFN yield in

LVR-2 cell culture was 4 times lower, suggesting more rapid synthesis of IFN mRNA in LVR-2 cells. These data suggest an accelerated IFN response in antiviral cell mutants after induction with NDV, and a later drop in IFN production due to blocking of virus replication. These findings were supported by other experiments in which total RNAs were extracted from L929B and LVR-2 cells 10 h after induction with NDV and microinjected into fish oocytes (HOU and YANG 1981). The translation product in oocytes injected with RNA from induced LVR-2 cells showed twice the IFN activity of that from L929B cells.

Thus, analysis of virus-resistant mutants has contributed to the understanding of how IFN synthesis is regulated. It is hoped that this approach as well as others discussed here will soon lead to a more complete picture of the control of IFN expression.

B. Regulatory Control of IFN Action

I. Introduction

The mechanisms which mediate IFN's antiviral action are only partially elucidated and those underlying the nonantiviral actions of IFN even less clear. Thus, it is not surprising that knowledge regarding the regulation of these mechanisms is rather limited. Nevertheless, some insight into the regulatory control of IFN action has been gained. Theoretically, any stage in the development or decay of IFN-induced antiviral activity is susceptible to regulation, for example: (a) interaction of IFN at the plasma membrane with a putative receptor; (b) transmission of the resulting signal (or signals) to the cell nucleus; (c) derepression of genes coding for the mediators of IFN action; (d) translation of these mRNAs into proteins; (e) interaction of the newly synthesized proteins with cellular and/or viral components; and (f) turnover of the mRNAs and proteins induced by IFN.

Sensitivity to IFN may be determined to a large degree by the putative IFN receptor. Although such an entity has not yet been isolated, the gene possibly coding for it has been mapped to human chromosome 21 and mouse chromosome 16. Little is known about the transmission of an IFN-induced signal to the cell interior, although it may involve the cytoskeleton and microtrabeculae. On the other hand, some progress has recently been made regarding the detection and identification of newly synthesized mRNAs and proteins in IFN-treated cells. Finally, experiments including some involving the use of metabolic inhibitors (as in studies on the regulation of IFN synthesis, itself) have shed light on the transient nature of components mediating the antiviral state. The evidence supporting these findings on regulation of IFN action and those factors enhancing or suppressing IFN activity will be reviewed. Some conclusions relating to the clinical use of IFN will also be discussed.

II. Genetic Factors Controlling Sensitivity to IFN

1. Human Chromosome 21

A gene (or genes) on human chromosome 21 appears to play a pivotal role in determining the sensitivity of cells to most of IFN's effects.

a) Antiviral Activity

One of the first pieces of evidence regarding genetic control of development of antiviral activity was provided in 1969 by the new technique of somatic cell hybridization. Using human/mouse cell hybrids, NABHOLZ (1969) found that development of the antiviral state was asyntenic with IFN production. CASSINGENA et al. (1971) showed that development of the antiviral state in mouse/monkey cell hybrids was asyntenic with IFN production and possibly correlated with a very small subtelocentric chromosome. In 1973, TAN et al. showed that, in mouse/human cell hybrids, sensitivity to human IFN and the cytoplasmic form of superoxide dismutase segregated concordantly and that both phenotypes correlated with the presence of human chromosome 21. The role of chromosome 21 in establishing the antiviral state was further supported by the observation that fibroblasts trisomic for chromosome 21 were more sensitive to IFN than were cells containing two copies of this chromosome (TAN et al. 1974b). In fact, a similar study which included monosomic 21 cells indicated that the inducibility of the antiviral state increased logarithmically as the number of chromosomes 21 increased linearly (TAN 1975). Several other laboratories also using aneuploid cell lines obtained similar results (CHANY et al. 1975; EPSTEIN and EPSTEIN 1976; WIRANOWSKA-STEWART and STEWART 1977). In order to determine the location of the gene (or genes) on chromosome 21 controlling sensitivity to IFN, TAN and GREENE (1976) obtained several fibroblast cell lines containing different translocations of parts of this chromosome. They found that the gene (or genes) governing sensitivity to IFN-α was localized in the long arm of chromosome 21. EPSTEIN and EPSTEIN (1976) confirmed this subregional localization and showed that this gene (or genes) resided in the distal region of the long arm of chromosome 21. Moreover, they showed that the same gene (or genes) involved in sensitivity to the classical IFN-α and -β was implicated in the antiviral response of cells to IFN-γ as well.

More recent evidence confirms that chromosome 21 alone is sufficient to render hybrid cells sensitive to IFN (SLATE et al. 1978). On the other hand, several lines of evidence indicate that genes residing on other chromosomes modulate chromosome 21-directed sensitivity to IFN. The observation that a linear increase in chromosome 21 dosage results in an exponential increase in sensitivity led TAN (1975) to postulate that regulator gene elements for induction of the antiviral state are present on another chromosome (or chromosomes). For example, chromosome 16 may bear one or more negative regulatory elements since some cell lines trisomic for this chromosome are significantly less sensitive to IFN than normal diploid cell (CHANY et al. 1975). Similarly, positive regulatory elements may reside on chromosomes 4 and 22, since human/mouse somatic cell hybrids retaining these as the only human chromosomes in addition to chromosome 21 are markedly more sensitive to IFNs-α and -β than are hybrids harboring only chromosome 21 (SLATE et al. 1978). Thus, the nonlinear dosage effect of chromosome 21 on sensitivity to IFN can be interpreted as an imbalance between one or more chromosome 21 gene products and products of regulatory genes on other chromosomes. Indeed, triploid cells, which contain three copies of chromosome 21, but a normal interchromosomal ratio, display a sensitivity to IFN equal to that of diploid cells (CHANY et al. 1975).

b) Nonantiviral Activities

Although some investigators reported contradictory evidence (LUBINIECKI et al. 1979; DE CLERCQ et al. 1976), chromosome 21 has been shown to confer sensitivity to some of the nonantiviral effects of IFN. For example, FRANKFORT et al. (1978) have shown that sensitivity to the priming activity of human IFN in mouse/human cell hybrids is highly correlated with the presence of chromosome 21. Studies of the dosage effect of this chromosome indicate that chromosome 21 also governs sensitivity of cells to the cell multiplication inhibitory (CMI) activity to IFN (TAN 1976). Closely related to IFN's CMI activity is its ability to alter rRNA metabolism; the ratio of newly synthesized 28 to 18 *S* rRNA is decreased (MAROUN 1978). This ratio is significantly more sensitive to the influence of IFN in trisomic 21 fibroblasts than in diploid cells (MAROUN 1979).

The genetic control of the response of immunocompetent cells to IFN has also been examined. CUPPLES and TAN (1977) reported that the mitogen-stimulated blastogenesis of lymphocytes from individuals with Down's syndrome is inhibited by much lower concentrations of IFN-β than are cells from normal donors. GURARI-ROTMAN et al. (1978) confirmed this finding with IFN-α as well as IFN-β. Recently, EPSTEIN and EPSTEIN (1980) also described an enhanced sensitivity of mitogen-stimulated trisomic 21 lymphocytes to inhibition by IFN whereas the production of IFN-γ by these cells was normal. Thus, the sensitivity of lymphocytes to the antiproliferative action of IFN displays a dosage response to chromosome 21. Similar results were reported recently by MATHESON et al. (1981) for both IFN-α and IFN-β. In addition, these investigators showed that both IFNs exert an enhancing, rather than inhibitory, effect on B-cell mitogenesis and that the sensitivity of lymphocytes to the positive effect of IFN on proliferation is also controlled by one or more genes on chromosome 21.

SMITH-JOHANNSEN et al. (1979) have described a case which suggests a chromosome 21-directed sensitivity to the antitumor effect of IFN. They studied the effect of IFN-β on peripheral white blood cells isolated from a diploid acute myelogenous leukemia (AML) patient whose leukemic cells carried an extra copy of chromosome 21. Compared with blast preparations of normal karyotype and cells from healthy donors, the trisomic 21 lymphocytes were much more sensitive to the inhibitory effects of IFN. When this AML patient received IFN-β in a phase I clinical trial, his blast count was reduced from 59% to 0% (MCPHERSON and TAN 1980).

Recently it has been shown that IFN inhibits the maturation of monocytes to macrophages (LEE and EPSTEIN 1980). Peripheral blood monocytes from Down's syndrome individuals were 3.7-fold more sensitive to the inhibitory effect of IFN-α compared with cells from diploid individuals (L. B. EPSTEIN et al. 1980a). Thus, the inhibition of monocyte maturation represents another IFN activity controlled by chromosome 21.

One nonantiviral activity of IFN, the development of which may not be under the control of chromosome 21, is the recruitment of natural killer (NK) cells. MATHESON et al. (1981) were unable to demonstrate any significant dosage effect of this chromosome on the enhancement of NK cell activity by IFN-α or IFN-β. However, the large variation inherent in this type of assay may not permit detection of such a dosage effect.

c) Nature of Chromosome 21-Coded Product

Although not the only interpretation (TAN 1975), perhaps the most direct explanation of the chromosome 21 dosage effect on sensitivity to IFN is that it bears a gene (or genes) which codes for IFN receptors localized in the cell membrane. The putative IFN receptors, like receptors for some glycoprotein hormones, may consist of two distinct sites, one for binding IFN and another for causing cell activation. This concept was first proposed by CHANY (1976) and has been reviewed and further developed by CHANY and others (CHANY et al. 1977; BESANÇON and ANKEL 1977; FRIEDMAN et al. 1977; FRIEDMAN 1978; GROLLMAN et al. 1978). This hypothesis remains unproven, but evidence is mounting for the existence of IFN receptors and some data is consistent with their being coded by one or more genes on chromosome 21.

α) Evidence of IFN Receptor. That IFN must bind to the external cell surface in order to elicit a response has been amply demonstrated by several different types of experiment. For example, FRIEDMAN (1967) showed that trypsin-sensitive chick IFN bound to chick embryo fibroblasts at 10 °C can induce an antiviral state in the cells when the temperature is elevated to 37 °C. Also, molecules of mouse IFN covalently bound to agarose beads and thus unable to enter cells can still elicit an antiviral response in murine fibroblasts (ANKEL et al. 1973; KNIGHT 1974). An acknowledged weakness of this experimental approach is that, considering the high specific activity of IFN, only a few molecules spontaneously released from the agarose beads could trigger an antiviral state. Moreover, it is difficult to rule out the possibility that, despite attachment to an agarose bead, an IFN molecule could still penetrate the cell membrane and initiate its antiviral activity internally. Such problems were avoided in a more definitive experiment reported by VENGRIS et al. (1975) who showed that human fibroblasts producing IFN in response to poly(I) · poly(C) fail to develop viral resistance if antiserum to IFN-β is present in the medium. Also, cells which do not bind detectable amounts of IFN are resistant to the antiviral effects of IFN (GRESSOR et al. 1974).

Gangliosides have been strongly implicated as the chemical entities in the cell membrane involved in the binding of IFN. Gangliosides GM_2 and GT_1, in particular, have been shown to neutralize the antiviral activity of mouse IFN in vitro (BESANÇON and ANKEL 1974; BESANÇON et al. 1976). Similarly, gangliosides GM_2, GT_1, GM_1, and GD_{1a} inactive human IFN-α and IFN-β in vitro (VENGRIS et al. 1976). VENGRIS et al. (1976) were able to confer sensitivity to IFN on a poorly responding glycolipid-deficient mouse cell line by incorporating exogenous gangliosides into the cell membranes. Pretreatment of MSV-BALB/c cells with sodium butyrate, which has been shown to stimulate the synthesis of gangliosides (FISHMAN et al. 1976; FISHMAN and ATIKKAN 1979), can also increase the sensitivity to IFN's antiviral effect (BOURGEADE and CHANY 1979). Recently, it has been reported that gangliosides can also inhibit the IFN-induced augmentation of murine NK cell activity (KRISHNAMURTI and ANKEL 1981).

Although gangliosides bind IFN, their role in receptor function remains obscure. Molecules which are known to interact with gangliosides such as cholera toxin and thyrotropin (KOHN et al. 1976) do not mimic IFN activity. Also, gangliosides bind IFNs from different species with comparable efficiency. On the other hand, early experiments suggested that IFN receptors are proteinaceous on the basis of their trypsin sensitivity CHANY 1976). More recently, GROLLMAN et al. (1978), working with membrane extracts from mouse Ly cells, obtained indirect evidence that the IFN receptor is a glycoprotein. They have proposed that the IFN receptor may be analogous to that of thyrotropin which consists of a low affinity ganglioside component and a high affinity glycoprotein component. However, BECKNER et al. (1981), using normal rat thyroid cells instead of isolated membranes, have obtained evidence which indicates that gangliosides may not be involved as a component of the thyrotropin receptor.

The most direct evidence for the existence and nature of IFN receptors is based on experiments carried out in the murine system by AGUET and his colleagues using ^{125}I-labeled pure mouse IFN. The radiolabeled probe is bound specifically to IFN-sensitive L1210 cells, but binding is only nonspecific to an IFN-resistant subline of L1210 cells and to heterologous chick embryo fibroblasts (AGUET 1980). The degree of binding of IFN to sensitive cells is directly correlated with the magnitude of subsequent antiviral activity or growth inhibition (AGUET and BLANCHARD 1981). Scatchard analysis indicates that the receptors have a very high affinity and bind IFN in a noncooperative manner. The results also suggest that IFN-α and IFN-β bind to the same receptor, but further studies will be required to confirm this. Binding is reduced in cells treated with trypsin or cycloheximide, indicating that the receptor involves a protein or glycoprotein component. In contrast to other work cited here, however, AGUET and BLANCHARD (1981) have found preliminary evidence that gangliosides do not play a role in specific binding of IFN. The reason for this discrepancy is unclear. The receptors for IFN appear to be quite different from those for some polypeptide hormones in that their number is not influenced by exposure to ligand and that they release intact IFN molecules after formation of the receptor–ligand complex. This release is energy dependent since it occurs only at 37 °C and not at 4 °C (AGUET and BLANCHARD 1981). It is interesting to note that specific binding of IFN to cells does not ensure a biologic response. Mouse EC cells bind ^{125}I-labeled IFN, but are IFN resistant (ARGUET et al. 1981). Presumably, the failure of these cells to respond to IFN is due to a defect elsewhere in the cell such as a lack of RNase F (EPSTEIN et al. 1981; PANET et al. 1981).

Although mouse IFN-α and IFN-β appear to bind to a common site, IFN-γ may have a distinct receptor. Mouse IFN-γ does not bind to gangliosides and is active on cells which are resistant to the action of IFN-α and IFN-β (ANKEL et al. 1980; FALCOFF et al. 1980; HOVANESSIAN et al. 1980). Also, mouse IFN-γ does not appear to compete with ^{125}I-labeled IFN-α or IFN-β (AGUET and BLANCHARD 1981). Furthermore, it has been reported that receptors for human IFN-γ may be distinct from those for IFN-α and IFN-β. BRANCA and BAGLIONI (1981) found that human IFN-γ does not compete with ^{125}I-labeled IFN-α for binding to Daudi cells.

β) Chromosome 21 and the IFN Receptor. The hypothesis that chromosome 21 codes for an IFN receptor was proposed by CHANY et al. (1975) to explain the dosage effect of chromosome 21 on sensitivity to IFN. The dosage effect, however, has alternative interpretations, as discussed by DE CLERCQ et al. (1976) who favored the view that the chromosome 21 gene product was not a receptor constituent per se, but probably a molecule serving to communicate the recognition of IFN from the surface of the cell to its interior. This conclusion was based on several findings, including the observation that monosomic, disomic, and trisomic 21 fibroblasts bound similar amounts of either IFN-α or IFN-β and that trisomic 21 fibroblasts were no more sensitive to the nonantiviral functions of IFN, such as priming and toxicity enhancement, than were diploid cells.

Other data, however, are consistent with the chromosome 21-coded receptor hypothesis. WIRANOWSKA-STEWART and STEWART (1977) reported that, in contrast to the findings of DE CLERCQ et al. (1976), the sensitivity and amount of IFN bound to human fibroblasts was correlated to the number of copies of chromosome 21. The discrepancy in the results of the two groups may be explained by the inability of the investigators to discriminate between nonspecific and specific binding of IFN to the cell surface. Valid quantitative data on the binding of IFN to the membrane can come only from studies employing a pure labeled ligand such as described for murine IFN by AGUET (1980). More compelling evidence for the hypothesis comes from studies utilizing mouse antisera directed against mouse/human somatic cell hybrids containing chromosomes 4, 21, and 22 (REVEL et al. 1976) or chromosome 21 (SLATE and RUDDLE 1978) as the only human genetic material. These antisera, which contain antibodies to determinants coded by chromosome 21, block induction of the antiviral response of cells treated with IFN. Recently, KAMARCK et al. (1981) reported generation of monoclonal antibodies of chromosome 21-coded determinants which inhibit development of the IFN-induced antiviral state. On the other hand, rabbit antisera directed against the cell surface of human fibroblasts failed to prevent expression of the antiviral state in human fibroblasts treated with IFN (VENGRIS et al. 1975). However, IFN receptors probably represent a small fraction of the total membrane antigens on fibroblasts and antibodies to these sites may have been present in the rabbit antisera in correspondingly small amounts or may have been absent.

Recently, BLALOCK and his colleagues (BLALOCK 1979a, b; BLALOCK and BARON 1979; BLALOCK et al. 1980a) have reported evidence indicating that sensitivity of a cell population to IFN may not necessarily be mediated by response of each individual cell to IFN, but rather by communication of a signal from relatively few IFN-sensitive cells to the majority. Gap junctions have been suggested as the channels through which this communication may be achieved. SLATE et al. (1981) have proposed an interesting experiment to test this possibility. Whether any relationship exists between chromosome 21 and the transfer mechanism for conveying sensitivity to IFN is unclear.

Definitive proof as to the nature of the chromosome 21-coded product (or products) controlling the sensitivity of cells to IFN awaits further investigation. The putative IFN receptor must first be isolated and characterized. Since pure, labeled active IFN is available, this could be accomplished soon using techniques similar to those used in the characterization of, for example, the insulin receptor (CUATRECASAS and HOLLENBERG 1976). Recombinant DNA methodology and nucleic acid hybridization could then be applied to determine eventually whether the receptor gene is located on chromosome 21.

2. Mouse Genes for Sensitivity to IFN

The influence of genetic disposition on IFN action has been studied in the mouse system. Strain differences in sensitivity to IFN have been described and the responsible loci subjected to genetic analysis. Recent evidence indicates that at least one of the genes influencing sensitivity to IFN in the mouse is located on chromosome 16.

a) Strain Differences in Sensitivity to IFN

LINDENMANN and his colleagues have shown that certain mice are highly resistant to specific viruses such as influenza virus and that this resistance is abolished when the mice are treated with anti-IFN serum (HALLER et al. 1980a; HALLER et al. 1981). The resistance cannot be explained by an exceptionally high output of IFN by these mice since their serum levels of antiviral activity are relatively low. Also, their resistance is not general, but restricted to the orthomyxovirus group. Therefore, these investigators have deduced the existence of a mouse gene *Mx* which confers a high degree of sensitivity to the antiviral effect of IFN on orthomyxoviruses. In vitro studies of macrophages (HALLER et al. 1980b) and hepatocytes (ARNHEITER et al. 1980) isolated from *Mx*/*Mx* and +/+ mice confirmed that the gene is virus specific and also indicated that it is dominant. The mechanism through which the *Mx* gene can selectively enhance the action of a general antiviral agent such as IFN toward a specific group of viruses is unclear. However, it is known that the IFN-induced block to influenza viral replication occurs at the translational level after virus attachment and penetration (HORISBERGER et al. 1980).

Studies carried out be DEMAEYER and DEMAEYER-GUIGNARD on various strains of mice (BALB/c, C57BL/6, B6-C-H-28^c, and recombinant inbred strains) have provided evidence for the existence of genes influencing IFN's immunomodulatory actions (DEMAEYER and DEMAEYER-GUIGNARD 1979, 1980a, b). They have shown that IFN can either enhance or inhibit the delayed hypersensitivity reaction of sensitized mice as measured by footpad swelling, depending on the time of IFN administration. The magnitude of the enhancing effect of IFN on delayed hypersensitivity was found to be significantly greater in C57BL/6 mice than in BALB/c mice. On the other hand, the degree of inhibition of this immune response by IFN was greater in BALB/c mice than in C57BL/6 mice. The possibility that these effects were related to different levels of serum IFN was ruled out. Preliminary evidence from DEMAEYER and DEMAEYER-GUIGNARD (1979) suggests those genes modulating the suppressive effect of IFN are located in or near the H-2 complex. Of course, one must be cautious in interpreting the results of experiments conducted in whole animals where other interpretations are possible. However, recent in vitro experiments on the effects of pure murine IFN on the proliferation of committed erythroid precursor cells derived from different mouse strains tend to support the in vivo results. GALLIEN-LARTIGUE et al. (1980) found that the proliferation of cells from BALB/c mice was tenfold more sensitive to the inhibitory effect of IFN than were cells from C57BL/6 mice. Similarly, the proliferation of macrophages derived from bone marrow of BALB/c mice was more sensitive to IFN than those of cells from C57BL/6 mice (DANDOY et al. 1981).

b) Chromosome Assignment

Recently, two laboratories have independently demonstrated that sensitivity to murine IFN is associated with mouse chromosome 16. RUDDLE and his colleaguses analyzed mouse/human somatic cell hybrids for their response to IFN and the presence of cytoplasmic superoxide dismutase. They found the two characteristics to be syntenic and to map to chromosome 16 (LIN et al. 1980). Cox et al. (1980) obtained similar findings using normal hamster/mouse somatic cell hybrids and also hybrids derived from a hamster cell line containing the robertsonian translocation which involves chromosome 16. As these investigators point out, mice trisomic for chromosome 16 will prove extremely useful as a model in which to study the relationship between enhanced sensitivity to IFN and developmental aberrations. This model system is particularly relevant to the question of whether IFN plays a role in the birth defects associated with the human trisomic 21 condition, Down's syndrome (TAN et al. 1974b; MAROUN 1980).

It is interesting to note that in both mice and humans, the genes coding for cytoplasmic superoxide dismutase and sensitivity to IFN are located on the same chromosome. Evidence that the physical relationship of the two phenotypes reflects a close functional relationship was reported by POTTATHIL et al. (1981). They found that inhibition of superoxide dismutase resulted in inhibition of IFN-induced antiviral activity.

III. Other Factors Influencing IFN Action

Cells cultured in vitro display a wide range of sensitivities to IFN, presumably reflecting differences in their expression and/or regulation of IFN action. In vivo the response of cells to IFN is probably also modulated by substances originating outside the cell such as hormones, drugs, and even other species of IFN.

1. Antiviral Activity

Within the last 5 years, several laboratories have identified enzymes which increase in activity significantly in IFN-treated cells. Thus, 2′,5′-oligodenylate [oligo(A)] synthetase (also referred to as 2-5A polymerase), a phosphokinase, and a phosphodiesterase are implicated as molecular mediators of IFN action. Details concerning the nature of these enzymes and the mechanism of IFN action can be found elsewhere (see reviews by BAGLIONI 1979; REVEL 1979; and other chapters in this Handbook). The product of the synthetase, 2′,5′-oligo(A), has been shown to exert an antiviral effect in intact cells in the absence of IFN (LIU et al. 1980 and Figs. 4–6).

Recently, the regulation of the induction of mRNAs associated with antiviral activity, including that for 2′,5′-oligo(A) synthetase, has been studied. Apparently, a single interaction of IFN-α or IFN-β with the cell membrane is sufficient to initiate development of the antiviral state (GARDNER and VILĆEK 1979). In L-cells, there is a 3-h lag after the beginning of IFN treatment before mRNA supporting the translation of 2′,5′-oligo(A) synthetase is detected (SHULMAN and REVEL 1980). Also, from experiments employing antibodies to IFN, continuous interaction of IFN molecules with the membrane is apparently required for maximal induction of this mRNA in mouse cells. In both mouse and human cells, the transcription of mRNAs responsible for antiviral activity induced by type I IFN (IFN-α and

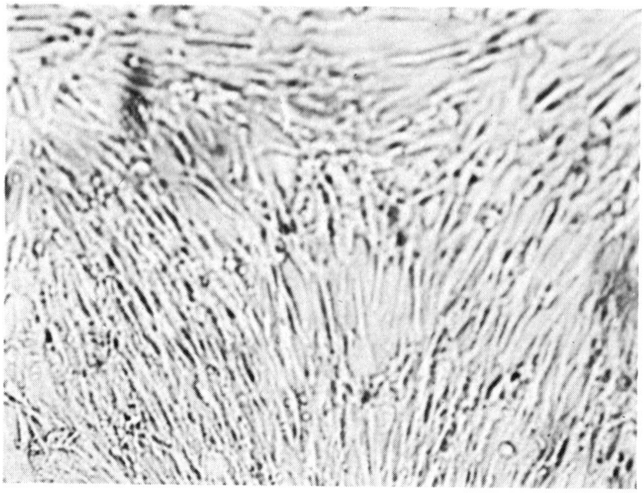

Fig. 4. Human embryo lung fibroblasts: no VSV, no 2′,5′-oligo(A)

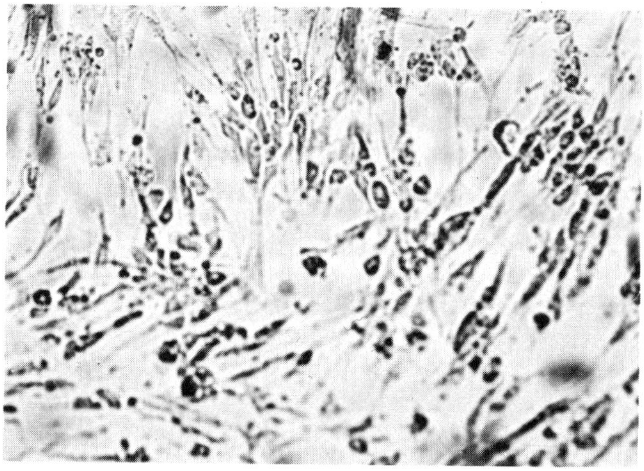

Fig. 5. Unprotected cells: VSV, no 2′,5′-oligo(A)

IFN-β) can proceed in the absence of protein synthesis (BAGLIONI and MARONEY 1980; DIANZANI et al. 1980). However, concurrent protein synthesis is required for the induction of these mRNAs by type I IFN (IFN-γ) (BAGLIONI and MARONEY, 1980; DIANZANI et al. 1980). This finding, together with the observation that the kinetics of appearance of mRNA for 2′,5′-oligo(A) synthetase are slower for immune IFN than for viral IFN (BAGLIONI and MARONEY 1980), suggests that the induction of antiviral activity by immune IFN differs fundamentally from that by viral IFN and involves the participation of intermediary proteins.

The turnover of mRNAs coding for antiviral activity has also been investigated. In experiments where newly synthesized proteins were detected in IFN-treated human fibroblasts by radiolabeling, RUBIN and GUPTA (1980) found in-

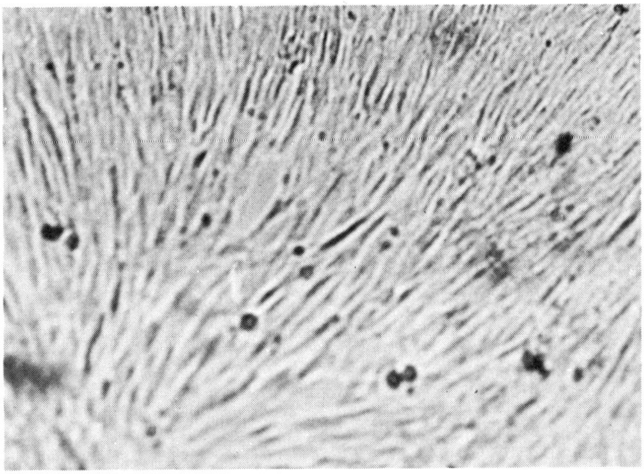

Fig. 6. Cells challenged with VSV and treated with 1 μM 2′,5′-oligo(A) in hypertonic medium to increase permeability of the cells to the oligonucleotide

direct evidence for the transient existence of some mRNAs, despite the continual presence of IFN. GORDON and STEVENSON (1980) treated mouse L929 cells with DRB, an inhibitor of RNA chain elongation, for varying periods following a 1-h exposure of the cells to IFN. Their results indicated that the IFN-induced mRNAs have a lifetime of 5–6 h. Whether the decay of these transcripts is due to an inhibition of synthesis, degradation, or some other phenomenon was not determined.

There is some evidence suggesting that one or more factors dependent on RNA and protein synthesis play a role in the turnover of the components of the antiviral state. For example, CHANY et al. (1971) reported that, when L-cells were exposed to actinomycin D 6 h after IFN was added, the antiviral state increased about ten fold. More recently, superinduction of 2′,5′-oligo(A) synthetase and protein kinase in L-cells by actinomycin D added 4 h after IFN has been reported (KIMCHI et al. 1979). Similar results have been found in human fibroblasts (GUPTA et al. 1981). LAB and KOEHREN (1972, 1976) showed that treatment of chick embryo fibroblasts with cycloheximide after establishment of the antiviral state can also potentiate IFN action. In experiments with chick cells enucleated by cytochalasin B, RADKE et al. (1974) demonstrated that protection against virus was significantly more stable in enucleated than in nucleated cells. These studies indicate the decay of mRNAs and proteins involved in antiviral activity is controlled by a dynamic process. The data of LAB and KOEHREN (1976) led these investigators to postulate the existence of a protein capable of reversibly inactivating one or more components of the antiviral state. However, it is perhaps premature to postulate the precise nature of the regulatory factors controlling IFN action, since much of the evidence derives from experiments involving metabolic inhibitors of other drastic interventions. Clearly, other approaches are desirable to identify the factors responsible for regulating IFN action at the molecular level.

Numerous examples of cells which display a range of sensitivity to IFN have been described in the literature and may provide model systems in which to study the mechanisms controlling IFN action. For instance, the human endometrial cancer cell line HEC-1 is totally insensitive to IFN, but contains high levels of both 2′,5′-oligo(A) synthetase and phosphokinase activities, even in the absence of IFN. To explain this observation, Verhaegen et al. (1980) suggested these enzymes are not sufficient in themselves to develop an antiviral state or that, although active in vitro, these enzymes are subjected to further regulatory control in vivo. Such a regulatory mechanism apparently does not involve inhibition of 2′,5′-oligo(A) synthetase, however, since in inhibitor of this enzyme was not detected in extracts of the HEC-1 cells.

EC cells are resistant to the protective effects of IFN against certain viruses, but their differentiated counterparts are sensitive (Burke et al. 1978; Nilsen et al. 1980). Since both the differentiated and nondifferentiated EC cells display an enhanced 2′,5′-oligo(A) synthetase activity in response to IFN (Wood and Hovanessian 1979), their different abilities to develop an antiviral state must be due to other factors. Perhaps the stimulation of phosphokinase activity in only the differentiated lines accounts for their IFN sensitivity. Regardless of the mechanism conferring antiviral activity, the observation of the transition from an insensitive to sensitive state in EC cells is a clear demonstration of the existence of regulatory factors controlling the ability to develop antiviral activity.

Among IFN-sensitive cells, there is variability in the degree of the induced antiviral state. For example, Tan et al. (1975) reported that fibroblasts from older donors (64 years) are 2–3-fold more sensitive to IFN than are cells from younger individuals (0–29 years). Harmon et al. (1980) found that the IFN dose–response curves for human foreskin fibroblasts and nasal epithelial cells were different. Ball (1980) suggested that the variations in response of cells to IFN may be related to corresponding differences in the extent of expression of components of the antiviral state. For example, he observed that, in chick cells, IFN stimulated a large increase in 2′,5′-oligo(A) synthetase activity without enhancing the activity of 2′-phosphodiesterase which is usually augmented in other cells treated with IFN (Schmidt et al. 1979). A lower than normal level of 2′-phosphodiesterase may also explain the enhanced sensitivity of DNA synthesis to 2′,5′-oligo(A) in a virus-resistant L-cell mutant recently isolated by Hou et al (to be published).

Expression of 2′-phosphodiesterase activity may play a key role in regulating IFN action. This enzyme increases up to five fold in IFN-treated cells (Schmidt et al. 1979). Breakdown of 2′,5′-oligo(A) by 2′-phosphodiesterase may reduce local concentrations of the oligonucleotide and prevent massive degradation of cellular RNA by RNase F (Schmidt et al. 1978; Williams and Kerr 1978; Minks et al. 1979). The enzyme may also play a role in inhibiting protein synthesis by degrading the CCA terminus of tRNA (Schmidt et al. 1979).

In addition to the regulatory mechanisms operating in the cell itself, the nature of the infecting virus can influence the expression of IFN-induced antiviral activity. Cells pretreated with IFN exhibit different degrees of protection, depending on the type of virus used as challenge (Samuel et al. 1980). Some viruses which are resistant to IFN may cause the synthesis of molecules which block IFN-induced activity during the course of infection. There is some evidence that Mengo virus infection in L-cells escapes inhibition by IFN for this reason (Fout and Simon 1981).

Moreover, the multiplicity of infection (m.o.i.) also appears to be an important factor with the degree of antiviral activity inversely proportional to the m.o.i.

(STITZ and SCHELLEKENS 1980). These phenomena may be related to the possibility that dsRNA plays a key role in the expression of antiviral activity in IFN-treated cells. Much evidence from studies on both extracts and intact cells indicates that dsRNA activates IFN-induced 2′,5′-oligo(A) synthetase (see BAGLIONI 1979; REVEL 1979; MINKS et al. 1980; GORDON and MINKS 1981). BAGLIONI et al. (1978) postulated that the localized activation of 2′,5′-oligo(A) synthetase by dsRNA might account for the preferential degradation of viral over cellular mRNA by 2′,5′-oligo(A)-activated nuclease. This hypothesis was supported by an experiment in which single-stranded RNA (ssRNA) tagged with dsRNA was degraded more rapidly than untagged RNA (NILSON and BAGLIONI 1979). Recently, WALLACH and REVEL (1980) found 2′,5′-oligo(A) synthetase bound to the ribonucleoprotein core of RNA viruses in IFN-treated infected cells. Although some investigators have reported that the IFN-induced phosphokinase also requires dsRNA to phosphorylate initiation factor elF-2 (FARRELL et al. 1978), others claim that the activity of this enzyme is independent of dsRNA (HOVANESSIAN and KERR 1979). If the kinase does require dsRNA, its interaction with the nucleic acid appears to be quite different from that of the synthetase (BAGLIONI and MARONEY 1981). Some evidence indicates dsRNA may also act to inhibit a phosphoprotein phosphatase (D. A. EPSTEIN et al. 1980).

Besides dsRNA, other agents can exert a stimulatory effect on the IFN-induced antiviral state. For example, the drug acyclovir (2-hydroxyethoxymethylguanine) has been reported to enhance the antiviral activity of IFN-α in human fibroblasts (LEVIN and LEARY 1981). The resistance of cells treated with both acyclovir and IFN to herpes simplex was greater than the protection predicted from treating cells with the two substances separately. A synergistic effect of acyclovir combined with IFN-β against herpes simplex types 1 and 2 has also been demonstrated (STANWICK et al. 1981). STANWICK et al. (1981) suggest that acyclovir may act by blocking the activity of an inhibitor of IFN generated as a result of herpes infection.

Different types of IFN interact to produce a positive synergistic effect on antiviral activity. This has been demonstrated in the murine system with mixtures of IFN-β and IFN-γ on L-cells. The resulting antiviral activity was 5–20-fold greater than predicted for an additive effect (FLEISCHMANN et al. 1979a; FLEISCHMANN et al. 1980). Thus, the regulatory mechanisms controlling the action of either IFN-β, IFN-γ, or both may be perturbed in favor of increasing the vigor of the antiviral state. Elevated temperature can also potentiate IFN-induced antiviral activity. HERON and BERG (1978) found the protective effect of IFN-α and IFN-β on human embryonic lung cells against VSV was at least three times greater at 40 °C than at 37 °C. Controls ruled out the possibility that the greater inhibition of infection was a direct effect of higher temperature on viral replication.

Some inhibitors of IFN-induced antiviral activity have been identified. For example, a product released by mitogen-stimulated mouse spleen cells reduces the potency of mouse IFN-β and IFN-γ (FLEISCHMANN et al. 1979b). The inhibitor has been partially purified and its molecular weight determined to be 8,000–10,000. Agents which inhibit the activity of fatty acid cyclooxygenase, an enzyme involved in the early stages of prostaglandin synthesis, also suppress development of IFN-mediated antiviral activity (POTTATHIL et al. 1980). Thus, a number of anti-inflammatory substances, including aspirin, were found to prevent the induction of antiviral activity in mouse L-cells by murine IFN. Although the end product of the reactions initiated by fatty acid cyclooxygenase is prostaglandin, addition of various prostaglandins failed to reverse the suppressive effect of cyclooxygenase inhibitors and further diminished IFN-mediated protection against viral challenge. The sensitive step in the induction of antiviral activity susceptible to cyclooxygenase inhibitors was determined to be a very early event. POTTATHIL et al. (1980) suggest that this early event may require an unstable intermediate of prostaglandin synthesis. Exogenous prostaglandins such as PGE_2, on the other hand, block development of the antiviral state (POTTATHIL et al. 1980; TROFATTER and DANIELS 1980). It is unlikely that this block is a consequence of prostaglandin-stimulated adenylate cyclase activity, but may result from competition between exogenous prostaglandin and the putative prostaglandin intermediate for a common site involved in expression of IFN action (POTTATHIL et al. 1980). Consistent with the results of these studies is the recent finding that the IFN-resistant cells, L1210R are essentially devoid of fatty acid cyclooxygenase activity (CHANDRABOSE et al. 1981).

INGLOT et al. (1980) have proposed that certain hormones and IFN may be antagonistic. For example, these investigators found that mouse or human IFN abolished the mitogenic effect of platelet growth factor and that platelet growth factor suppressed IFN-induced antiviral activity. The importance of such phenomena in vivo remains to be determined.

2. Nonantiviral Activities

a) CMI Activity

Recent evidence indicates that the CMI effect of IFN is separable from its antiviral action. Cells resistant to IFN's CMI activity, but sensitive to its antiviral action have been derived from both mouse (BORECKY et al. 1980) and human (KUWATA et al. 1980) cell lines. Conversely, Moloney murine leukemia virus- (M-MLV)-infected NIH 3T3 cells have been described which are resistant to IFN-mediated CMI but, sensitive to IFN-induced protection against M-MLV, although not EMCV, replication (CZARNIECKI et al. 1981). Moreover, among cells which respond to the CMI effect of IFN there is a trememdous range of sensitivity (CREASY et al. 1980; LUNDGREN et al. 1980; HILFENHAUS and MAULER 1980). For example, the proliferation of Daudi cells can be retarded by exceedingly low concentrations of IFN (ADAMS et al. 1975).

These observations indicate that distinct mechanisms and/or regulatory factors exist for IFN's anticellular action. This conclusion is supported by the finding that in an IFN-treated human transformed fibroblast line resistant to the CMI effect, but sensitive to the antiviral action of IFN, the activities of the two major enzyme systems associated with IFN action are induced to levels similar to those observed in fibroblasts sensitive to both aspects of IFN activity (VANDENBUSSCHE et al. 1981). On the other hand, it is likely that the regulation of IFN's antiviral and anticellular activities share at least some common mechanisms since both activities are often lost concurrently (L1210 cells) and both are potentiated at elevated temperature (HERON and BERG 1978).

b) Immunomodulatory Activity

Lymphocytes from different sources vary in their sensitivity to IFN. THORLEY-LAWSON (1981) recently reported that whereas the Epstein–Barr virus-induced transformation of B-cells obtained from adults was suppressed by IFN, even high concentrations of IFN failed to suppress the virus-induced stimulation of neonatal B-lymphocytes. Thus, human neonatal cells, or at least B-lymphocytes, appear to be insensitive to IFN. In contrast, the primary antibody response of young suckling mice is very sensitive to IFN, which inhibitis the response. On the other hand, in adult mice, IFN does not suppress antibody synthesis, but rather enhances it when given after the antigen (VIGNAUX et al. 1980).

The stimulatory action of IFNs on cell-mediated cytotoxicity in vitro (PERUSSIA et al. 1980; HERBERMAN et al. 1980) is subject to both enhancing and suppressive effects. HERBERMAN et al. (1980) has shown that Fc receptors may play an important role in determining the sensitivity of effector cells to this IFN action. They found that NK cells, Killer cells, monocytes, and some lectin-induced cytotoxicity cells which respond to IFN treatment bear Fc receptors, whereas other effector cells which are relatively insensitive to IFN lack these receptors.

Just as antiviral and anticellular activities of IFN are enhanced at elevated temperatures, the stimulatory effect of IFN on NK activity is also increased. HERON and BERG (1978) demonstrated a three fold increase in the augmentation of cytotoxicity induced by IFN in human lymphocytes at 39 °C compared with that at 37 °C. On the other hand, IFN-induced enhancement of NK activity is inhibited by prostaglandins (SCHULTZ et al. 1978; HOLDEN et al. 1980) and estradiol (SEAMAN et al. 1979).

Corticosteroids reverse the IFN-mediated stimulation of macrophage cytotoxicity. CHIRIGOS et al. (1980) found that dexamethasone, and to a lesser extent hydrocortisone and prednisone, severely inhibited the in vitro and in vivo tumoricidal activity of IFN-stimulated macrophages on murine MBL-2 leukemia cells. Similarly, prostaglandins of the E series abrogated the IFN-induced stimulation of macrophage cytotoxicity (CHIRIGOS et al. 1980). Since activated macrophages reportedly release significant amounts of PGE_2 (BRAY et al. 1974), this prostaglandin may play an important role in regulating the activity of these cells by negative feedback (SCHULTZ 1980). However, the precise mechanism or mechanisms by which prostaglandins and also corticosteroids suppress the enhancing effects of IFN on immune effector cells are obscure.

c) Antitumor Activity

An area of great practical interest is the modulation of IFN's antitumor action, but current knowledge regarding this subject is poor. Investigators are not even certain whether IFN's antitumor effects are direct or host mediated, although various combinations of both mechanisms may be in operation, depending on the conditions (TAYLOR-PAPADIMITRIOU 1980). Although human neoplastic cells may be more sensitive to IFN than normal cells (ATTALLAH et al. 1980), the response of different tumor cell lines to IFN is variable (CARTER and HOROSZEWICZ 1980). Also, ascites tumor cells are more sensitive to IFN than are those comprising solid tumors (L. B. EPSTEIN et al. 1980b). Some tumors may produce prostaglandins (HONG et al. 1977). Since it is known that these substances counteract other IFN-mediated effects, prostaglandins may subvert the antitumor effect of endogenous or administered IFN on neoplastic cells (SCHULTZ 1980).

IV. Clinical Considerations

1. IFN Therapy

The therapeutic value of IFN in the treatment of viral and neoplastic disease remains controversial. Aside from the scarcity of IFN itself, a major problem in designing clinical trials for IFN has been the lack of knowledge regarding the regulation of its action as well as the actual mechanisms by which IFN mediates its multiple effects. One recurrent observation in many recent studies on IFN action which is relevant to the clinical use of IFN is the variability in sensitivity of different cells to its antiviral, anticellular, immunomodulatory, and antitumor effects. This is most likely related to differences in the physiologic states of these cells and to the complexity of the regulatory mechanisms governing the activity of such a potent molecule as IFN. Thus, it would not be surprising if considerable variation occurred in the response of different patients, depending on their genetic background, the nature of their disease, and other factors. In view of this situation, the utility of rapid in vitro screening tests for selecting patients with a high chance of responding to IFN therapy should not be underestimated. Various assay systems have been described (L. B. Epstein et al. 1980b; Sikora et al. 1980; Bradley and Ruscetti 1981).

The observation that IFN enhanced the level of NK cell activity in patients (Einhorn et al. 1978; Huddlestone et al. 1979) suggested at first that this effect of IFN mediated at least partly its antitumor action. However, more recently, an IFN-induced decline in NK activity in lymphocytes from patients has been reported (Matheson et al. 1982; Herberman et al. 1980; Ho et al. 1981). Thus, the response of this class of cells to IFN appears to be quite variable. Recently, Ziegler et al. (1981) found that IFN-β stimulated NK activity in preparations from early stage chronic lymphocytic leukemia patients, but not in preparations from late stage patients. The reasons for the variable response of NK cells to IFN in different patients and its significance with respect to the therapeutic effect of IFN remain unclear.

Some of the studies discussed here indicate the possibility that administration of certain drugs to patients receiving IFN would compromise the results of such treatment. For example, both corticosteroids (Chirigos et al. 1980) and aspirin (Pottathil et al. 1980) may abrogate the effects of IFN treatment. Phenacetin apparently could be used as a substitute for aspirin by a patient receiving IFN (see Pottathil et al. 1980). On the other hand, in view of the suppressive effect of prostaglandins on IFN action and the fact that tumors and macrophages release these substances, administration of aspirin, which inhibits prostaglandin synthesis (see Goodman and Gilman 1980), may actually facilitate the action of IFN in some cases. Since many potential IFN recipients may have had previous drug treatment, the patient's chemotherapy history would also be an important consideration for the clinician.

The observation that immune IFN can enhance the action of virally induced IFN synergistically (Baron et al. 1980) suggests the administration of different IFNs simultaneously for clinical purposes. Another approach to combination IFN therapy might be to alternate IFN-α or IFN-β with IFN-γ. Falcoff et al. (1980) have suggested that such a regime would minimize the possibility of selecting for cells resistant to one or the other type of IFN. The use of IFN-γ alone also appears to have some advantages. For example, the anticellular activity of purified human IFN-γ is 20–100 times more potent than that of IFN-α or IFN-β (BLALOCK et al. 1980b; RUBIN and GUPTA 1980b). Also, IFN-γ does not bind to gangliosides (ANKEL et al. 1980), which are often found at elevated levels in the circulation of some cancer patients (KLOPPEL et al. 1977) and which could neutralize IFN-α or IFN-β (VENGRIS et al. 1976).

2. Combination Therapy

It is possible that IFN therapy combined with other drugs may produce an enhanced or even synergistic effect. Indeed, some drugs have been found to improve the clinical effect of IFN treatment. For example, MERIGAN (1981) has observed an improved therapeutic effect of IFN-α when combined with adenosine arabinoside in the treatment of chronic hepatitis B. A synergistic effect has been reported for acyclovir and IFN-α and IFN-β in the treatment of herpes simplex (LEVIN and LEARY 1981; STANWICK et al. 1981).

More recently, INOUE and TAN (1982) have reported that human IFN enhances cell killing by actinomycin D and *cis*-platinum. The magnitude of this enhancement is of the order of 2–3 logarithmic units. It would be useful to test this respect to other chemotherapeutic drugs and whether this in vitro phenomenon has relevance in vivo.

3. "Misregulation" of IFN Action

It has been proposed that certain diseases may arise from defects in the regulation of IFN production or action (SKURKOVICH 1981). It has been suggested, for example, that the immunosuppressed state of individuals with Down's syndrome may be related to the extreme sensitivity of their trisomic 21 lymphocytes to IFN (L. B. EPSTEIN et al. 1980a). Down's syndrome itself may result from the extreme sensitivity of a developing trisomic 21 fetus to IFN (TAN et al. 1974b); TAN and INOUE 1982). In contrast, an inability of NK cells to respond to IFN may be a contributing factor in some diseases such as subacute sclerosing panencephalitis and multiple sclerosis which are thought to be caused by viruses (BENCZUR et al. 1980; MINATO et al. 1980). Alternative explanations are that individuals suffering from these diseases fail to produce IFN in response to the infecting virus or that their infected cells escape the cytotoxicity of a normal NK cell system. Since it is likely that IFNs play an important role in modulating the proliferation and activity of immunocompetent cells (TAYLOR-PAPADIMITRIOU 1980), it is also possible that autoimmune disease, such as systemic lupus erythematosus (RICH 1981) and also some non-Hodgkin lymphomas (HABESHAW 1979) may result from defects in the regulation of IFN production or action.

From the foregoing section, it is clear that our understanding of how IFN's actions are regulated is still relatively primitive. However, the answers to some important questions such as what the identity and nature of the putative IFN receptor are may soon be forthcoming. Also, one can anticipate that the regulation of activity mediated by each or some of the IFN molecular subspecies may have unique features. Research in the area of regulation of the IFN system will help to provide not only the basis for more efficient use of IFN in the clinic, but also a more profound understanding of eukaryotic gene regulation in general.

Acknowledgments. We wish to thank Dr. REGINA HAARS and Dr. MORLEY HOLLENBERG for critical reading of the manuscript and the MRC of Canada for support. Y.H.T. is a PCHB of Alberta Research Scientist.

References

Adams A, Strander H, Cantell K (1975) Sensitivity of the Epstein-Barr virus transformed human lymphoid cell lines to interferon. J Gen Virol 28:207–217

Aguet M (1980) High-affinity binding of ^{125}I-labelled mouse interferon to a specific cell receptor. Nature 284:459–461

Aguet M, Blanchard B (1981) High-affinity binding of ^{125}I-labelled mouse interferon to a specific cell surface receptor II. Analysis of binding properties. Virology 115 (2):249–261

Aguet M, Gressor I, Hovanessian AG, Bandu M-T, Blanchard B, Blangy D (1981) Specific high-affinity binding of ^{125}I-labelled mouse interferon to interferon resistant embryonal carcinoma cells in vitro. Virology 114:585–588

Ankel H, Chany C, Galliot B, Chevalier MJ, Robert M (1973) Antiviral effect of interferon covalently bound to sepharose. Proc Natl Acad Sci USA 70:2360–2363

Ankel H, Krishnamurti C, Besançon F, Stefanos S, Falcoff E (1980) Mouse fibroblast (type I) and immune (type II) interferons: pronounced differences in affinity for gangliosides and in antiviral and antigrowth effects on mouse leukemia L-1210 R cells. Proc Natl Acad Sci USA 77:2528–2532

Armstrong JA (1970) Control of interferon production in rabbit cells treated with polyI.C. J Gen Physiol 56:97s–98s

Arnheiter H, Haller O, Lindenmann J (1980) Host gene influence on interferon action in adult mouse hepatocytes: specificity for influenza virus. Virology 103:11–20

Attallah AM, Fleisher T, Khalil R, Noguchi PD, Irritia-Shaw A (1980) Proliferative and functional aspects of interferon-treated human normal and neoplastic T and B cells. Br J Cancer 42:423–429

Baglioni C (1979) Interferon-induced enzymic activities and their role in the antivirale state. Cell 17:255–264

Baglioni C, Maroney PA (1980) Mechanisms of action of human interferons. Induction of 2′5′-oligo (A) synthetase. J Biol Chem 255:8390–8393

Baglioni C, Maroney PA (1981) Inhibition of double-stranded ribonucleic acid activated protein kinase and 2′,5′ oligo (adenylic acid) polymerase by ethidium bromide. Biochemistry 20:758–762

Baglioni C, Minks MA, Maroney PA (1978) Interferon action may be mediated by activation of a nuclease by pppA2′p5′A2′p5′A. Nature 273:684–687

Ball AL (1980) Induction, purification and properties of 2′5′ oligo-adenylate synthethase. Ann NY Acad Sci 350:486–496

Baron S, Blalock JE, Dianzani F, Fleishmann JR WR, Georgiades JA, Johnson HM, Stanton GJ (1980) Immune interferon: some properties and functions. Ann NY Acad Sci 350:130–144

Beckner SK, Brady RO, Fishman PH (1981) Reevaluation of the role of gangliosides in the binding and action of thyrotropin Proc Natl Acad Sci 78:4848–4852

Bencyzur M, Petrányl GG, Pálffy G, Varga M, Tálas M, Kotsy B, Földes I, Hollan SR (1980) Dysfunction of natural killer cells in multiple sclerosis: a possible pathogenic factor. Clin Exp Immunol 39:657–662

Besançon F, Ankel H (1974) Binding of interferon to gangliosides. Nature 252:478–480

Besançon F, Ankel H (1977) Membrane receptors for interferon. Tex Rep Biol Med 35:282–289

Besançon F, Ankel H, Basu S (1976) Specificity and reversibility of interferon ganglioside interaction. Nature 259:576–578

Billiau A, Joniau M, Desomer P (1973) Mass production of human interferon in diploid cells stimulated by polyI.C. J Gen Virol 19:1–8

Blalock JE (1979a) A small fraction of cells communicates the maximal interferon sensitivity to a population. Proc Soc Exp Biol Med 162:80–84
Blalock JE (1979b) Cellular interactions determine the rate and degree of interferon action. Infect Immun 23:496–501
Blalock JE, Baron S (1979) Mechanisms of interferon induced transfer of viral resistance between animal cells. J Gen Virol 42:363–372
Blalock JE, Weigent DA, Langford MP, Stanton GJ (1980a) Transfer of interferon-induced viral resistance from human leukocytes to other cell types. Infect Immun 29:356–360
Blalock JE, Georgiades JA, Langford MP, Johnson HM (1980b) Purified human immune interferon has more potent anticellular activity than fibroblast or leukocyte interferon. Cell Immunol 49:390–394
Borecký L, Hajnicka V, Fushberger N, Kontsek P, Lacković V, Russ G, Ćapková J (1980) The cell growth inhibitory and antiviral effects of interferon in cloned transformed mouse cells. Ann NY Acad Sci 350:188–207
Bourgeade MF, Chany C (1979) Effect of sodium butyrate on the antiviral and anticellular action of interferon in normal and MSV-transformed cells. Int J Cancer 24:314–318
Brack C, Nagata S, Mantei N, Weissman C (1981) Molecular analysis of the human interferon-α gene family. Gene 15:279–394
Bradley EC, Ruscetti FW (1981) Effect of fibroblast, lymphoid and myeloid interferons on human tumor colony formation in vitro. Cancer Res 41:244–249
Branca AA, Baglioni C (1981) Evidence that types I and II interferons have different receptors. Nature 294:768–770
Bray MA, Gordon D, Morley J (1974) Role of prostaglandins in reactions of cellular immunity. Br J Pharm 52:453P
Burke DC, Graham CF, Lehman JM (1978) Appearance of interferon inducibility and sensitivity during differentiation of murine teratocarcinoma cells in vitro. Cell 13:243–248
Carter WA, Horoszewicz JS (1980) Production, purification and clinical application of human fibroblast interferon. Pharmacol Ther 8:359–377
Carver DH, Seto DY, Migeon BR (1968) Interferon production and action in mouse, hamster and somatic hybrid mouse-hamster cells. Science 160:558–559
Cassingena R, Chany C, Vignal M, Suarez H, Estrade S, Lazar P (1971) Use of monkey-mouse hybrid cells for the study of the cellular regulation of interferon production and action. Proc Natl Acad Sci USA 68:580–584
Chandrabose KA, Cuatrecasas P, Pottathil R, Lang DJ (1981) Interferonresistant cell line lacks fatty acid cyclooxygenase activity. Science 212:329–331
Chany C (1976) Membrane-bound interferon specific cell receptor system: role in the establishment and amplification of the antiviral state. Biomedicine 24:148–157
Chany C, Fournier F, Rousset S (1971) Potentiation of the antiviral activity of interferon by actinomycin D. Nature New Biol 230:113–114
Chany C, Pauloin A, Chany-Fournier F (1977) Role of the membrane-bound receptor system in the biological activity of interferon. Tex Rep Biol Med 35:330–335
Chany C, Vignal M, Couillin P, Van Cong N, Boué J, Boué A (1975) Chromosomal localization of human genes governing the interferoninduced antiviral state. Proc Natl. Acad Sci USA 72:3129–3133
Chany C, Finaz C, Weil D, Vignal M, Van Cong N, de Grouchy J (1981) Investigations on the chromosomal localizations of the human and chimpanzee interferon genes: possible role of chromosomes 9 and 13. Ann Genet 23:201–207
Chirigos MA, Schultz RM, Stylos WA (1980) Interaction of interferon, macrophage and lymphocyte tumoricidal activity with prostaglandin effect. Ann NY Acad Sci 350:91–101
Colby C, Morgan MJ, Hulse JLN, Loza T (1975) Isolation and preliminary characterization of virus-resistant mouse embryo fibroblasts. In: Geraldes A (ed) Effect of interferon on cells, viruses and the immune system. Academic, New York, p 267
Cox DR, Epstein LB, Epstein CJ (1980) Genes coding for sensitivity to interferon (IfRec) and soluble superoxide dismutase (SOD-1) are linked in mouse and man and map to mouse chromosome 16. Proc Natl Acad Sci USA 77:2168–2172

Creasy AA, Bartholomew JC, Merigan TC (1980) Does human leukocyte interferon influence the restriction point control in cultured cells? Ann NY Acad Sci 350:207–208
Cuatresasas P, Hollenberg MD (1976) Membrane receptors and hormone action. Adv Prot Chem 30:250–450
Cupples CG, Tan YH (1977) Effect of human interferon preparations on lymphoblastogenesis in Down's syndrome. Nature 267:165–167
Czarniecki CW, Sreevalsan T, Friedman RM, Panet A (1981) Dissociation of interferon effects on murine leukemia virus and encephalomyocarditis virus replication in mouse cells. J Virol 37:827–831
Dandoy F, DeMaeyer E, DeMaeyer-Guignard J (1981) The antiproliferative action of interferon on murine bone-marrow derived macrophages is influenced by the genotype of the marrow-donor. Interferon Scientific Memoranda
Darlington GH, Bernhard HP, Ruddle FH (1974) Human serum albumin phenotype activation in mouse hepatoma human leukocyte cell hybrids. Science 185:859–862
De Clercq E, Edy VG, Cassiman JJ (1976) Chromosome 21 does not code for an interferon receptor. Nature 264:249–251
Degrave W, Derynck R, Tavernier J, Haegeman G, Fiers W (1981) Nucleotide sequence of the chromosomal gene for human fibroblast (β_1) interferon and of the flanking regions. Gene 14:137–143
DeMaeyer E, DeMaeyer-Guignard J (1979) Considerations on mouse genes influencing interferon production and action. Interferon 1:75–100
DeMaeyer E, DeMaeyer-Guignard J (1980a) Immunoregulatory action of type I interferon in the mouse. NY Acad Sci 350:1–11
DeMaeyer E, DeMaeyer-Guignard J (1980b) Host genotype influences immunomodulation by interferon. Nature 284:173–175
Derynck R, Content J, DeClercq E, Volckaert G, Tavernier J, Devos R, Fiers W (1980) Isolation and structure of a human fibroblast interferon gene. Nature 285:542–547
Desmyter J, Melnick JL, Rawls WE (1968) Defectiveness of interferon production and of rubella virus interference in a line of African green monkey kidney cells (Vero). J Virol 2:955–961
Dianzani F, Zucca M, Scupham A, Georgiades JA (1980) Immune and virusinduced interferons may activate cells by different derepressional mechanisms. Nature 283:400–402
Dianzani F, Monohan TM, Jordan CA, Langford MP (1981) Inhibition of RNA synthesis in human lymphoid cells induces interferon production. Proc Soc Exp Biol Med 167:338–342
Einhorn S, Blomgren H, Strander H (1978) Interferon and spontaneous cytotoxicity in man. Acta Med Scand 204:477–483
Epstein DA, Torrence PF, Friedman RM (1980) Double-stranded RNA inhibits a phosphoprotein phosphatase present in interferon-treated cells. Proc Natl Acad Sci USA 77:107–111
Epstein DA, Czarniecki CW, Jakobsen H, Friedman RM, Panet A (1981) A mouse cell line, which is unprotected by interferon against lytic virus infection, lacks ribonuclease F activity. Eur J Biochem 118:9–15
Epstein LB, Epstein CJ (1976) Localization of the gene AVG for the antiviral expression of immune and classical interferon to the distal portion of the long arm of chromosome 21. J Infect Dis 133 suppl:A56–A62
Epstein LB, Epstein CJ (1980) T-lymphocyte function and sensitivity to trisomy 21. Cell Immunol 51:303–318
Epstein LB, Lee SHS, Epstein CJ (1980a) Enhanced sensitivity of trisomy 21 monocytes to the maturation-inhibiting effect of interferon. Cell Immunol 50:191–194
Epstein LB, Shen JT, Abele JS, Reese CC (1980b) Further experience in testing the sensitivity of human ovarian carcinoma cells to interferon in an in vitro semisolid agar culture system: comparison of solid and ascitic forms of the tumor. Prog Clin Biol Res 48:277–290
Falcoff E, Wietzerbin J, Stefanos S, Lucerno M, Bellardon C, Catinot L, Besançon F, Ankel H (1980) Properties of mouse immune T-interferon (type II). Ann NY Acad Sci 350:145–156

Farrell PJ, Sen GC, Dubois MF, Ratner L, Slattery E, Lengyel P (1978) Interferon action: two distinct pathways for inhibition of protein synthesis by double-stranded RNA. Proc Natl Acad Sci USA 75:5893–5897
Fishman PH, Atikkan EE (1979) Induction of cholera toxin receptors in cultured cells by butyric acid. J Biol Chem 254:4342–4344
Fishman PH, Bradley RM, Henneberry RC (1976) Butyrate-induced glycolipid biosynthesis in HeLa cells: properties of the induced sialyltransferase. Arch Biochem Biophys 172:618–626
Fleischmann WJ Jr, Georgiades JA, Osborne LC, Johnson HM (1979a) Potentiation of interferon activity by mixed preparations of fibroblast and immune interferon. Infect Immun 26:248–253
Fleischmann WR Jr, Georgiades JA, Osborne LC, Dianzani F, Johnson HM (1979b) Induction of an inhibitor of interferon action in a mouse lymphokine preparation. Infect Immun 26:949–955
Fleischmann WR Jr, Kleyn KM, Baron S (1980) Potentiation of antitumour effect of virus-induced interferon by mouse immune interferon preparations. J Natl Cancer Inst 65:963–966
Fout GS, Simon EH (1981) Studies on an interferon-sensitive mutant of mengovirus: effects on host RNA and protein synthesis. J Gen Virol 52:391–394
Frankfort HM, Havell EA, Croce CM, Vilćek J (1978) The synthesis and actions of mouse and human interferons in mouse-human hybrid cells. Virology 89:45–52
Friedman RM (1967) Interferon binding: the first step in establishment of antiviral activity. Science 156:1760–1761
Friedman RM (1978) The mechanism of action of interferon: possible primary effects on membranes. Horiz Biochem Biophys 5:281–313
Friedman RM, Grollman EF, Chang EH, Kohn LD, Lee G, Jay FT (1977) Interferon and glycoprotein hormones. Tex Rep Biol Med 35:326–329
Gallien-Lartique O, Correz D, DeMaeyer E, DeMaeyer-Guignard J (1980) Strain dependence of the antiproliferative action of interferon on murine erythroid precursors. Science 209:292–293
Gardner LJ, Vilćek J (1979) Initial interaction of human fibroblast and leukocyte interferons with FS-4 fibroblasts. J Gen Virol 44:161–168
Goeddel DV, Leung DW, Dull TJ, Gross M, Lawn RM, McCandliss R, Seeburg PH, Ullrich A, Yelverton E, Gray P (1981) The structure of eight distinct cloned human leukocyte interferon cDNAs. Nature 290:20–25
Goodman LS, Gilman A (1980) The pharmacological basis of therapeutics. Macmillan, New York
Gordon I, Stevenson D (1980) Kinetics of decay in the expression of interferon-dependent mRNAs responsible for resistance to virus. Proc Natl Acad Sci USA 77:452–456
Gordon J, Minks MA (1981) The interferon renaissance: molecular aspects of induction and action. Microbiol Rev 45:244–266
Gray PW, Leung DW, Pennica D, Yelverton E, Najarian R, Simonsen C, Derynck R, Sherwood PJ, Wallace DM, Berger SL, Levinson AD, Goeddel DV (1982) Expression of human immune interferon cCNA in E. coli and monkey cells. Nature 293:503–508
Greene JJ, Dieffenbach CW, Yang LC, Ts'O POP (1980) Species-specific posttranscriptional regulation of interferon synthesis. Biochem 19:2485–2491
Gresser I, Bandu MT, Brouty-Boyé D (1974) Interferon and cell division IX. Interferon-resistant L_{1210}cells: characteristics and origin. J Natl Cancer Inst 52:553–559
Grollman EF, Lee G, Ramos S, Lazo PS, Kaback HR, Friedman RM, Kohn LD (1978) Relationships of the structure and function of the interferon receptor to hormanone receptors and establishment of the antiviral state. Cancer Res 38:4712–4185
Gross G, Mayr U, Bruns W, Grosveld F, Dahl HHM, Collins J (1981) The structure of a thirty-six kilobase region of the human chromosome including the fibroblast interferon gene IFN-β. Nucleic Acids Res 9:2495–2507
Grossberg SE, Smith AJ, Sedmak JJ (1975) Control of the interferon mechanism in hamster-mouse heterokaryons. In: Geraldes A (ed) Effects of interferon on cells, viruses and the immune system. Academic, New York, pp 33–43

Gupta SL, Rubin BY, Holmes SL (1981) Regulation of interferon action in human fibroblasts: transient induction of specific proteins and amplification of the antiviral response by actinomycin D. Virology 111:331–340

Gurari-Rotman D, Revel M, Tartakovsky B, Segal S, Hahn T, Handzel Z, Levin S (1978) Lymphoblastogenesis in Down's Syndrome and its inhibition by human interferon. FEBS Lett 94:187–190

Habeshaw JA (1979) Hypothesis: Non-Hodgkin lymphomas are abnormal immune responses. Cancer Immunol Immunother 7:37–42

Haller O, Arnheiter H, Horisberger MA, Gressor I, Lindenmann J (1980a) Interaction between interferon and host genes in the antiviral defense. Ann NY Acad Sci 350:558–565

Haller O, Arnheiter H, Lindenmann J, Gressor I (1980b) Host gene influences sensitivity to interferon action selectively for influenza virus. Nature 283:660–662

Haller O, Arnheiter H, Gressor I, Lindenmann J (1981) Virus-specific interferon action. Protection of newborn Mx carriers against lethal infection with influenza virus. J Exp Med 154:199–203

Harmon MW, Greenberg SB, Johnson PE (1980) Rapid onset of the interferon-induced antiviral state in human nasal epithelium and foreskin fibroblast cells. Proc Soc Exp Biol Med 164:146–152

Hauser H, Mayr U, Bruns W, Gross G, Lindemaier W, Collins J (1981) Studies on the regulation of the human interferon-β gene. Second annual international congress for interferon research, San Francisco

Havell EA, Vilćek J (1974) Production of high titred IFN in cultures of human diploid fibroblasts. Antimicrob Agents Chemother 2:47–53

Herberman RB, Ortaldo JR, Djeu, JY, Holden HT, Jett J, Lang NP, Rubinstein M, Pestka S (1980) Role of interferon in regulation of cytotoxicity by natural killer cells and macrophages. Ann NY Acad Sci 350:63–71

Heron I, Berg K (1978) The actions of interferon are potentiated at elevated temperature. Nature 274:508–510

Hilfenhaus J, Mauler R (1980) Human fibroblast and human leukocyte interferon: Their differences in cell growth inhibition activities on lymphoblastoid cells. Ann NY Acad Sci 350:626

Ho M, Tan YH, Armstrong JA (1972) Accentuation of production of human interferon by metabolic inhibitors. Proc Soc Exp Biol Med 193:295–299

Ho M, Armstrong JA, Ke YH, Tan YH (1973) Interferon production. US Patent Office 3773924

Ho M, White LT, Haverkos HW, Breining MC, Pazin GJ, Armstrong JA (1981) Depression of natural killer cell activity by interferon. J Infect Dis 144:605

Ho M, Pazin GJ, Wechsler H, White L, Breinig MK (to be published) Effect of interferon-α on multiple warts and NK cells, TNO converence, Rotterdam, April 1981. Elsevier, Amsterdam

Hoffman RA, Robinson PF, Magalhaes H (1968) The golden hamster. Its biology and use in medical research. Iowa State University Press, Ames, p 545

Holden HT, Djeu JY, Brunda MJ, Herberman RB (1980) In: DeWeck AL, Kristensen F, Landy M (eds) Biochemical characterization of lymphokines. Academic, New York

Hong SCL, Wheless CM, Levine L (1977) Elevated prostaglandin synthetase activity in methylcholanthrene-transformed mouse BALB/3T3. Prostaglandins 13:271–279

Horisberger MA, Haller O, Arnheiter H (1980) Interferon-dependent genetic resistance to influenza virus in mice: virus replication in macrophages is inhibited at an early step. J Gen Virol 50:205–210

Hou YT, Yang CT (1981) Translation of human fibroblast interferon mRNA in African fish ova. Methods Enzymol 79:72–76

Hou YT, Yang CT, Zhang AQ (to be published) Selection and characterization of virus-resistant L cell mutants with changed interferon gene expression. J Interferon Res

Houghton M, Jackson IJ, Porter AG, Doel SM, Catlin GH, Barber C, Carey NH (1981) The absence of introns within a human fibroblast interferon gene. Nucleic Acids Res 9:247–266

Hovanessian AG, Kerr IM (1979) The (2′–5′)oligoadenylate(pppA2′–5′A2′–5′A) synthetase and protein kinase(s) from interferon-treated cells. Eur J Biochem 93:515–526

Hovanessian AG, LaBonnardiere C, Falcoff E (1980) Action of murine γ (immune) interferon on β (fibroblast)-interferon-resistant L_{1210} and embryonal carcinoma cells. J Interferon Res:125–134

Hu YW, Xue GX, Haars R, Wong TK, Mark D, Colby C, Tan YH (1982) The processing of human interferon-β mRNA. In: Merigan TC, Friedman RM (eds) Molecular and cellular biology, UCLA somposia, vol 25. Academic, New York, pp 249–252

Huang RC, Tan YH (to be published) Transient effect on cellular RNA metabolism during interferon induction. 2nd international workshop on interferons, April 1979, New York. Rockefeller University Press, New York

Huddlestone JR, Merigan TC Jr, Oldstone MB (1979) Induction and kinetics of natural killer cells in humans following interferon therapy. Nature 282:417–419

Inglot AD, Oleszak E, Kisielow B (1980) Antagonism in action between mouse or human interferon and platelet growth factor. Arch Virol 63:291–296

Inoue M, Tan YH (1981) Radioimmunoassay for human beta interferon. Infect Immun 33:763–768

Inoue M, Tan YH (1982) Human interferon enhances cell killing by actinomycin D and cisplatinum. In: Proceedings of the 3rd congress on interferon research (Abstract)

Jarvis AP, Colby C (1978) Murine interferon system regulation: isolation and characterization of a mutant 3T6 cell engaged in the semiconstitutive synthesis of interferon. Cell 14:355–363

Kamarck ME, Slate DL, D'Eustachio P, Barel B, Ruddle FH (1981) Monoclonal antibodies to human cell surface components which block the response to human interferon. Fed Proc 40:1051

Kimchi A, Shulman L, Schmidt A, Chernajovsky Y, Fradin A, Revel M (1979) Kinetics of the induction of three translation-regulatory enzymes by interferon. Proc Natl Acad Sci USA 76:3208–3212

Kloppel TM, Keenan TW, Freeman, MJ, Morré DJ (1977) Glycolipid-bound sialic acid in serum: increased levels in mice and humans bearing mammary carcinomas. Proc Natl Acad Sci USA 74:3011–3013

Knight E Jr (1974) Interferon-Sepharose: induction of the anti-viral state. Biochem Biophys Res Comm 56:860–864

Knight E Jr, Hunkapillar MW, Korant BD, Hardy RWF, Hood LE (1980) Human fibroblast interferon: amino acid analysis and amino terminal amino acid sequence. Science 207:525–526

Kohn LC, Friedman RM, Holmes JM, Lee G (1976) Use of thyrotropin and cholera toxin to probe the mechanism by which interferon initiates its antiviral activity. Proc Natl Acad Sci USA 73:3695–3699

Krishnamurti C, Ankel H (1981) Inhibition of β-interferon augmentation of murine natural killer cytotoxicity by gangliosides 2nd annual international congress of interferon research, San Francisco

Kuwata T, Fuse A, Takayama N, Morinaga N (1980) Effects of concanavalin A on the antiviral and cell growth inhibitory action of human interferons. Ann NY Acad Sci 350:211–227

Lab M, Koehren F (1972) Potentiation of the antiviral action of interferon by cycloheximide. Ann Inst Pasteur 122:567–573

Lab M, Koehren F (1976) Maintenance and recovery of the interferoninduced antiviral state. Proc Soc Exp Biol Med 153:112–118

Lawn RM, Adelman J, Dull TJ, Gross M, Goeddel D, Ullrich A (1981 a) DNA sequence of two closely linked human leukocyte interferon genes. Science 212:1159–1162

Lawn RM, Gross M, Houck CM, Franke AE, Gray PV, Goeddel DV (1981 b) DNA sequence of a major human leukocyte interferon gene. Proc Natl Acad Sci USA 78:5435–5439

Lawn RM, Adelman J, Franke AE, Houck CM, Gross M, Najarian R, Goeddel DV (1981 c) Human fibroblast interferon gene lacks introns. Nucleic Acids Res 9:1045–1052

Lee SHS, Epstein LB (1980) Reversible inhibition by interferon of the maturation of human peripheral blood monocytes to macrophages. Cell Immunol 50:177–190

Levin MJ, Leary PL (1981) Inhibition of human herpes viruses by combinations of acyclovir and human leukocyte interferon. Infect Immun 32:995–999

Lin P-F, Slate DL, Lawyer F, Ruddle FH (1980) Assignment of the murine interferon sensitivity and cytoplasmic superoxide dismutase genes to chromosome 16. Science 209:285–287

Liu XY, Lou YC, Wang TP (1980) Biochem Comm Chinese Biochem Soc 5:66

Lubiniecki AS, Jones V, Eatherly C (1979) Cytogenetic analysis of the sensitivity to antiviral and anti-cell growth activities of human fibroblast interferon in aneuploid human tumor cell lines. Arch Virol 60:341–346

Lundgren E, Hillörn W, Holmberg D, Lenner P, Roos G, Strannegård Ö (1980) Comparative study on the effects of fibroblast and leukocyte interferon on short-term cultures of leukemic cells. Ann NY Acad Sci 350:628

Maroun LE (1978) Interferon-mediated effect on ribosomal RNA metabolism. Biochim Biophys Acta 517:109–114

Maroun LE (1979) Interferon effect on ribosomal ribonucleic acid related to chromosome 21 ploidy. Biochem J 179:221–225

Maroun LE (1980) Interferon action and chromosome 21 trisomy. J Theor Biol 86:603–606

Matheson DS, Green B, Tan YH (1981) The enhancement of B cell mitogenesis by human interferon is controlled by chromosome 21. Cell Immunol 65:366–372

Matheson DS, McPherson TA, Tan YH, Green B (1982) Alteration in immune response in patients receiving human fibroblast interferon. Fed Proc 41:406

McPherson TA, Tan YH (1980) Phase I pharmaco-toxicology study of human fibroblast interferon in human malignancy. J Natl Cancer Inst 65:75–79

Meager A, Graves HE, Walker JR, Burke DC, Swallow DM (1979) Involvement of a gene on chromosome 9 in human fibroblast interferon production. Nature 280:493–495

Minato N, Reid L, Neighbor A, Bloom VR, Holland J (1980) Interferon, NK cells and persistant virus infection. Ann NY Acad Sci 350:42–52

Minks MA, West DK, Benvin S, Baglioni C (1979) Structural requirements of double-stranded RNA for the activation of 2′5′-oligo(A)polymerase and protein kinase of interferon-treated HeLa cells. J Biol Chem 254:10180–10183

Minks MA, Benvin S, Baglioni C (1980) Mechanism of $pppA(2'p5'A)_n2'p5'A_{OH}$ synthesis in extracts of interferon-treated HeLA cells. J Biol Chem 255:5031–5035

Morgan MJ, Faik P (1977) The expression of the interferon system in clones of Chinese hamster/human hybrid cells. Br J Cancer 35:254

Morgan MJ, Colby C, Hulse JDN (1973) Isolation and characterization of virus-resistant mouse embryo fibroblasts. J Gen Virol 20:377–385

Nabholz M (1969) Studies on somatic cell hybridization as a tool for the genetic analysis of man. PhD thesis, Stanford University

Nagata S, Mantei N, Weissman C (1980) The structure of one of the eight or more distinct chromosomal genes for human interferon-α. Nature 287:401–408

Ng WS, Ng MH, Inoue M, Tan YH (1981) Kinetics of human immune interferon production and blastogenesis. Clin Exp Immunol 44:594–602

Nilson TW, Baglioni C (1979) Mechanism for discrimination between viral and host mRNA in interferon-treated cells. Proc Natl Acad Sci USA 76:2600–2604

Nilsen TW, Wood DL, Baglioni C (1980) Virus-specific effects of interferon in embryonal carcinoma cells. Nature 286:178–180

Nyari LJ, Tan YH, Erlich HA (1982) Monoclonal antibodies directed against Hu IFN-beta: characterization and functional studies. Hybridoma

Ohno S, Taniguchi T (1981) Structure of a chromosomal gene for human interferon. Proc Natl Acad Sci (USA) 78:5305–5309

Okamura H, Berthold W, Hood L, Hunkapillar M, Inoue M, Smith-Johannsen H, Tan YH (1980) Human fibroblastoid interferon: immunosorbent column chromatography and N-terminal amino acid sequence. Biochemistry 19:3831–3835

Owerbach D, Rutter WJ, Shows TB, Gray P, Goeddel DV, Lawn RM (1981) Leukocyte and fibroblast interferon genes are located on human chromosome 9. Proc Natl Acad Sci USA 78:3132–3127

Panet A, Czarniecki CW, Falk H, Friedman RM (1981) Effect of 2′5′-oligoadenylic acid on a mouse cell line partially resistant to interferon. Virology 114:567–572

Peries J, Alves-Cardoso E, Canivet M, Debons Guillemin MC, Lasneret J (1977) Lack of multiplication of ecotropic murine C-type virus in mouse teratocarcinoma primitive cells. J Natl Cancer Inst 59:463–465

Perussia B, Santoli D, Trinchieri (1980) Interferon modulation of natural killer cell activity. Ann NY Acad Sci 350:55–62

Pickering LA, Kronenberg LH, Stewart II WE (1980) Spontaneous production of human interferon. Proc Natl Acad Sci USA 77:5938–5942

Pottathil R, Chandrabose K, Cuatrecasas P, Lang DJ (1980) Establishment and maintenance of the interferon-induced antiviral state: role of fatty acid cyclooxygenase. Proc Natl Acad Sci USA 77:5437–5440

Pottathil R, Chandrabose KA, Cuatrecasa P, Lang DJ (1981) Establishment of the interferon-mediated antiviral state: Possible role of superoxide dismutase. Proc Natl Acad Sci USA 78:3343–3347

Radke KL, Colby C, Kates JR, Krider JM, Prescott DM (1974) Establishment and maintenance of the interferon-induced antiviral state: studies in enucleated cells. J Virol 13:623–645

Raj NB, Pitha P (1981) Analysis of interferon mRNA in human fibroblast cells induced to produce interferon. Proc Natl Acad Sci USA 78:7426–7430

Revel M (1979) Molecular mechanisms involved in the antiviral effects of interferon. Interferon 1:102–141

Revel M, Bash R, Ruddle FH (1976) Antibodies to a cell-surface component coded by human chromosome 21 inhibit action of interferon. Nature 260:139–141

Rich SA (1981) Human lupus inclusions and interferon. Science 213:772–775

Rubin BY, Gupta SL (1980) Interferon-induced proteins in human fibroblasts and development of the antiviral state. J Virol 34:446–454

Rubin BY, Gupta SL (1981) Differential efficacies of human type I and type II interferons as antiviral and anti-proliferative agents. Proc Natl Acad Sci USA 77:5928–5932

Samuel CE, Kingsman SM, Melamed RW, Farris DA, Smith MD, Miyamot NG, Lasky SR, Knutson GS (1980) Mechanisms of interferon-mediated inhibition of protein synthesis. Ann NY Acad Sci 350:473–485

Schmidt A, Chernajovsky Y, Shulman L, Federman, P, Berissi H, Revel M (1978) Interferon action: isolation of nuclease F, a translation inhibitor activated by interferon-induced (2′–5′)oligo-isoadenylate. FEBS Lett 95:257–264

Schmidt A, Chernajovsky Y, Shulman L, Federman P, Berissi H, Revel M (1979) An interferon-induced phosphodiesterase degrading (2′–5′oligoisoadenylate and the C-C-A terminus of tRNA. Proc Natl Acad Sci USA 76:4788–4792

Schultz RM (1980) E-type prostaglandins and interferons: ying-yang modulation of macrophage tumoricidal activity. Med Hypotheses 6:831–843

Schultz RM, Povlidis NA, Stylos WA, Chirigos MA (1978) Regulation of macrophage tumoricidal function: a role for prostaglandins of the E series. Science 202:320–321

Seaman WE, Merigan TC, Talal N (1979) Natural killing in estrogen-treated mice responds poorly to polyI·C despite normal stimulation of circulating interferon. J immunol 123:2903–2905

Sehgal PB (1981) Heterogeneity and regulation of expression of human β (fibroblast) interferon messenger RNA species. Antiviral Res 1:4

Sehgal PB, Sagar AD, Braude IA (1981) Further heterogeneity of human α interferon mRNA species. Science 214:803–805

Shulman L, Revel M (1980) Interferon-dependent induction of mRNA activity for (2′–5′)oligo-isoadenylate synthetase. Nature 288:98–100

Sikora K, Basham T, Dilley J, Levy R, Merigan T (1980) Inhibition of lymphoma hybrids by human interferon. Lancet 2:891–893

Skurkovich SV (1981) The possible participation of interferon inhibitor in the formation of the remission in autoimmune diseases and allergy (hypersensitivity of the immediate type). Med Hypotheses 7:1189–1191

Slate DL, Ruddle FH (1978) Antibodies to chromosome 21 coded cell surface components can block response to human interferon. Cytogenet Cell Genet 22:265–269

Slate DL, Ruddle FH (1979) Fibroblast interferon in man is coded by two loci on separate chromosomes. Cell 16:171–180

Slate DL, Shulman L, Lawrence JB, Revel M, Ruddle FH (1978) Presence of human chromosome 21 alone is sufficient for hybrid cell sensitivity to human interferon. J Virol 25:319–325

Slate DL, Ruddle FH, Tan YH (1981) Genetic control of the interferon system. Interferon 3:65–76

Smith-Johannsen H, McPherson A, Tan YH (1979) Genetics of the antitumour effect of interferon. 2nd international workshop on interferons, April 1979, New York, Rockefeller University Press, New York

Stanwick TL, Schinazi RF, Campbell DE, Nahmias AJ (1981) Combined antiviral effect of interferon and acyclovir on herpes simplex virus types 1 and 2. Antimicrob Agents Chemother 19:672–674

Stein S, Kenny C, Friesen H-J, Shively J, Del Valle U, Pestka S (1980) NH_2-terminal amino acid sequence of human fibroblast interferon. Proc Natl Acad Sci USA 77:5716–5719

Stewart II WE (ed) (1979) The interferon system. Springer, Berlin Heidelberg New York, p 421

Stitz, L, Schellekens H (1980) Influence of input multiplicity of infection of the antiviral activity of interferon. J Gen Virol 46:205–210

Tan YH (1975) Chromosome-21-dosage effect on inducibility of antiviral gene(s). Nature 253:280–282

Tan YH (1976) Chromosome 21 and the cell growth inhibitory effect of interferon preparations. Nature 260:141–143

Tan YH (1981) Induction and production of human interferon with a continous line of modified fibroblasts. Methods Enzymol 78:120–125

Tan YH, Berthold W (1977) A mechanism for the induction and regulation of human fibroblastoid interferon genetic expression. J Gen Virol 34:401–411

Tan YH, Greene AE (1976) Subregional localization of the gene(s) governing the human interferon induced antiviral state in man. J Gen Virol 32:153–155

Tan YH, Armstrong JA, Ke YH, Ho M (1970) Regulation of cellular interferon production: enhancement by antimetabolites. Proc Natl Acad Sci USA 67:464–471

Tan YH, Armstrong JA, Ho M (1971) Accentuation of interferon production by metabolic inhibitors and its dependence on protein synthesis. Virology 41:503–509

Tan YH, Tischfield, Ruddle FH (1973) The linkage of genes for the human interferon-induced antiviral protein and indophenoloxidase-B traits to chromosome G-21. J Exp Med 137:317–330

Tan YH, Creagan RP, Ruddle FH (1974a) The somatic cell genetics of human interferon: assignment of human interferon loci to chromosomes 2 and 5. Proc Natl Acad Sci USA 71:2251–2255

Tan YH, Schneider EL, Tischfield J, Epstein CJ, Ruddle FH (1974b) Human chromosome 21 dosage: effect on the expression of the interferon induced antiviral state. Science 186:61–63

Tan YH, Chou EL, Lundh N (1975) Regulation of chromosome 21-directed anti-viral gene(s) as a consequence of age. Nature 251:310–312

Tan YH, Tan C, Berthold W (1977) Genetic control of the interferon system. Tex Rep Biol Med 35:63–68

Tavernier J, Derynck R, Fiers W (1981) Evidence for a unique human fibroblast interferon (IFN-β) chromosomal gene, devoid of intervening sequences. Nucleic Acids Res 9:461–471

Taylor-Papidimitriou J (1980) Effects of interferons on cell growth and function. Interferon 2:13–46

Taylor-Papadimitriou J, Stoker M (1971) Effect of interferon on some aspects of transformation by polyoma virus. Nature New Biol 230:114–117
Teich NM, Weiss RA, Martin GR, Lowy DR (1977) Virus infection of murine teratocarcinoma stem cell lines. Cell 12:973–982
Thorley-Lawson DA (1981) The transformation of adult but not newborn human lymphocytes by Epstein Barr virus and phytohaemagglutinin is inhibited by interferon: the early suppression by T cells of Epstein Barr infection is mediated by interferon. J Immunol 126:829–833
Trofatter KF Jr, Daniels DA (1980) Effect of prostaglandins and cyclic adenosine 3′,5′-monophosphate modulators on herpes simplex virus growth and interferon response in human cells. Infect Immun 27:158–167
Vandenbussche P, Divizia M, Verhaegen M, Fuse A, Kuwata T, DeClercq E, Content J (1981) Enzymatic activities induced by interferon in human fibroblast cell lines differing in their sensitivity to the anticellular activity of interferon. Virology 111:11–22
Vengris VE, Stollar BD, Pitha PM (1975) Interferon externalization by producing cell before induction of antiviral state. Virology 65:410–417
Vengris VE, Reynolds FH Jr, Hollenberg MD, Pitha P (1976) Interferon action: role of membrane gangliosides. Virology 72:486–493
Verhaegen M, Divizia M, Vandenbussche P, Kuwata T, Content J (1980) Abnormal behavior of interferon-induced enzymatic activities in an interferon-resistant cell line. Proc Natl Acad Sci USA 77:4479–4483
Vignaux F, Gressor I, Fridman WH (1980) Effect of virus-induced interferon on the antibody response of suckling and adult mice. Eur J Immunol 10:767–772
Vilćek J, Ng MH (1971) Post-transcriptional control of interferon synthesis. J Virol 7:588–594
Wallach D, Revel M (1980) An interferon-induced cellular enzyme is incorporated into virions. Nature 287:68–70
Weissenbach J, Chernajovsky Y, Zeevi M, Schulman L, Soreq H, Nir U, Wallach D, Perricaudet M, Tiollais P, Revel M (1980) Two interferon mRNAs in human fibroblasts: in vitro translation and E. coli cloning studies. Proc Natl Acad Sci USA 77:7152–7156
Williams BRG, Kerr IM (1978) Inhibition of protein synthesis by 2′–5′ linked adenine oligonucleotides in intact cells. Nature 276:88–90
Wiranowska-Stewart M, Stewart WE (1977) The role of human chromosome 21 in sensitivity to interferons. J Gen Virol 37:629–633
Wood JN, Hovanessian AG (1979) Interferon enhances 2–5A synthetase in embryonal carcinoma cells. Nature 282:74–76
Wu SH, Li Y, Hou YT (1979) Some factors affecting the superinduction of interferon in human diploid cell cultures. Acta Acad Med Sinicae 1:14–20
Ziegler HW, Kay NE, Zarling JM (1981) Deficiency of natural killer cell activity in patients with chronic lymphocytic leukemia. Int J Cancer 27:321–327

CHAPTER 7

Application of Recombinant DNA Technology to Expression of Human Interferon Genes

S. PANEM

A. Introduction

Interferon (IFN) has captured the imagination of the virologic community (and only more recently those concerned with cancer therapy), since its discovery in 1957. However, the lack of adequate quantities of high purity IFN has hampered basic research on the biology of IFN as well as the conduct of clinical trials to determine IFN's practical efficacy. Both problems – quantity and purity – have been addressed and solved by the application of recombinant DNA (rDNA) technology to IFN production. In addition to allowing the production of pure IFN in copious quantity, experimental use of cloned IFN genes has generated fundamental information which has radically altered our conception of IFN's physiologic role and has explained apparent contradictions within the literature.

In this chapter, I shall attempt to describe the experimental strategies devised to clone IFN-α and IFN-β and to direct their synthesis in bacteria. I will also illustrate the potential of using recombinant IFNs in elucidating the biology of the IFN phenomenon. The literature review upon which the bulk of this chapter is based was completed in May, 1981; Sect. B.III was added in February, 1983. By the time of publication, additional recombinant IFNs will have been developed which supersede those described here. This chapter can therefore be viewed only as an interim report and as an indication of the power of genetic engineering in solving traditional biologic problems and raising new questions.

B. General Comments on the Experimental Strategies for Cloning IFNs

With minor modifications, two strategies have been successfully employed for cloning the IFN-α and IFN-β (Tables 1 and 2) and are currently being used to clone IFN-γ genes. The general strategy used for IFN-α and IFN-β cloning can be summarized as six sequentail steps as follows. Detailed citations are given in the tables and the sections on specific comments on cloning strategies.

1. Induction of IFN: human cells in vitro were superinduced to produce IFN. The particular cells and inducer were chosen to select for either IFN-α or IFN-β production.

2. Selection of IFN mRNA: polyadenylated messenger RNA [poly(A) mRNA] was isolated from IFN-producing cells and size-fractionated on sucrose velocity gradients. A population of mRNA enriched in IFN mRNA was chosen by functional criteria. Each size fraction was tested for its ability to direct synthesis of IFN

activity in a *Xenopus laevis* oocyte translation assay. The test for IFN in this assay is to demonstrate IFN activity in an oocyte extract by standard plaque reduction bioassay.

3. Preparation of IFN cDNA and plasmid construction: double-stranded complementary DNA (cDNA) was prepared to RNA in IFN mRNA-enriched fractions using avian myeloblastosis virus reverse transcriptase. The primer for the reverse transcriptase was either nonselective [oligo(dt)] and therefore mediated copies of any mRNA, or selective (a synthetic primer designed from knowledge of an IFM amino acid sequence), and therefore mediated only copies of IFN mRNAs. Double-stranded cDNA (or in some cases DNA:RNA hybrids) were then elongated using terminal transferase to allow insertion into the *Pst* I restriction endonuclease site of the plasmid vector pBR322. The resulting plasmid DNA population was then used to transform bacteria.

4. Selection of cDNA clones with IFN inserts: the most difficult part of IFN cloning was the selection of clones carrying IFN-specific sequences. Following primary selection of transformants based on antibiotic sensitivities, several approaches were employed to distinguish plasmids with inserted IFN sequences from those with inserts which were specific for non-IFN mRNAs which had copurified with IFN mRNA.

a) In situ filter hybridizations of plasmid-containing bacteria were performed with isotopically labeled cDNA made to size-selected mRNA from IFN-producing and uninduced cells. This allowed selection of clones which carry copies of mRNAs augmented or found only in IFN-producing cells.
b) In situ filter hybridization of DNA from plasmid-containing bacteria was performed using isotopically labeled cDNA prepared to IFN-producing cell mRNA made with synthetic primers. The primers were designed using knowledge of NH_2 terminal amino acids of purified IFN. Such primers allow synthesis of only a select fraction of mRNA and therefore mediate selection of colonies with inserts which share sequence homology with IFN.
c) Colonies were screened for IFN inserts by using preparations of the cloned DNAs in hybridization arrest studies. Plasmid DNA was prepared from pools of 12–100 colonies and then hybridized to mRNA which had previously been shown to direct IFN synthesis in *X. laevis* oocytes. If the plasmid pool contained an IFN insert, then IFN mRNA entered into a hybrid. When used in oocyte translation assays, the RNA which did not enter into hybrids did not direct IFN synthesis, whereas RNA recovered from hybrids did. Once a pool of plasmids was shown to contain an IFN insert, plasmids were individually examined to identify IFN clones. The final test that a clone contained an IFN gene was therefore its ability to select by hybridization, translatable IFN mRNA from hetergeneous RNA populations.

5. Selection of genomic IFN clones: cDNA clones represent copies of functional mRNA. As the mRNA of many genes undergoes processing, noncoding portions of the gene (control sequences, introns) will not occur in cDNA clones. Furthermore, the reverse transcriptase reaction used to make cDNA may be inaccurate and the sequence of cDNA clones may therefore deviate from the authentic sequence. It is therefore desirable to clone the genomic IFN sequences. A different approach from that used for cDNA cloning was employed to isolate genomic IFN

sequences following the acquisition of cDNA clones. Inserted DNA representing partial or complete IFN genes was excised from IFN cDNA plasmids, isotopically labeled, and used in situ in filter hybridization assays with bacteria infected with phage λ carrying random pieces of human DNA, i.e., a phage λ library. This procedure allowed isolation of genomic sequences on the basis of cross-hybridization with IFN cDNA. Cloned genomic DNAs, selected by this method, were then utilized in hybridization arrest studies to confirm their IFN nature.

6. Selection of colonies containing complete IFN sequences: the procedures described assured selection of cDNA or genomic clones which cross-hybridize with IFN mRNA as determined by hybridization arrest experiments. Plasmids carrying sequences of a portion of an IFN gene or a pseudointerferon gene would be as effectively chosen by these procedures as clones of complete coding sequences. The ultimate test that a colony contained a functional IFN gene sequence would be its direction of mRNA synthesis which in turn directs IFN protein synthesis. In several cases, the primary cDNA clones and genomic clones directed IFN synthesis in bacteria without manipulation.

It is of interest to note that the general cloning strategy was first to prepare cDNAs of IFN mRNAs and examine them for IFN coding potential, as opposed to using cDNA to screen genomic libraries directly. This approach was chosen to avoid problems which occur with genes which contain introns. Introns are sequences located within genomic structural genes which do not code for amino acids found in the mature proteins. In retrospect, this caution was not needed, as no currently known IFN-α and IFN-β_1 contain introns. The cloning strategies also presumed that IFN heterogeneity was due to differential glycosylation and therefore predicted that a single IFN-α mRNA and a single IFN-β mRNA would be found. Knowing about the multiplicity of IFN-α (rapidly discovered as a result of cloning studies) has altered the cloning strategies for IFN-γ. A great deal of effort has been directed to determine the heterogeneity or homogeneity of IFN-γ and its mRNA (or mRNAs) prior to IFN-γ mRNA isolation and cloning.

I. Specific Comments on Cloning IFN-β

Historically, the cDNA cloning of IFN-β_1 by Taniguchi et al. (1979), was the first successful cloning of any IFN gene. The first IFN-β_1 clone represented only a portion of the IFN-β gene and therefore did not direct IFN-β synthesis. Yet it was active in hybridization arrest studies (Taniguchi et al. 1979), and was used to select full length cDNA clones (Taniguchi et al. 1980a, b). Tenfold more IFN-β_1 clones were identified when the partial IFN-β_1 insert from the first cloning attempt was used to screen a library of cDNA clones as compared with using labeled cDNA preparations for screening. The general approach used by Taniguchi et al. (1979) war also successfully employed by several other groups (Table 1). Table 1 lists the cloning strategies for IFN-β. The highest rate of IFN-β_1 clone selection from a cDNA library was achieved by Goeddel et al. (1980a), using an IFN-β_1 cDNA clone for the screening probe. As in Taniguchi's experience, using a specific IFN-β probe increased identification of IFN clones tenfold (Goeddel et al. 1980a). It can be estimated that 1%–8% of 12 S mRNA in IFN-β-producing cells is IFN-β_1 specific, as judged from the frequencies reported for IFN-β_1 cloning in the references noted in Table 1.

Table 1. Strategies for the isolation of human fibroblast interferon (IFN-β) by rDNA techniques

Plasmid name	Source of IFN mRNA	Selection of mRNA to clone	Method of selection of IFN-β clones
TpIF319	DIP2 human fibroblasts, 12 *S* poly(A) mRNA from poly(I) · poly(C)-induced cells	*Xenopus* oocyte translation and IFN bioassay	cDNA to mRNA from induced and uninduced cells
TpIF319-13	DIP2 human fibroblasts, 12 *S* poly(A) mRNA from poly(I) · poly(C)-induced cells	*Xenopus* oocyte translation and IFN bioassay	TpIF319 nick-translated DNA
pHFIF (1 – 21)	VGS human fibroblasts, 12 *S* poly(A) mRNA from poly(I) · poly(C)-induced cells	*Xenopus* oocyte translation and IFN bioassay	Plasmid DNA selection of induced cell mRNA which is active in *Xenopus* oocyte translation, e.g., hybridization arrest
pFIF-526	GM-2504A human fibroblasts, 12 *S* poly(A) mRNA from cells, superinduced with poly(I) · poly(C)	*Xenopus* oocyte translation and IFN bioassay – cDNA prepared using synthetic primer	cDNA to 12 *S* mRNA using 16 synthetic primers cycled against uninduced cell mRNA
pFIF-313	GM-2504A human fibroblasts, 12 *S* poly(A) mRNA from cells superinduced with poly(I) · poly(C)	*Xenopus* oocyte translation and IFN bioassay – cDNA prepared using synthetic primer	Selected with pFIF-526 DNA
A341	FS-11 human fibroblasts 14 *S* poly(A) mRNA	*Xenopus* oocyte translation and IFN bioassay – cDNA prepared using synthetic primer	cDNA to 14 *S* mRNA from induced and uninduced cells
I-6-5 and 4E1	FS-11 and FS-4 human fibroblasts, 11 *S* poly(A) mRNA from induced cells	*Xenopus* oocyte translation and IFN bioassay – cDNA prepared using synthetic primer	cDNA to 11 *S* mRNA from FS-11 induced cells using synthetic primer
C15	Charon 4A phage λ library of ECoRI restricted DNA from human peripheral blood leukocytes		Plasmid DNA of I-6-5 and 4E1 nick-translated probes

Two populations of mRNA 11 *S* and 14 *S*, from FS-11 and FS-4 human fibroblasts were reported by WEISSENBACH et al. (1980), to be active in *Xenopus* translation assays for IFN-β. Other workers have reported detecting at least two size classes of IFN mRNA in human fibroblasts (SEHGAL and SAGAR 1980). IFN-β_2, as described by MORY et al. (1981), differs from IFN-β_1 in that: (1) it does not cross-hybridize with IFN-β_1; (2) it does not direct translation of an IFN-like protein which can be specifically neutralized by IFN-β_1 or IFN-α sera; and (3) genomic IFN-β_2 clones contain introns which IFN-β_1 does not. Whether IFN-β_2 represents

IFN-β-transformants	IFN-β-specific transformants (%)	Comment	Reference
1/3600	0.027	Not a full length coding sequence	TANIGUCHI et al. (1979)
15/4000	0.37	Full length coding sequence	TANIGUCHI et al. (1980b)
21/1700	1.23	Only pHFIF-21 is both a full length coding sequence and free of sequence inversion	DERNYCK et al. (1980a)
1/600	0.16	16 Synthetic primers representing all possible combinations for the first 4 NH_2 terminal amino acids were employed	GOEDDEL et al. (1980a)
16/200	8.0	16 Synthetic primers representing all possible combinations for the first 4 NH_2 terminal amino acids were employed	GOEDDEL et al. (1980a)
25/3000	0.83	14 *S* mRNA is a minor species coding for IFN-β_2; 11 *S* mRNA for IFN-β_1	WEISSENBACH et al (1980)
14/3500	0.40	DNA:RNA hybrids from reverse transcription reaction were used for cloning	WEISSENBACH et al (1980)
		IFN-β_1 has no introns; IFN-β_1 and IFN-β_2 do not significantly hybridize with each other	MORY et al. (1981)

a second type of virally induced fibroblast IFN or a pseudogene remains to be determined.

II. Specific Comments on Cloning IFN-α

The same general strategies used to clone IFN-β have been applied to the isolation of IFN-α genes. The first publication of successful IFN-α cloning was by NAGATA et al. (1980a), whose IFN-α cDNA clone spontaneously produced active IFN-α_1. When this cloned IFN-α cDNA was used to screen a cDNA library made to 12 *S*

Table 2. Strategies for isolating human leukocyte interferon (IFN-α) genes by rDNA techniques

Plasmid name (IFN-α gene)	Source of mRNA for cDNA preparation or DNA library	Selection procedure for mRNA	Selection of IFN-α clones
Hif-2H ($IFN-\alpha_1$)	12 *S* poly(A) mRNA from pooled human peripheral leukocytes induced to produce IFN with Sendai virus	*Xenopus* oocyte translation	Plasmid DNA selection of IFN mRNA from poly(A) RNA is active in *Xenopus* oocytes
Hif-SN206 ($IFN-\alpha_2$)	12 *S* poly(A) mRNA from pooled human peripheral leukocytes induced to produce IFN with Sendai virus	*Xenopus* oocyte translation	Screen cDNA clone library from line 1 with Hif-4/cDNA, a plasmid isolated in parallel with Hif-2H
pL1 → pL30	12 *S* poly(A) mRNA from human KG-1 cells induced with Sendai virus	*Xenopus* oocyte translation	Spot hybridization of plasmid DNA preparations of 500 nutritionally selected transformants – screen with cDNA to induced cell 12 *S* mRNA or to cell mRNA using synthetic templates or packed cDNA clone (p1FL104)
pL31 → pL39	12 *S* poly(A) mRNA from human KG-1 cells induced with Sendai virus	*Xenopus* oocyte translation	
chr1, 3, 10, 12 13, 16, 23, 26, 30, 35	Hae III and Alu I library of human chromosomal DNA inserted into λ charon 4A with ECoRI linkers		^{32}P-labeled $IFN-\alpha_1$ (Hif-2HO to screen phage by in situ hybridization)

mRNA from Sendai virus-induced leukocytes, 3.7% of 5,000 colonies was found to be IFN-α specific. Restriction endonuclease mapping of several full length IFN-α cDNA clones rapidly indicated that the IFN-α comprise a multigene family with 10%–30% sequence diversity (STREULI et al. 1980). The multigene nature of IFN-α was confirmed in parallel cDNA cloning experiments in other laboratories (GOEDDEL et al. 1980b), and by direct examination of genomic DNA (GOEDDEL et al. 1981; NAGATA et al. 1980b; see Sect. D.I). The multigene nature of IFN-α explains the increased frequency of successful cloning attempts of IFN-α when compared with the parallel methodology used for $IFN-\beta_1$ (Tables 1 and 2).

Two groups have defined at least ten distinct IFN-α genes in human genomic DNA (GOEDDEL et al. 1981; NAGATA et al. 1980b). In addition, several pseudogenes have been described (WEISSMANN 1981). The IFN-α gene named $IFN-\alpha_3$ by

IFN-α plasmids plasmids screened	IFN-α plasmids (%)	Comment	Reference
			NAGATA et al. (1980a)
185/5000	3.7	1. IFN-α_1 and -α_2 have different species specificity in vitro; 2. IFN-α_1 and -α_2 differ 20% based on cDNA sequence analysis and 17% amino acid divergence	STREULI et al. (1980)
30/500	6	1. cDNA product sized on agarose gel before addition of poly(G) and poly(C) residues (GC tailing) to the cDNA termini which facilitates the generation of a restriction site for insertion into pBR322 2. Four synthetic templates designed from IFN-α tryptic peptide data used to make cDNA for screening	GOEDDEL et al. (1980b)
9/400	2.25	1. pL31 chain for length (1000 base pairs) strong reaction in synthetic template spot hybridization and reaction with a partial IFN-α cDNA clone; 2. Using pL31 detect 10 IFN-α genes in genomic DNA; 3. Sequences of cDNA clones	GOEDDEL et al. (1981)
16/240,000	0.116	1. chr 35 corresponds to IFN-α_1; 2. at least 8, but as many as 15 distinct IFN-α in genomic human DNA	NAGATA et al. (1980b)

WEISSMANN'S group, the LeIF F of GOEDDEL'S group and the lymphoblastoid IFN from Namalwa cells whose NH_2 terminal amino acid sequence has been reported (ZOON et al. 1980), appear to be the same gene. A common nomenclature for IFN-α isolated by different laboratories has not yet been codified.

III. Cloning IFN-γ

The successful cloning of IFN-γ was accomplished using cDNA (DEVOS et al. 1982). Facilitating these experiments were protocols for the enhanced production of IFN-γ and the subsequent isolation of IFN-γ-enriched mRNA as a 16 *S* peak of RNA in sucrose velocity gradients (TANIGUCHI et al. 1981). Based on Southern blot hybridization analysis, there is only one chromosomal human IFN-γ (GRAY et al. 1982). Unlike the IFN-α and IFN-β genes which do not contain introns, IFN-γ is split into four coding regions (exons) which are separated by three untranslated, but transcribed, introns (GRAY and GOEDDEL 1982). The gene for IFN-γ has been expressed in *Escherichia coli*, monkey cells and in yeast.

C. Comments on Strategies for IFN Production in rDNA Hosts

Utilization of DNA technology to produce pure IFN in quantity requires solution of two problems. First, the isolation of IFN structural genes and second, the translation of IFN mRNA in rDNA hosts. Solutions to the first problem have been described in Sect. B. The approach for solving the second is the same as for achieving elevated production of any cloned eukaryotic gene in bacteria and/or yeast. For a detailed discussion of protein production of eukaryotic genes in recombinant vectors, the reader is referred to definitive sources on methodology, with the caveat that the technology is continually evolving. The following discussion illustrates several approaches which have recently resulted in greatly increased yields of pure IFN in bacteria. Although there has been speculation of IFN production in yeast, to date no accounts have been published and therefore the following remarks are remarks are restricted to bacterial systems.

When a recombinant IFN clone contains one or more promoters and initiation codons which can be utilized by bacterial RNA polymerase and ribosomes, and when the clone contains the complete coding sequence for an IFN polypeptide, IFN should be synthesized within the bacteria. Several, but not all of the original cDNA clones spontaneously made IFN owing to fortuitous cloning of complete coding sequences (NAGATA et al. 1980a). However, these spontaneous producers synthesized IFN at levels less than can be achieved by induction of IFN in human cells in vitro. To achieve augmented IFN production, the clones were modified via "recombinant constructions." Table 3 illustrates several successful strategies for achieving IFN expression plasmids, which are described, as follows.

1. Placing IFN structural genes, under strong prokaryotic promotors: expression of cloned genes requires a configuration of regulatory sequences (promotor, initiation codon, distance between promotor, and initiation coding) which can be maximized for efficient transcription. A commonly used strategy is to place a eukaryotic sequence adjacent to strong prokaryotic control sequences. This strategy was employed for, generating the IFN-β_1 expression plasmids (entries 1–7) and for IFN-α (entries 9–12) shown in Table 3. The promotors employed were those from the *Escherichia coli* "lac" operon, the "tryp" operon or the phage lambda P_L promotor. An example of how the final IFN concentration can be manipulated by the choice of promotor is shown in the case were IFN-β_1 was placed next to three tandem-linked tryp promotors (GOEDDEL et al. 1980a). When the final levels of IFN-β_1 were measured, plasmids containing the tandem-linked promotors produced an order of magnitude more IFN-β_1 than plasmids placed next to the *E. coli* lac promotor. Table 3 shows the levels of IFN for each construction as reported in the appropriate reference. Because of nonuniformity in the manner of reporting IFN activity, it is almost impossible to compare the results of different groups directly. However, an increase of not less than 8–10 log IFN production has been

Table 3. Expression plasmids for IFN-α and IFN-β

Plasmid	Translation product in *Escherichia coli*	Product molecular mass (daltons)	Promotor	Activity[a]	Reference
IFN-β plasmids					
1. pLG104R	Pre-IFN-β_1	23,000	*E. coli* lac	Inactive	Taniguchi et al. (1979, 1980a)
2. pLG117R	Mature	20,000	*E. coli* lac	50 per Molecules per bacterium	Taniguchi et al. (1980a)
3. pPla-HFIF-67-12△	Mature IFN-β_1; and IFN-β_1 fused with β-lactamase	15,000–18,000 28,000	Phage lambda P_L	100 U per 5×10^8 cells per ml	Dernyck et al. (1980b)
4. pPlc-HFIF-6-8	Mature IFN-β_1; and mature IFN-β_1 fused with	15,000–18,000 33,000	Phage lambda P_L	100 U per 5×10^8 cells per ml	Dernyck et al. (1980b)
5. pFIF-lac9	Mature IFN-β_1[b]	N.D.	*E. coli* lac	9×10^6 U/l	Goeddel et al. (1980a, b)
6. pFIF-tryp^{3}69	Mature IFN-β_1[b]	N.D.	3 *E. coli* tryp in tandem	8.1×10^7 U/l	Goeddel et al. (1980a, b)
7. CI 5	IFN-β_1	N.D.	Phage lambda p_L or human	7×10^6 U/l	Mory et al. (1981)
IFN-α plasmids					
8. Hif-2H	IFN-α_1		Human IFN-α		Nagata et al. (1980a)
9. Hif-SN206 (IFN-α_2)	IFN-α_1 and/or pre-IFN-α_2	N.D.	Human IFN-α	3–5 $\times10^3$ U per gram wet cells	Streuli et al. (1980)
10. Hif-5N35-AH-L6 (IFN-α_1)	IFN-α_1 and/or Pre-IFN-α_1	17,000–18,000	lac UV5	4.2×10^3 U per milligram protein after partial purification	Masucci et al. (1980)
11. Hif-5N35-AH-L6 (IFN-α_1)	IFN-α_2			1.2×10^4 U per 4×10^8 mini cells	Stewart et al. (1980)
12. pLeIFA25	Mature IFN-αA	20,000	*E. coli* tryp	2.5×10^8 U/l; active in vivo, EMC infection of squirrel monkeys	Goeddel et al. (1980a, b)

[a] Bioactivity of bacterial extracts as measured by inhibition of virus-induced cytopathology in parallel with NIH IFN standards
[b] Translation product identified as mature IFN-α or IFN-β by sequence analysis, reaction with antibody, pH stability, and bioactivity
[c] N.D. not determined

conservatively achieved by a combination of construction and choice of bacterial hosts, when compared with IFN levels in bacteria carrying cDNA plasmids which contain their natural human control sequences and spontaneously produced IFN.

2. Generating fused proteins: a second strategy is to insert an IFN structural gene into a plasmid within the coding sequence for a bacterial protein which is very efficiently synthesized (BACKMAN et al. 1976). This results in synthesis of a "fused" or hybrid protein containing part of a bacterial protein and all of an IFN protein. While this approach avoids problems of choosing transcription and translation control sequences, the final product needs to be processed to eliminate the bacterial component because fused proteins may have altered bioactivities and may be pyogenic. Table 3 shows generation of IFN-β_1 fused to either β-lactamase or MS2 polymerase (entries 2 and 3). IFN-α_1 or -α_2 have also been made as fused proteins (STREULI et al. 1981).

3. Use of bacteria which predominantly produce plasmid proteins: certain bacterial strains preferentially transcribe and translate plasmid gene products (MERTENS and REEVE 1977). Such strains are useful because the quantity of the desired cloned protein in the bacterial protein population is elevated and therefore facilitates purification. Use of bacterial strains with low protease activity is also useful.

4. Activity of the product: IFN, like many secretory proteins, is synthesized in human cells as a precursor protein which requires proteolytic cleavage and in some cases glycosylation, before achieving its mature form (STEWART 1979). It is therefore necessary to ask whether the bacterial product represents a mature or intermediate IFN and whether the product is active. To date, both pre-IFN and IFN synthesized in bacteria are active in vitro challenge assay, even though they are not glycosylated (Table 3). While it is now known that not all natural IFNs are glycosylated (ALLEN and FANTES 1980), some are, and it therefore remains to be determined how essential glycosylation is for specific IFN activity in vivo.

At the time of writing this chapter, production of bacterial IFN was sufficient to allow crystallization of IFN-α. However, the optimum constructions for high production are not public knowledge.

D. Examples of Findings Directly Derived from Cloning Experiments

I. Multigene Families

Several provocative early results of cloning studies were that the IFN-α represent a multigene family of at least ten members (GOEDDEL et al. 1981; NAGATA et al. 1981), that the IFN-β are more restricted with perhaps only two members (MORY et al. 1981; SEHGAL and SAGAR 1980), and that IFN-α and IFN-β_1 share a common genetic pedigree (TANIGUCHI et al. 1980c). These conclusions follow directly from hybridization studies where single IFN-α cDNA probes were used to detect cross-hybridizing genomic sequences and by comparison of nucleotide sequences of individual IFN-α and IFN-β_1. The details and implication of these experiments are discussed elsewhere in this volume. The demonstration that IFN-α are a family of proteins encoded by genes with both constant and variable regions explains the physical heterogeneity of IFN preparations which showed conservation of NH_2

terminal amino acids (ZOON et al. 1980). Originally attributed to differential glycosylation (STEWART 1979), IFN-α heterogeneity is now clearly interpreted as due to the presence of multiple IFN-α genes.

II. Chromosomal Clustering of IFN-α and IFN-β

Cross-species somatic cell hybrids or aneuploid human cells have previously been employed to study the chromosomal location of genes required for IFN expression (TAN 1980; SLATE and RUDDLE 1979). In general, karyotypically defined cells were examined for qualitative and quantitative responses to IFN treatment and IFN inducers. Studies have reported that the presence of human chromosomes 2, 5, 9, and 21 are obligatory for the interferon response (TAN et al. 1974; SLATE and RUDDLE 1979; MEAGER et al. 1979a, b; STEWART 1979). These experiments do not allow the assignment to individual chromosomes of the different genes involved in the IFN response, e.g., IFN structural genes, IFN cell surface receptors, structural genes for IFN-induced enzymes. The chromosomal location of IFN-α and IFN-β_1 have recently been resolved by employing cloned probes in Southern blot hybridization experiments with DNAs isolated from somatic cell hybrids (OWERBACH et al. 1981).

High molecular weight DNA was isolated from human virgule mouse hybrids with known karyology and digested with the restriction endonuclease, ECoRI. Following agarose electrophoresis of digests and their transfer to nitrocellulose filters, replicate blots were hybridized to nick-translated inserts from a IFN-β_1 clone, pFiF3 (GOEDDEL et al. 1980a), and two IFN-α clones, pleIF-A and pleIF-D (GOEDDEL et al. 1980a, 1981). IFN-α and IFN-β_1 probes reacted only with DNA from hybrid cells which contained human chromosome 9 marker enzymes, adenylate kinase-1 and aconitase-1. The correlation of chromosome 9 with IFN-α and IFN-β_1 sequences occurred even in hybrids carrying a 9/X translocation. Furthermore, the number of bands detected in enzyme-restricted DNA indicated that IFN-β_1 and at least eight of the IFN-α are present in cells where chromosome 9 is the only human chromosome. Therefore, these data demonstrate that the majority, if not all IFN-α and IFN-β_1 are located on chromosome 9. The linkage relationship of the individual IFN-α and IFN-β_1 have not yet been reported. As these genes do not contain introns, their genetic fine map will be of great interest, especially as it relates to speculations on the origin of multigene families.

III. Absence of Introns in IFN-α and IFN-β_1

To date, the majority of eukaryotic genes which have been examined in detail are not encoded in genomic DNA as uninterrupted, contiguous sequences, but contain introns, or sequences which do not code for amino acids found in mature proteins. An unexpected finding with each of the ten IFN-α and IFN-β_1 is that their genomic sequences do not contain introns (NAGATA et al. 1980b; MORY et al. 1981; STREULI et al. 1981; HOUGHTON et al. 1981; TAVERNIER et al., to be published; T. TANIGUCHI 1981, personal communication). Using labeled IFN-α_1 from a cDNA clone, NAGATA et al. (1980b), selected IFN-α containing genomic DNA sequences from a human library. A detailed comparison of the restriction map of one of these genomic fragments with that of IFN-α_1 cDNA showed colinearity of the maps, thereby indicating that a genomic IFN-α did not contain introns. This observation is consistent with the restriction maps and sequence data available for each of the ten IFN-α (HOUGHTON 1980 a, b).

Similar findings are reported for IFN-β_1 (MORY et al. 1981). Nicktranslated inserts of two IFN-β_1 cDNA clones were used to select genomic sequences by filter hybridization from a charon phage library of human DNA. A 17 kilobases fragment was selected which, on restriction, yielded a 1.84 kilobases fragment which hybridized to the IFN-β_1 cDNAs. After subcloning into pBR322, the 1.84 kilobases fragment revealed an identical restriction map to that of the IFN-β_1 cDNA clones. In addition, the genomic fragment directed IFN-β_1 synthesis in *E. coli*. Therefore, IFN-β_1 does not contain introns. This finding was independently confirmed by two other groups in similarly designed studies using independently isolated IFN-β_1 clones (TAVERNIER et al., to be published). Futhermore, direct nucleotide sequence analysis of an IFN-β_1 cDNA clone and the genomic IFN-β_1 sequence confirmed their colinearity (HOUGHTON 1980 a, b). IFN-γ differs from IFN-α and IFN-β in that it contains four exons separated by three introns (GRAY and GOEDDEL 1982).

IV. Species and Tissue Specificity of IFNs

One of the early IFN dogmas was that IFN was "species specific", e.g., chicken IFN was active only on chicken cells and human IFN was active only on human cells (STEWART 1979). This concept has been altered by studies of human IFN-α synthesized in bacteria which have a broad spectrum of IFN activity in in vitro challenge assays on cells of many species. In fact, some human IFN-α are more active on nonhuman cells than on human cells.

When activities of two different IFN-α made in bacteria were compared with a mixed natural IFN preparation on human, monkey, hamster, rabbit, and mouse cells, each displayed a distinctive spectrum of effectiveness (GOEDDEL et al. 1980 b). The mixed population was most active on monkey cells, threefold less active on human cells, and inactive on mouse cells. One cloned IFN-α showed highest activity on hamster cells and least activity (40-fold less) on rabbit cells; whereas a second cloned IFN-α had equal activity in human and monkey cells, but 50-fold less activity in hamster cells. Unique patterns for species effectiveness for cloned IFN-α has been a reproducible finding (STREULI et al. 1980; STEWART et al. 1980) and differences in titer of more than 70-fold for a single cloned IFN-α preparation on different human cell strains has also been reported (STREULI et al. 1981).

A fascinating observation is the report of differential inhibition of viruses in a single cell strain by cloned IFN-α preparations (GOEDDEL et al. 1981). pLE-preIFA2 was tenfold more active in inhibiting Sindbis virus-mediated cytopathology than vesicular stomatitis virus- (VSV)-mediated cytopathology in human WISH cells; whereas pLE-preIFB4 was tenfold more active in inhibiting VSV as compared with Sindbis virus in the same cells. These experiments demonstrate specific diversity of IFN-α bioactivity, the mechanisms for which have yet to be delineated.

In contrast to studies with cloned IFN-α, tests of recombinant IFN-β_1 activity in different cells report 5–3000-fold greater activity of IFN-β_1 activity in human cells as compared with monkey, rabbit, cattle, mouse, and cat cells (HOUGHTON et al. 1980a; MORY et al. 1980; DERNYCK et al. 1980b). However, these studies also showed that a single IFN-β_1 had variable protective activity on different human cells.

Differential titration of individual IFNs as a function of assay cell most probably reflects variable binding of IFN to cell receptors. Support of this interpretation comes from using chimeric IFNs generated by linking portions of two IFN-α together (STREULI et al. 1981). In virus challenge assays using human WISH and mouse L929 cells, IFN-α_1 was slightly more active on human than on mouse cells. Recombinant IFNs were generated which contained the COOH proximal half of IFN-α_1 and the NH_2 proximal half of IFN-α_2. The reciprocal hybrid IFN was also constructed, and when the activities of these hybrids were compared with the parental IFNs, it was found that: (1) the activity for mouse cells resides with the COOH proximal portion of IFN-α_1; and (2) the hybrids showed individual and distinctive patterns of effectiveness when tested on cells of different species. These data suggest that at least two domains, one in the COOH proximal half of the IFN-α molecule and one in the NH_2 proximal half of the molecule, determine binding for one or more IFN cell surface receptors. It is not unreasonable, in view of the known 10%–30% sequence divergence of IFN-α, to conceive of an extensive pattern of binding affinities of IFN-α for different cells, even if there is a restricted number of IFN receptor types. If IFN receptor types are numerous, the specific tissue binding patterns for IFNs may be very complex.

Experiments on the binding specificities of cloned IFN-α therefore replaces the previous concept of species specificity by one which focuses on the specific IFN binding site configuration on cells of different tissues regardless of species. As individual IFNs have differential effectiveness on a variety of human cells, the interesting questions now focus on understanding the physiologic importance of multiple IFNs, each with exquisite binding specificities and their tissue tropisms. The experiments with chimeric IFNs (STREULI et al. 1981) also indicate that genetic engineering can produce IFNs with new biologic potential and open the possibility for the generation of "superinterferons."

Acknowledgments. This chapter was supported by USPHS CA 19264-06. Mrs. JANE WEIL provided excellent assistance. I thank my colleagues in the interferon field for generously sharing their data prior to publication.

References

Allen G, Fantes KH (1980) A family of structural genes for human lymphoblastoid (leukocyte-type) interferon. Nature 287:408–411

Backman K, Ptashne M, Gilbert W (1976) Construction of plasmids carrying the cI gene of bacteriophage λ. Proc Natl Acad Sci USA 73:4174–4178

Dernyck R, Content J, DeClercq E, Volckaert G, Tavernier J, Devos R, Fiers W (1980a) Isolation and structure of a human fibroblast interferon gene. Nature 285:542–577

Dernyck R, Remaut E, Saman E, Stanssens P, DeClercq E, Content J, Fiers W (1980b) Expression of human fibroblast interferon gene in E. coli. Nature 287:193–197

Devos R et al. (1982) Molecular cloning of human immune interferon cDNA and its expression in eucaryotic cells. Nucleic Acids Res 10:2847–2501

Goeddel DV, Shepard HM, Yelverton E, Leung D, Crea R (1980a) Synthesis of human fibroblast interferon by E. coli. Nucleic Acids Res 8:4057–4074

Goeddel DV, Yelverton E, Ullrich A, Heymeker NL, Miozzari G, Holmes W, Seeburg TD, Dull T, May L, Stebbing N, Crea R, Maeda S, McCandliss R, Sloma A, Tabor JM, Gross M, Familletti P, Pestka S (1980b) Human leukocyte interferon produced by E. coli is biologically active. Nature 287:411–416

Goeddel DV, Leung D, Dull T, Gross M, Lawn R, McCandliss R, Seeburg P, Ullrich A, Yelverton E, Gray PW (1981) The structure of eight distinct cloned human leukocyte interferon cDNAs. Nature 290:20–26

Gray PW, Goeddel DV (1982) Structure of the human immune interferon gene. Nature 298:859–863

Gray PW et al. (1982) Expression of human immune interferon CDNA in E. coli and monkey cells. Nature 295:503–508

Houghton M (1980) Human interferon gene sequences. Nature 285:536–540

Houghton M, Eaton MAW, Stewart AG, Smith JC, Doel SM, Catlin GH, Lewis HM, Patel TP, Emtage JS, Carey NH, Porter AG (1980a) The complete amino acid sequence of human fibroblast interferon as deduced using synthetic oligodeoxyribonucleotide primers of reverse transcriptase. Nucleic Acids Res 8:2885–2894

Houghton M, Jackson IJ, Porter AG, Doel SN, Catlin GH, Barber C, Carey NH (1981) The absence of introns within a human fibroblast interferon gene. Nucleic Acids Res 9:247–265

Houghton M, Stewart AG, Dowl SM, Emtage JS, Eaton MAW, Smith JC, Patel TP, Lewis HM, Porter AG, Birch JR, Cartwright T, Carey NH (1980b) The aminoterminal sequence of human fibroblast interferon as deduced from reverse transcripts obtained using synthetic oligonucleotide primers. Nucleic Acids Res 8:1913–1931

Masucci MG, Szigeti R, Klein E, Klein G, Gruest J, Montagnier L, Taira H, Hall A, Nagata S, Weissmann C (1980) Effect of Interferon-αl from E. coli on some cell functions. Science 209:1431–1435

Meager A, Graves H, Burke DC, Swallow DM (1979a) Involvement of a gene on chromosome 9 in human fibroblast interferon production. Nature 280:493–494

Meager A, Graves HE, Walker JR, Burke DC, Swallow DM, Westerveld A (1979b) Somatic cell genetics of human interferon production in human-rodent cell hybrids. J Gen Virol 45:309–321

Mertens G, Reeve JB (1977) Synthesis of cell envelope components by anucleate cells (minicells) of Bacillus subtilis. J Bacteriol 129:1198–1207

Mory Y, Chernajovsky Y, Feinstein SI, Chen L, Nir U, Weissenbach J, Tiollais P, Marks D, Ladner M, Colby C, Revel M (1981). Synthesis of human interferon-β_1 in E. coli infected by a lambda phage recombinant containing a human genomic fragment. Eur J Biochem 120:197–202

Nagata S, Taira H, Hall A, Johnsrud L, Streuli M, Ecsodi J, Boll W, Cantell K, Weissmann C (1980a) Synthesis in E. coli of a polypeptide with human leukocyte interferon activity. Nature 284:316–319

Nagata S, Mantei N, Weissmann C (1980b) The structure of one of the eight or more distinct chromosomal genes for human interferon-α. Nature 287:401–408

Nagata S, Brack C, Henco K, Schambock A, Weissmann C (1981) J Interferon Res 1: 333–336

Overbach D, Hutter WJ, Shows TB, Gray P, Goeddel DV, Lawn RM (1981) The leukocyte and fibroblast interferon genes are located on human chromosome 9. Proc Natl Acad Sci USA 78:3123–3127

Sehgal PB, Sagar AD (1980) Heterogeneity of poly (l)-poly (C)-induced human fibroblast interferon mRNA species. Nature 288:95–97

Slate DL, Ruddle FH (1979) Fibroblast interferon in man is coded by two loci on separate chromosomes. Cell 16:171–180

Stewart WE II (ed) (1979) The interferon system. Springer, Berlin Heidelberg New York, pp 187–190

Stewart, WE II, Sarkar FH, Taira H, Hall A, Nagata S, Weissmann C (1980) Comparison of several biological and physiochemical properties of human leukocyte interferons produced by human leukocytes and by E. coli. Gene 11:181–186

Streuli M, Nagata S, Weissmann C (1980) At least three human type α interferons: Structure of α2. Science 209:1343–1349
Streuli M, Hall A, Boll W, Stewart WE II, Nagata S, Weissmann C (1981) Target cell specificity of two species of human interferon-α produced in E. coli and of hybrid molecules derived from them. Proc Natl Acad Sci USA 78:2848–2852
Tan YH (1980) In: Stewart WE (ed) Interferons and their actions. CRC, Cleveland, pp 73–90
Tan YH, Creagan RP, Ruddle FH (1974) The somatic cell genetics of human interferon: Assignment of human interferon loci to chromosomes 2 and 5. Proc Natl Acad Sci USA 71:2251–2255
Taniguchi T, Sakal M, Fujii-Kuriyama Y, Muramatsu M, Kobayashi S, Sudo T (1979) Construction and identification of a bacterial plasmid containing the human fibroblast interferon gene sequence. Proc Jpn Acad Sci B55:464–469
Taniguchi T, Buarente L, Roberts TM, Kimelman D, Douhan J III, Ptashne M (1980a) Expression of the human fibroblast interferon gene in E. coli. Proc Natl Acad Sci USA 77:5230–5233
Taniguchi T, Fujii-Kuriyama Y, Muramatsu M (1980b) Molecular cloning of human interferon cDNA. Proc Natl Acad Sci USA 77:4003–4006
Taniguchi T, Mantei N, Schwarzstein M, Nagata S, Muramatsu M, Weissmann C (1980c) Human leukocyte and fibroblast interferons are structurally related. Nature 285:547–549
Taniguchi T, Ohno S, Fujii-Kuriyama Y, Muramatsu M (1980d) The nucleotide sequence of human fibroblast interferon cDNA. Gene 10:11–15
Taniguchi T, Pang RHL, Yip YK, Henriksen D, Vilček J (1981) Partial characterization of gamma (immune) interferon mRNA extracted from human lymphocytes. Proc Natl Acad Sci USA 78:3469–3472
Tavernier J, Dernyck R, Fiers W (to be published) Evidence for a unique human fibroblast interferon (IFN-β_1) chromosomal gene, devoid of intervening sequences
Weissenbach J, Charnajovsky Y, Zeevi M, Shulman L, Soreo H, Nir U, Wallach D, Perricaudet M, Tiollais P, Revel M (1980) Two interferon mRNAs in human fibroblasts: In vitro translation and E. coli cloning studies. Proc Natl Acad Sci USA 77:7152–7156
Weissmann C (1981) The cloning of interferon and other mistakes. In: Gresser I (ed) Interferon B. Academic, New York
Yip YK, Pang RHL, Oppenheim JD, Nachbar MS, Henriksen D, Zerebeckyj-Eckhardt I, Vilček J (1981) Stimulation of human gamma (immune) interferon production by diterpene esters. Infect Immun 34:131–139
Zoon KC, Smith ME, Bridgen PJ, Anfinsen CB, Hunkapiller MW, Hood LE (1980) Human fibroblast interferon: Amino acid analysis and amino terminal amino acid sequence. Science 207:527–529

CHAPTER 8

The Molecular Mediators of Interferon Action

C. BAGLIONI

A. Introduction

The molecular mediators of interferon action are those cellular components which change in relative amount upon treatment with interferon. The mediators to be discussed in this chapter are enzymes which are synthesized at an increased rate in interferon-treated cells (BAGLIONI 1979). It should be pointed out that interferon induces the synthesis of several proteins in mammalian cells (GUPTA et al. 1979; KNIGHT and KORANT 1979). These proteins can be identified as polypeptides with characteristic electrophoretic mobility by labeling the cells with radioactive amino acids and fractionating cell extracts by electrophoresis. The increase in these proteins is inhibited by actinomycin D, indicating that RNA synthesis is required for their induction by interferon (FARRELL et al. 1980). The synthesis of these proteins begins a few hours after tissue culture cells are exposed to interferon, but is is transient, even in the continuous presence of this antiviral agent (RUBIN and GUPTA 1980). These proteins, however, have not been identified with specific enzymatic activities or cellular components and it is unclear at this time whether or how they are involved in the different activities of interferon.

Interferon induces the synthesis of two enzymes which have been extensively purified and well characterized (LENGYEL 1982). These enzymes are an oligoadenylate polymerase (sometimes referred to as a synthetase) and a protein kinase. The first enzyme forms short chains of adenosines linked by a highly unusual 2′–5′ phosphodiester bond (all natural polynucleotides have a 3′–5′ phosphodiester bond), and is therefore designated 2′,5′-oligo(A) or, for short, 2–5A polymerase. The other enzyme phosphorylates with high specificity the eukaryotic initiation factor eIF-2. These enzymes are inactive in cells or cell extracts untill activated by binding to double-stranded RNA (dsRNA). This chapter will review in detail our present understanding of the mechanism of action of these enzymes and of their role as molecular mediators of interferon action.

Some metabolic changes have also been described in interferon-treated cells. MAHESHWARI et al. (1980a) reported, for example, a decrease in the synthesis of *N*-acetylglucosaminylphosphoryldolichol; DE FERRA and BAGLIONI (1981b) observed an elevation of the *S*-adenosylmethionine (AdoMet) and *S*-adenosylhomocysteine (AdoHcy) concentrations with a significant increase in the AdoHcy: AdoMet ratio. These metabolic changes may have profound effects on the glycosylation of proteins and on the methylation of RNA. Since the enzymes responsible for these metabolic changes have not been identified, these effects of interferon will only be briefly reviewed in this chapter.

B. The Inhibition of Protein Synthesis by Double-Stranded RNA

In experiments designed to investigate the shutoff of host protein synthesis in cells infected with poliovirus, EHRENFELD and HUNT (1971) identified viral dsRNA as a potent inhibitor of in vitro protein synthesis. This finding was of interest to investigators working on the mechanism of action of interferon, who were aware of the potent interferon-inducing activity of viral or synthetic dsRNA (FIELD et al. 1967). KERR et al. (1974) discovered that dsRNA inhibits protein synthesis in extracts of interferon-treated cells much more than in extracts of untreated cells. This was the starting point for a successful series of observations by KERR and collaborators, which led to the discovery of a low molecular weight inhibitor of protein synthesis (HOVANESSIAN et al. 1977) and to the identification of this inhibitor with 2–5A (KERR and BROWN 1978). These investigators established that 2–5A is synthesized from ATP by an enzymatic activity, which can be absorbed onto the synthetic dsRNA poly(I)·poly(C) covalently bound to agarose beads. The enzyme is activated in this way and synthesizes large amounts of 2–5A. This ingenious procedure allowed the isolation of 2–5A and the determination of its chemical structure (KERR and BROWN 1978).

At about the same time, LENGYEL and collaborators observed that reovirus mRNA was degraded in extracts of interferon-treated cells at a rate faster than in extracts of untreated cells (BROWN et al. 1976). This cleavage was found to be dependent on the presence of dsRNA in the mRNA preparation. Subsequent studies showed that addition of synthetic dsRNA resulted in the degradation of cellular and viral mRNAs and that ATP was required for the activation of this nuclease activity (SEN et al. 1976).

These observations led to the subsequent discovery by CLEMENS and WILLIAMS (1978) that addition of 2–5A reduces the amount of translatable mRNA in an in vitro protein-synthesizing system and by BAGLIONI et al. (1978) that 2–5A activates an endonuclease activity which cleaves both cellular and viral mRNA in cell extracts at apparently similar rates. RATNER et al. (1978) fractionated the cell extracts into two enzymatic components, one responsible for the synthesis of 2–5A and the other for the endonuclease activity. Similar observations were also reported by SCHMIDT et al. (1978). One mechanism for the inhibition of protein synthesis by dsRNA was therefore clarified by these studies.

Another mechanism, however, was discovered by investigating the inhibition of protein synthesis by dsRNA in rabbit reticulocyte lysates. These cells contain a protein kinase which, in the presence of dsRNA, phosphorylates the eukaryotic initiation factor eIF-2 (FARRELL et al. 1977). The phosphorylated eIF-2 is inactive and cannot catalyze the first step in the initiation of protein synthesis, namely the formation of the ternary complex between eIF-2, Met-tRNA, and GTP. The same kinase activity was found to be present in elevated levels in extracts of interferon-treated cells by several investigators (LEBLEU et al. 1976; ZILBERSTEIN et al. 1978; ROBERTS et al. 1976). It should be pointed out that there is as yet no evidence that this dsRNA-dependent protein kinase is activated in intact cells, whereas it was clearly shown that 2–5A is formed in interferon-treated cells infected with some viruses and that an endonuclease cleaves cellular and viral RNA in these cells (WILLIAMS et al. 1979; KNIGHT et al. 1980; Wreschner et al. 1981; NILSEN et al. 1982).

For this reason, the synthesis of 2–5A and the activation of the endonuclease will be discussed in great detail in the following section, whereas little will be said about the dsRNA-dependent protein kinase.

C. 2′–5′-Oligo(A)

The analysis of the oligonucleotides synthesized by the enzymatic activity bound to dsRNA–agarose beads (Hovanessian et al. 1977) led to the discovery that an oligomeric series of adenylates was formed from ATP and to the elucidation of the structure of these oligoadenylates (Kerr and Brown 1978). The members of the oligomeric series were separated by chromatography on DEAE–cellulose and their structure was determined. The major components of the oligomeric series are the triadenylate and the tetraadenylate, but small amounts of the diadenylate and of larger oligomers are also formed. The reaction can be described as follows:

$$\text{pppA} + \text{pppA} \rightarrow \text{pppA2'pA} + \text{pp} \quad (1)$$

$$\text{pppA2'pA} + (\text{pppA})_n \rightarrow \text{pppA(2'pA)}_n + (\text{pp})_n \quad (2)$$

(where pppA = ATP and pp = pyrophosphate).

The 2–5A polymerase adds stepwise adenylate residues to the "acceptor" end of ATP, oligoadenylate, or even other compounds such as NAD or AppppA, which have a free 2′-OH (Ball and White 1978; Minks et al. 1980). The probability of addition of an adenylate decreases as the "acceptor" oligomer is elongated, resulting in the preferential synthesis of short chains (Minks et al. 1980).

I. 2′,5′-Oligo(A) Polymerase

The original assay for 2–5A synthesis was based on the incubation of the enzyme bound to dsRNA–agarose beads with radioactive ATP and on the separation by chromatography of the labeled 2–5A formed (Hovanessian et al. 1977). A faster assay with dsRNA in solution was subsequently developed by Minks et al. (1979 a). By increasing the concentration of the substrate ATP in reactions with extracts prepared from interferon-treated HeLa cells, it was observed that the yield of 2–5A increased much more than expected from a simple substrate concentration effect. This was explained by the observation that high concentrations of ATP inhibited an enzymatic activity (2′-phosphodiesterase), which degraded 2–5A as it was being synthesized (Minks et al. 1979 b). The formation of 2–5A could be conveniently measured with dsRNA in solution and the structural requirements of dsRNA for the activation of the 2–5A polymerase could be easily studied.

The increase in 2–5A polymerase activity was measured in cells treated with different amounts of interferon or treated for increasing times (Baglioni et al. 1979; Ball 1979). After an initial lag of 3–6 h, this enzymatic activity increases progressively for up to 24–30 h; this increase is correlated with a concomitant inhibition of virus replication in infected cells (Baglioni et al. 1979). The relative increase in enzymatic activity at the end of this "induction" is a function of the basal level of 2–5A polymerase in the cells before treatment with interferon. This basal activity was found to vary greatly in cells of different species and to be influenced by the stage of differentiation of the cells (STARK et al. 1979) or by hormonal treatment (KRISHNAN and BAGLIONI 1980). The 2–5A polymerase activity can increase several thousandfold in chick fibroblasts, which have a very low basal level of this enzyme (BALL and WHITE 1978), whereas it is much lower in HeLa cells, which have a high basal activity (BAGLIONI et al. 1979). When these cells are transferred to interferon-free medium, the 2–5A polymerase activity decreases with the growth of the cells; it is apparently a stable enzyme in these cells, which is diluted out by the increase in cell mass (MINKS et al. 1979a). In quiescent human fibroblasts, however, even in the continuous presence of interferon, the 2–5A polymerase activity decreases after a few days and these cells become susceptible to viral infections (KRISHNAN and BAGLIONI 1981). The increase in 2–5A polymerase, therefore, is transient and the level of this enzyme appears to be regulated by the cells and to return to a basal level within a few days after exposure to interferon.

The 2–5A polymerase was partially purified from mouse cells by HOVANESSIAN and KERR (1979) and was recently completely purified by DOUGHERTY et al. (1980). The synthesis of 2–5A was investigated with the pure enzyme and SAMANTA et al. (1980) observed that over 97% of the ATP added to a reaction can be converted into 2–5A, with production of an equivalent amount of pyrophosphate and no apparent end product inhibition in the reaction.

1. Activation of 2′,5′-Oligo(A) Polymerase

In a systematic series of experiments, MINKS et al. (1979c) investigated the structural requirements of dsRNA for the activation of the 2–5A polymerase. Double-stranded DNA or DNA:RNA hybrids are inactive and only dsRNA longer than 30 base pairs can activate the enzyme. Moreover, the presence of mismatched base pairs reduces the activation of the 2–5A polymerase or even abolishes it above a certain level of mismatch (MINKS et al. 1979c). These studies indicate that only well-base-paired dsRNA of a certain minimum size can activate the 2–5A polymerase. Interestingly, the structural requirements of dsRNA for the induction of interferon synthesis are very similar to those for activation of the 2–5A polymerase, though some exceptions to this rule were recently found for some synthetic dsRNAs by BAGLIONI et al. (1981a). It appears unlikely at this time that synthesis of 2–5A is directly involved in the induction of interferon synthesis, whereas it seems quite possible that both this induction and the activation of the 2–5A polymerase rely on a similar recognition mechanism, which is triggered by the presence of replicating viral RNA in infected cells.

The 2–5A polymerase can be activated by the replicative complexes of the encephalomyocarditis virus (EMCV) (NILSEN et al. 1979). The replicative complexes were isolated from infected cells by velocity and isopyknic sedimentation; they contain viral RNA which is being transcribed by a viral replicase from a template strand. Both RNA strands maybe associated with protein, but stretches of dsRNA must be available for the 2–5A polymerase binding and activation. It seems quite likely that these viral structures are responsible for the activation of the 2–5A polymerase in infected cells.

2. 2′,5′-Oligo(A) in Intact Cells

WILLIAMS et al. (1979) reported the isolation of 2–5A from mouse L-cells treated with interferon and infected with EMCV. The 2–5A was identified by high pressure liquid chromatography and by its biologic activity in inhibiting protein synthesis. The concentration of 2–5A in these cells was subsequently measured by a sensitive competition binding assay (KNIGHT et al. 1980). This assay is based on the synthesis of a highly radioactive 2–5A derivative, obtained by ligating radioactive ^{32}pCp to the terminal 3′-OH with T4 RNA ligase (SILVERMAN et al. 1981), and on the binding of this derivative to the endonuclease present in unfractionated cell extracts. As will be discussed in detail later, the binding of 2–5A to the endonuclease is required for the activation of this enzyme. This is a very high affinity binding and this assay, therefore, can measure subnanomolar concentrations of 2–5A (KNIGHT et al. 1980). A modification of this assay was used by NILSEN et al. (1981 a) to show that 2–5A is formed in interferon-treated cells incubated with dsRNA. In this modification, the endonuclease was separated from the 2′-phosphodiesterase activity because this latter enzyme is present at such high concentrations in HeLa cells that it degrades the 2–5A during the binding assay with unfractionated cell extract. It should be pointed out that NILSEN et al. (1981 a) were unable to detect 2–5A in cells just treated with interferon, whereas KNIGHT et al. (1980) had found 60 n*M* 2–5A in L-cells treated with interferon, but uninfected. More recently, such high levels of 2–5A were not detected in L-cells just treated with interferon (I. M. KERR 1981, personal communication) and no explanation was found to account for the early findings.

Nanomolar amounts of 2–5A were also detected by NILSEN et al. (1982) in interferon-treated HeLa cells infected with reovirus. This virus has a dsRNA genome, which is found in the cytoplasm of infected cells 3 h after infection. At about this time, 2–5A is present in cells infected at high multiplicity, but not in infected cells not treated with interferon or in cells infected at low multiplicity. The 2–5A concentration increases in interferon-treated cells up to 6 h after infection with reovirus, but declines afterwards. Since the level of 2–5A formed is related to the multiplicity of infection, it seems likely that the dsRNA genomme of infecting virions contributes proportionally to the activation of the 2–5A polymerase. At low multiplicity, very small amounts of 2–5A may be formed which are undetectable by the competition binding assay.

II. 2′,5′-Oligo(A)-Activated Endonuclease (RNAse L)

The only known biologic activity of 2–5A is the activation of an endonuclease, which is designated RNase L (L for latent). There are specific structural requirements of 2–5A for the activation of RNase L; only oligoadenylates with two or three 5′-terminal phosphates are active (MARTIN et al. 1979). Moreover, triadenylates or longer oligomers activated the human or murine enzyme, whereas tetraadenylates or longer oligomers are required to activate a corresponding enzyme obtained from rabbit reticulocytes (WILLIAMS et al. 1979). The activation is reversible; when the 2–5A dissociates, the enzyme returns to the latent or inactive state, but can again be activated by new additions of 2–5A (SLATTERY et al. 1979). This activation–deactivation mechanism makes the enzyme completely dependent on the 2–5A concentration for activity. The affinity constant K_a of RNase L for 2–5A was measured by binding experiments and analysis of the data by Scatchard plots (NILSEN et al. 1981 b). From these data it can be calculated that the human RNase L is 50% activated at a 0.3 n*M* concentration of 2–5A, whereas the murine enzyme is comparably activated at an even lower concentration of 2–5A. These values are well in agreement with those shown to inhibit protein synthesis in cell-free systems (WILLIAMS et al. 1979).

The RNase L was partially purified by CHERNAJOVSKY et al. (1979) and by FLOYD-SMITH et al. (1981). These latter authors and WRESCHNER et al. (1981) showed that the activated RNase L cleaves RNA preferentially at UA, UG, and UU sequences, yielding products terminating with a 3′-phosphate. The RNase L does not cleave dsRNA or DNA (NILSEN et al. 1980). The RNase L does not show substrate specificity, but cleaves cellular and viral RNAs equally well. In fact, the activated RNase L can cleave specific sequences of 28 *S* ribosomal RNA in intact cells (WRESCHNER et al. 1981).

III. Degradation of 2′,5′-Oligo(A)

The 2–5A is resistant to hydrolysis by many nucleases which cleave 3′–5′ phosphodiester bonds, such as RNase T2 (KERR and BROWN 1978). WILLIAMS et al. (1978), MINKS et al. (1979 b), and CHERNAJOVSKY et al. (1979) discovered that 2–5A is rapidly degraded in cell extracts. The enzyme responsible for this degradation cleaves preferentially 2′–5′ phosphodiester bonds and has been partially purified from murine cells (SCHMIDT et al. 1979). The 2–5A is cleaved to ATP and AMP, as expected for a phosphodiesterase. The presence of a phosphate group at the 3′-terminal end of 2–5A effectively prevents its degradation by this enzyme (SCHMIDT et al. 1979). This indicates that 2–5A is cleaved stepwise from the 2′-terminus. Synthetic analogs of 2–5A methylated at the terminal 3′-OH are resistant to degradation by the 2′-phosphodiesterase and activate efficiently the RNase L (BAGLIONI et al. 1981 b). Analogs methylated at all 3′-OH residues, however, are inactive.

The 2–5A is degraded very rapidly in cell extracts. This degradation can be effectively prevented by the addition of high concentrations of ATP (MINKS et al. 1979 b). It is not clear whether 2–5A is rapidly degraded in intact cells, but it seems likely that this is the case. The concentration of ATP in intact cells may be too low to inhibit the 2′–5′ phosphodiesterase activity effectively and the 2–5A synthesized by the activated polymerase may have a relatively short half-life. If this is the case, the RNase L remains active only when 2–5A is continuously synthesized.

D. Degradation of Viral RNA in Infected Cells

The pathway for the activation of the 2–5A polymerase and RNase L is summarized in Fig. 1. The effect of interferon is to increase the level of 2–5A polymerase in the cell. Without formation of an activator, however, this increase has no detectable effect on the RNase L activity. It should be pointed out that all the other enzymes in this pathway are constitutive and are present in a relatively constant amount in all cells, whether treated with interferon or not. Each reaction shown in the pathway is reversible and this allows a fine tuning of RNase L activity. More-

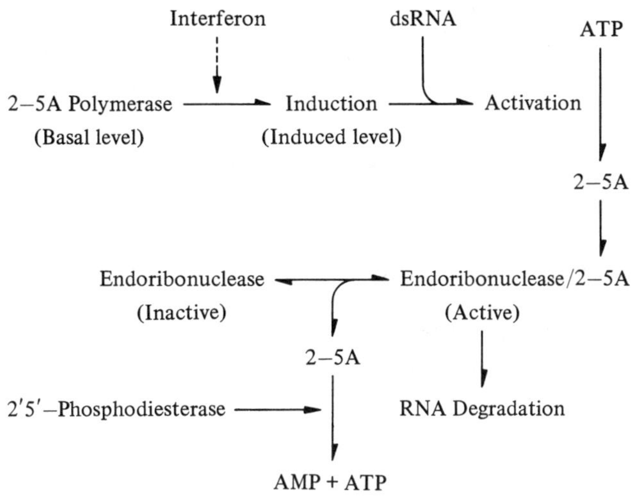

Fig. 1. Schematic representation of the induction of the synthesis of 2–5A polymerase by interferon, of the activation of this enzyme by dsRNA, of the activation of the RNase L by 2–5A, and of the degradation of 2–5A

over, this nuclease is transiently activated as long as 2–5A is being produced, but returns to an inactive state when 2–5A synthesis ceases. Ultimately, the extent of RNA degradation is a direct function of the amounts of 2–5A polymerase and its activator present. In interferon-treated cells infected at high multiplicity with reovirus, there is a measurable 2–5A concentration, but in untreated cells infected in the same way, 2–5A is not detectable (NILSEN et al. 1982). This difference in 2–5A concentration can best be explained by the presence of elevated levels of 2–5A polymerase in the interferon-treated cells.

In cells treated with interferon and infected with reovirus at low multiplicity, however, there is no detectable 2–5A in the cytoplasm and there is no evidence for the degradation of cellular mRNA (NILSEN et al. 1982). Since these cells are better protected by the treatment with interferon than are cells infected at high multiplicity, the presence of nanomolar concentrations of 2–5A is not necessary to prevent viral replication. When cells treated with interferon are infected at low multiplicity, the pathway shown in Fig. 1 functions in a discriminative way, with preferential degradation of viral RNA and little cleavage of cellular RNA.

I. The Localized Activation of 2′,5′-Oligo(A) Polymerase–RNAse L

To explain the preferential degradation of viral RNA in interferon-treated cells, NILSEN and BAGLIONI (1979) carried out some suggestive experiments with the replicative intermediate of EMCV isolated from infected cells. This replicative intermediate contains double-stranded regions which can activate the 2–5A polymerase (NILSEN et al. 1979), and single-stranded nascent viral RNA chains which are synthesized by a viral RNA polymerase. These single-stranded chains are preferentially cleaved when the replicative intermediate is incubated with an extract prepared from interferon-treated cells, but not when incubated with an extract of untreated cells. Other viral RNAs present in the same incubation, which do not contain double-stranded regions, are not degraded (NILSEN and BAGLIONI (1979). The essential element to obtain degradation of the replicative intermediate is the dsRNA present in this viral structure. Evidence for this role of dsRNA was provided by experiments with model substrates formed by annealing synthetic polyribonucleotides, such as poly(U), with the poly(A) of cellular or viral mRNA. Only mRNA which contains a double-stranded region is degraded in extracts of interferon-treated cells, whereas the same mRNA without the double-stranded region is not degraded even when included in the same incubation. This finding provides a clear example of "localized" activation of the 2–5A polymerase–RNase L system. Only the RNA which is covalently linked to double-stranded regions is cleaved by the combined action of these two enzymes, whereas other RNAs are unaffected.

The localized degradation of RNA requires formation of 2–5A. This was shown by experiments with inhibitors of the synthesis of 2–5A (NILSEN et al. 1980). Two inhibitors, which act by different mechanisms, suppress the degradation of single-stranded RNA covalently linked to dsRNA. They are 2′-dATP, which competes with ATP, the substrate of the 2–5A polymerase (MINKS et al. 1980), and ethidium bromide, which intercalates into dsRNA and prevents the activation of the 2–5A polymerase (BAGLIONI and MARONEY 1981).

The main consequence of the localized activation of the 2–5A polymerase–RNase L system is the discrimination between viral and cellular RNA. Under conditions where viral RNA in replicative complexes is degraded, the cellular RNA may not be cleaved. This discrimination is directly dependent on the concentration of 2–5A present. This was shown in in vitro experiments by incubating increasing amounts of mRNA annealed to poly(U) with extract of interferon-treated cells; at high input of this RNA which contains a double-stranded region, other RNAs are also degraded (NILSEN and Baglioni 1979). The same result is obtained by directly adding 2–5A to the incubations. These findings in vitro are the exact counterpart of the observations with intact cells treated with interferon and infected with reovirus. At a low multiplicity of infection, small amounts of 2–5A are formed and predominantly viral RNA is degraded; at high multiplicity, nanomolar amounts of 2–5A are formed and both viral and cellular RNA are degraded.

The localized activation of RNA by the 2–5A polymerase–RNase L system was clearly shown in experiments with cells extracts by NILSEN and BAGLIONI (1979). However, it has been very difficult to demonstrate this mechanism in intact cells. In early experiments by KNIGHT et al. (1980), the aim of the investigators was to demostrate the formation of 2–5A in infected cells. The conditions of infection were chosen accordingly to favor the formation of measurable levels of 2–5A, i.e., high multiplicity of infection of cells treated with large doses of interferon. Under these conditions, there is little synthesis of viral RNA and there is substantial cleavage of cellular RNA (WRESCHNER et al. 1981). At low multiplicity of infection, there is even less synthesis of viral RNA in interferon-treated cells and it is quite difficult to establish whether the viral RNA is cleaved in the absence of detectable degradation of cellular RNA. Evidence for the preferential degradation of viral RNA under these conditions was recently obtained by T.W. NILSEN and P.A. MARONEY (1982, unpublished work) in interferon-treated HeLa cells infected with

EMCV. Fragments of viral RNA, presumably resulting from cleavage of nascent RNA strands, were detected by a very sensitive hybridization assay (Northern blot). Viral RNA of the correct size was shown by this technique in infected cells not treated with interferon, but not in interferon-treated cells. Predominantly, fragments of viral RNA were found in these cells.

II. The Requirement for Double-Stranded RNA

The activation of the 2–5A polymerase requires the presence of dsRNA, the same polynucleotide which induces interferon synthesis. It seems likely that, in the absence of this activator, the 2–5A polymerase, which is present in elevated amounts in interferon-treated cells, does not impair the metabolism of these cells. The cells are alerted by circulating interferon of an ongoing viral infection and prepare the defenses necessary to fight this infection. These defenses, however, are only activated when the virus enters the cell and starts replicating. In the case of RNA viruses with a cytoplasmic replicative cycle, the formation of viral dsRNA activates the line of defense based on the 2–5A polymerase–RNase L system. The viral dsRNA is a signal of the presence of a replicative virus which induces the cells to produce interferon, but it is also the site of action of this line of defense, because of the binding of the 2–5A polymerase to double-stranded regions and of the consequent activation of the RNase L by the 2–5A produced.

Not all viruses, however, form replicative complexes containing dsRNA. This is most likely the case for DNA viruses, but it is also true for at least some RNA viruses such as vesicular stomatitis virus. This was established by NILSEN et al (1981 c), who developed an assay for the presence of viral dsRNA in infected cells. Viral RNA is specifically labeled in these cells, which are then treated with aminomethyltrioxsalen, a psoralen derivative which intercalates into double-stranded regions of nucleic acids and cross-links them upon irradiation. Cross-linked viral RNA can be recovered from cells infected with EMCV and it is found in replicative intermediates. The cross-linking is demostrated by the snapback reassociation of heat-denatured viral RNA. When HeLa cells infected with different viruses were examined with this assay, no dsRNA could be demonstrated in cells infected with vesicular stomatitis virus (NILSEN et al. 1981 c). Moreover, the presence of 2–5A in these cells could not be detected (C. BAGLIONI and T. W. NILSEN 1982, unpublished work). It seems unlikely that the 2–5A polymerase-RNase L system is involved in preventing the replication of vesicular stomatitis virus or of DNA viruses in interferon-treated cells. Since these cells are protected from infection with these viruses, the requirement for formation of dsRNA during a viral infection is not an obligatory one. Other antiviral mechanisms which do not require this activator are presumably responsible for preventing the replication of these viruses.

E. Other Antiviral Mechanisms

It has become clear in recent years that the antiviral state is comprised of several different mechanisms, each presumably contributing to the inhibition of virus replication. Therefore, there are some mediators of interferon action which are yet to be discovered.

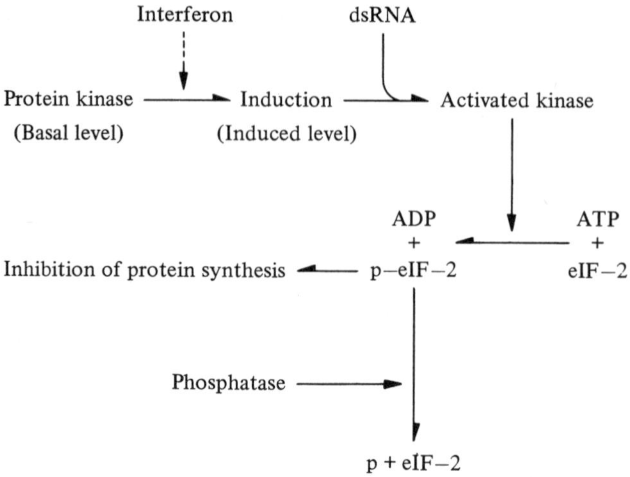

Fig. 2. Schematic representation of the induction of the synthesis of a protein kinase by interferon, of the activation of this enzyme by dsRNA, of the phosphorylation of initiaton factor eIF-2, and of the consequent inhibition of protein synthesis

I. Protein Kinase Activated by Double-Stranded RNA

The synthesis of the protein kinase activated by dsRNA is induced by interferon (BAGLIONI 1979). The increase in the activity of this kinase is 3- to 10-fold, much less therefore than that of the 2–5A polymerase. The kinase has been extensively purified from mouse cells treated with interferon (SEN et al. 1978; KIMCHI et al. 1979). All interferons induce the synthesis of this protein kinase (HOVANESSIAN et al. 1980). The purified protein kinase contains a protein of molecular weight 67,000 as the major component (LENGYEL et al. 1980), when isolated from mouse cells. The corresponding protein from human cells has a slightly larger molecular weight, abouth 72,000 (WEST and BAGLIONI 1979). In the presence of dsRNA and ATP, this protein is phosphorylated. This may be due to an autophosphorylation which leads to the activation of the kinase. The activated kinase phosphorylates the α subunit of initiation factor eIF-2 (FARRELL et al. 1978).

The phosphorylation of eIF-2 causes inhibition of protein synthesis in cell-free systems (Fig. 2). The phosphate moiety, however, can be removed from eIF-2 by a phosphoprotein phosphatase present in cell extracts (KIMCHI et al. 1979). Since the activity of this phosphatase is inhibited by dsRNA (EPSTEIN et al. 1980), in the presence of this polynucleotide there is accumulation of phosphorylated eIF-2 and inhibition of protein synthesis. This inhibition has not been observed, however, in interferon-treated cells infected by viruses which activate the 2–5A polymerase, such as EMCV or reovirus. There is no evidence, therefore, that the protein kinase activated by dsRNA plays a defined role among the antiviral mechanisms elicited by interferon. It is also difficult to understand how an inhibition of the function of eIF-2 could be selective with regard to the synthesis of viral proteins. A "localized" activation of the kinase at the level of viral replicative intermediates may possibly inactivate eIF-2, but it is not known whether this phosphorylated initiation factor could bind to viral mRNA and form a stable complex inactive in protein synthesis. The binding of eIF-2 to mRNA was reported by KAEMPFER et al. (1978), but it is not known whether phosphorylated eIF-2 binds to mRNA and whether such eIF-2 would become resistant to dephosphorylation by the phosphatase. In any event, the role of dsRNA-activated protein kinase as a mediator of interferon action remains to be demonstrated.

II. Other Metabolic Changes in Interferon-Treated Cells

All cellular and most viral mRNAs contain at the 5′-terminus a cap structure, a 7-methyl guanosine (m^7G) linked to the penultimate nucleotide methylated in the 2′-OH position of the ribose moiety; the only exception is represented by picornavirus mRNA, which does not have a cap with methylated nucleotides (BANERJEE 1980). The m^7G is required for efficient translation of cellular and viral mRNAs. SEN et al. (1975, 1977) discovered that the methylation of reovirus mRNA is inhibited in extracts from interferon-treated L-cells or HeLa cells. This impairment in methylation is due to an inhibitor, which could not be purified owing to a marked instability in vitro.

Other defects in the methylation of viral mRNAs have been observed in intact interferon-treated cells infected with different viruses. The mRNS synthesized by reovirus and vaccinia virus in cells treated with interferon has a reduced 2′-O methylation, but an apparently normal m^7G methylation (DESROSIERS and LENGYEL 1977; KROATH et al. 1978). This defect in methylation has apparently no effect on the translatability of these mRNAs. DE FERRA and BAGLIONI (1981 a), however, reported that a fraction of vesicular stomatitis virus mRNA synthesized in HeLa cells treated with interferon is unmethylated in the 5′-terminal guanosine. This mRNA does not associate with polysomes and is therefore untranslated. The defects in methylation of viral mRNAs can be explained by a change in the cytoplasmic concentration of AdoMet and AdoHcy. The methylation of the viral mRNAs is carried out by viral enzymes which have a characteristic K_m for AdoMet and K_i for AdoHcy (this is an inhibitor of the transmethylases). In the case of vesicular stomatitis virus, the viral enzymes (L-protein) methylates preferentially the 2′-OH position at low AdoMet concentration or at elevated AdoHcy concentration; under these conditions the 5′-terminal guanosine is poorly methylated in reactions in vitro (TESTA and BANERJEE 1977). The opposite is true for the transmethylases of reovirus and vaccinia virus. In this case, the 2′-methylation is impaired when the AdoMet:AdoHcy ratio decreases. The AdoMet and AdoHcy levels are significantly altered in HeLa cells treated with interferon (DE FERRA and BAGLIONI 1981 b). The change in the concentration of these metabolites occurs after a few hours of treatment with interferon and is dependent on the dose of this antiviral agent. The cause of this effect of interferon has not yet been identified.

A defect in protein glycosylation was also reported in cells treated with interferon by MAHESHWARI et al. (1980 a). Mouse L-cells treated with interferon show decreased transfer of *N*-acetylglucosamine from UDP-*N*-acetylglucosamine into glycolipid with properties of dolichol derivatives. These dolichol-bound oligosaccharides serve as intermediates in protein glycosylation. A defect in glycosylation might explain the observation by MAHESHWARI and FRIEDMAN (1980) that interferon-treated cells produce vesicular stomatitis virus particles with low infectivity and reduced content of the glycosylated viral G-protein (MAHESHWARI et al. 1980 b). Recent results of OLDEN et al. (1982), however, indicate that interferon does not inhibit the glycosylation of cellular or viral glycoproteins in mouse cells.

F. Conclusions

The remarkable progress of the last 5 years in understanding the mechanism of action of interferon has led to the discovery of the molecular mediators. More recently, many investigators have attempted to explain the role of these mediators in preventing the replication of viruses. This has proved to be a somewhat elusive task and convincing evidence, so far, has been obtained only for the role of one mediator, 2–5A. It should be stressed, however, that synthesis of 2–5A and activation of RNase L may play an important role in only some viral infections, while other mechanisms may be involved in infections by different viruses. There is agreement today that the antiviral state is comprised of several mechanisms, each contributing in some way to stop viral replication. The details of these antiviral mechanisms remain to be explained and we presently have only some useful research leads. The investigation of the antiviral mechanisms is complicated by the number of variables involved. Different viruses may be fought by different mechanisms in different cells. At this time, we can only analyze those situations where a specific antiviral mechanism is predominantly responsible for preventing the replication of a given virus. To do this, we have to study model systems that present the investigator with a relatively simple situation. The elucidation of more complex systems may have to wait for a better knowledge of each antiviral mechanism involved. The study of the molecular mediators of interferon action is no longer in its infancy, but has yet to reach a level of understanding sufficient to explain fully the inhibition of virus replication of the molecular level. If the rate of progress in the last 5 years is an indication of future developments in this field, we should be able to witness substantial progress in the next few years.

References

Baglioni C (1979) Interferon induced enzymatic activities and their role in the antiviral state. Cell 17:255–264

Baglioni C, Maroney PA (1981) Inhibition of double-stranded RNA activated protein kinase and 2′5′-oligo(A) polymerase by ethidium bromide. Biochemistry 20:758–765

Baglioni C, Minks MA, Maroney PA (1978) Interferon action may be mediated by activation of a nuclease by pppA2′p5′A2′p5′A. Nature 273:684–687

Baglioni C, Maroney PA, West DK (1979) 2′5′-oligo(A) polymerase activity and inhibition of viral RNA synthesis in interferon-treated HeLa cells. Biochemistry 18:1765–1770

Baglioni C, Minks MA, De Clercq E (1981 a) Structural requirements of polynucletides for the activation of (2′–5′)A_n polymerase and protein kinase. Nucleic Acids Res 19:4939–4950

Baglioni C, D'Alessandro SB, Nilsen TW, Den Hartog JA, Crea R, Van Boom JH (1981 b) Analogs of (2′–5′)oligo(A): Endonuclease activation and inhibition of protein synthesis in intact cells. J Biol Chem 256:3253–3257

Ball LA (1979) Induction of 2′Π′oligoadenylate synthetase activity and a new protein by chick interferon. J Virol 94:282–296

Ball LA, White CN (1978) Oligonucleotide inhibitor of protein synthesis made in extracts of interferon-treated chick embryo cells: Comparison with the mouse low molecular weight inhibitor. Proc Natl Acad Sci USA 75:1167–1171

Ball LA, White CN (1979) Induction, purification and properties of 2′5′-oligoadenylate synthetase. In: Koch G, Richter D (eds) Regulation of macromolecular synthesis by low molecular weight mediators. Academic, New York, pp 304–317

Banerjee AK (1980) 5′-Terminal cap structure in eukaryotic messenger ribonucleic acids. Microbiol Rev 44:175–205

Brown GE, Lebleu B, Kawakita M, Shaila S, Sen GC, Lengyel P (1976) Increased endonuclease activity in an extract from mouse Ehrlich ascites tumor cells which had been treated with a partially purified interferon preparation: Dependence on double-stranded RNA. Biochem Bophys Res Commun 69:114–121

Chernajovsky Y, Kimchi A, Schmidt A, Zilberstein A, Revel M (1979) Differential effects of two interferon-induced translational inhibitors on initiation of protein synthesis. Eur J Biochem 96:35–41

Clemens MJ, Williams BRG (1978) Inhibition of cell-free protein synthesis by pppA2′-p5′A2′p5′A: a novel oligonucleotide synthesized by interferon-treated L cell extracts. Cell 13:565–572

De Ferra F, Baglioni C (1981 a) Viral messenger RNA unmethylated in the 5′-terminal guanosine in interferon-treated HeLa cells infected with vesicular stomatitis virus. Virology 112:426–435

De Ferra F, Baglioni C (1981 b) Changes in the level of the methyl donor S-adenosylmethionine and its antagonist S-adenosylhomocysteine in HeLa cells treated with interferon. Abstr of the 2nd international congress for interferon research, San Francisco, Oct 1981

Desrosiers RC, Lengyel P (1977) Impairment of reovirus mRNA cap methylation in interferon-treated L cells. Fed Proc 36:812

Dougherty JP, Samantha H, Farrell PJ, Lengyel P (1980) Interferon, double-stranded RNA, and RNA degradation. J Biol Chem 255:3813–3816

Ehrenfeld E, Hunt T (1971) Double-stranded poliovirus RNA inhibits initiation of protein synthesis by reticulocyte lysates. Proc Natl Acad Sci USA 68:1075–1078

Epstein DA, Torrence PF, Friedman RM (1980) Double-stranded RNA inhibitis a phosphoprotein phosphatase in interferon-treated cells. Proc Natl Acad Sci USA 77:107–111

Farrell PJ, Balkow K, Hunt T, Jackson R (1977) Phosphorylation of initiation factor eIF-2 and the control of reticulocyte protein synthesis. Cell 11:187–200

Farrell PJ, Sen GC, Dubois MF, Ratner L, Slattery E, Lengyel P (1978) Interferon action: Two distinct pathways for the inhibition of protein synthesis by double-stranded RNA. Proc Natl Acad Sci USA 75:5893–5897

Farrell PJ, Broeze RJ, Lengyel P (1980) Interferon induced mRNA and proteins in Ehrlich ascites tumor and HeLa cells. Ann NY Acad Sci 350:615–616

Field AK, Tytell AA, Lampson GP, Hilleman MR (1967) Inducers of interferon and host resistance. II. Multistranded synthetic polynucleotide complexes. Proc Natl Acad Sci USA 58:1004–1009

Floyd-Smith G, Slattery E, Lengyel P (1981) Interferon action: RNA cleavage pattern of a (2′–5′)oligoadenylate-dependent endonuclease. Science 212:1030–1032

Gupta SL, Rubin BY, Holmes SL (1979) Interferon action: Induction of specific proteins in mouse and human by homologous interferons. Proc Natl Acad Sci USA 76:4817–4821

Hovanessian AG, Brown RE, Kerr IM (1977) Synthesis of low molecular weight inhibitor of protein synthesis with enzyme from interferon-treated cells. Nature 268:537–540

Hovanessian AG, Kerr IM (1979) The (2′–5′)oligoadenylate (pppA2′–5′A2′5′A) synthetase and protein kinase(s) from interferon-treated cells. Eur J Biochem 93:515–526

Hovanessian AG, La Bonnardiere C, Falcoff E (1980) Action of murine γ (immune)-interferon on β (fibroblast)-interferon resistant L 1210 and embryonal carcinoma cells. J Interferon Res 1:125–136

Kaempfer R, Rosen H, Israeli R (1978) Translational control. Recognition of the methylated 5′-end and an internal sequence in eukaryotic mRNA by the initiation factor that binds methionyl-$tRNA_f^{met}$. Proc Natl Acad Sci USA 75:650–654

Kerr IM, Brown RE (1978) pppA2′p5′A2′p5′A: An inhibitor of protein synthesis synthe-

sized with an enzyme fraction from interferon-treated cells. Proc Natl Acad Sci USA 75:256–260
Kerr IM, Brown RE, Ball LA (1974) Increased sensitivity of cell-free protein synthesis to double-stranded RNA after interferon-treatment. Nature 250:57–59
Kimchi A, Zilberstein A, Schmidt A, Shulman L, Revel M (1979) The interferon induced protein kinase PK-i from mouse L cells. J Biol Chem 254:9846–9853
Knight E Jr, Korant BD (1979) Fibroblast interferon induces synthesis of four proteins in human fibroblast cells. Proc Natl Acad Sci USA 76:1824–1827
Knight M, Cayley PJ, Silverman RH, Wreschner DH, Gilbert CS, Brown RE, Kerr IM (1980) Radioimmune, radiobinding and HPLC analysis of 2–5A and related oligonucleotides from intact cells. Nature 288:189–192
Krishnan I, Baglioni C (1980) Increased levels of (2′–5′)oligo(A) polymerase activity in human lymphoblastoid cells treated with glucocorticoids. Proc Natl Acad Sci USA 77:6506–6510
Krishnan I, Baglioni C (1981) Regulation of 2′5′-oligo(A) polymerase activity in quiescent human fibroblasts treated with interferon. Virology 111:666–670
Kroath H, Gross HJ, Jungwirth C, Bodo G (1978) RNA methylation in vaccinia virus-infected chick embryo fibroblasts treated with homologous interferon. Nucleic Acids Res 5:2441–2454
Lebleu B, Sen GC, Shaila S, Cabrer B, Lengyel P (1976) Interferon, doublestranded RNA and protein phosphorylation. Proc Natl Acad Sci USA 73:3107–3111
Lengyle P (1982) Biochemistry of interferons and their action. Ann Rev Biochem 51:251–282
Lengyel P, Desrosiers R, Broeze R, Slattery E, Taira H, Dougherty J, Samantha H, Pichon J, Farrell P, Ratner L, Sen G (1980) Biochemistry of the interferon system. In: Schlessinger D (ed) Microbiology. American Society of Microbiology, Bethesda, pp 219–226
Maheshwary RK, Friedman RM (1980) Effect of interferon treatment on vesicular stomatitis virus (VSV). Release of unusual particles with low infectivity. Virology 101:399–407
Maheshwari RK, Banerjee DK, Waechter CJ, Olden K, Friedman RM (1980a) Interferon treatment inhibits glycosylation of a viral protein. Nature 287:454–456
Maheshwary RK, Demsey AE, Mohanty SB, Friedman RM (1980b) Interferon treated cells release vesicular stomatitis virus particles lacking glycoprotein spikes: Correlation with biochemical data. Proc Natl Acad Sci USA 77:2284–2287
Martin EM, Birsdall NJM, Brown RE, Kerr IM (1979) Enzymic synthesis, characterization and nuclear magnetic resonance spectra of pppA2′p5′A2′p5′A and related oligonucleotides: Comparison with chemical synthesized material. Eur J Biochem 95:295–307
Minks MA, Benvin S, Maroney PA, Baglioni C (1979a) Synthesis of 2′5′oligo(A) in extracts of interferon-treated HeLa cells. J Biol Chem 254:5058–5064
Minks MA, Benvin S, Maroney PA, Baglioni C (1979b) Metabolic stability of 2′5′oligo(A) and activity of 2′5′oligo(A)-dependent endonuclease in extracts of control and interferon-treated HeLa cells. Nucleic Acids Res 6:767–780
Minks MA, West DK, Benvin S, Baglioni C (1979c) Structural requirements of double-stranded RNA for the activation of 2′5′oligo(A) polymerase and protein kinase of interferon-treated HeLa cells. J Biol Chem 254:10180–10183
Minks MA, Benvin S, Baglioni C (1980) Mechanism of $pppA(2'p5'A)_n2'p5'A_{OH}$ synthesis in extracts of interferon-treated HeLa cells. J Biol Chem 255:5031–5035
Nilsen TW, Baglioni C (1979) A mechanism for discrimination between viral and host mRNA in interferon-treated cells. Proc Natl Acad Sci USA 76:2600–2604
Nilsen TW, Maroney PA, Baglioni C (1979) 2′5′oligo(A): a mediator of viral RNA cleavage in Interferon-treated cells? In: Koch H, Richter D (eds) Regulation of macromolecular synthesis by low molecular weight mediators. Academic, New York, pp 329–339
Nilsen TW, Weissman SG, Baglioni C (1980) Role of 2′5′-oligo(A) polymerase in the degradation of RNA linked to double-stranded RNA by extracts of interferon-treated cells. Biochemistry 19:5574–5579
Nilsen TW, Maroney PA, Baglioni C (1981a) Double-stranded RNA causes synthesis of

2′,5′-oligo(A) and degradation of messenger RNA in interferon-treated cells. J Biol Chem 256:7806–7812

Nilsen TW, Wood DL, Baglioni C (1981 b) 2′5′-oligo(A)-activated endoribonuclease. Tissue distribution and characterization with a binding assay. J Biol Chem 256:10751–10754

Nilsen TW, Wood DL, Baglioni C (1981 c) Cross-linking of viral RNA by 4′-aminomethyl-4, 5′,8-trimethylpsoralen in HeLa cells infected with Encephalomyocarditis virus and the tsG114 mutant of vesicular stomatitis virus. Virology 109:82–93

Nilsen TW, Maroney PA, Baglioni C (1982) Synthesis of (2′–5′)oligo(A) and activation of an endoribonuclease in interferon-treated HeLa cells infected with reovirus. J Virol 42:1039–1045

Olden K, Bernard BA, Turner W, White SL (1982) Effect of interferon on protein glycosylation and comparison with tunicamycin. Nature 300:290–292

Ratner L, Wiegand RC, Farrell PJ, Sen GC, Cabrer B, Lengyel P (1978) Interferon, double-stranded RNA and RNA degradation, fractionation of the endonuclease system into two macromolecular components; Role of a small molecule in nuclease activation. Biochem Biophys Res Commun 81:947–954

Roberts WK, Hovanessian A, Brown RE, Clemens MJ, Kerr IM (1976) Interferon-mediated protein kinase and low-molecular weight inhibitor of protein synthesis. Nature 264–477–480

Rubin BY, Gupta SL (1980) Differential efficacies of human type I and type II interferons as antiviral and antiproliferative agents. Proc Natl Acad Sci USA 77:5928–5932

Samantha H, Dougherty JP, Lengyel P (1980) Synthesis of (2′–5′)A_n from ATP. J Biol Chem 255:9807–9813

Schmidt A, Zilberstein A, Shulman L, Federman P, Berissi H, Revel M (1978) Interferon action: isolation of nuclease F, a translation inhibitor activated by interferon-induced (2′–5′)oligo-isoadenylate. FEBS Lett 95:257–264

Schmidt A, Chernajovsky Y, Shulman L, Federman P, Berissi H, Revel M (1979) An interferon-induced phosphodiesterase degrading (2′–5′)oligoisoadenylate and the C-C-A terminus of tRNA. Proc Natl Acad Sci USA 76:4788–4792

Sen GC, Lebleu B, Brown GE, Rebello MA, Furuichi H, Morgan M, Shatkin AJ, Lengyel P (1975) Inhibition of reovirus messenger RNA methylation in extracts of interferon-treated Ehrlich ascites tumor cells. Biochem Biophys Res Commun 65–427–434

Sen GC, Lebleu B, Brown GE, Kawakita M, Slattery E, Lengyel P (1976) Interferon, double-stranded RNA and mRNA degradation. Nature 264:370–372

Sen GC, Shaila S, Lebleu B, Brown GE, Desrosierd RC, Lengyel P (1977) Impairment of reovirus mRNA methylation in extracts of interferon-treated Ehrlich ascites tumor cells: further characteristics of the phenomenon. J Virol 21:69–83

Sen GC, Taira H, Lengyel P (1978) Characteristics of a double-stranded RNA-activated protein kinase system partially purified from interferon-treated Ehrlich ascites tumor cells. J Biol Chem 253:5915–5921

Silverman RH, Wreschner DH, Gilbert CS, Kerr IM (1981) Synthesis, characterization and properties of ppp(A2′p)$_n$ApCp and related high specificactivity ^{32}P-labelled derivatives of ppp(A2′p)A_n. Eur J Biochem 115:79–85

Slattery E, Ghosh N, Samantha H, Lengyel P (1979) Interferon, double-stranded RNA, and RNA degradation: Activation of an endonuclease by (2′–5′)A_n. Proc Natl Acad Sci USA 76:4778–4782

Stark GR, Dower WJ, Schimke RT, Brown RE, Kerr IM (1979) pppA2′p5′A2′p5′A synthetase: Convenient assay, species and tissue distribution and variation upon withdrawal of oestrogen from chick oviducts. Nature 278: 471–473

Testa D, Banerjee AK (1977) Two methyltransferase activities in the purified virions of vesicular stomatitis virus. J Virol 24:786–793

West DK, Baglioni C (1979) Induction by interferon of a protein kinase activated by double-stranded RNA in HeLa cells. Eur J Biochem 101:461–468

Williams BRG, Kerr IM, Gilbert CS, White CN, Ball LA (1978) Synthesis and breakdown auf pppA2′p5′A2′p5′A and transient inhibition of protein synthesis in extracts from interferon-treated and control cells. Eur J Biochem 92:455–462

Williams BRG, Golgher RR, Brown RE, Gilbert CS, Kerr IM (1979) Natural occurrence of 2–5A in interferon-treated EMC virus-infected L cells. Nature 282:582–586

Wreschner DH, James TC, Silverman RH, Kerr IM (1981) Ribosomal RNA cleavage, nuclease activation and 2–5A (ppp(A2′p)$_n$A in interferon-treated cells. Nucleic Acids Res 9:1571–1581

Zilberstein A, Kimchi A, Schmidt A, Revel M (1978) Isolation of two interferon-induced translational inhibitors: a protein kinase and an oligoisoadenylate synthetase. Proc Natl Acad Sci USA 75:4743–4738

CHAPTER 9

The Cellular Effects of Interferon

J. L. TAYLOR, J. L. SABRAN, and S. E. GROSSBERG

A. Introduction

Although interferon (IFN) was discovered by virtue of its antiviral effect, an activity which indeed defines it, a large body of literature now documents that IFN can also have significant effects on uninfected cells. The range of these effects is extensive; the largest number of reports deals with the ability of IFN to inhibit cell growth in culture (see reviews by GRESSER and TOVEY 1978; DAHL 1977b; BARON et al. 1979; GRESSER 1977; HOVANESSIAN 1979; HO and ARMSTRONG 1975). Published reports describe the inhibition of growth of cells of human (see Table 1) and mouse (see Table 2) origin. In this chapter we shall limit our discussion to the effects of IFN on cells grown in culture. Such effects may be involved in the antitumor and immunomodulatory activities of IFN in vivo described in other chapters of this book.

This chapter attempts to describe the many different effects of IFN that appear to be qualitatively different; these effects appear to be inhibitory or stimulatory, dependent in part upon the metabolic or physiologic state of the cells or their ability to express specialized functions. We have tried to document IFN dosage, since cellular alterations seem to require more than is needed to exert antiviral effects; the difficulty in making comparisons of dosages should be lessened in the future by the use of international standards (for at least human, mouse, rabbit, and chicken IFNs) that will permit the reporting of activities in international units (IU). Tabular summaries have been provided of the multiple effects of IFN on human cells as well as mouse cells, the most commonly employed models (see Tables 3 and 4). In the concluding section, we attempt to relate the possible threads of commonality among the seemingly bewildering varieties of IFN effects to potential mechanisms of action.

The volume of work generated about the cellular (nonantiviral) effects of IFN reflects in large part the large number of variables which can be tested, including assay method, cell type, nature and dose of the IFN preparation, the conditions of IFN treatment, as well as the varieties of expression of specialized cell function. We shall therefore discuss first the methodology used, since approaches taken to study these effects impose certain constraints upon the kinds of information obtainable.

B. Cell Growth Inhibition by IFN

I. Assay Systems

1. Viable Cell Counts

Perhaps the most common assay for cell growth inhibitory activity is that of viable cell counting. Cells are subcultured at a sufficiently low density to allow subsequent adequate cell growth, and the cells are enumerated at various times in cultures grown in the presence or absence of IFN. Viable counts can be made either by direct enumeration of cells in the presence of a vital stain, such as trypan blue, or by mechanical means in a Coulter counter. Viable cell counting, used in the first studies on cell growth inhibition by IFN (PAUCKER et al. 1972), has allowed investigation of the effects of IFN on growth rate, saturation density, and cell viability.

2. Colony Formation

A second assay system has been used with cells which will form discrete colonies attached to a solid surface or in agar. Cells are plated with IFN present in the medium, and colony number and size monitored. BALKWILL et al. (1978 a) found that colony formation at low plating density was a more sensitive assay than population growth (as described in Sect. B.I.1) for their system, i.e., human breast cells from normal and cancerous tissue. This technique has been modified to examine the growth inhibitory action of IFN on bone marrow cells in plasma clots under agar (for example, by LUDWIG and SWETLY 1980). Because these cells can be grown at very low densities it becomes possible to examine primary tissue samples, such as from biopsy, where small cell numbers may make population growth studies difficult, if not impossible.

MONTAGNIER and GRUEST (1980) usefully modified the agar colony formation method by suspending the human Daudi lymphoblastoid line of cells in semisolid agar and then adding IFN to a filter disc placed on the agar surface. After incubation, a zone of inhibition of cell growth surrounded the disc containing IFN and the width of the zone was directly proportional to the concentration of IFN added.

3. Measurement of Macromolecular Synthesis

Because a decrease in cell growth rate generally correlates with a decrease in macromolecular synthesis, especially that of DNA, incorporation of radioactive precursors into DNA, RNA, or protein has been used as a method of determining inhibition of cell growth. LEVY and MERIGAN (1966) found that at a dose of 300 U/ml IFN had no effect on protein or RNA synthesis in dividing chicken embryo fibroblasts. BORECKY et al. (1972, 1973) observed that fractions eluted from pH 4.3 polyacrylamide gel electrophoresis of IFN [induced in mouse peritoneal macrophage or L-cells with Newcastle diesease virus (NDV)] having antiviral activity, did not inhibit protein synthesis, while some fractions without antiviral activity either decreased or increased amino acid incorporation. L-cell IFN enhanced the rate of degradation of protein in Ehrlich ascites tumor cells without affecting the overall rate of protein synthesis (PANNIERS and CLEMENS 1980). IFN has been shown to enhance diphtheria toxin-mediated inhibition of protein synthesis in mouse NIH/3T3 (MLV) cells carrying Moloney leukemia virus and in human HeLa cells; the IFN-modulated effect was species and dose dependent (ABOUD et al. 1980).

Uridine transport and phosphorylation in Daudi cells were unaffected by treatment with HuIFN-α at doses which did cause inhibition of thymidine incorporation (GEWERT and CLEMENS 1980; GEWERT et al. 1981). The synthesis of 28 *S* ribosomal RNA was inhibited by treatment of trisomy 21 cells (CCL-84) with 500 U/ml HuIFN-β whereas the synthesis of 18 *S* rRNA was not affected. IFN-treated CCL-84 cells contained 50%–75% less cytoplasmic RNA than did control cells (MAROUN 1978).

Inhibition of DNA synthesis has been frequently used as an assay for growth inhibition. MATSUZAWA and KAWADE (1974) pointed out that incorporation of labeled precursors into DNA often does not distinguish among a decrease in cell number in the sample, a decrease in uptake of the label, or a true decrease in incorporation of the label into DNA. They felt that since all three situations represent a decrease in cellular activity the use of DNA precursors provides a valid assay for the cellular effects of IFN, although not necessarily of antiproliferative effect. TOVEY et al. (1975) demonstrated that IFN treatment caused a decrease in uptake of labeled thymidine into L1210 mouse leukemia cells cultured in a chemostat, a change first detectable between 2 and 8 h after IFN treatment and reaching a maximum between 8 and 24 h. Whereas the level of *uptake* of thymidine ^3H was maximally inhibited 20%–40% by IFN treatment, the amount of *incorporation* decreased 50%–70% from controls at 8–12 h. In a batch cell growth method, TOVEY (1981) showed that the inhibition of incorporation of thymidine ^3H was not detected until 18 h, much later than in the chemostat-grown cultures, suggesting that culture conditions greatly affect this response to IFN treatment.

In concanavalin A- (con A)-stimulated mouse spleen cell cultures, WEINSTEIN et al. (1977) found a decrease in incorporation of thymidine ^3H. The effect was maximal 44 h after simultaneous treatment with con A and IFN, at a time when DNA synthesis of con A-stimulated controls was maximum and synthesis of RNA and protein was inhibited. GLASGOW et al. (1978a, b) compared the inhibition of cell growth and inhibition of incorporation of labeled thymidine into murine osteogenic sarcoma cells by IFN produced in C243 mouse cells. At 3 days after treatment cells treated with 10 U IFN showed a 50% decrease in cell growth; to show a similar decrease in incorporation of label at the same time required 300–30,000 U IFN, suggesting again that decrease in incorporation of DNA precursor is less sensitive a measure than is inhibition of cell growth.

CZARNIECKI et al. (1981) compared two clones of Swiss 3T3 cells, D8 and H2 chronically infected with Moloney murine leukemia virus (MLV). The H2, clone was 5 times more sensitive to the growth inhibitory effects of IFN than the D8 clone, which however required 45 times the dose of IFN to inhibit thymidine incorporation than was required for H2. The incorporation of radioactively labeled thymidine was less sensitive than the cell growth assay for both clones. These clones were found to be similar in their sensitivity to inhibition of MLV production by IFN, but encephalomyocarditis virus (EMCV) replication in the H2 clone was inhibited by IFN more than it was in the D8 clone. This study illustrates the variability in sensitivity to IFN's actions in cells within a single population.

Effects on DNA synthesis by IFN have also been demonstrated in human cells. In virus-transformed human fibroblasts, RSa cells, incubated with human leukocyte IFN (500 U/ml) during the G1 and early S phases of the cell cycle, the uptake and incorporation of thymidine were decreased whereas the uptake and incorporation of amino acids were not affected (FUSE and KUWATA 1978). VANDENBUSSCHE et al. (1981), also using RSa cells, found that thymidine incorporation was inhibited more than 60%–80% by treatment with IFN at doses of 100 and 1,000 U/ml, respectively.

HuIFN-α and HuIFN-γ have been effective in inhibiting thymidine uptake and incorporation by human diploid fibroblasts, FS-4, with incorporation inhibited more than 50% by 400 U/ml HuIFN-α or 25 U/ml purified HuIFN-γ induced by staphylococcal enterotoxin A (RUBIN and GUPTA 1980). Thymidine uptake was inhibited in Daudi lymphoblastoid cultures by both HuIFN-α and HuIFN-β (HILFENHAUS and MAULER 1980). Exposure of Daudi cells to IFN for 48 h resulted in up to 90% inhibition of thymidine incorporation with a reduction in cell number by 30%–40% compared with untreated cultures; IFN apparently inhibited both the transport and phosphorylation of thymidine (GEWERT and CLEMENS 1980; GEWERT et al. 1981). HALLINAN et al. (1977) reported a seemingly paradoxical circumstance in which cell growth was inhibited but DNA synthesis was stimulated by treatment of mouse L929 cells with 0.8–80 U/ml IFN followed by arginine starvation.

EIFE et al. (1981) attempted to measure antiviral and cell growth inhibitory actions of IFN simultaneously in HeLa cells infected with vesicular stomatitis virus (VSV). Cells treated with a range of doses of IFN were infected with VSV, and 24 h later the cells were labeled with thymidine ^{3}H for 3 h. The antiviral titer was determined by inhibition of cytopathic effect (CPE), but could also be defined as the reciprocal of that dilution which gives counting rates two standard deviations above the amount of incorporation of labeled thymidine into VSV-infected controls not treated with IFN, inasmuch as IFN at this dosage level prevented the virus disruption of cellular metabolism, i.e., DNA synthesis. The anticellular dose was defined as the reciprocal of the dilution giving the maximum incorporation of thymidine ^{3}H. This seems to be a paradox since the anticellular dose is the point at which anticellular activity is really at its lowest detectable level. This assay measures the extent to which IFN can be diluted to give a defined effect, but the shape of the dose–response curve is not considered. For example HuIFN-α and HuIFN-β decrease thymidine uptake by less than 5,000 cpm at the dilution defined as the antiproliferative titer, while HuIFN-γ having the same antiproliferative titer, because it also has a peak of incorporation at the same dilution, decreased uptake of label by approximately 17,000 cpm. The sensitivity of this assay was such that it was able to detect the assigned value of the reference standard for HuIFN-α, but tenfold lower for the HuIFN-β standard. Determination of titers by cpm correlated with those by CPE.

The previous examples of the effects that IFN has on the synthesis of macromolecules in treated cells demonstrate the need for properly controlled conditions of assay. Since an effect varies with the growth state of the cell, the time of assay, etc., caution must be exercised when trying to draw correlations between the ability of IFN to inhibit growth and its ability to affect macromolecular synthesis. Studies on the inhibition of cell growth by examining effects on the stages in the cell cycle by means of radiolabeling of cellular nuclei, flow cytometry and microcinematography are discussed in Sect. C.

II. Variables in Analysis of Growth Inhibition by IFN

1. Cell Type

a) Transformed Cells

Comparisons of different cells in culture have shown differing sensitivity to the growth inhibitory activity of IFN. Clones were chosen by BORECKY et al. (1981) and HAJNICKA and BORECKY (1979) from C3H cells transformed by simian virus 40 (SV40), murine sarcoma virus (MSV), or 20-methylcholanthrene (MCH) and tested for sensitivity to mouse IFN. SV40-transformed cell clones were grouped as: (a) very sensitive, requiring 110 U IFN or less to inhibit cell growth by 30%; (b) sensitive, requiring 1,400–2,000 U; or (c) relatively insensitive, requiring more than 3,000 U for inhibition. MCH-transformed cell clones also showed a considerable range of sensitivities; while MSV-transformed cultures were all inhibited by IFN doses of 750–1,500 U. This study demonstrates the variability of IFN sensitivity found within some cell populations.

Various lymphoblastoid cell lines have been compared for sensitivity to IFN growth inhibition. Daudi cells were found to be very sensitive to inhibition by HuIFN-α (ADAMS et al. 1975; HILFENHAUS et al. 1977; HILFENHAUS and KARGES 1976a, b); other lines were less sensitive to IFN (P3HR-1 and Diehl I) while the growth of RPMI 1788 cells was only weakly inhibited by IFN. Inasmuch as the IFN dose–response curves for growth of these various cell lines were markedly different (HILFENHAUS and KARGES 1976a, b), the effect ot treatment of different cell lines with a single dosage of IFN may not be representative of cell response; for example, Raji cells give a sigmoidal dose–response curve with a sharp drop in cell number at doses of 250 U/ml while other cells give a linear response with different slopes. To complicate the interpretation of these results further, mock IFN preparations inhibited the growth of some cell lines to a limited extent while other lines were unaffected.

There was no inhibition of growth of primary human amnion cells, spontaneously transformed human amnion FL cells, and HeLa cells by IFN doses up to 1,000 U. SV40-transformed amnion cells were sensitive, such that 50 U/ml resulted in 45% inhibition, although higher doses did not increase inhibition (GAFFNEY et al. 1973). It is not clear whether the response of SV40-transformed cells represents an antiviral or strictly anticellular action of IFN.

BALKWILL and OLIVER (1977) compared the sensitivity to inhibition by IFN of cells from 12 acute myelogenous leukemia patients. There was a wide range of effects with 10,000 U/ml resulting in 7%–93% inhibition of growth. Similarly, cells from pleural effusions of breast cancer patients varied in sensitivity to HuIFN-α(Ly) (BALKWILL et al. 1978a, b) as did a variety of other human tumor cells (BRADLEY and RUSCETTI 1981; ITO and BUFFET 1981). STRANDER and EINHORN (1977) found osteosarcoma cell lines from patients' tumor suspectible to IFN, with normal fibroblastic and glial cells less sensitive than tumor cells. Tumor cells were sensitive to as little as 10 U/ml IFN, well within the levels obtainable in patients' serum after intramuscular injection (10–100 U/ml). EPSTEIN et al. (1980a, b) found no correlation between responsiveness to IFN and histologic grade of tumor cells taken from ascites fluid of patients with ovarian carcinoma.

b) Cells from Different Stages of Embryonic Development

Many of these studies have sought to compare normal cells with cells from tumors in the hope that some selective advantage in the inhibition of tumor growth could be found. Other studies have compared normal cells at various stages of development to determine whether there is a change in susceptibility during this process. DRASNER et al. (1979) studied sensitivity to IFN of primary cultures of cells taken from mouse embryos of different ages. At 10–12 days there was maximum inhibition of thymidine ^{3}H incorporation due to IFN treatment, whereas IFN (3,000 U/ml) had no inhibitory effects on cultures from embryos up to 7 days old. Cells from 8- to 9-day-old embryos showed some inhibition of thymidine incorporation. GROSSBERG and MORAHAN (1971) had made similar observations earlier, showing that cells from early chicken embryos were far less sensitive to the action of IFN than cells from older embryos. BURKE et al. (1979) showed that two undifferentiated teratocarcinoma cell lines were insensitive to the antiviral action of mouse IFN whereas differentiated cell lines were sensitive. No effect of the IFN on growth or differentiation of any of these cells was described.

c) Cells from Patients with Erythropoietic Disorders

The effect of IFN on the colony forming ability of bone marrow and peripheral blood cells from patients with disorders of erythropoiesis was examined by LUTTON and LEVERE (1980). Bone marrow cells from anemic patients with idiopathic erythroid hyperplasia were very sensitive to both HuIFN-α and -β, such that doses of 10 U/ml resulted in 50% inhibition. The response of bone marrow cells from patients with hemolytic anemia was similar to cells from normal individuals in that 100 U/ml resulted in 66%–80% inhibition. Patients those with nutritional anemia were inhibited only 25%–51% by 200 U/ml. Peripheral blood cells were found to be at least as sensitive as bone marrow cells to inhibition by IFN. Cells from sickle cell anemia patients were more sensitive than those from normal individuals.

2. Type of IFN

a) Mouse IFNs

Investigators have been interested in the relative anticellular activities of different types of IFN in relation to their antiviral potency. GRESSER et al. (1970a) examined IFNs induced in L1210 or MSV-Ia cells with ultraviolet inactivated NDV, mouse brain IFN induced by West Nile virus, or mouse serum IFN induced with NDV or poly(I)·poly(C). All of the IFN preparations had comparable antiproliferative effects against L1210 cells when used at equivalent antiviral activity. In a similar study, OHWAKI and KAWADE (1972) found NDV-induced L-cell or mouse serum IFN and Japanese encephalitis virus-induced mouse brain IFN equal in their growth inhibitory activity on L-cells.

b) Human IFNs

The majority of studies comparing IFNs have been done with human IFNs, generally, comparing HuIFN-α and HuIFN-β. In bone marrow cells, HuIFN-α and -β were equivalent in their ability to inhibit colony formation (VAN'T HULL et al.

1978). Similar effects were also found in Daudi cells, with the 50% inhibitory doses not significantly different. However, in this system HuIFN-α and HuIFN-β showed different dose–response curves (HILFENHAUS et al. 1976a, b). HuIFN-β has been found to be more inhibitory than HuIFN-α in certain cell systems, including astrocytoma (SLIMMER et al. 1981), several human tumor cell cultures (BRADLEY and RUSCETTI 1981), RSa and RSb, human embryonic fibroblast cell lines doubly transformed by Rous sarcoma virus and SV40 (KUWATA et al. 1979, 1980), and human embryo fibroblasts (LUNDGREN et al. 1979).

Conversely, LUDWIG and SWETLY (1980) have shown that bone marrow cells from multiple myeloma patients were inhibited to a greater extent by HuIFN-α than HuIFN-β. EINHORN and STRANDER (1977) suggest that the difference in sensitivity may be due to a tissue specificity of IFN. They found that HuIFN-α was significantly more inhibitory than HuIFN-β for lymphoblastoid cells, both Daudi and P3HR-1. For two osteosarcoma cell lines, HuIFN-β was more inhibitory than HuIFN-α. The reasons for these differences on Daudi cells are not clear since, as mentioned previously, HILFENHAUS et al. (1976a, b) found no difference between HuIFN-α and -β. Because the dose–response curves of HuIFN-α and -β are different, it is possible that the antiproliferative effects were measured at different portions of the curve. Comparing HuIFN-γ with HuIFN-α and HuIFN-β, BLALOCK et al. (1980) found that HuIFN-γ had 10–20 times as much activity on WISH or Hep-2 cells as HuIFN-α and HuIFN-β. HuIFN-γ also showed greater antiproliferative activity in human fibroblast (FS-4), HeLa, U amnion, and osteogenic sarcoma cells than did HuIFN-α (RUBIN and GUPTA 1982).

3. Conditions of IFN Treatment

The exact experimental conditions under which the antiproliferative action of IFNs has been tested vary, even when a similar type of assay has been used. These variations might result in differences in assay sensitivity. LEANDERSSON and LUNDGREN (1980) found that for P3HR-1 cells, a lymphoblastoid cell line, addition of IFN to stationary phase cells either 24 h before or at the time of dilution into fresh growth medium gave equivalent inhibition of cell growth, but if IFN was added to cells that were already growing exponentially, the inhibition of growth was diminished. HOROSZEWICZ et al. (1979) had similar findings with Daudi cells, with the level of inhibition ten times less when IFN was added to actively growing cells.

WEINSTEIN et al. (1977) had similar findings with con A-stimulated mouse spleen cells. The inhibitory effects were greatest when IFN was added at the time of con A addition and decreased in effectiveness over the next 18 h. This early period corresponds to the time prior to the beginning of DNA synthesis, which occurs at 18–24 h in this system. Resting cells were unaffected by IFN treatment at doses up to 2,000 U/ml as measured by DNA, RNA, or protein synthesis.

The time of treatment required for IFNs to initiate their antiproliferative action appears to vary considerably in different cell systems. Mouse L1210 cells required more than 8 h exposure (GRESSER et al. 1970b) and human bone marrow cells more than 4 h (GREENBERG and MOSNEY 1977). GLASGOW et al. (1978a) found murine osteogenic sarcoma cells required more than 24 h treatment to achieve inhibition of growth and the degree of inhibition increased as time of exposure increased. BORECKY et al. (1973) compared the time to establishment of antiviral and antiproliferative activities of IFN in L-cells; antiviral action was detected when cells were exposed for 2–4 h, but inhibition of cell growth was not seen unless cells were exposed for more than 16 h. In contrast, BRADLEY and RUSCETTI (1981) examined 55 fresh human tumor isolates, 10 tumor cell lines, and normal bone marrow cells from 12 individuals to find that 1 exposure to HuIFN-α, -β, or -γ, was equivalent to continuous prolonged exposure to IFN when tested by colony formation in soft agar. Human cells from breast cancer patients (SHIBATA and TAYLOR-PAPADIMITRIOU 1981) and RSb, a doubly transformed human cell line (KUWATA et al. 1976), were more sensitive to IFN when plated at low density than at high density

Reports vary as to the effect of serum concentration on the antiproliferative effect of IFNs. KADING et al. (1978) found that, as serum concentration increased, the effect of IFN on colony formation by L929 cells decreased. However, RATNER et al. (1980) found that the antiproliferative effect of IFN on S91 cells was independent of serum concentration. Other reports of factors affecting the antiproliferative effect of IFN include a report (MOEHRING and STINEBRING 1971) that trypsinization of cells before treatment reduces cell sensitivity, perhaps due to IFN receptor destruction. GRESSER et al. (1970 b) found that agitated cultures of L1210 cells were more susceptible to inhibition by IFN than stationary cultures.

4. Reversibility of IFN Effect

The question of whether the antiproliferative effects of IFN are reversible, or whether treated cells remain inhibited in growth after IFN is removed, reflecting some permanent cell effect, has been repeatedly investigated. Most workers have found that the effects are reversible. ADAMS et al. (1975) studying human lymphoblastoid cells, and GRESSER et al. (1970b) in L1210 cells, showed that a lag of 24 h or more occurs between the time of removal of IFN and the time when cell growth rate returns to normal. The extent of recovery may depend upon the conditions of initial treatment. Human RSb cells completely recover from 3 days of treatment with 500 U/ml IFN, but if the dosage is increased to 1,000 U/ml the cells do not recover (KUWATA et al. 1976). Incomplete recovery of growth potential was also reported for human rhabdosarcoma cells treated for 5 days with HuIFN-β (WHITMAN et al. 1980). If human breast cells were removed from IFN and plated at a relatively high density, recovery was complete, but if plated at a low density, as for a colony formation assay, recovery was limited (BALKWILL et al. 1978 a).

III. Proof That Cell Growth Inhibitor Is IFN

1. Physical/Chemical Proof

Since the first reports of inhibition of cell growth by preparations of IFN apeared in the literature, workers have tried to determine if this activity resides in the same molecule as the antiviral activity. In the first report of this activity, PAUCKER et al. (1962) found that the cell growth inhibitory activity of the mouse IFN preparation they used was trypsin sensitive, did not sediment after centrifugation at 40,000 rpm for 4 h, and showed some species specificity, since no similar activity on L-cells was detectable with a chicken IFN preparation. Other standard treatments which have been used to define a preparation as IFN in the past have also been used routinely to compare anticellular and antiviral actions of IFN preparations including pH 2 stability, relative sensitivity to heat, nondialyzable character, etc. Also common is the demonstration that a mock IFN preparation has no antiviral or anticellular effect (for example, HILFENHAUS et al. 1976; TOVEY et al. 1975).

2. Neutralization by Antiserum

A number of workers (ADAMS et al. 1975; GREENBERG and MOSNEY 1977; GLASGOW et al. 1978a, b; EPSTEIN et al. 1980c; BART et al. 1980; DEGRE and ROLLAG 1980) have demonstrated that the addition of antiserum prepared against IFN preparations can eliminate the anticellular effects of IFN. However, the specificity of this effect, of course, depends upon the purity of the antibody preparation; this in turn depends upon the purity of the IFN preparation used as antigen to induce the antibody and the degree to which the antibody is subsequently absorbed or purified away from cellular antigens. Despite the impurity of most IFN preparations, these important facts are often not presented in the papers, making evaluation of the significance of the data presented difficult.

3. Purification

Studies correlating antiviral and antiproliferative activity through the stages of purification have been useful, e.g., those studies by DAHL and her co-workers. In 1975, DAHL and DEGRE examined human IFN-α preparations ranging in specific activity from 6×10^2 to 7×10^5 U per milligram protein. Using HeLa cells or human embryonic lung cells, they assayed fractions from albumin–agarose column chromatography and found two peaks of activity, one with antiviral activity and no antiproliferative activity, and a second that inhibited cell growth but had little antiviral activity. The cell growth inhibitory peak was further characterized as dialyzable, having a molecular weight of 3,200 by Sephadex G-25 chromatography, and destroyed by 1 *M* NaCl or 4 *M* urea. Further studies (DAHL 1977a) showed that the cell growth inhibitory activity of crude HuIFN-α was not stable at pH 2, was not trypsin sensitive, and was enhanced with heating at 37° or 56 °C for 1 h. Clearly, this antiproliferative activity found in crude HuIFN-α preparations, which was also active on mouse cells, did not have the characteristics of an IFN. Another publication (DAHL 1978) confirmed these previous data, but also reported that when tested on Daudi cells, a lymphoblastoid cell line reported by others to be very sensitive to the growth inhibitory activities of IFN, the peak from the albumin–agarose column which had antiviral activity, but no anticellular activity in other cells, did inhibit proliferation. In addition, the second peak which inhibited growth of Hela and mouse cells did not inhibit Daudi cell growth. This factor merits further characterization. These studies exemplify the need for critical analysis of actions attributed to IFN in relatively crude preparations and the difficulties in comparing results from different systems.

Further purification of HuIFN-α has confirmed that the anticellular and antiviral activities are found in the same molecular fractions. HuIFN-α was separated into two peaks by SDS gel electrophoresis, of 15,000 and 20,000 daltons, each having antiviral and cell growth inhibitory action (STEWART et al. 1976). Under reducing conditions, achieved by treatment with mercaptoethanol, antiviral and anticellular activities of the 15,000 daltons species were lost simultaneously. Similar results were also reported for mouse IFN.

BERG and HERON (1980) purified HuIFN-α through several steps, including concentration by potassium thiocyanate precipitation, gel filtration, copper chelate chromatography, Blue Sepharose chromatography, antibody affinity chromatography, and finally SDS–polyacrylamide gel electrophoresis. Five peaks of activity in the resulting preparation had a total specific activity of 10^8 U per milligram protein. All five peaks had anticellular activity that correlated with antiviral activity. Further separation of HuIFN-α by high pressure liquid chromatography resolved HuIFN-α into ten peaks with anticellular activity, some of which had no antiviral activity, and some with both antiviral and anticellular activities (EVINGER et al. 1981). These peaks could correspond to the products of numerous genes detected for HuIFN-α (ALLEN and FANTES 1980) in human cells.

MASUCCI et al. (1980) were able to produce HuIFN-α from *Escherichia coli* into which they had introduced a plasmid containing a HuIFN-α gene. These authors compared the rDNA-derived IFN product with HuIFN-α from human leukocytes and found that both inhibited replication of Daudi cells. The anticellular and antiviral activities of HuIFN-β purified together (WHITMAN et al. 1980).

Mouse IFNs have also been characterized by copurification of antiviral and cell growth inhibitory actions. OHWAKI and KAWADE (1972) and BORECKY et al. (1972) purified MuIFN from L-cells and peritoneal leukocytes, respectively, separating these IFNs into two components by pH 4.3 polyacrylamide gel electrophoresis. Both groups found that the fast moving component (probably-α) had a proportionately lower anticellular: antiviral ratio than the slower moving component (probably-β). Further studies of these two components of L-cell IFN showed that the slow component had ten times the anticellular activity of the fast component (MATSUZAWA and KAWADE 1974). Storage at −20 °C resulted in a loss of antiviral activity in the fast component, but no loss in growth inhibitory action, resulting in equal anticellular: antiviral activity ratios of the fast and slow components after storage.

FUCHSBERGER et al. (1975) found that the fast component had more cell growth inhibitory activity on 16-h-old cultures of L-cells than on 3-day-old cultures and suggested that the cells may change in binding capacity with age. IWAKURA et al. (1978) purified L-cell IFN and attained fast and slow peaks with specific activities of 3×10^8 and 2×10^8 U/mg, respectively. They did not detect the differences in antiviral and anticellular activity seen in earlier, less purified, preparations. Separating L-cell IFN preparations by a different method from that used by the previous workers, i.e., SDS treatment followed by gel filtration of sephadex G-25, DEGRE (1980) found two peaks of cell growth inhibitory activity, one with antiviral activity and one without. GRESSER et al. (1973) compared four NDV-induced L-cell IFN preparations and one MM virus-induced preparation, all purified by different methods to achieve specific activities $\geqq 1.6 \times 10^7$ U/mg. These workers found that not only were the dose–response curves for antiviral and anticellular actions parallel, but the kinetics of appearance of these two activities were similar.

4. Cell Mutants Resistant to IFN

Cells which show resistance to the antiproliferative effects of IFN have been isolated. GRESSER et al. (1974) selected two subclones of L1210 cells, one sensitive to the antiproliferative action of IFN, L1210S, and one resistant, L1210R. L1210R cells were shown to be resistant to 400,000 U in 0.2 ml. They were also resistant to the antiviral action of IFN. When these cells were treated with IFN and then disrupted, no detectable IFN could be recovered from L1210R cells, but a very small fraction of the original dose was recovered from L1210S cells, suggesting that L1210R cells do not efficiently bind IFN. ANKEL et al. (1980) confirmed the IFN resistance of L1210R cells and showed that this resistance was not due to any factor produced by these cells and shed into the medium. KUWATA et al. (1976) isolated a resistant line of human RSa cells (IFr) the growth of which was not inhibited by HuIFN-α. However, these cells were similar to the original RSa line in sensitivity to antiviral action. As with L1210R, fewer units of IFN could be recovered from these cells after treatment. In addition, a second resistant line was isolated, F-IFr, which was less resistant to HuIFN-β than to HuIFN-α.

Attempts have been made to determine what accounts for resistance by comparing IFN-resistant cells with normally sensitive cells. RSa IFr cells were found to be similar in agglutinability by con A; however, HuIFN-α or -β was found to enhance the binding of con A to control RSa cells, but not to resistant IFr cells (KUWATA et al. 1980). FUSE and KUWATA (1979) showed that cholera toxin reduced the antiviral action of IFN when given simultaneously to RSa cells, but had no effect on the cell growth inhibition by IFN. A cell line resistant to both antiviral and anticellular effects of IFN (IFr-V1) reacted similarly, merely requiring more IFN to give the same results. There was no correlation found between sensitivity to IFN and sensitivity to cholera toxin.

The growth inhibition of IFN in RSa cells was enhanced by treatment with ouabain, a cardiac glycoside which inhibits Na^+, K^+-ATPase, protein synthesis, and DNA synthesis (KUWATA et al. 1977a). Ouabain action was reversible and if it was removed from IFr cells simultaneously treated with IFN, growth recovered. This agent reduced the antiviral action of IFN in both control and resistant cells (KUWATA et al. 1977a and DAHL 1980). ITO and BUFFET (1981) found some human tumor cell lines to be very resistant to the antiproliferative action of IFN while being quite sensitive to the antiviral action. Relative sensitivities to these two activities varied greatly from one cell line to another; for example, thymidine uptake in RT-4 cells from urinary bladder carcinoma was inhibited by 50% by 28 U/ml HuIFN-β, while colon adenocarcinoma cells, HT-29, did not show this inhibition at 5,000 U/ml. Yet for these two cell lines, the amounts of IFN which reduced CPE due to VSV by 50% were similar, i.e., 9.4 and 18.6 U/ml, respectively.

C. Effects of IFN on Cell Cycle

Several methods have been used to evaluate what effect IFN treatment has on the progression of cells through the cell cycle. MACIEIRA-COELHO et al. (1971) compared incorporation of thymidine ^3H in untreated L1210 cells with IFN-treated cells. The fraction of interphase cells that were labeled after 48 h of IFN treatment showed a slower increase than in controls not treated with IFN. In addition, the rate of cells entering mitosis, as detected in colicimid-blocked cells, was similar in

Table 1. Inhibition of cell growth by human interferon

Cells	Interferon	Assay	Reference
Epstein–Barr virus-transformed lymphoblastoid	HuIFN-α (Le)	Cell count	Adams et al. (1975) Attallah et al. (1981) Dahl (1978) Dahl and Degre (1976) Einhorn and Strander (1977) Evinger and Pestka (1980) Evinger et al. (1981) Hilfenhaus and Karges (1976) Masucci et al. (1980) Stewart et al. (1976)
		DNA synthesis	Berg and Heron (1980) Hilfenhaus et al. (1976, 1977) Hilfenhaus and Karges (1976) Leandersson and Lundgren (1980)
	HuIFN-α (Ly)	Cell count	Gewert et al. (1981)
	HuIFN-β	Cell count	Dahl and Degre (1976) Einhorn and Strander (1977) Hilfenhaus et al. (1976) Hilfenhaus and Karges (1976) Horoszewicz et al. (1979) Knight (1976)
Normal lymphocytes	HuIFN-α (Le)	Cell count and DNA synthesis	Balkwill and Oliver (1977)
B- and T-cells	HuIFN-α (Ly)	DNA and RNA synthesis	Attallah et al. (1980 a, b)
Bone Marrow	HuIFN-α (Le)	Cell count and DNA synthesis	Balkwill and Oliver (1977) Greenberg and Mosney (1977) Nissen et al. (1977) Van't Hull et al. (1978)
	HuIFN-α (Ly)	Colony formation	Bradley and Ruscetti (1981) Ludwig and Swetly (1980) Nagano and Saito (1979 a)
	HuIFN-β	Colony formation	Bradley and Ruscetti (1981) Nagano and Saito (1979 a) Van't Hull et al. (1978)
Leukemia cells	HuIFN-α (Le)	Cell count and DNA synthesis	Balkwill and Oliver (1977)
RPMI 1196	HuIFN-α (Ly)	Cell count	Cantell (1970)
Primary tumor cells and tumor cell lines	HuIFN-α (Ly), -β	Colony formation	Bradley and Ruscetti (1981)
Pleural effusions and breast tissue	HuIFN-α (Ly)	Cell count and colony formation	Balkwill et al. (1978 a, b) Shibata and Taylor-Papadimitriou (1981)
Prostatic cells	HuIFN-β	DNA synthesis	Chawda et al. (1979)
Melanoma cells	HuIFN-α (Ly)	Cell count	Creasy et al. (1980 a, b, 1981)

Table 1 (continued)

Cells	Interferon	Assay	Reference
RSa, RSb	HuIFN-α (Le)	Cell count and DNA synthesis	DAHL (1980) KUWATA et al. (1976, 1977a, b, 1979, 1980) FUSE and KUWATA (1979)
	HuIFN-β	Cell count	KUWATA et al. (1977b, 1980)
Osteosarcoma	HuIFN-α (Le)	Cell count	EINHORN and STRANDER (1977) STRANDER and EINHORN (1977)
	HuIFN-β	Cell count	EINHORN and STRANDER (1977) ITO and BUFFET (1981)
Ovarian carcinoma	HuIFN-α (Le)	Colony formation	EPSTEIN et al. (1980b, c)
Amnion	HuIFN-α (Le)	Cell count	DAHL (1978) DAHL and DEGRE (1976)
	HuIFN-β	Cell count	DAHL and DEGRE (1976)
Transformed amnion	HuIFN-α (Le) or amnion	Cell count or DNA synthesis	GAFFNEY et al. (1973)
T98G, glioblastoma multiforme	HuIFN-α (Le)	Cell count	INGLOT et al. (1980)
RT-4, urinary bladder carcinoma and HT-29, colon adenocarcinoma	HuIFN-β	Cell count	ITO and BUFFET (1981)
Rhabdomyosarcoma	HuIFN-β	Cell count	WHITMAN et al. (1980)
Astrocytoma	HuIFN-α (Le)	Cell count	SLIMMER et al. (1981)
U 937, macrophage-like	HuIFN-α (Ly), -β	DNA synthesis	ATTALLAH et al. (1981)
Embryonic lung	HuIFN-α (Le)	Cell count	DAHL (1977a) DAHL and DEGRE (1975, 1976)
	HuIFN-α (Le)	DNA synthesis	FUSE and KUWATA (1979)
	HuIFN-β	Cell count	DAHL and DEGRE (1976)
Foreskin fibroblast	HuIFN-α (Le), -γ	Cell count and DNA synthesis	RUBIN and GUPTA (1980)
	HuIFN-β	Cell count	ITO and BUFFET (1981) KNIGHT (1976) MOEHRING and STINEBRING (1971) PFEFFER et al. (1979) RUBIN and GUPTA (1980)
Embryonic fibroblast	HuIFN-α (Le)	Cell count and DNA synthesis	LEE et al. (1972) LUNDGREN et al. (1979)
	HuIFN-β	Cell count and DNA synthesis	LUNDGREN et al. (1979)

Table 1 (continued)

Cells	Interferon	Assay	Reference
HeLa	HuIFN-α (Le)	Cell count	LEE et al. (1972)
	HuIFN-α (Le)	DNA synthesis	EIFE et al. (1981)
WISH and Hep-2	HuIFN-α (Le), -γ	Colony formation	BLALOCK et al. (1980)
Mouse myeloma/human lymphoma B-lymphocyte hybrids	HuIFN-α (Le)	Cell count	SIKORA et al. (1980)

Table 2. Inhibition of cell growth by mouse interferon

Cells	Interferon	Assay method	Reference
L1210 mouse leukemia cells	C243	Cell count	AUGET and BLANCHARD (1981) GRESSER et al. (1979) STEWART et al. (1976) TOVEY et al. (1975)
	MSV-Ia	Cell count	GRESSER et al. (1974a) MACIEIRA-COEHLO et al. (1971) GRESSER et al. (1970a, b)
	Mouse serum	Cell count	GRESSER et al. (1970a)
	L-cell	Cell count	GRESSER et al. (1974) GRESSER et al. (1973)
	L-cell	Colony formation	GRESSER et al. (1973)
	MSV-Ia	Colony formation	GRESSER et al. (1971)
L-cells	L-cell	Cell count	FUCHSBERGER et al. (1975) IWAKURA et al. (1978) KNIGHT (1973) OHWAKI and KAWADE (1972) PAUKER et al. (1962) KADING et al. (1978)
	L-cell	DNA synthesis	MATSUZAWA and KAWADE (1974)
	MSV-Ia	Cell count	LINDAHL-MAGNUSSON et al. (1971)
	Mouse serum	Cell count	BARON et al. (1966)
	Peritoneal macrophage	Protein synthesis	BORECKY et al. (1972) BORECKY et al. (1973)
L929	C243	Cell count	INGLOT et al. (1980)
B16 melanoma	L-cell	Cell count	BART et al. (1980) FISHER et al. (1981) JAMESON et al. (1981)
S91	Ehrlich ascites	Cell count	RATNER et al. (1980)

Table 2 (continued)

Cells	Interferon	Assay method	Reference
C3H transformed	L-cell	Cell count	BORECKY et al. (1980, 1981) HAJNICKA and BORECKY (1979)
Embryonic cells	L-cell	DNA synthesis	BOURGEADE and CHANY (1979)
	L-cell	Cell count	OHWAKI and KAWADE (1972)
	C243	DNA synthesis	DRASNER et al. (1979)
	MSV-Ia or brain	Cell count	LINDAHL-MAGNUSSON (1971)
Fibroblast	L-cell	DNA synthesis	BUFFET et al. (1978) CZARNIECKI et al. (1981) KIMCHI et al. (1981 a) SOKAWA et al. (1977) WATANABE and SOKAWA (1978)
		Cell count	BUFFET et al. (1978) CZARNIECKI et al. (1981)
		Colony formation	BUFFET et al. (1978)
Osteosarcoma	L-cell	Cell count and DNA synthesis	DEGRE (1980)
	C243	Colony formation	GLASGOW et al. (1978 a, b)
		DNA synthesis	GLASGOW et al. (1978 b)
EMT6	C243	Cell count	D'HOOGHE et al. (1977)
Bone marrow cells	Serum	Colony formation	FLEMING et al. (1972) MCNEIL and FLEMING (1971) MCNEIL and GRESSER (1973)
	L-cell	Colony formation	MCNEIL and GRESSER (1973) VAN'T HULL et al. (1978)
	Brain	Colony formation	MCNEIL and GRESSER (1973)
Peritoneal macrophage	L-cell	Cell count	FUCHSBERGER et al. (1974) ROLLAG and DEGRE (1981)
	Peritoneal macrophage	Cell count	FUCHSBERGER et al. (1974)
	Serum	Cell count	ROLLAG and DEGRE (1981)
CSVp	L-cell	Cell count	FUCHSBERGER et al. (1975)
3T3	L-cell	Cell count	KNIGHT (1973) OHWAKI and KAWADI (1972)
Friend leukemia		Cell count and DNA synthesis	MATARESE and ROSSI (1977)
Ehrlich ascites	L-cell	Cell count	NAGANO and SAITO (1979 a, 1981) PANNIERS and CLEMENS (1981)
S180 and myeloblasts	L-cell	Cell count	NAGANO and SAITO (1979 a)
Lymphocytes	L-cell	DNA synthesis	WEINSTEIN et al. (1977)

treated and control cells for approximately 4 h, after which the rate leveled off in treated cells. These results indicate that IFN delays entry of cells into the growth cycle.

SOKAWA et al. (1977) found similar effects in BALB/c3T3 cells, in which the labeling index, the number of cells with thymidine ^{3}H-labeled nuclei, in IFN-treated cultures as detected by autoradiography, was decreased. These authors showed that the addition of IFN at different times after serum stimulation of cells had different effects. If added within 4 h of stimulation, the effect was maximal, decreasing the probability of a cell entering S phase from 0.13/h in controls to 0.036/h in treated cells. If IFN was added after cells were beginning to enter S phase, no effects were detected. MATARESE and ROSSI (1977) also reported decreased entry into S phase of IFN-treated Friend leukemia cells. Total cell cycle time, normally 16 h, was increased by approximately 4 h.

BALKWILL et al. (1978a), using autoradiography of labeled cell nuclei and cytofluorimetry in cells from human breast tissue, found approximately 20% fewer cells in S phase in IFN-treated cultures and a small increase in both G1 and G2 phases after IFN treatment, with all phases of the cell cycle increasing in duration. BALKWILL and TAYLOR-PAPADIMITRIOU (1978) examined mouse and human cells synchronized by serum depletion followed by serum stimulation. The peak of labeling index and mitotic index, number of cells with labeled mitotic figures, were both delayed 4–8 h by IFN treatment, indicating a delayed entry into both S and M phases. The duration of this delay was dose dependent. Confirmation of these findings for both HuIFN-α and HuIFN-β was obtained by LUNDGREN et al. (1979) using synchronized human embryonic fibroblast cells; the greatest effects were found when IFN was added early in G1 phase. Similar observations were made in BALB/c3T3 cells (WATANABE and SOKAWA 1978), Ehrlich ascites, and S180 cells (NAGANO and SAITO 1979a). D'HOOGHE et al. (1977) and PFEFFER et al. (1979) used cinematography to study the effects of IFN on individual cells. Doubling times were increased by 10%–40%, with the effects becoming evident only after several days of incubation.

Creasy et al. (1981) examined the effects of IFN on cell cycle using microfluorometry, in which cells are heat and acid treated to cause denaturation, and stained with acridine orange (cells in G0 give a red fluorescence and those in G1 give a green fluorescence). Some of the human melanoma cell lines they studied were resistant to IFN inhibition of growth and these cells had no G0 phase in their normal cell cycle. They interpreted their results to mean that the duration of G0 phase or number of cells present in G0 at any time did not correlate with sensitivity, but that a G0 phase was necessary for IFN inhibition.

In summary, it appears that IFN is most active when contact with cells is during a gap period (G0, G1, or G2 phases) and that cells rapidly synthesizing DNA (S phase) or undergoing mitosis (M phase) are least sensitive to growth inhibition by IFN.

D. Other Cellular Effects of IFN

For a summary of the effects of IFN on a variety of cell functions see Table 3.

I. Morphology

RICH (1981) reported a morphological alteration in IFN-treated cells. Treatment of Raji lymphoblastoid cells with HuIFN-α or -β resulted in the appearance of lupus inclusions, abnormal microtubule structures found in the reticuloendothelial cells of patients suffering from autoimmune disease, neoplasias, immunodeficiencies, or systemic lupus erythematosus. No inhibition of cellular growth was detected in cells showing these inclusions. The morphological changes which normally accompany the differentiation of 3T3-L1 fibroblasts to adipocytes, i.e., changes in microfilaments and accumulation of lipids in vacuoles are inhibited by IFN (GROSSBERG et al. 1981). Other effects on cell cytoskeleton and cell membrane changes are described in Sect. D.VIII.

II. Mobility

Cellular mobility has also been reported to be inhibited by IFN. The mobility of bovine endothelial cells, stimulated to move by extracts from tumor cells, was inhibited by as little as 6.4 U IFN (BROUTY-BOYE and ZETTER 1980). The movement of human fibroblast cells, studied by cinemicrography, was decreased to 44% of controls after 24–36 h of IFN treatment (TAMM et al. 1981).

III. Physiologic Cell Responses to IFN

The beat frequency of cultured mouse myocardial cells treated with 0.3–33 U/ml mouse IFN was increased relative to untreated cells (BLALOCK and STANTON 1980). LAMPIDIS and BROUTY-BOYE (1981) report opposite findings with postmitotic rat cardiac cells in culture; the beat rate was decreased in a dose-dependent manner by rat or mouse IFN. Several differences between conditions used in these two studies may help to explain the findings. BLALOCK and STANTON (1980) studied cells 24 h after trypsinization at room temperature and at high pH. LAMPIDIS and BROUTY-BOYE (1981) allowed cells to grow and stabilize for 7 days after trypsinization before IFN treatment. Temperature and pH were maintained at physiologic conditions. LAMPIDIS and BROUTY-BOYE were able to prevent increased beating rate with antibody to mouse IFN. Rat neurons, upon exposure to rat IFN exhibited an increase in the frequency of discharges CALVERT and GRESSER (1979).

IV. Phagocytosis

Phagocytosis by macrophages is enhanced by IFN (HUANG 1977). IFN-treated cells stimulated to phagocytize colloidal carbon particles (HUANG et al. 1971), latex particles (IMANISHI et al. 1975), or nonopsonized *E. coli* (ROLLAY and DEGRE 1981) ingest more particles than do untreated cells.

V. Interaction with Chemicals or Factors Affecting Growth

The interaction of IFN with colony stimulating factor has been examined by several workers. This factor, found in conditioned medium from several cell sources, stimulated bone marrow cells to grow in soft agar. IFN has been shown in several studies to inhibit this stimulation (MCNEIL and FLEMING 1971; FLEMING et al. 1972; MCNEIL and GRESSER 1973; and GREENBERG and MOSNEY 1977). IFN was found to act in opposition to platelet growth factor in mouse or human cells (INGLOT et al. 1980). Stimulation of L929 mouse or T986, human glioblastoma multiforme cells with this growth factor was reduced by IFN; and at the same time treatment with growth factor reduced the antiviral and cell growth inhibitory actions of IFNs.

The interaction of IFN with additional chemical agents which affect cellular activities has been studied to a limited extent. FISHER et al. (1981) found that, in clone C3 of B16 mouse melanoma, tumor promoters decreased the initiation of melanin production. IFN was found to inhibit this cellular change and the effect was additive with the tumor promoters, 12-O-tetradecanoylphorbol-B-acetate (TPA) and phorbol-12,13-didecanoate (PDD). As with most other effects, IFN was most effective when treatment of cells was begun early. The interaction of IFN and sodium butyrate on normal and MSV-transformed embryonic mouse cells was examined by BOURGEADE and CHANY (1979). Butyrate decreased the multiplication of transformed cells. IFN alone had little effect on these cells, but in combination with butyrate, DNA synthesis was greatly reduced. In normal embryonic cells, IFN decreased DNA synthesis to a limited extent, but the extent of this decrease was unaltered by butyrate treatment.

VI. Anticellular Effects of 2′,5′-Oligonucleotide

In view of the considerable evidence (KERR et al. 1981) that the antiviral action of IFN is mediated to some degree by the oligonucleotide, 2′,5′-oligo-(A) (2-5A) some studies have been done on the growth inhibitory potential of this compound. HOVANESSIAN and WOOD (1980) showed that 2-5A inhibited protein synthesis within 30 min of treatment, RNA and DNA synthesis was inhibited later, but by 48 h all macromolecular synthesis had returned to normal. DNA synthesis in serum-stimulated, synchronized BALB/c3T3 cells was delayed by treatment with 2-5A (KIMCHI et al. 1981 a). Like IFN, 2-5A was most effective when added early in G1. NIH/3T3 clone 1 cells which lack RNase F, the endonuclease stimulated by IFN, were found to be resistant to the antiviral and cell growth inhibitory actions of IFN. KIMCHI et al. (1981 b) have also reported that 2-5A inhibits the con A-induced mitogenesis of mouse spleen cells. Other effects of 2-5A are discussed in Chap. 8.

VII. Effect on Synthesis of Specific Proteins

Alterations in the expression of specific proteins as a result of exposure to IFN have also been reported. Cells treated with 500 U/ml HuIFN-α or -β expressed more β_2-microglobulin than untreated cells, but the levels of IgM and T-lymphocyte antigens were not altered (HERON et al. 1978). FELLOWS et al. (1981) found that human IFN-α treatment of Ramos cells, a Burkitt's lymphoma cell line sensitive to the antiviral action of IFN, caused increased levels of β_2-microglobulin in the culture medium and membrane extracts. In contrast, treatment of Namalwa cells, which are insensitive to HuIFN-α antiviral action, did not cause an increase in β_2-microglobulin in either the culture medium or cell membrane extracts (FELLOWS et al. 1981).

Carcinoembryonic antigen (CEA) expression was stimulated by a dose of 500 U IFN in a human colon cell line, but RNA synthesis was not affected. Although the increase in CEA was variable at this dose, ranging from 20% to 400%, with

5,000 U IFN a constant 200% to 300% increase in CEA expression was observed (ATTALLAH et al. 1979).

The induction of ornithine decarboxylase, a critical enzyme in the synthesis of polyamines, in quiescent serum-stimulated cultures of Swiss mouse 3T3 cells was inhibited by mouse IFN in a dose-dependent manner (SREEVALSAN et al. 1981). In addition, increases in *S*-adenosylmethionine decarboxylase activity resulting from serum stimulation was also inhibited by addition of mouse IFN at the time of serum addition.

The hormonal induction of glutamine synthetase in chicken embryo neuroretina in vitro is also inhibited by IFN treatment while the levels of lactate dehydrogenase and acetylcholinesterase were not affected (MATSUNO et al. 1976). The mechanism by which this suppression takes place has been analyzed in detail (MATSUNO and SHIRASAWA 1978; SHIRASAWA and MATSUNO 1979). Immunoprecipitation of radiolabeled glutamine synthetase was reduced in hydrocortisone-induced cultures treated with IFN. IFN treatment resulted in an inhibition of biosynthesis and accumulation of glutamine synthetase. However, there was no inhibition of generalized protein synthesis, as monitored by leucine ^{3}H incorporation into trichloroacetic acid-precipitable material (MATSUNO and SHIRASAWA 1978). The inhibition of enzyme synthesis in IFN-treated, hydrocortisone-induced neuroretinal cultures has been related to decreased levels of glutamine synthetase mRNA associated with polysomes (SHIRASAWA and MATSUNO 1979). However, it still is not clear whether there is a reduction in the total number of mRNA molecules, indicative of inhibition by IFN at the level of transcription. The addition of dimethylsulfoxide (DMSO) to logarithmic phase cultures of Friend leukemia cells results in a 5- to 10-fold increase in ornithine decarboxylase activity. The addition of IFN at a dose which will inhibit erythroid differentiation of these cells (50,000 U/ml) inhibited the increase of the decarboxylase normally seen 3 h after inducer addition (GAZITT and FRIEND 1980).

VIII. Cell Membrane-Associated Changes

Several studies suggest that plasma membrane changes occur in cells treated with IFN. The release of budding virus by RNA tumor virus-transformed cells is inhibited by IFN and appears to be mediated at the membrane level (FRIEDMAN 1981). In addition, an alteration in the binding of cholera toxin to mouse Ly cells is altered after exposure to IFN (CHANG et al. 1978). Terminal galactose residues in the oligosaccharide of some membrane glycoproteins were apparently exposed after IFN treatment in the absence of an effect on ganglioside pattern as determined by thin layer chromatography (CHANG et al. 1978).

Cap formation (i.e., the lateral movement of membrane-bound lectin to accumulate at one site in the membrane) by con A phytohemagglutinin or soybean agglutinin on mouse splenocytes or lymph node cells was found to be inhibited more than 50% by treatment with 300 U/ml L-cell IFN. This inhibition was rapidly reversible and capping occurred normally within 60 min of IFN removal. The effect was apparently mediated by IFN binding to the cell membrane. Heterologous species IFN or heat-inactivated IFN did not inhibit capping (MATSUYAMA 1979).

The level of expression of H-2 antigens was altered on the surface of IFN-treated lymphoid and nonlymphoid cells (KILLANDER et al. 1976; VIGNAUX and GRESSER 1978). Whereas the multiplication of mouse L1210 cells upon exposure to 600 U/

ml mouse IFN was inhibited by more than 50%, the histocompatibility antigen expression was stimulated (KILLANDER et al. 1976). In addition, the expression of H-2 antigens on the surface of mouse embryo fibroblasts was enhanced by exposure to C243 mouse IFN (10,000 U/ml). Human and rabbit IFNs did not cause any enhancement of H-2 antigen expression by these cells (VIGNAUX and GRESSER 1978). Both the mixture MuIFN-α/β and MuIFN-γ stimulated mouse thymus and spleen cell expression of H-2Dd antigen. MuIFN-γ induced by BCG in vivo stimulated expression of H-2Ks antigen up to fivefold at a dose of 300 U per culture; the H-2 antigen enhancement activity by IFN was shown to be pH 2 labile and stable at 56 °C. MuIFN-α/β did not affect H-2Ks expression (SONNENFELD et al. 1981).

IFN-treated cells undergo ultrastructural changes (PFEFFER et al. 1980; WERENNE et al. 1980; GROSSBERG et al. 1981). The cytoskeleton of human fibroblasts, FS and ME, was dramatically altered by exposure to 640 U/ml HuIFN-β. The proportion of cells with prominent actin fibers was increased to more than 40% in IFN-treated cells. Less than 5% of the control cells had obvious actin cables. The number of actin fibers per cell was increased compared with control cells. In addition, the distribution of fibronectin was altered in IFN-treated cells, with fibronectin being found in long filaments over the entire cell surface in contrast to control cells, where the network is located primarily at points of cell–cell contact. These changes were correlated with a reduction in cell motility and intracellular movement by ME cells after IFN treatment (PFEFFER et al. 1980).

Further ultrastructural characterization of IFN action on cell surfaces indicates that attachment of HuIFN-β to human carcinoma KB cells results in a decrease in receptors on the cell surface for diphtheria toxin, although IFN and the toxin do not share receptors (KUSHNARYOV et al. 1982). Lysosome fragility in IFN-treated mouse cells resulted in the release of lysosomal hydrolases (HALBACH et al. 1978; WERENNE et al. 1980). The uptake and release of horseradish peroxidase by IFN-treated L1210 cells was altered, leading to the conclusion that exocytosis, i.e., the externalization of the contents of phagocytic vacuoles, accompanied by a recycling of membrane components, was affected by treatment with IFN (WERENNE et al. 1980).

In addition to its effects on proteins associated with the cell membrane and proteins comprising the cytoskeleton, IFN has been shown to affect the composition of the cell membrane itself (APOSTOLOV and BARKER 1981; CHANDRABOSE et al. 1981). Human MRC-5 cells, bovine kidney cells, and chicken embryo fibroblasts were exposed to appropriate IFNs and changes in the ratio of fatty acids separated by gas–liquid chromatography were determined (APOSTOLOV and BARKER 1981). Increases in saturated fatty acid content of MRC-5 membranes occurred 10–12 h after addition of IFN. A decrease in saturated fatty acid content followed 20–22 h after addition. By 72 h after addition of IFN, the ratio of saturated to unsaturated fatty acids in the cell membranes returned to control values. The effect appeared to be mediated by IFN as antibody to HuIFN-α (Ly) inhibited the effect of HuIFN-α by 98%. Increasing doses of IFN resulted in a greater increase in the ratio of saturated to unsaturated fatty acids 12 h after addition of IFN (APOSTOLOV and BARKER 1981). The fatty acid composition of S180 cell phospholipids was also altered to a more saturated state by treatment with mouse IFN (CHANDRABOSE et al. 1981).

IX. IFN Effects on Cyclic Nucleotides

Tovey et al. (1979) using steady state cultures of L1210 mouse leukemia cells treated with IFN, measured intracellular cyclic nucleotide concentrations. Steady state cultures of L1210 cells are characterized by constant intracellular concentrations of cAMP, cGMP, DNA, RNA, and protein and constant rates of incorporation of thymidine, uridine, and amino acids. Tovey et al. (1979) and Tovey and Rochette-Egly (1980) found that within 10 min after IFN addition, a 2- to 4-fold increase in intracellular cGMP was detected. The cGMP concentration returned to the steady state level between 10 and 30 min later. No increase in cAMP concentration was found during the first 5 h of exposure to IFN (Tovey et al. 1979). However, a 2- to 3.8-fold increase in cAMP concentration was found 24 h after addition of IFN concomitant with the inhibition of cell multiplication.

X. IFN Effects on Prostaglandin Synthesis

Human fibroblasts treated with 100 U/ml human fibroblast IFN produced 15-fold more prostaglandin E (PGE) than untreated cells (Yaron et al. 1977). The increase in PGE production was noted within 3 h after addition and peaked at 24 h after addition. HuIFN-α (Ly) was also effective in stimulating prostaglandin synthesis by human foreskin fibroblast cell lines. Mouse IFN did not stimulate PGE production in either primary human fibroblasts or foreskin fibroblast cell strains.

XI. IFN Effects on Steroidogenesis

The Y-1 cell line (mouse adrenal tumor) ketosteroid secretion increases 2.5- to 3-fold upon treatment of these cells with mouse IFN (5,000 U) (Chany et al. 1980b). At doses of IFN ranging from 2,500 to 10,000 U, cell rounding was induced (Chany et al. 1980b; Blalock and Harp 1981). An increase in cAMP concentration was also induced within 1 h after exposure to IFN (Chany et al. 1980a, b). Chany et al. (1980a) also reported a dissociation between antiviral activity of IFN and its effect on steroid production: the maximal antiviral effect was observed with doses of IFN ranging from 62 to 15,000 U, but in contrast, steroid production was stimulated by doses of IFN ranging from 3,800 to 15,000 U.

G. Effects of IFN on Cellular Differentiation

As can be seen from Table 4, IFN may affect cellular differentiation in several ways.

I. Fibroblast–Adipocyte Conversion

The mouse 3T3-L1 clonal derivative isolated from the 3T3 fibroblast line (Green and Kehinde 1974; Green 1978) normally differentiates into lipid-containing adipocytes upon cessation of cell growth. IFN treatment of insulin-stimulated 3T3-L1 cells resulted in morphological arrest at the fibroblast stage (Keay and Grossberg 1980) and marked decreases in the rates of synthesis and accumulation of triglycerides, cholesterol esters, and cholesterol compared with insulin-stimulated con-

Table 3. Effects of interferon on cell function

Effects on	Cells	Reference
Cellular membrane	Ly cells	Chang et al. (1978)
	AKR, C-cells, L-cells	Friedman (1981)
	Lymph node cells	Matsuyama (1979)
Fatty acid composition	S180 cells	Chandrabose et al. (1981)
	MRC-5 cells	Apostolov and Barker (1981)
	Chick fibroblasts	Apostolov and Barker (1981)
Steroidogenesis	Y-1 mouse adrenal tumor	Blalock and Harp (1981)
		Chany et al. (1980a, b)
CEA expression	WiDr human colon carcinoma cell line	Attallah et al. (1979)
Beat frequency	Mouse myocardial cells	Blalock and Stanton (1980)
		Lampidis and Brouty-Boye (1981)
Neuron excitability	Kitten neurons	Calvet and Gresser (1979)
Prostaglandin synthesis	Human fibroblasts	Yaron et al. (1977)
	L929 cells	Fitzpatrick and Stringfellow (1980)
	Hamster cells	Fitzpatrick and Stringfellow (1980)
	Chicken kidney cells	Fitzpatrick and Stringfellow (1980)
β_2-Microglobulin	Ramos (Burkitt's lymphoma cell line)	Fellows et al. (1981)
	BJAB (Burkit's lymphoma cell line)	Heron et al. (1978)
Lysosome fragility	L929 mouse cells	Halbach et al. (1978)
Histocompatibility antigens	L1210 mouse cells	Killander et al. (1976)
H-2 antigens	Mouse embryo fibroblasts	Vignaux and Gresser (1978)
	Mouse thymus and spleen cells	Sonnenfeld et al. (1981)
Ornithine decarboxylase	3T3 mouse cells	Lee et al. (1980)
		Sreevalsan et al. (1980)
		Sreevalsan et al. (1981)
Erythroid colony formation	Bone marrow cells	Lutton and Levere (1980)
		McNeil and Fleming (1977)
Cytochrome P-450	Rat or mouse (in vivo)	Mannering et al. (1980)
Cytoskeleton	FS-4 human fibroblasts	Pfeffer et al. (1980)
	ME human fibroblasts	Pfeffer et al. (1980)
Cylic nucleotides	L1210 mouse leukemia cells	Tovey et al. (1979)
		Tovey and Rochette-Egly (1980)
	RSa cells	Fuse and Kuwata (1978)
Gangliosides	L-cells	Vengris et al. (1980)
	BALB/c3T3 cells	Vengris et al. (1980)
Granulopoiesis	Bone marrrow cells	Verma et al. (1979)
Cell motility	L1210 cells	Werenne et al. (1980)
	FS-4 human fibroblasts	Pfeffer et al. (1980)
	ME human fibroblasts	Pfeffer et al. (1980)
rRNA metabolism	Human fibroblasts (trisomy 21)	Maroun (1978)

Table 3 (continued)

Effects on	Cells	Reference
Protein synthesis and degradation	Ehrlich ascites tumor cells	PANNIERS and CLEMENS (1980)
DNA synthesis	RSa-transformed human fibroblasts	FUSE and KUWATA (1978) VANDENBUSSCHE et al. (1981)
	3T3 mouse fibroblasts	SREEVALSAN et al. (1980)
	Thymocytes (rat or mouse)	SELA and GURARI-ROTMAN (1978)
	FS-4 human cells	RUBIN and GUPTA (1980)
	L929 cells	HALLINAN et al. (1977)
	Mouse embryo cells	DRASNER et al. (1979)
	WiDr human colon carcinoma cells	ATTALLAH et al. (1979)
	Daudi cells (human lymphoblastoid)	GEWERT and CLEMENS (1980) GEWERT et al. (1981) HILFENHAUS and MAULER (1980)
Uptake of iodide	FRTL cells (rat thyroid)	FRIEDMAN et al. (1981)

trol cultures. The degree of inhibition of acetate ^{14}C incorporation into lipids was linearly dependent upon the dose of IFN used, and less than 1 IU (antiviral) was inhibitory. In addition, neither heterologous IFN preparations nor mock IFN nor IFN which had been neutralized by exposure to specific antibody or inactivated by trypsin had an inhibitory effect on lipid synthesis by insulin-stimulated cultures. The identity between antiviral and antidifferentiation activities has been more conclusively established by using isoelectrically focused samples of purified IFN (S. KEAY and S. E. GROSSBERG 1981, unpublished work); fractions of isoelectric focusing gels which contained antiviral activity also contained antidifferentiation activity.

Treatment of insulin-stimulated 3T3-L1 cells with low doses of IFN resulted in an inhibition of the differentiation-associated cytoskeletal alterations and accumulation of lipid (GROSSBERG et al. 1981). In addition, collagen formation, as demonstrated by electron microscopy and incorporation of proline ^{3}H into salt-extractable soluble collagen, continued in the cultures treated with both insulin and IFN, whereas collagen synthesis diminishes in insulin-stimulated 3T3-L1 cells as the fibroblasts (which characteristically produce collagen) differentiate to adipocytes (which characteristically do not) (GROSSBERG et al. 1981).

The patterns of proteins synthesized by differentiating adipocytes was distinctly different from that obtained from undifferentiated fibroblasts (SPIEGELMAN and GREEN 1980; GROSSBERG et al. 1981). The protein profile of 3T3-L1 cells treated with IFN and insulin resembled that of the unstimulated control fibroblasts. IFN treatment thus inhibited changes in synthesis of specific proteins while total protein synthesis was not affected (KEAY and GROSSBERG 1980).

The inhibition by IFN of adipocyte conversion of fibroblasts has also been reported using another cell line, BALB/c3T3 (CIOE et al. 1980). A dose-dependent inhibition by IFN of the appearance of lipid-containing cells was established by microscopic examination of BALB/c3T3 cultures at various times after insulin addition. The inhibition of conversion could be reversed by removal of IFN from the culture medium.

II. Myoblast–Myotube Conversion

IFN inhibits the normal differentiation of chicken embryo myoblasts, as demonstrated by inhibition of both creatine kinase (CK) isozyme transition and multinucleated myotube formation (LOUGH et al. 1982). Proliferation of the myogenic cells was not inhibited. A dose-dependent inhibition of the appearance of the mature muscle-specific MM-CK isozyme was demonstrated, concomitant with an increase in the embryonic BB-CK isozyme. The time of initial application of IFN to cultures was a determining factor in the extent of inhibition of differentiation observed, with the greatest inhibition observed when IFN was first added to the cells at the time of plating; addition of IFN to cultures 24 h after plating resulted in less inhibition of MM-CK activity, while addition of IFN 48 h after plating resulted in a negligible inhibition of the CK transition. As myogenic cell commitment to differentiate usually occurs during the first 40 h in vitro and cellular fusion is extensive by 48 h, it would appear that IFN inhibits cellular differentiation at the commitment step (LOUGH et al. 1982; GROSSBERG and SABRAN 1982).

III. Erythroid Differentiation

1. Friend Leukemia Cells

The regulation of expression of erythroid cell differentiation has been studied extensively in the murine erythroleukemia cell system, Friend leukemia cells. These cells are established cell lines, grow in suspension and are chronically infected by Friend leukemia virus. Friend leukemia cells are erythroid precursors which are blocked in the differentiation pathway at the proerythroblast stage. Spontaneous differentiation of various clones of Friend leukemia cells occurs with low frequency (0.5%–2%). Differentiation can be induced in these cells by exposure to DMSO, resulting in the synthesis of heme, hemoglobin, and globin mRNA by 70%–90% of the cell population.

IFN appears to affect the differentiation process induced in Friend leukemia cells by DMSO in a "pendulum" fashion (ROSSI et al. 1980). Low doses of IFN (5–250 U) have been shown to enhance the DMSO-induced differentiation of Friend leukemia cells as quantitated by benzidine staining of hemoglobin-producing cells (BELARDELLI et al. 1980). The increase in hemoglobin-producing cells has been related to increases in globin mRNA and hemoglobin content in DMSO-stimulated cultures treated with IFN (LUFTIG et al. 1977; DOLEI et al. 1979a, b). ROSSI et al. (1980) have suggested that IFN treatment results in a more efficient induction of differentiation by DMSO.

These results contrast with those obtained upon exposure of DMSO-stimulated cultures to high doses of IFN (1,000–90,000 U). ROSSI et al. (1977b) have shown that growth and differentiation of DMSO-stimulated Friend leukemia cells were inhibited in a dose-dependent fashion by IFN. The inhibition could be reversed by transferring the cells into fresh growth medium lacking IFN. Inhibition of the appearance of benzidine-staining cells was accompanied by a reduction in the amount of globin mRNA which accumulated in IFN-treated, DMSO-stimulated cells (ROSSI et al. 1977b, 1980). Synthesis of globin in DMSO-stimulated cultures was almost completely inhibited upon IFN addition (ROSSI et al. 1977b).

Table 4. Interferon-modulated effects on cellular differentiation

Cells	Interferon	Effect	References
Friend leukemia cells	Mouse (50–100 U/ml)	Enhance DMSO-induced appearance of hemoglobin-producing cells	LIEBERMAN et al. (1974) DOLEI et al. (1979) BELARDELLI et al. (1980) ROSSI et al. (1980)
	Mouse (50 U/ml)	Enhance DMSO-induced globin mRNA production	LUFTIG et al. (1977)
	Mouse (50,000 U/ml)	Inhibit DMSO-induced increase in ornithine decarboxylase activity	GAZITT and FRIEND (1980)
	Mouse (1,000 U/ml)	Inhibition of appearance of hemoglobin-producing cells	ROSSI et al. (1977a) ROSSI et al. (1977b)
	Mouse (300–900 U/ml)	No inhibition of appearance of hemoglobin-producing cells	SWETLY and OSTERTAG (1974) SWETLY and OSTERTAG (1976)
BALB/c3T3	Mouse (50–200 U/ml)	Inhibition of appearance of lipid-containing cells	CIOE et al. (1980)
3T3-L1	Mouse (1–1,000 U/ml)	Inhibition of lipid synthesis and accumulation induced by insulin	GROSSBERG and KEAY (1980) KEAY and GROSSBERG (1980)
	Mouse (30 U/ml)	Inhibition of cytoskeletal changes associated with adipocyte conversion	GROSSBERG et al. (1981)
Chicken embryo neural retina	Chicken (30–1,000 U)	Inhibit hydrocortisone-induced increase in glutamine synthetase	MATSUNO et al. (1976) MATSUNO and SHIRASAWA (1978) SHIRASAWA and MATSUNO (1979)
Myeloid leukemia cells (M1)	Mouse (10,000 U)	Stimulate appearance of phagocytic cells	NAGANO and SAITO (1979b) TOMIDA et al. (1980a, b)
Monocytes	Human (30–300 U/ml)	Inhibit maturation into monocytes	EPSTEIN et al. (1980a) LEE et al. (1980)

2. Myeloid Leukemia Cells

The M1 cell line, established from a spontaneous myeloid leukemia of SL strain mouse, can be induced to differentiate in vitro by a number of differentiation-stimulating so-called D-factors (ICHIKAWA 1969, 1970). In the absence of these factors, the morphology of M1 cells is that of a myeloblast, and these cells are neither phagocytic nor motile. Differentiation into macrophages and granulocytes in vitro has been induced by D-factor, lipopolysaccharide, glucocortocoid hormones and poly(I) (TOMIDA et al. 1980a, b). Poly(I) · poly(C) also stimulated the induction of differentiation of M1 cells by D-factor in vitro (YAMAMOTO et al. 1979). While poly(I) · poly(C) itself did not induce phagocytic activity in the M1 cells, the exposure of cultures to both poly(I) · poly(C) and conditioned medium resulted in a tenfold increase of phagocytic activity compared with cultures exposed to conditioned medium. Poly(A) · poly(U) addition to cultures also stimulated the induction of differentiation, as measured by phatogytosis, by conditioned medium. The inclusion of poly(I) and conditioned medium in the culture medium resulted in a comparable stimulation of differentiation. It was shown that dsRNA induced IFN in the M1 cells, as did poly(I).

H. Conclusions and Epilogue

From the variegated effects that IFNs can have on vastly different cell types, both specialized and relatively undifferentiated, it is not yet possible to discern a basis for a common mode of action on cells. There are two well-accepted pathways activated in IFN-treated cells that interfere with viral protein synthesis: (1) the phosphorylation of initiation factor 2 by an induced protein kinase; and (2) the cleavage of RNA by an endoribonuclease activated by 2–5A. Both pathways require dsRNA; whether dsRNA of requisite size and quantity is present in normal cells remains uncertain. How such inhibition of cellular protein synthesis can cause the many changes described in IFN-treated cells has not been determined. Clearly, some effects such as those on the differentiation of fibroblasts to adipocytes or myoblasts to skeletal muscle occur without inhibition of generalized protein synthesis. EPSTEIN et al. (1981) have reported that at least twelve new proteins occur in HuIFN-α-treated human diploid cells, a circumstance which represents an apparent switching on of synthesis of cellular proteins in the face of a mechanism that possibly inhibits protein synthesis. It would be helpful to know the kinetics of the appearance and disappearance of these proteins in relation to the 2–5A-activated ribonuclease and kinase systems. It may be that some classes of messengers are more susceptible to such regulation than others. In systems which have been studied, IFN treatment inhibits the synthesis or expression of many proteins (e.g., enzymatic functions or isozymes characteristic of differentiated cells) and apparently increases others, such as related isozymes or structural proteins (actin). What contribution dsRNA might make toward shutting off synthesis of some proteins while switching on others may need to be explored. It is tempting to speculate that IFN can act to control gene expression by some action at the level of transcription. Such effects might be exerted by altering the methylation patterns of DNA (perhaps by means of the methylase found in IFN-treated cells) or differentially phosphorylating histones, by the induced protein kinase.

Do the cellular effects of IFN depend upon alterations of cell membranes? Although this idea is an attractive one, there is no conclusive evidence to indicate if such alterations are primary, secondary to other metabolic activities, or nonspecific and achievable only by high concentrations of IFN. Alterations in surface properties of IFN-treated cells may be responsible for other demonstrated actions, such as the changes in uptake of thymidine. Secondary effects resulting from changes in cell membranes are just beginning to be explored. It is known that binding of various ligands at the cell surface may cause rearrangement of membrane components, an action that might be considered to be nonspecific. Such alterations may affect the cytoskeleton, which does appear to be sensitive to cell signals received via the membrane: profound effects on protein and RNA synthesis and cell mobility can occur after normal cells come in contact with one another. The mechanism by which messages are transmitted from the cell surface to the nucleus, where expression of specific genes is controlled, remains unclear. Recent studies on gene regulation by hormones may provide some clues as to how such activities occur.

While a number of intriguing questions about how IFN affects cellular activities are currently being investigated, one must be cautious in interpreting results obtained with impure IFNs or inadequate mock IFN controls. Until very recently even the most highly purified IFNs in common use were 1%–10% pure; rDNA technology now permits the production of large quantities of IFN that make the use of pure IFN feasible to help determine the true effects of IFN on cellular processes. However, HuIFN-α constitutes a multigene family of about 14 types, representing as many genes. Initial studies with products from some of these genes show that they differ in antiviral activity on human and other cells. Therefore, it is likely that these gene products may also vary in their cellular effects. In addition, because in vivo production of more than one kind of IFN has been shown to occur simultaneously, i.e., not only as mixtures of HuIFN-α gene products, but also as mixtures of HuINF-α with either HuIFN-γ or HuIFN-β, combinations of IFNs in different proportions should also be tested for specific cell effects. The current status of work in the field would suggest that the further study of the cellular effects of IFN may offer a means of examining the control of a wide range of cellular activities, including mechanisms of host defense, growth, differentiation, and gene expression in general.

References

Aboud M, Michalski-Stern T, Nizan Y, Salzberg S (1980) Enhancement of cellular protein synthesis sensitivity of diphtheria toxin by interferon. Infect Immun 28:11–16

Adams A, Strander H, Cantell K (1975) Sensitivity of Epstein-Barr virus transformed human lymphoid cell lines to interferon. J Gen Virol 28:207–217

Aguet M, Blanchard B (1981) High affinity binding of ^{125}I-labeled mouse interferon to a specific cell surface receptor II Analysis of binding properties. Virology 115:249–261

Allen G, Fantes KH (1980) A family of structural genes for human lymphoblastoid (leukocyte-type) interferon. Nature 287:408–411

Ankel H, Krishnamurti C, Besancon F, Stefanos S, Falcoff E (1980) Mouse fibroblast (type I) and immune (type II) interferons: pronounced differences in affinity for gangliosides and in antiviral and antigrowth effects on mouse leukemia L-1210R cells. Proc Natl Acad Sci USA 77:2528–2532

Apostolov K, Barker W (1981) The effects of interferon on the fatty acids in uninfected cells. FEBS Lett 126:261–264

Attallah AM, Needy CF, Noguchi PD, Elisberg BL (1979) Enhancement of carcinoembryonic antigen expression by interferon. Int J Cancer 24:49–52

Attallah AM, Fleischer T, Khalil R, Noguchi PD, Urritia-Shaw A (1980a) Proliferative and functional aspects of interferon-treated human normal and neoplastic T and B cell. Br J Cancer 42:423–429
Attallah AM, Fleischer T, Neefe JR, Kazakis A, Yeatman TJ (1980b) Differential effects of human interferon on normal and neoplastic T- and B-cell lymphocytes. Ann NY Acad Sci 350:245–253
Attallah AM, Zoon K, Folks T, Huntington J, Yeatman TJ (1981) Multiple biological activities of homogeneous human alpha interferon. Infect Immun 34:1068–1070
Balkwill FR, Oliver RTD (1977) Growth inhibitory effects of interferon on normal and malignant human haemopoetic cells. Int J Cancer 20:500–505
Balkwill FR, Taylor-Papadimitriou J (1978) Interferon affects both G1 and S+G2 in cells stimulated from quiescence to growth. Nature 274:798–800
Balkwill FR, Watling D, Taylor-Papadimitriou J (1978a) Inhibition by lymphoblastoid interferon of growth of cells derived from the human breast. Int J Cancer 22:258–265
Balkwill FR, Watling D, Taylor-Papadimitriou J (1978b) The effect of interferons on cell growth and cell cycle. In: Chandra P (ed) Antiviral mechanisms in the control of neoplasia. Plenum, New York, p 719
Baron S, Merigan TC, McKerlie ML (1966) Effect of crude and purified interferons on the growth of uninfected cells in culture. Proc Soc Exp Biol Med 121:50–52
Baron S, Brunell PA, Grossberg SE (1979) Mechanism of action and pharmacology: the immune and interferon system. In: Galasso G, Merigan TC, Buchanan RA (eds) Antiviral agents and viral diseases of man. Raven, New York, pp 151–208
Bart RS, Porzio NR, Kopf AW, Vilcek JT, Cheng EH, Farcet Y (1980) Inhibition of growth of B16 murine malignant melanoma by exogenous interferon. Cancer Res 40:614–619
Belardelli F, Ausiello C, Tomasi M, Rossi GB (1980) Cholera toxin and its B subunit inhibit interferon effects on virus production and erythroid differentiation of Friend leukemia cells. Virol 107:109–120
Berg K, Heron I (1980) SDS-polyacrylamide gel electrophoresis of purified human leukocyte interferon and the antiviral and anticellular activities of different interferon species. J Gen Virology 50:441–446
Blalock JE, Harp C (1981) Interferon and adrenocorticotropic hormone induction of steroidogenesis, melanogenesis and antiviral activity. Arch Virol 67:45–49
Blalock JE, Stanton JD (1980) Common pathways of interferon and hormonal action. Nature 283:406–408
Blalock JE, Georgeades JA, Langford MP, Johnson HM (1980) Purified human immune interferon has more potent anticellular activity than fibroblast or leukocyte interferon. Cell Immunol 49:390–394
Borecky L, Fuchsberger N, Hajnicka V, Stanlek D, Zemla J (1972) Distribution of antiviral and cell-inhibitory activity in interferon preparations. Acta Virol 16:356–358
Borecky L, Fuchsberger N, Hajnicka V, Lackovic V (1973) Antiviral and cell-growth inhibitory effect of interferon. Biomedicine 19:281–286
Borecky L, Hajnicka V, Fuchsberger N, Kontsek P, Lackovic V, Russ G, Capkova J (1980) The cell growth inhibitory and antiviral effects of interferon in cloned transformed mouse cells. Ann NY Acad Sci 350:188–207
Borecky L, Hajnicka V, Kontsek P, Lackovic V, Russ G, Peknicova J, Capkova J, Rajcani J, Fuchsberger N (1981) Growth inhibitory effect of mouse interferon in transformed cells. Acta Microbiol Acad Sci Hung 28:271–282
Bourgeade MF, Chany C (1979) Effect of sodium butyrate on the antiviral and anticellular action of interferon in normal and MSV-transformed cells. Int J Cancer 24:314–381
Bradley EC, Ruscetti FW (1981) Effect of fibroblast, lymphoid, and myeloid interferons on human tumor colony formation in vitro. Cancer Res 41:244–249
Brouty-Boye D, Zetter B (1980) Inhibition of cell mobility by interferon. Science 208:516–518
Buffet RF, Ito M, Cairo AM, Carter WA (1978) Antiproliferative activity of highly purified mouse interferon. J Natl Cancer Inst 60:243–246
Calvet MC, Gresser I (1979) Interferon enhances the excitability of cultured neurones. Nature 278:558–560

Cantell K (1970) Attempts to prepare interferon in continuous cultures of human leukocytes. Ann NY Acad Sci 173:160–168
Chandrabose K, Cuatrescasas P, Pottahil R (1981) Changes in fatty acyl chains of phospholipids induced by interferon in mouse sarcoma S-180 cells. Biochem Biophys Res Commun 98:661–668
Chang EH, Grollman EF, Jay FT, Lee G, Kohn LD, Friedman RM (1978) Membrane alterations following interferon treatment. Adv Exp Med Biol 110:85–99
Chany C, Rousset S, Boutgeade MF, Mathew D, Gregoire A (1980a) Role of receptors and the cytoskeleton in reverse transformation and steroidogenesis induced by IFN. Ann NY Acad Sci 350:254–265
Chany C, Mathiew D, Gregoire A (1980b) Induction of delta 43 ketosteroid synthesis by interferon in mouse adrenal tumor cell cultures. J Gen Virol 50:447–450
Chawda R, Job L, Horoszewicz JS, Carter WA, Arya SK (1979) Effect of bromodeoxyuridine and interferon on cellular and viral functions in human prostatic cells. Oncology 36:35–39
Cioe L, O'Brien TG, Diamond L (1980) Inhibition of adipose conversion of BALB/c3T3 cells by interferon and 12-0-tetradecanoylphorbol-13-acetate. Cell Biol Int Rep 4:255–264
Creasey AA, Bartholomew JC, Merigan TC (1980a) Does human leukocyte interferon influence the restriction point control in cultured cells? Ann NY Acad Sci 350:208–210
Creasey AA, Bartholomew JC, Merigan TC (1980b) Role of G0 and G1 arrest in the inhibition of tumor cell growth by interferon. Proc Natl Acad Sci USA 77:1471–1475
Creasey AA, Bartholomew JC, Merigan TC (1981) The importance of G0 in the site of action of interferon in the cell cycle. Exp Cell Res 134:155–160
Czarniecki CW, Sreevalsan T, Friedman RM, Panet A (1981) Dissociation of interferon effects on murine leukemia virus and encephalomyocarditis virus replication in mouse cells. J Virol 37:827–831
Dahl H (1977a) Human interferon and cell growth inhibition II Biological and physicochemical properties of the growth inhibitory component. Acta Path Microbiol Scand B85:54–60
Dahl H (1977b) Differentiation between antiviral and anticellular effects of interferons. Tex Rep Biol Med 35:381–387
Dahl H (1978) Human interferon and cell growth inhibition III Separation of activities by treatment with sodium dodecyl sulphate. Biochem Biophys Res Commun 82:6–12
Dahl H (1980) Human interferon and cell growth inhibition V Effect of ouabain on interferon activities. Biochem Biophys Res Commun 92:586–590
Dahl H, Degre M (1975) Separation of antiviral activity of human interferon from cell inhibitory effect. Nature 257:799–802
Dahl H, Degre M (1976) Human interferon and cell growth inhibition I Inhibitory effect of human interferon on the growth rate of cultured human cells. Acta Path Microbiol Scand B84:285–292
Degre M (1980) Antiviral and cell multiplication inhibitory activites of mouse interferon preparations tested on an interferon sensitive murine sarcoma cell line. Acta Path Microbiol Scand B88:219–223
Degre M, Rollag H Jr (1980) Influence of interferon on phagocytic activity in vitro and in vivo. In: Khan A, Hill NO, Doran GL (eds) Interferon: properties and clinical uses. Leland Fikes Foundation, Dallas
D'Hooghe MC, Brouty-Boye D, Malaise EP, Gresser I (1977) Interferon and cell division XII Prolongation by interferon in the intermitotic time of mouse mammary tumor cells in vitro, Microcinematographic analysis. Exp Cell Res 105:73–77
Dolei A, Capobranchi MR, Cioe L, Colletta G, Vecchio G, Rossi GB, Affabris E, Belardelli (1979a) Possible role of the Friend virus life cycle in differentiating Friend leukemia cells treated with interferon. Hamatol Bluttransfus 23:307–311
Dolei A, Capobranchi MR, Cioe L, Colletta G, Vecchio G, Rossi, GB, Affrabris E, Belardelli F (1979b) Effects of interferon on the expression of cellular and integrated viral genes in Friend erythroleukemia cells. In: Chandra P (ed) Antiviral mechanisms in the control of neoplasia. Plenum, New York, pp 729–739

Drasner K, Epstein CJ, Epstein LB (1979) Antiproliferative effects of interferon on murine embryonic cells. Proc Soc Exp Biol Med 160:46–49

Eife R, Hahn T, DeTavera M, Schertel F, Holtmann H, Eife G, Levin S (1981) A comparison of the antiproliferative and antiviral activities of alpha, beta, and gamma-interferons: Description of a unified assay for comparing both effects simultaneously. J Immunol Meth 47:339–347

Einhorn S, Strander H (1977) Is interferon tissue specific? – Effect of human leukocyte and fibroblast interferons on the growth of lymphoblastoid and osteosarcoma cells. J Gen Virol 35:573–577

Epstein LB, Lee SHS, Epstein CJ (1980 a) Enhanced sensitivity of trisomy 21 monocytes of the maturation-inhibiting effect of interferon. Cell Immunol 50:191–194

Epstein LB, Shen JT, Abele JS, Reese CC (1980 b) Further experience in testing the sensitivity of human ovarian carcinoma cells to interferon in an in vitro semisolid agar culture system: Comparison of solid and ascites forms of the tumor. In: Salmon SE (ed) Cloning of human tumor stem cells. Liss, New York, pp 277–290

Epstein LB, Shen JT, Abele JS, Reese CC (1980 c) Sensitivity of human ovarian carcinoma cells to interferon and other antitumor agents as assessed by an in vitro semi-solid agar technique. Ann NY Acad Sci 350:228–244

Epstein LB, Weil J, Lucas DO, Cox DR, Epstein CJ (1981) The biology and properties of interferon-gamma: an overview, studies of production by T lymphocyte subsets, and analysis of peptide synthesis and antiviral effects in trisomy 21 and diploid human fibroblasts. In: DeMayer E, Galasso G, Schelleken H (eds) The biology of the interferon system. Elsevier, Amsterdam

Evinger M, Pestka S (1981) Assay of growth inhibition in lymphoblastoid cell cultures. Meth Enzymol 79:362–368

Evinger M, Rubinstein, Pestka S (1980) Growth-inhibitory and antiviral activity of purified leukocyte interferon. Ann NY Acad Sci 350:399–404

Evinger M, Rubinstein M, Pestka S (1981) Antiproliferative and antiviral activities of human leukocyte interferons. Arch Biochem Biophys 210:319–329

Fellows M, Bono R, Hyafil F, Gresser I (1981) Interferon enhances the amount of membrane-bound B2-microglobulin and its release from human Burkitt cells. Eur J Immunol 11:524–526

Fisher PB, Mufson RA, Weinstein IB (1981) Interferon inhibits melanogenesis in B-16 mouse melanoma cells. Biochem Biophys Res Commun 100:823–830

Fitzpatrick FA, Stringfellow DA (1980) Virus and interferon effects on cellular prostaglandin biosynthesis. J Immunol 125:431–437

Fleming WA, McNeill TA, Killen M (1972) The effects of an inhibiting factor (interferon) on the in vitro growth of granulocyte-macrophage colonies. Immunology 23:429–437

Friedman RM (1981) Cell surface alterations induced by interferon. Meth Enzymol 79:458–461

Friedman RM, Kohn LD, Lee G, Epstein D, Jacobsen H (1981) Stimulating activity by mouse interferon on the uptake of iodide by rat thyroid cells. In: DeMayer E, Galasso G, Schelekens H (eds) The biology of the interferon system. Elsevier, Amsterdam

Fuchsberger N, Borecky, Hajnicka V (1974) Effect of prolonged interferon treatment on "L" mouse fibroblast cells. Acta Virol 18:85–87

Fuchsberger N, Hajnicka V, Borecky L (1975) Antiviral and cell-growth inhibitory activities of highly purified L-cell interferon. An analysis of quantitative disproportions. Acta Virol 19:59–66

Fuse A, Kuwata T (1978) Inhibition of DNA synthesis and alteration of cyclic adenosine 3′,5′-monophosphate levels in RSa cells by human leukocyte interferon. J Natl Cancer Inst 60:1227–1232

Fuse A, Kuwata T (1979) Effect of cholera toxin on the antiviral and anticellular activities of human leukocyte interferon. Infect Immun 26:235–239

Gaffney EV, Picciano PT, Grant CA (1973) Inhibition of growth and transformation of human cells by interferon. J Natl Cancer Inst 50:871–878

Gazitt Y, Friend C (1980) Polyamine biosynthesis enzymes in the induction and inhibition of differentiation in Friend erythroleukemia cells. Cancer Res 40:1727–1732

Gewert DR, Clemens MJ (1980) Inhibition by interferon of thymidine uptake and deoxyribonucleic acid synthesis in human lymphoblastoid cells. Biochem Soc Trans 8:353–354

Gewert DR, Shah S, Clemens MJ (1981) Inhibition of cell division by interferons: changes in the transport and intracellular metabolism of thymidine in human lymphoblastoid (Daudi) cells. Eur J Biochem 116:487–492

Glasgow LA, Crane JL Jr, Kern ER (1978a) Antitumor activity of interferon against murine osteogenic sarcoma cells in vitro. J Natl Cancer Inst 60:659–666

Glasgow LA, Crane JL, Kern ER, Youngner JS (1978b) Antitumor activity of interferon against murine osteogenic sarcoma in vitro and in vivo. Cancer Treat Rep 62:1881–1888

Green H (1978) The adipose conversion of 3T3 cells. In: Ahmad F, Schultz J, Russell TR, Werner R (eds) Differentiation and development, Miami winter symposia, vol 15. Academic, New York, pp 13–36

Green H, Kehinde O (1974) Sublines of mouse 3T3 cells that accumulate lipid. Cell 1:113–116

Greenberg PL, Mosney SA (1977) Cytotoxic effects of interferon in vitro on granulocytic progenitor cells. Cancer Res 37:1794–1799

Gresser I (1977) On the varied biological effects of interferon. Cell Immunol 34:406–415

Gresser I, Tovey MG (1978) Antitumor effects of interferon. Biochim Biophys Acta 516:231–247

Gresser I, Brouty-Boye D, Thomas MT, Macieria-Coelho A (1970a) Interferon and cell division I Inhibition of the multiplication of mouse leukemia L1210 cells in vitro by interferon preparations. Proc Natl Acad Sci USA 66:1052–1058

Gresser I, Brouty-Boye D, Thomas MT, Macieria-Coelho A (1970b) Interferon and cell division II Influence of various experimental conditions on the inhibition of L1210 cell multiplication in vitro by interferon preparations. J Natl Cancer Inst 45:1145–1153

Gresser I, Thomas MT, Brouty-Boye D, Macievia-Coelho A (1971) Interferon and cell division V Titration of the anticellular action of interferon preparations. Proc Soc Exp Biol Med 137:1258–1261

Gresser I, Bandu MT, Tovey M, Bodo G, Paucker K, Stewart W III (1973) Interferon and cell division VII Inhibitory effect of highly purified interferon preparations on the multiplication of leukemia L1210 cells. Proc Soc Exp Biol Med 142:7–10

Gresser I, Bandu MT, Brouty-Boye D (1974) Interferon and cell IX Interferon-resistant L1210 cells: characteristics and origin. J Natl Cancer Inst 52:553–559

Gresser I, DeMaeyer-Guignard J, Tovey MG, DeMaeyer E (1979) Electrophoretically pure mouse interferon exerts multiple biologic effects. Proc Natl Acad Sci USA 76:5308–5312

Grossberg SE, Morahan PS (1971) Repression of interferon action: induced dedifferentiation of embryonic cells. Science 171:77–79

Grossberg SE, Keay S (1980) The effects of interferon on 3T3-L1 cell differentiation. Ann NY Acad Sci 350:294–300

Grossberg SE, Sabran JL (1982) Interferon inhibition of cellular differentiation. Tex Rep Biol 41:332–335

Grossberg SE, Keay S, Kushnaryov V, Sabran JL (1981) Interferon inhibition of 3T3-L1 adipocyte differentiation: alterations of cytoskeleton and cell protein profiles. In: DeMaeyer E, Galasso G, Schellekens H (eds) The biology of the interferon system. Elsevier, Amsterdam, pp 153–156

Hajnicka W, Borecky L (1979) Antiviral and anticellular effects of interferon on the mouse embryonic cells transformed by viruses and/or chemical carcinogen. Acta Biol Med Germ 38:821–827

Halbach M, Koschell K, Jungwirth C (1978) Interferon enhances the fragility of lysosomes in L-929 mouse fibroblasts. J Gen Virol 39:387–390

Hallinan FM, Bishop J, Lee SHS, Rozee K (1977) The characteristics of enhanced DNA synthesis in L cells treated with interferon and arginine-deprived. Exp Cell Res 110:283–288

Heron I, Hokland M, Berg K (1978) Enhanced expression of B2-microglobulin and HLA antigens on human lymphoid cells by interferon. Proc Natl Acad Sci USA 75:6215–6219

Hilfenhaus J, Karges HE (1976) Growth inhibition of human lymphoblastoid cells by human interferon preparation. In: Deutsch E, Moser K, Rainer H, Stacher A (eds) Molecular base of malignancy, new clinical and therapeutic evidence. Thieme, Stuttgart
Hilfenhaus J, Mauler R (1980) Human fibroblast and human leukocyte interferon: their differences in cell growth inhibition activities on lymphoblastoid cells. Ann NY Acad Sci 350:626–627
Hilfenhaus J, Damm H, Karges HE, Manthey KF (1976) Growth inhibition of human lymphoblastoid Daudi cells in vitro by interferon preparations. Arch Virol 51:87–97
Hilfenhaus J, Damm H, Johannsen R (1977) Sensitivity of various human lymphoblastoid cells to the antiviral and anticellular activity of human leukocyte interferon. Arch Virol 54:271–277
Ho M, Armstrong JA (1975) Interferon. Ann Rev Microbiol 29:131–161
Horoszewicz JS, Leong SS, Carter WA (1979) Noncycling tumor cells are sensitive targets for antiproliferative activity of human interferon. Science 206:1091–1093
Hovanessian AG (1979) Intracellular events in interferon-treated cells. Differentiation 15:139–151
Hovanessian AG, Wood JN (1980) Anticellular and antiviral effects of pppA(2′p5′A)n. Virology 101:81–90
Huang K (1977) Effect of interferon on phagocytosis. Tex Rep Biol Med 35:350–356
Huang SY, Donahoe RM, Gordon FB, Dressler HR (1971) Enhancement of phagocytosis by interferon-containing preparations. Infect Immun 4:581–588
Ichikawa Y (1969) Differentiation of a cell line of myeloid leukemia. J Cell Physiol 74:223
Imanishi J, Yokota Y, Kishida T, Mukainaka T, Matsuo A (1975) Phagocytosis-enhancing effect of human leukocyte interferon preparation of human peripheral monocytes in culture. Acta Virol 19:52–58
Inglot AD, Oleszak E, Kisielow B (1980) Antagonism in action between mouse or human interferon and platelet growth factor. Arch Virol 63:291–296
Ito M, Buffet RF (1981) Cytocidal effect of purified human fibroblast interferon on tumor cells in vitro. J Natl Cancer Inst 66:819–825
Iwakura Y, Yonehara S, Kawade Y (1978) Purification of mouse L cell interferon, essentially pure preparation with associated cell growth inhibitory activity. J Biol Chem 253:5074–5079
Jameson P, Taylor JL, Grossberg SE (1981) Bluetongue virus induction of interferon: Potential for cancer therapy. Prog Cancer Res Ther 16:193–203
Kading VH, Blalock JE, Gifford GE (1978) Effect of serum on the antiviral and anticellular activities of mouse interferon. Arch Virol 56:237–242
Keay S, Grossberg SE (1980) Interferon inhibits the conversion of 3T3-L1 mouse fibroblasts into adipocytes. Proc Natl Acad Sci USA 77:4099–4103
Kerr IM, Weschner DH, Silverman RH, Cayley PJ, Knight M (1981) The 2-5A (pppA2′-p5′A2′p5′A) and protein kinase systems in interferon-treated and control cells. Adv Cyclic Nucleotide Res 14:469–478
Killander D, Lindahl P, Lundin L, Leary P, Gresser I (1976) Relationship between the enhanced expression of histocompatibility antigens on interferon-treated L1210 cells and their position in the cell cycle. Eur J Immunol 6:56–59
Kimchi A, Shure H, Lapidot Y, Rapoport S, Panet A, Revel M (1981 a) Antimitogenic effects of interferon and (2′-5′)-oligoadenylate in synchronized 3T3 fibroblasts. FEBS Lett 134:212–216
Kimchi A, Shure H, Revel M (1981 b) Anti-mitogenic function of interferon-induced (2′-5′) oligo (adenylate) and growth-related variations in enzymes that synthesize and degrade this oligonucleotide. Eur J Biochem 114:5–10
Knight E Jr (1973) Interferon: Effect on the saturation density to which mouse cells will grow in vitro. J Cell Biol 56:846–849
Knight E Jr (1976) Antiviral and cell growth inhibitory activities reside in the same glycoprotein of fibroblast interferon. Nature 262:302–303
Kushnaryov VM, Sedmak JJ, Bendler JW III, Grossberg SE (1982) Ultrastructural localization of interferon receptors on the surfaces of cultured cells and erythrocytes. Infect Immun 36:811–821

Kuwata T, Fuse A, Morinaga N (1976) Effect of interferon on cell and virus growth in transformed human cell lines. J Gen Virol 33:7–15
Kuwata T, Fuse A, Morinaga N (1977a) Effects of ouabain on the anticellular and antiviral activities of human and mouse interferon. J Gen Virol 34:537–540
Kuwata T, Fuse A, Morinaga N (1977b) Effects of cycloheximide and puromycin on the antiviral and anticellular activities of human interferon. J Gen Virol 37:195–198
Kuwata T, Fuse A, Suzzuki N, Morinaga N (1979) Comparison of the suppression of cell and virus growth in transformed human cells by leukocyte and fibroblast interferon. J Gen Virol 43:435–439
Kuwata T, Fuse A, Takayama N, Morinaga N (1980) Effects of concanavalin A on the antiviral and cell growth inhibitory action of human interferons. Ann NY Acad Sci 350:211–227
Lampidis TJ, Brouty-Boye D (1981) Interferon inhibits cardiac cell function in vitro. Proc Soc Exp Biol Med 166:181–185
Leandersson T, Lundgren E (1980) Antiproliferative effect of interferon on a Burkitt's lymphoma cell line. Exp Cell Res 130:421–426
Lee SHS, Epstein LB (1980) Reversible inhibition by interferon of the maturation of human peripheral blood monocytes to macrophages. Cell Immunol 50:177–190
Lee SHS, O'Shaughnessy MV, Rozee KR (1972) Interferon induced growth depression in diploid and heteroploid human cells. Proc Soc Exp Biol Med 139:1438–1440
Lee EJ, Larkin PC, Sreevalsan T (1980) Differential effect of interferon on ornithine decarboxylase activation in quiscent Swiss 3T3 cells. Biochem Biophy Res Comm 97:301–308
Levy HB, Merigan TC (1966) Interferon and uninfected cells. Proc Soc Exp Biol Med 121:53–55
Lieberman D, Voloch Z, Aviv H, Nudel U, Revel M (1974) Effects of interferon on hemoglobin synthesis and leukemia virus production in Friend cells. Mol Biol Rep 1:447–451
Lindahl-Magnusson P, Leary P, Gresser I (1971) Interferon and cell division VI Inhibitory effect of interferon on the multiplication of mouse embryo and mouse kidney cells in primary cultures. Proc Exp Biol Med 138:1044–1050
Lough J, Keay S, Sabran JL, Grossberg SE (1982) Inhibition of chicken myogenesis in vitro by partially purified interferon. Biochem Biophys Res Commun 109:92–99
Ludwig H, Swetly P (1980) In vitro inhibitory effect of interferon on colony formation of myeloma stem cells. Cancer Immunol Immunother 9:139–143
Luftig RB, Conscience J, Skoultchi A, McMillan P, Revel M, Ruddle FH (1977) Effect of interferon on dimethyl sulfoxide-stimulated Friend erythroleukemia cells: ultrastructural and biochemical study. J Virol 23:799–810
Lundgren E, Larson I, Miorner H, Strannegard O (1979) Effects of leukocyte and fibroblast interferon on events in the fibroblast cell cycle. J Gen Virol 42:589–595
Lutton JD, Levere RD (1980) Suppressive effect of human interferons on erythroid colony growth in disorders of erythropoiesis. J Lab Clin Med 96:328–333
Macieira-Coelho A, Brouty-Boye D, Thomas MT, Gresser I (1971) Interferon and cell division III Effect of interferon on the division cycle of L1210 cells in vitro. J Cell Biol 48:415–419
Mannering GJ, Renton KW, et Azhary R, Deloria LB (1980) Effects of interferon-inducing agents on hepatic cytochrome P-450 drug metabolizing systems. Ann NY Acad Sci 350:314–331
Maroun LE (1978) Interferon-mediated effect on ribosomal RNA metabolism. Biochim Biophys Acta 517:109–114
Masucci MG, Szigeti R, Klein E, Klein G, Gruest J, Montagnier L, Taira H, Hall A, Nagata S, Weismann C (1980) Effect of interferon-alpha-1 from E. coli on some cell functions. Science 209:1431–1435
Matarese GP, Rossi GB (1977) Effect of interferon on growth and division cycle of Friend erythroleukemic murine cells in vitro. J Cell Biol 75:344–354
Matsuno M (1979) Action of interferon on cell membrane of mouse lymphocytes. Exp Cell Res 124:253–259

Matsuno T, Shirasawa N (1978) Interferon suppresses steroid-inducible glutamine synthetase biosynthesis in embryonic chick neural retina. Biochim Biophys Acta 538:188–194

Matsuno T, Shirasawa N, Kohno S (1976) Interferon suppresses glutamine synthetase induction in chick embryonic neural retina. Biochem Biophys Res Commun 70:310–314

Matsuyama M (1979) Action of interferon on cell membrane of mouse lymphocytes. Expt Cell Res 124:253–259

Matsuzawa T, Kawade Y (1974) Cell growth inhibitory activity of electrophoretic functions of L-cell interferon preparation. Acta Virol 18:383–390

McNeill TA, Fleming WA (1971) The relationship between serum interferon and an inhibitor of mouse haemopoietic colonies in vitro. Immunology 21:761–766

McNeil TA, Fleming WA (1977) Effect of interferon on hemopoietic colony-forming cells. Tex Rep Biol Med 35:343–349

McNeil TA, Gresser I (1973) Inhibition of haemopoietic colony growth by interferon preparations from different sources. Nature 244:173–174

Moehring JM, Stinebring WR (1971) Prolonged application of interferon and "aging" of human diploid fibroblasts. Proc Soc Exp Biol Med 137:191–193

Montagnier L, Gruest G (1980) Disc-agarose assay of interferon and cytostatic drugs on malignant cells. Ann Virol 131:247–253

Nagano Y, Saito H (1979a) Effet du facteur inhibiteur des virus ou interferon sur la multiplication in vitro des cellules malignes murines. CR Soc Biol 173:20–25

Nagano Y, Saito H (1979b) Effet du facteur inhibiteur des virus su interferon sur la division et la differenciation de cellules leucemiques murines. CR Soc Biol 173:967–972

Nagano Y, Saito H (1981) Procedures to study the cytostatic effects of interferon on Ehrlichs ascites cells. Meth Enzymol 79:360–361

Nissen C, Speck B, Emodi G, Iscove NM (1977) Toxicity of human leukocyte interferon preparations in human bone marrow cultures. Lancet 1 (8004):203–204

Ohwaki M, Kawade Y (1972) Inhibition of multiplication of mouse cells in culture by interferon preparations. Acta Virol 16:477–486

Panniers LRV, Clemens MJ (1980) Interferon enhances protein degradation in Ehrlich ascites-tumor cells. Biochem Soc Trans 8:352–353

Panniers LRV, Clemens MJ (1981) Inhibition of cell division by interferon: Changes in cell cycle characteristics and in morphology of Ehrlich ascites tumour cells in culture. J Cell Sci 48:259–279

Paucker K, Cantell K, Henle W (1962) Quantitative studies on viral interference in suspended L cells III Effect of interfering viruses and interferon on the growth rate of cells. Virology 17:324–334

Pfeffer LM, Murphy JS, Tamm I (1979) Interferon effects on the growth and division of human fibroblasts. Exp Cell Res 121:111–120

Pfeffer LM, Wang E, Tamm I (1980) Interferon effects on microfilament organization, cellular fibronectin distribution, and cell motility in human fibroblasts. J Cell Biol 85:9–17

Ratner L, Nordlund JJ, Lengyel P (1980) Interferon as an inhibitor of cell growth: Studies with mouse melanoma cells. Proc Soc Exp Biol Med 163:267–272

Rich SA (1981) Human lupus inclusions and interferon. Science 213:772–775

Rollag H, Degre M (1981) Effect of interferon preparations on the uptake of non-opsonized Escherichia coli by mouse peritoneal macrophages. Acta Path Microbiol Scand B89:153–159

Rossi GB, Dolei A, Cioe L, Benedetto A, Matarese GP, Belardelli F, Rita G (1977a) Interferon and Friend cells in culture. Tex Rep Biol Med 35:420–428

Rossi GB, Matarese GP, Grappelli C, Belardelli F, Bendetto A (1977b) Interferon inhibits dimethyl sulphoxide-induced erythroid differentiation of Friend leukaemia cells. Nature 267:50–52

Rossi GB, Dolei A, Capobianchi MR, Peschle C, Affabris E (1980) Interactions of interferon with in vitro model systems involved in hematopoietic cell differentiation. Ann NY Acad Sci 350:279–293

Rubin RY, Gupta SL (1980) Differential effacacies of human type I and type II interferons as antiviral and antiproliferative agents. Proc Natl Acad Sci USA 77:5928–5932

Sela BA, Gurari-Rotman D (1978) Interferon abrogates the arrest of DNA synthesis in heterologous thymocytes treated with lectins. Biochem Biophys Res Commun 84:550–556
Shibata H, Taylor-Papadimitriou J (1981) Effects of human lymphoblastoid interferon on cultured breast cancer cells. Int J Cancer 28:447–453
Shirasawa N, Matsuno T (1979) Suppression of the accumulation of steroid-inducible glutamine synthetase mRNA on embryonic chick retinal polysomes by interferon preparation. Biochim Biophys Acta 562:271–280
Sikora K, Dilley J, Basham T, Levy T, Merigan T (1980) Inhibition of lymphoma hybrid by human interferon. Lancet 2(8200):891–893
Slimmer S, Masui H, Kaplan NO (1981) Antiproliferative assay for human interferons. Meth Enzymol 79:419–422
Sokawa Y, Watanabe Y, Watanabe Y, Kawade Y (1977) Interferon suppresses the transition of quiescent 3T3 cells to a growing state. Nature 268:236–238
Sonnenfeld G, Muruelo D, McDevitt HO, Merigan TC (1981) Effect of type 1 and type II interferons on murine thymocyte surface antigen expression: induction or selection? Cell Immunol 57:427–439
Spiegelman BM, Green H (1980) Control of specific protein biosynthesis during adipose differentiation of 3T3 cells. J Biol Chem 255:8811
Sreevalsan T, Rozengurt E, Taylor-Papadimitriou J, Burchell J (1980) Differential effect of interferon on DNA synthesis, 2-deoxyglucose uptake and ornithine decarboxylase activity in 3T3 cells stimulated by polypeptide growth factors and tumor promoters. J Cell Physiol 104:1–9
Sreevalsan T, Lee E, Friedman RM (1981) Assay of effect of interferon on intracellular enzymes. Meth Enzymol 79:342–349
Stewart WE II, Gresser I, Tovey MG, Bandu MT, LeGoff S (1976) Identification of the cell multiplication inhibitory factors on interferon preparations as interferons. Nature 262:300–302
Strander H, Einhorn S (1977) Effect of human leukocyte interferon on the growth of human osteosarcoma cells in tissue culture. Int J Cancer 19:468–473
Swetly P, Ostertag W (1974) Friend virus release and induction of haemoglobin synthesis in erythroleukaemic cells respond differently to interferon. Nature 251:642–644
Swetly P, Ostertag W (1976) Interferon; action and induction in Friend virus transformed erythroleukemia cells during erythropoietic differentiation. In: Deutsch E, Moser K, Rainer H, Stache A (eds) Molecular basis of malignancy. New clinical and therapeutic evidence. Thieme, Stuttgart
Tamm I, Pfeffer LM, Murphy JS (1981) Assay of the inhibitory activities of human interferons on the proliferation and locomotion of fibroblasts. Meth Enzymol 79:404–413
Tomida M, Yamamoto Y, Hozumi M (1980 a) Stimulation by interferon of induction of differentiation of mouse myeloid leukemic cells. Cancer Res 40:2919–2924
Tomida M, Yamamoto Y, Hozumi M (1980 b) Inhibition of the leukemogenicity of myeloid leukemic cells in mice and in vivo induction of normal differentiation of the cells by poly(I)-poly(C). Gann 71:457–463
Tovey MG (1981) Use of chemostat culture for the study of the effect of interferon on tumor cell multiplication. Meth Enzymol 79:391–404
Tovey MH, Rochette-Egly C (1980) The effect of interferon on cyclic nucleotides. Ann NY Acad Sci 350:266–278
Tovey M, Brouty-Boye D, Gresser I (1975) Early effect of interferon on mouse leukemia cells cultivated in a chemostat. Proc Natl Acad Sci USA 72:2265–2269
Tovey MG, Rochette-Egly C, Castagna M (1979) Effect of interferon on concentrations of cyclic nucleotides in cultured cells. Proc Natl Acad Sci USA 76:3890–3893
Vandenbussche P, Divizio M, Verhaegen-Lewalle M, Fuse A, Kuwata T, DeClercq E, Content J (1981) Enzymatic activities induced by interferon in human fibroblast cell lines differing in their sensitivity to the anticellular activities of interferon. Virology 111:11–22
Van't Hull E, Schellekens H, Lowenberg B, De Vrie MJ (1978) Influence of interferon preparations on the proliferative capacity of human and mouse bone marrow cells in vitro. Cancer Res 38:911–914

Vengris VE, Fernie BF, Pitha PM (1980) Interaction between gangliosides and interferon. Adv Exp Med Biol 125:479–486

Verma DS, Spitzer G, Dicke KA (1980) Human leukocyte interferon: a possible regulation of myelopoietic differentiation. In Khan A, Hill NO, Dores GL (eds) Interferon: properties and clinical uses. Leland Fikes Foundation, Dallas, pp 543–558

Verma DS, Spitzer G, Gutterman JU, Zander AR, McCredie KB, Dicke KA (1979) Human leukocyte interferon preparation blocks granulopoietic differentiation. Blood 54:1423–1427

Vignaux F, Gresser I (1978) Enhanced expression of histocompatibility antigens on interferon-treated mouse embryonic fibroblasts. Proc Soc Exp Biol Med 157:456–460

Watanabe Y, Sokawa Y (1978) Effect of interferon on the cell cycle of BALB/c3T3 cells. J Gen Virol 41:411–415

Weinstein Y, Brodeur BR, Melmon KL, Merigan TC (1977) Interferon inhibition of lymphocyte mitogenesis. Immunology 33:313–319

Werenne J, Emonds-Alt X, Bartholeyns J (1980) Interferon regulates cell motility. Ann NY Acad Sci 350:623–624

Whitman JE, Crowley GM, Hung C (1980) Anti-proliferative activity of purified human fibroblast interferon on human tumor cells in vitro. In: Kahn A, Hill NO, Dorn GL (eds) Interferon: properties and clinical uses. Leland Fikes Foundation, Dallas

Yamamoto Y, Tomida M, Hozumi M (1979) Stimulation of differentiation of mouse myeloid leukemia cells and induction of interferon in the cells by double-stranded polyribonucleotides. Cancer Res 39:4170–4174

Yaron M, Yaron I, Gurari-Rotman D, Revel M, Lindner HR, Zor U (1977) Stimulation of prostaglandin E production in cultured human fibroblasts by poly(I)-poly(C) and human interferon. Nature 267:4557–4559

CHAPTER 10

Interferon Induction by Viruses

P. I. MARCUS

A. Introduction and Perspective

Interferon was discovered when ISAACS and LINDENMANN (1957) infected fragments of chick chorioallantoic membrane with heat-inactivated influenza virus. The viral component or components responsible for interferon induction were not identified then, and indeed the inducer remains unknown a quarter-century later. ISAACS et al. (1963) postulated that the molecular species responsible for interferon induction was "foreign nucleic acid". In 1967 that "foreign nucleic acid" took the form of double-stranded RNA (dsRNA) when FIELD et al. (1967) discovered that exogenously added synthetic polyribonucleotides were inducers of interferon. There followed a plethora of studies designed to relegate to viral dsRNA the comparable role of interferon inducer in the virus-infected cell. Many of the studies provided evidence in support of viral dsRNA as the interferon inducer moiety, yet many others suggested that dsRNA itself did not induce interferon and that some additional early viral replicative events were required. In the extreme, interferon induction was reported to occur in cells infected with inactivated viruses and under conditions where dsRNA was not detectable. In addition, the apparent lack of correlation between the replication of viral RNA and interferon induction in several systems again pointed to the possibility that the accumulation of viral dsRNA might not suffice to induce interferon. To complicate matters, some investigators reported inverse correlations between viral RNA replication and interferon induction. Even virions containing preformed dsRNA did not always function as inducers of interferon. Confronted with these apparently conflicting data, it was reasonable to conclude that either dsRNA was not the molecule responsible for interferon induction, or that additional factors were involved. JOHNSTON and BURKE (1973) and STEWART (1979) very succinctly review and astutely interpret these earlier studies. Against this background of conflicting reports we initiated a series of experiments designed to define the molecule or molecules of viral origin responsible for interferon induction (MARCUS and SEKELLICK 1977). We report these and related results herein.

Several reviews concerned, at least in part, with the mechanism of interferon induction by viruses have appeared over the past decade. These are cited here in chronological order to provide the reader with a comprehensive reference source to the literature and a sense of the evolving views of viruses as inducers of the interferon system: DE CLERCQ and MERIGAN (1970), LOCKART (1970), VILČEK (1970), COLBY and MORGAN (1971), FINTER (1973), JOHNSTON and BURKE (1973), SOLOV'EV and BEKTEMIROV (1973), BARON and DIANZANI (1977), DE MAEYER and DE

MAEYER-GUIGNARD 1979), STEWART (1979), MARCUS (1980), STRINGFELLOW (1980), YABROV (1980), GORDON and MINKS (1981), MARCUS (1981–1982).

We assume as firmly established that interferons are bona fide inducible cellular gene products. STEWART (1979, p 27) reviews a compelling list of data to support this conclusion. From that list we note that interferon induction/production requires new cellular RNA and protein synthesis, and that interferon mRNA is isolable only from induced cells. Stringent repression of expression of the interferon gene appears to characterize most cells although there are notable exceptions, as reviewed by STEWART (1979, p 55). Even these may reflect the presence of an adventitious inducer, although they may also mean that constitutive expression takes place at low levels (THANG et al. 1977). Cell mutants which spontaneously produce interferon (JARVIS and COLBY 1978) may be useful for defining regulatory events in interferon induction/production.

The interferon induction system can be considered to involve five elements: (1) the inducer molecule; (2) the cell's processing and recognition systems for inducer molecules; (3) derepression and transcription of the interferon gene (genes, or gene banks) and their regulation; (4) translation of interferon mRNA and its regulation; and (5) production of extracellular functional interferon. This chapter will address primarily the first of these elements as it relates to viruses as inducers of interferon. With the first element of the induction system defined (see Sect. B), the second becomes a subject for future study. Other aspects of the induction/production process will be reviewed in accompanying chapters in this volume.

This chapter will depart from the usual format by limiting its coverage primarily to reports which bear directly on two hypotheses promulgated by MARCUS and SEKELLICK (1977): that (1) the interferon inducer moiety of viruses is dsRNA; and (2) the threshold for interferon induction is one molecule of dsRNA per cell. Additional observations were subsequently added: (3) induction results in the production of a quantum (finite) yield of interferon per cell; (4) the kinetics of interferon production can be described by two types of dose(multiplicity)–response (interferon yield) curves; and (5) in one type of induction the simultaneous introduction of two or more molecules of dsRNA into the cell abrogates the induction/production of interferon (MARCUS and FULLER 1979; MARCUS and SEKELLICK 1980; FULLER and MARCUS 1980a, 1980b; WINSHIP and MARCUS 1980; MARCUS et al. 1981a, b).

B. A Quantitative Approach to Interferon Induction by Viruses: Defining the Interferon-Inducing Particle

Our study of interferon induction by viruses was initiated by first defining virus stocks quantitatively in terms of interferon-inducing particle (IFP) activity. This was done by generating dose (multiplicity)–response (interferon yield) curves for each virus stock, and analyzing the curves in terms of the number of particles capable of inducing interferon. This was achieved by examining the dose–response curve over a wide range of virus multiplicities, including the particularly critical portion of the curve where the amount of interferon produced is most responsive to changes in multiplicity. Because IFP activity often exceeds PFP (plaque-forming particle) activity by a large factor, it is important to test for IFP activity at multiplicities where $m_{PFP} \ll 1$. Once the dose–response curve has been established, the virus dilution which contains an average of 1 IFP can be determined based on the particular nature of the curve (see Sect. C). Knowing this multiplicity, the number of cells in the infected population, and the fraction of virus particles attached, the IFP titer of the virus stock can be calculated in a manner similar to that used to determine the number of cell-killing particles in a virus stock (MARCUS 1959; MARCUS and SEKELLICK 1974). Once defined, the sensitivity of IFP activity to various reagents (for example, UV radiation and heat) and its expression by different *ts* mutants at nonpermissive temperatures can be measured. Data acquired in this manner reveal the degree of integrity required for a virus particle and/or its genome to express IFP activity, thereby providing insight into the viral functions needed to create an interferon inducer moiety.

C. Dose(Multiplicity)–Response (Interferon Yield) Curves for Interferon Induction/Production

Interferon induction/production (dose–response) curves appear to fall into two general types. Representative examples are illustrated in Sects. C.I and C.II and each type is analyzed and discussed in the context in which it is used to define IFP activity.

I. Type $r \geqq 1$ Curves

In a type $r \geqq 1$ interferon induction/production curve, cells subjected to increasing multiplicities of virus respond by producing within a constant period of time (usually about 12–24 h), increasing amounts of interferon until a plateau is reached. Any further increase in multiplicity has little or no effect on the absolute yield of interferon, i.e., plateau levels of interferon production remain relatively constant. This type of induction curve shows a good fit to the theoretical curve generated by assuming that all cells infected with one or more ($\geqq 1$) virions produce a quantum (finite) yield of interferon. The plateau of this type of curve represents the yield (maximum) of interferon achieved when all the cells of the population have been infected. This theoretical curve is generated by plotting as a function of multiplicity m, the fraction of cells infected with one or more viruses $P_{(r \gg 1)}$, as calculated from the Poisson distribution:

$$P_{(r)} = (e^{-m} m^r / r!)$$

where $P_{(r)}$ = the fraction of cells receiving r particles when the multiplicity of infection is m (LURIA 1940; MARCUS 1959). According to this distribution, the value of m which induces 63% of the maximum yield (plateau value) of interferon, i.e., where 37% (e^{-1}) of the cells escape infection, represents an average of 1 IFP per cell in the population. The titer of IFPs can be calculated knowing the number of cells in the population, the fraction of virus adsorbed to the cells, and m (MARCUS 1959). As shown in Fig. 1 typical $r \geqq 1$ curves are generated when "aged" chick embryo cells are infected with avian reovirus (WINSHIP and MARCUS 1980) or as seen in Fig. 2 when mouse L(Y) cells (also referred to as Ly cells) are infected with a non-*ts* revertant, R1, of vesicular stomatitis virus (VSV) T1026 (MARCUS and SEKEL-

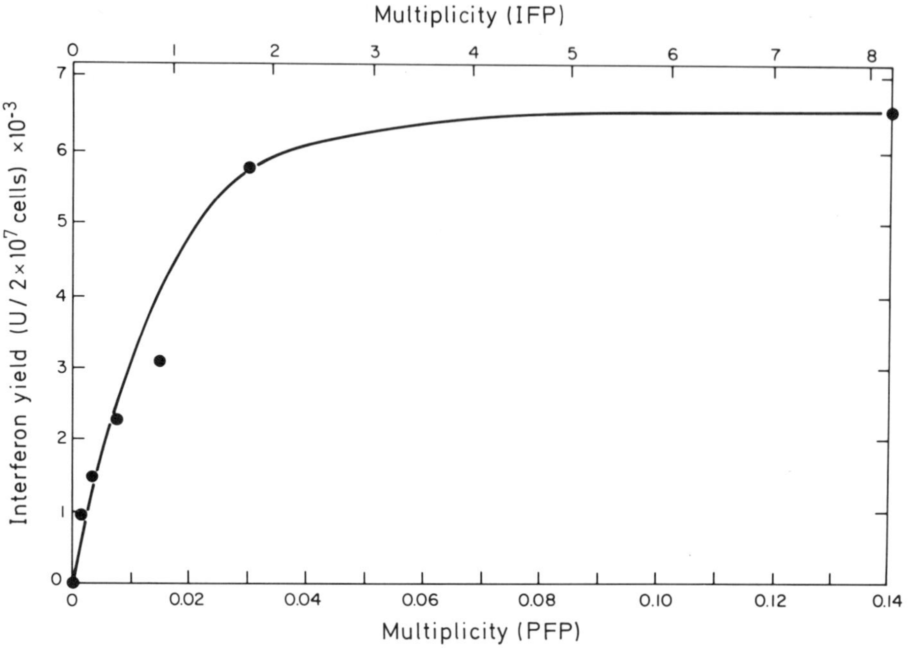

Fig. 1. Dose–response curve relating multiplicity of infectious particles of avian reovirus (S1133 vaccine) to interferon yield on "aged" primary (1°) chick embryo cells at 40.5 °C. The lower abscissa represents the multiplicity of infection in terms of PFPs. The upper abscissa represents the multiplicity of IFPs derived as described in the text. At the multiplicity of infection which induces 63% of the maximum (plateau value) yield of interferon the cell population contains on average 1 IFP per cell. WINSHIP and MARCUS (1980)

LICK 1980). In the former case the observed ratio of IFP:PFP ~ 60:1 means that the virus stocks contain a large excess of noninfectious reovirus particles capable of inducing interferon. In the latter case, there is still an excess of IFP to PFP in VSV R1 stocks since the ratio is about 6:1. The induction of interferon by human reovirus type 3 in chick embryo cells also assumes an $r \geqq 1$ curve when plotted appropriately (LONG and BURKE 1971).

II. Type $r=1$ Curves

In a type $r=1$ dose–response curve, a cell population infected with increasing multiplicities (m) of virus (IFP) responds by producing increasing amounts of interferon until a sharp peak in yield is reached – any further increase in m results in a marked decline in the amount of interferon produced. Curves of this type fit best a model in which cells infected with only one IFP (the $r=1$ class of cells in the Poisson distribution) produce a quantum yield of interferon, and cells infected with $\geqq 2$ particles produce little or no interferon. In a type $r=1$ curve the peak of the interferon yield corresponds to an effective multiplicity (m_{IFP}) of 1 IFP per cell, thus permitting a rapid determination of the IFP titer. As shown in Fig. 3 a typical $r=1$

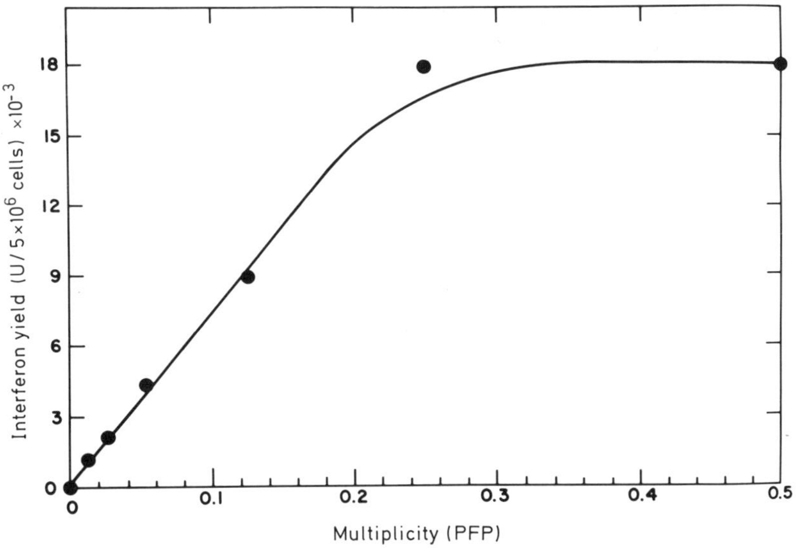

Fig. 2. Dose–response curve relating multiplicity of infection (*PFP*) of VSV non-*ts* revertant R1 (T1026) to the interferon yield on mouse L(Y) cells at 37.5 °C. MARCUS and SEKELLICK (1980)

curve is generated when "aged" chick embryo cells are infected with the [±]RNA DI-011 particle of VSV (MARCUS and SEKELLICK 1977), or when mouse L(Y) cells are infected with the *is*-1 mutant of Mengo virus (Fig. 4) (MARCUS et al. 1981a). In the former case, virtually every physical particle of VSV DI-011 functions as an IFP. In the latter instance, only infectious particles of Mengo virus mutant *is*-1 appear capable of inducing interferon. The dose–response curve described by SLATTERY et al. (1980) for interferon induction/production by Newcastle disease virus on mouse Ehrlich ascites cells also fits well a type $r=1$ response. The peak quantum yield of interferon ($m_{IFP}=1$) in their experiments was extremely high, namely, about 0.5–1 U/cell. The factors which control the absolute value of the interferon quantum yield produced in either a type $r \geqq 1$ or $r=1$ situation remain unknown.

D. dsRNA as the Interferon Inducer Moiety of Viruses: One Molecule as the Threshold for Induction

In spite of conflicting reports, it is generally accepted that dsRNA produced during virus replication or added to the cell as a preformed molecule in the virion constitutes the molecular species most likely responsible for interferon induction. However, the absence of demonstrable dsRNA under some experimental conditions where interferon is produced in abundance casts doubt on this view (reviewed in JOHNSTON and BURKE 1973; STEWART 1979). This apparent anomaly could be resolved were it possible to demonstrate interferon induction by dsRNA at levels below biochemical detection. Experiments we reported in 1977 bear on this point and

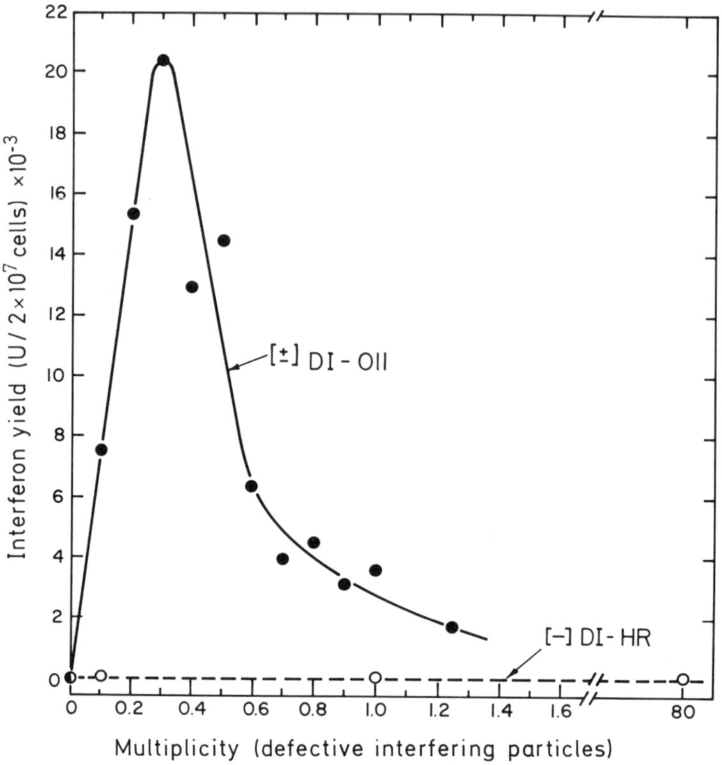

Fig. 3. Dose–response curves relating multiplicity of defective interfering particles of VSV to interferon yield on "aged" primary chick embryo cells. MARCUS and SEKELLICK (1977)

provided compelling evidence that: (1) viral dsRNA generated within a cell can induce interferon; and (2) that the threshold for induction consists of a single molecule of dsRNA pr cell (MARCUS and SEKELLICK 1977). We obtained this evidence by testing the interferon-inducing capacity of an unusual defective interfering particle of VSV, DI-011 (LAZZARINI et al. 1975). This particle contains one linear molecule of covalently linked totally self-complementary RNA of molecular weight 8×10^5. Deproteinization of this RNA permits rapid self-annealing (snapback) into a perfectly base paired helical form (SCHUBERT and LAZZARINI 1981).

Would this [±]RNA assume a helical structure within the cell and function as an interferon inducer? To answer this question we infected monolayers of "aged" chick embryo cells (these cells produce high levels of interferon upon induction; CARVER and MARCUS 1967) with increasing multiplicities of thrice-gradient-purified DI-011 particles. As a control we tested the interferon-inducing capacity of a conventional [−]RNA defective interfering particle prepared by using the same standard helper VSV (Indiana), thus insuring that the polypeptide composition of the two types of defective interfering particles was identical (WAGNER et al. 1969). As illustrated in Fig. 3 [±]DI-011 particles could induce high levels of interferon, whereas conventional [−]DI-HR particles lacked this capacity. Peak interferon

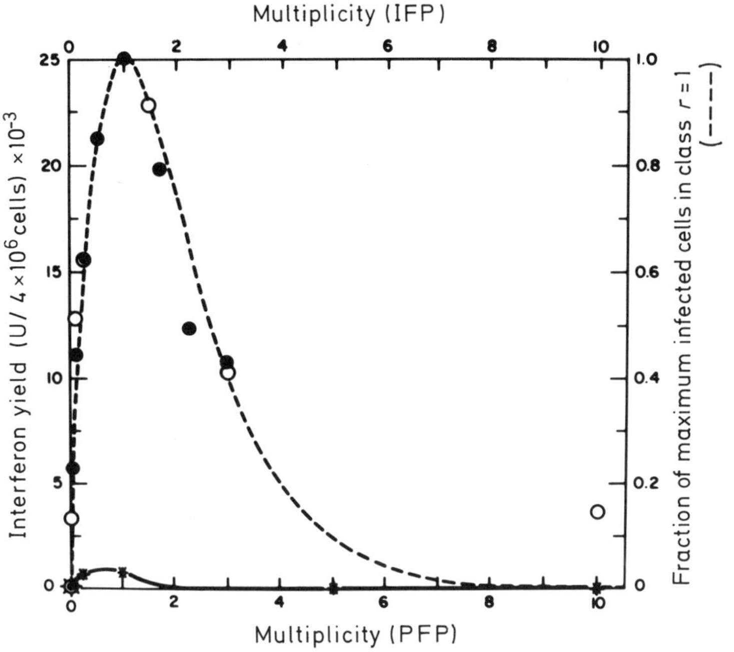

Fig. 4. Dose–response curve relating multiplicity of wild-type Mengo virus is^+ (*asterisks*) and mutant *is*-1 (*open circles* and *full circles* represent two experiments) to interferon yield on mouse l(Y) cells at 37 °C. The lower abscissa represents the multiplicity of infection in terms of PFPs on mouse L(SP) cells. The upper abscissa represents the multiplicity of IFPs calculated on the basis of $m_{IFP} = 1$ at the point of maximal interferon yield. The *broken curve* represents the Poisson distribution for cells infected with only 1 IFP, and fits best a model in which cells infected with 1 IFP produce maximal amounts (quanta) of interferon and those infected with $\geqq 2$ IFP produce little or no interferon. Marcus et al. (1981)

levels of over 20,000 U per monolayer of cells were induced by DI-011 particles, whereas [−]DI-HR particles induced <10 U. When the dose(multiplicity)–response (interferon yield) data for [±]DI-011 particles was analyzed, it fitted best an $r = 1$ curve for interferon induction/production. We concluded that infection with a single particle of DI-011 sufficed to induce a quantum yield of interferon – in effect, defining this particle as an IFP. The number of IFPs and physical particles was found to be equivalent, and hence we concluded that upon entry into the cell each defective interfering particle results in the generation of a dsRNA molecule of sufficient length and stability to trigger the cell's recognition system for interferon induction. Although we do not know whether specific interferon genes or gene banks are induced in "aged" chick embryo cells, the high reproducibility of the dose–response curves and their good fit to theoretical curves of type $r = 1$ require the production of a quantum yield of interferon per induction event.

Interferon induction by DI-011 particles displays all the attributes expected of a bona fide induction process: no interferon is induced in the presence of actinomycin D or cycloheximide. Also, when preparations of DI-011 particles were exposed to antiserum specific for the Indiana serotype of VSV they failed to induce interferon, from which we conclude that the molecule responsible for interferon induction in populations of these particles gains entry into the cell through a particle with the specificity of the Indiana serotype.

It is important to know whether the IFP activity of DI-011 particles results solely from the one molecule of dsRNA which is presumed to form when a single particle enters the cell, or if amplification of viral RNA is required. To determine this we used two means to inactivate the potential RNA-synthesizing capacity of DI-011 particles: (1) ultraviolet (UV) inactivation of the RNA genome; and (2) heat (50 °C) inactivation of the virion transcriptase (MARCUS and SEKELLICK 1975). We inactivated the RNA by delivering the equivalent of up to 50 lethal hits (as measured by PFP activity), representing about 10 lethal hits to the particle's capacity to function in homotypic interference (BAY and REICHMANN 1979). The high levels of UV radiation had virtually no effect on the IFP capacity of DI-011 (MARCUS and SEKELLICK 1977). This result is consistent with the "preformed" nature of the interferon inducer in the DI-011 virion and makes it appear very unlikely that the [±]RNA genome need be used as a template for RNA synthesis to produce an interferon inducer moiety. However, this dose range of UV radiation did not eliminate a role for the small target of leader-like RNA at the 3′ end of the defective interfering particle's genome and its possible transcription into a complementary 46-base sequence (EMERSON et al. 1977). Transcription of the leader-like sequence depends on the integrity of a relatively heat-labile transcriptase in the particle (SZILÁGYI and PRINGLE 1972). Consequently, we subjected the DI-011 particles to 50 °C for 20 min, a regimen which inactivates over 90% of virion-associated transcriptase activity as measured in vivo (MARCUS and SEKELLICK 1975). Particles heated in this manner were as effective as inducing interferon as were unheated particles (MARCUS and SEKELLICK 1977). Furthermore, these heated DI-011 particles lost much of their capacity to produce leader-like product as measured in an in vitro transcribing system (BALL and WHITE 1978; L. A. BALL 1980, personal communication).

In concert, these data provide substantial evidence that a single particle of DI-011 which contains a molecule with the potential of assuming a helical form in the cell, can, in the absence of any RNA replication, induce a quantum yield of interferon. This makes the DI-011 particle perhaps the most efficient inducer of interferon thus far described. The good fit of the dose–response curve to the $r=1$ term of the Poisson distribution establishes that the threshold for interferon induction is one molecule of dsRNA per cell. The shape of the dose–response curve suggests another important concept, namely, while one molecule of dsRNA suffices to turn on an interferon gene (or gene bank), the simultaneous addition of presumably a second molecule of dsRNA, delivered in the form of a second DI-011 particle, leads to virtually complete suppression of that gene and/or its expression. This novel concept seems applicable because the amount of interferon produced at $m_{IFP} > 1$ fits well that expected if only cells infected with 1 IFP produce a quantum yield (the $r=1$ class), leading us to conclude that cells infected with $\geqq 2$ IFP produce little or no interferon! Further study is required to identify the event or events which regulate so exquisitely the induction/production of interferon under $r=1$ conditions.

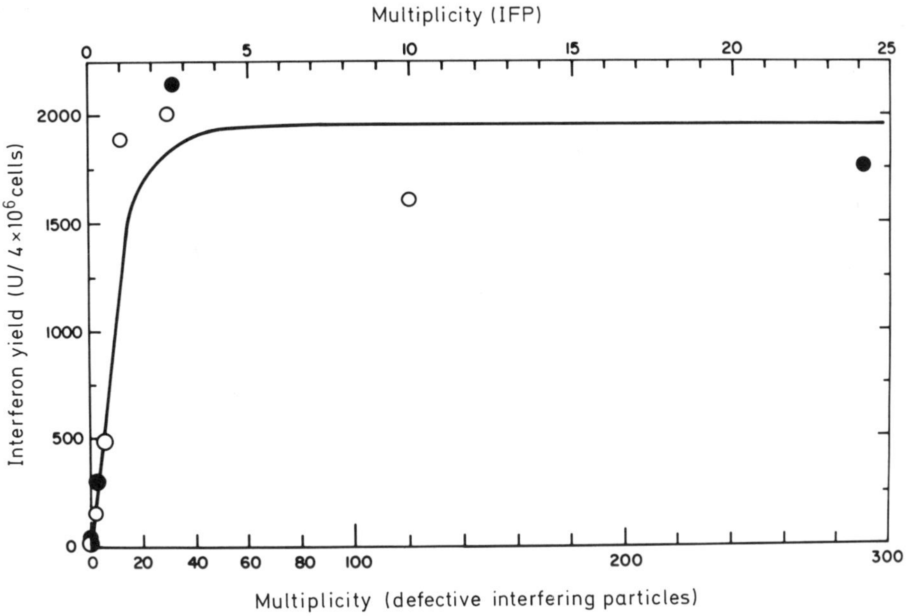

Fig. 5. Dose–response surve relating multiplicity of quadruply gradient-purified VSV DI-011 particles to interferon yield from mouse L(Y) cells at 37 °C. The lower abscissa represents m_{DIP} (assayed on GMK-Vero cells), and the upper abscissa represents m_{IFP} as determined from the dilution of DI-011 particles which induce 63% of the maximum yield of interferon. SEKELLICK and MARCUS (1980 b)

Interferon induction by DI-011 particles is not unique to "aged" primary chick embryo cells. We have demonstrated their interferon inducing capacity in mouse L(Y) and GMK-BSC cells (SEKELLICK and MARCUS 1978), and primary mouse embryo cells. In human FS-4 cells, little or no interferon was induced by DI-011 particles, yet a demonstrable multiplicity-dependent antiviral state developed as measured by yield reduction of Sindbis virus (MARCUS and SEKELLICK 1977). Also, when human MRC-5 cells were infected with DI-011 particles, the cells developed resistance to the lethal action of superinfecting Sindbis virus (P. I. MARCUS 1981, unpublished work) even though the interferon-inducible enzymes, 2–5A synthetase (also referred to as polymerase) and protein kinase, were presumably below detectable levels (MEURS et al. 1981). As expected, DI-011 particles failed to induce interferon in GMK-Vero or BHK cells, both of which are genetically incompetent for interferon induction (DESMYTER et al. 1968; MARCUS and SEKELLICK 1976; SEKELLICK and MARCUS 1978).

Induction of interferon by VSV DI-011 particles in mouse L(Y) cells is particularly significant since FREY et al. (1979, 1980) have questioned the capacity of such particles by themselves to induce interferon. However, we have found that a single particle of DI-011 is intrinsically capable of inducing interferon in mouse L(Y) cells, albeit the probability of doing so is 10–100-fold lower than in "aged" chick embryo cells (SEKELLICK and MARCUS 1982). As illustrated in Fig. 5, an $r \geqq 1$ type of induction curve was generated. In four successive gradient bandings of the DI-

011 particles, we observed no diminution of the IFP activity (or of homotypic interference) of the banded virus, in spite of a steady decrease in contaminating levels of infectious virus. Furthermore, heat treatment or UV irradiation sufficient to detroy virtually all virion-associated transcriptase activity or template function of all but a small portion of the parental genome, failed to diminish the IFP activity of the DI-011 stocks. Either of these inactivation conditions would destroy the ability of any "contaminating" standard virus to function as a helper and of the defective particle to function in homotypic interference. Also, when specific anti-VSV serum was added to cells after attachment and entry of VSV DI-011 particles in order to prevent cycling of infection by any contaminating standard virus, there was no adverse effect on the induction or production of interferon. It is difficult to conceive of amplification of a viral product under any of these circumstances or cooperative events leading to interferon induction. Consequently, we attribute the production of interferon in DI-011 particle-infected L(Y) cells to a property intrinsic to the particle itself, namely, its potential to form a dsRNA molecule. These results confute the conclusions of FREY et al. (1979, 1980).

E. One Molecule of dsRNA as the Interferon Inducer Moiety of Different Viruses

In this section we examine the virus–cell systems thus far analyzed for IFP activity interferon induction/production fitted to an $r=1$ or $r \geqq 1$ type dose–response curve, along with evidence for dsRNA as the common molecule responsible for interferon induction by these viruses.

I. Vesicular Stomatitis Virus

Vesicular stomatitis virus (VSV) is considered a poor inducer of interferon (reviewed in MARCUS 1980) and hence not a likely subject for studies on interferon induction. Yet, the reports of interferon in cultures persistently infected with VSV and the emergence of *ts*-mutants during persistent infection (reviewed in SEKELLICK and MARCUS 1980a) suggested a possible role for *ts* mutants as IFPs. We tested the interferon-inducing capacity of VSV *ts* mutants representing all five of the complementation groups of the Indiana serotype and found that all *ts* mutants which failed to turn off cellular protein synthesis, or kill cells at nonpermissive temperatures (MARVALDI et al. 1977) were excellent inducers of interferon, both in "aged" primary chick embryo cells and in mouse L(Y) cells (SEKELLICK and MARCUS 1979). Dose–response curves for these mutants in chick cells bore a striking similarity to that produced by VSV DI-011 particles, namely, an $r=1$ type of response; however, the *ts* mutants usually induced peak yields of interferon at $m_{PFP} \sim 0.1$, indicating there was an excess of IFPs over PFPs in stocks of VSV. One of the better inducers, *ts*G11(I), is defective in the L-protein: primary transcription is normal, but amplified RNA synthesis does not occur at 40.5 °C – conditions optimal for interferon induction (MARCUS and SEKELLICK 1980). This suggested that primary transcription may be required to form an interferon-inducing moiety. We tested this possibility by measuring the IFP activity of *ts*G11 heated at 50 °C to inactivate virion transcriptase. The IFP capacity of this mutant was lost at the same rate as PFP and transcriptase activity, confirming that transcription was a rate-limiting and requisite event for the formation of an interferon inducer by VSV (MARCUS and SEKELLICK 1980). UV irradiation of another excellent inducer of interferon, the non-*ts* revertant, R1, of T1026 (FRANCOEUR et al. 1978; SEKELLICK and MARCUS 1979) showed that its interferon-inducing capacity was lost at about one-tenth the rate of infectivity (MARCUS and SEKELLICK 1980). Taken in concert, these studies indicate that a single IFP of VSV suffices to induce a quantum yield of interferon, and that there are several times more IFP than PFP in stock preparations of VSV. Furthermore, while virus replication or amplified RNA synthesis is not required for IFP activity, there is a requirement for primary transcription. About one-tenth of the genome must remain intact and presumably be transcribed to synthesize an interferon-inducing moiety.

We conclude that in contrast to the [±]DI-011 particles, infectious VSV does not contain a preformed inducer of interferon. We proposed a model for interferon inducer formation in which the cumulative loss of N- (and/or NS- and L-) protein from the ribonucleoprotein (RNP) complex during primary transcription leads ultimately to extensive base pairing between the genome RNA and its complementary transcript. We suggest that the dsRNA thus formed constitutes the interferon-inducing molecule of VSV (MARCUS and SEKELLICK 1980). We also hypothesized that certain *ts* mutants of VSV were excellent inducers because defects in N-, NS-, or L-proteins increased the probability for dsRNA formation during primary transcription. One mutant, *ts*G31(III), an RNA^+ mutant defective in M-protein, did not appear to fit this hypothesis since it inhibited cellular protein synthesis and killed cells at nonpermissive temperature, but was nonetheless an excellent inducer of interferon (SEKELLICK and MARCUS 1979). However, HUGHES and JOHNSON (1981) have recently reported differences between the N-protein peptide maps of *ts*G31(III) and its wild-type parent. Possibly then, in addition to a defect in M-protein which confers temperature sensitivity, the N-protein of *ts*G31 may be altered sufficiently to enhance formation of the interferon-inducing moiety, though not enough to effect its function in transcription and replication. We interpret these results to mean that a subtle alteration in the conformation of N-protein may enhance interferon-inducer formation yet leave transcription and replication functionally equivalent to that achieved by the wild-type polypeptide. In this context we note that while most VSV wild-type strains (Glasgow, Massachusetts, Canada-HR, and MS) of the Indiana serotype VSV are poor inducers of interferon, the New Jersey serotype, Hazelhurst isolate, is an excellent inducer. Perhaps, with respect to interferon inducer formation the Hazelhurst N-protein is functionally like that of *ts*G31.

Our model for interferon induction by VSV requires that *ts* mutants capable of inducing interferon form dsRNA in cells, whereas wild-type virus (a poor inducer) might not. Experiments of NILSEN et al. (1981) provide direct evidence for the formation of dsRNA in cells infected with an interferon-inducing *ts* mutant of VSV and its absence in cells infected with wild-type VSV. These investigators were able to demonstrate dsRNA directly in infected cells by "capturing" base paired RNA in situ with 4′-aminomethyl-4,5′,8-trimethylpsoralen (AMT) and long wavelength UV radiation. AMT is an agent that cross-links between pyrimidine bases on opposite strands upon irradiation with long wavelength UV light. Wild-type VSV produced little or no "capturable" dsRNA in the cell, whereas the *ifp*$^{+}$ mutant *ts*G114(I) (SEKELLICK and MARCUS 1979) generated significant amounts of dsRNA within the infected cell (NILSEN et al. 1981). These results have other implications. They suggest that the failure of some viruses to induce interferon may not reside solely in their capacity to turn off cellular macromolecular synthesis as has been suggested (WERTZ and YOUNGNER 1970; NISHIYAMA et al. 1979), but instead, may be due to a failure to generate dsRNA. We think that the wild-type N- (NS- and/or L-) protein may remain bound more firmly to the transcribing nucleoprotein complex of VSV than defective N- (NS- and/or L-) of mutant virus, thus lowering the chances of base pairing between the [−]RNA genome strand and its newly synthesized [+]RNA complementary transcript. In a cell mixedly infected with wild-type virus and a mutant which is phenotypically positive for IFN induction (*ifp*$^{+}$), the expressed phenotype is invariably *ifp*$^{-}$ (P. I. MARCUS and M. J. SEKELLICK 1982, unpublished work). Conceivably this result might reflect the dominant expression of the wild-type ribonucleoproteins in the transcribing core (SCHNITZLEIN and REICHMANN 1977) and their ability to minimize or prevent base pairing.

II. Sindbis Virus

Realizing that a single molecule of dsRNA, when properly introduced or produced in a cell, could induce a quantum yield of interferon (MARCUS and SEKELLICK 1977), we were encouraged to reexamine a long-standing question regarding the interferon-inducing capacity of togaviruses, especially Sindbis virus, and its *ts* mutants (reviewed in STEWART 1979, p 73). In most instances there was no apparent correlation between dsRNA formation and interferon induction. Using the hyperresponsive "aged" primary chick embryo cells as host, we determined the interferon-inducing capacity of standard stocks of Sindbis virus prepared from low multiplicity infection. The dose–response curves for interferon induction were very similar to those observed with DI-011 particles, *ts* mutants of VSV, and Mengo virus mutant *is*-1 (Figs. 3 and 4), i.e., they fit the $r=1$ class of inducer curves. Peak yields of interferon occurred at $m_{PFP} \sim 1$, indicating that a single infectious particle of Sindbis virus was required to induce a quantum yield of interferon and that IFPs and PFPs were functionally equivalent (MARCUS and FULLER 1979). Nonetheless, the IFN-inducing capacity of Sindbis virus was four times more resistant to UV irradiation than was infectivity, indicating that only about 25% of the viral genome need be intact in order to induce interferon, and that viral replication per se was not a requisite event for interferon induction. Thus, 75% of the genome could be inactivated, destroying its capacity to amplify viral RNA synthesis, but its capacity to function as an IFP remained intact. We used the *ts* mutants of PFEFFERKORN and BURGE (1967) and of STRAUSS et al. (1976) to determine whether this quarter of the genome represented a unique portion. We reasoned that mutants unable to induce interferon at a nonpermissive temperature (40.5 °C) were defective in a function required for interferon inducer formation. We found that mutants from all three of the RNA^{+} complementation groups (groups C, D, and E) were capable of inducing interferon at 40.5 °C, as were two of the four RNA^{-} complementation

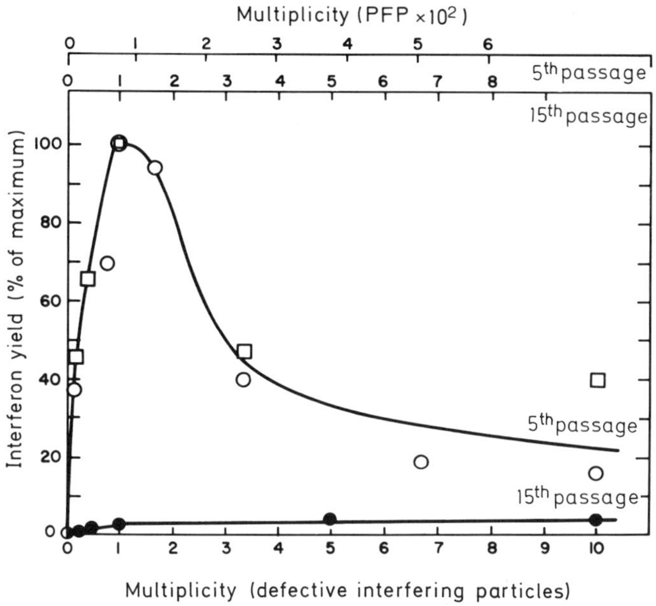

Fig. 6. Dose–response curves relating multiplicity of infection of Sindbis virus defective interfering particles, 5th and 15th passage, to interferon yield from "aged" primary chick embryo cells. Maximum yields of interferon at $m_{DIP} = 1$ for the 5th passage particles averaged 8,000 U per 10^7 cells. The upper abscissa indicates the level of "contaminating" PFP. FULLER and MARCUS (1980 a)

groups, B and F. However, mutants in groups G and A produced very little interferon. We concluded that no performed inducer of interferon is present in Sindbis virus and that genes G and A represent a special quarter of the genome which must be functional in order to synthesize an interferon-inducing moiety. We postulated that this moiety was a dsRNA molecule formed after synthesis of a segment of RNA complementary to the genome. By analogy with Semliki Forest virus (CLEWLEY and KENNEDY 1976) we think gene products G and A may function as a negative-strand polymerase (SAWICKI and SAWICKI 1980) to catalyze this synthesis, starting with the polyadenylate residues at the 3′ terminus of the virion RNA (FREY and STRAUSS 1978).

A significant portion of the viral genome proximal to the 5′ terminus is conserved in defective particles generated during early serial passages of Sindbis (and Semliki Forest) virus (GUILD and STOLLAR 1977; STARK and KENNEDY 1978), and this 5′ end contains genes G and A (FULLER and MARCUS 1980 c). If expression of Sindbis virus genes G and A represents the minimal information required for formation of an interferon-inducing molecule of dsRNA, then certain defective interfering particles might function as interferon inducers. We tested the interferon-inducing activity of early (5th) passage defective interfering particles which contained a segment of RNA sufficiently large (25 *S*, 1.6×10^6 daltons) to accommodate genes G and A. The 5th passage defective interfering particles were excellent inducers of interferon (Fig. 6). Analysis of the $r = 1$ type of dose–response curve

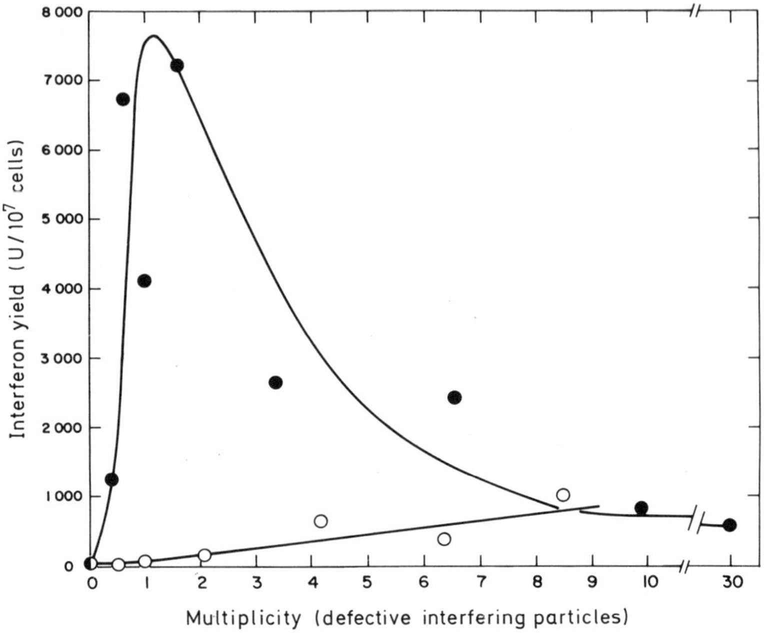

Fig. 7. Dose–response curve relating multiplicity of wild-type Sindbis virus (W^+) (*full circles*) and *ts*-24(A)-derived (*open circles*) defective interfering particles (5th passage) to interferon yield from "aged" primary chick embryo cells incubated at 40.5 °C. FULLER and MARCUS (1980 b)

they generated indicated that each defective interfering particle was also capable of functioning as an IFP! It is important to point out that interferon induction by defective interfering particles took place in the absence of "helper" virus. The IFP activity of early passage Sindbis virus defective interfering particles was sensitive to both UV radiation and low doses of interferon (FULLER and MARCUS 1980 a), suggesting that a preformed inducer is not indigenous to the particle, and that genes G and A have to be translated to produce the interferon inducer moiety. Late (15th) passage defective interfering particles provided a control since the RNA from these particles was too small (20 *S*, 1.0×10^6 daltons) to encode for both of these genes. Indeed, 15th passage particles did not induce IFN, even though they functioned efficiently as defective interfering particles (Fig. 6; FULLER and MARCUS 1980 a).

As a final test of our hypothesis for interferon induction by Sindbis virus we constructed a defective interfering particle which was temperature sensitive for gene A – deriving it from the parent mutant *ts*24(A). If the role we proposed for genes G and A in the formation of an interferon inducer moiety by Sindbis virus is correct, the *ts*24(A) defective interfering particles should display a phenotype which is temperature sensitive for interferon induction. This was indeed the case: this mutant induced interferon at a permissive temperature (30 °C), but not at 40.5 °C (Fig. 7), a nonpermissive temperature. Wild-type defective interfering particles induced IFN at both of these temperatures (FULLER and MARCUS 1980 b).

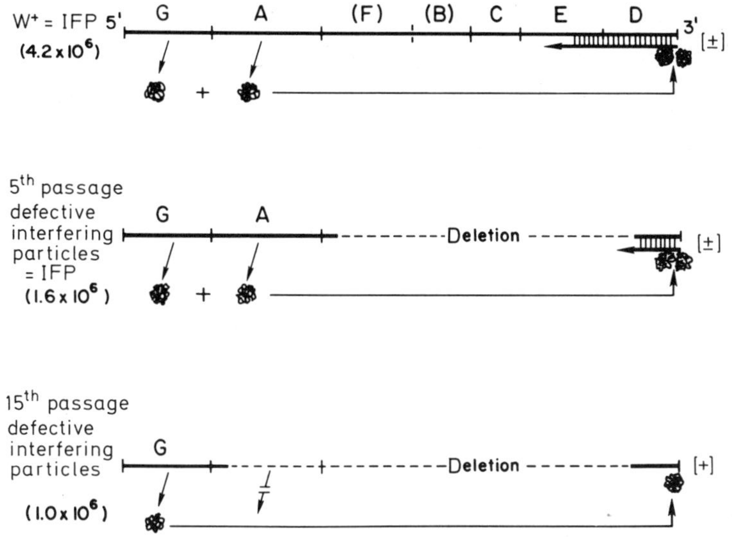

Fig. 8. A model for the formation of interferon inducer (dsRNA) by standard infectious virus (W^+) and 5th passage defective interfering particles. The placement of genes G and A at the 5′ end of the genome is based on the results of FULLER and MARCUS (1980c). Some aspects of the model are derived in part from and are consistent with schemes published by others. FULLER and MARCUS (1980a)

Figures 8 presents a schematic of our model for the formation of an interferon inducer molecule, dsRNA, by standard infectious Sindbis virus and its 5th passage defective interfering particles. Considering the data of FREY and STRAUSS (1978) and SAWICKI and SAWICKI (1980), we can update this model by postulating that the inducer dsRNA consists of the poly(A) tail at the 3′ end of the positive-strand genome base paired with its newly synthesized complement of poly(U). In that context, the 3′ terminus of the parenteral positive-strand does not bind ribosomes (reviewed in SAWICKI and SAWICKI 1980) and hence would be readily accessible as a template for the negative-strand polymerase. It is, of course, possible that the newly synthesized negative-strand itself assumes enough secondary structure to constitute an interferon-inducing moiety.

III. Reovirus

Members of the reoviridae family with their genome content of preformed dsRNA molecules might be expected to be excellent inducers of interferon. Yet, large numbers of physical particles of human reovirus are required for maximal levels of interferon induction (LONG and BURKE 1971; LAI and JOKLIK 1973). We suggest that this represents the small chance that even one genomic dsRNA segment becomes accessible to the cell's recognition system for interferon induction – most likely a reflection of the fact that human reovirion ds RNA has a low probability of being released free into the cytoplasm (SILVERSTEIN and DALES 1968). However, this low probability event per particle–cell encounter would become a high probability event per cell when infection is carried out at very high multiplicities of physical particles, and considering that each particle contains ten segments of dsRNA, only one of which may be required for induction of interferon.

Analyses of published dose–response curves reveal a type $r \geqq 1$ induction for human reovirus (type 3) on mouse L-cells (LAI and JOKLIK 1973) or chick embryo cells (LONG and BURKE 1971; WINSHIP and MARCUS 1980) and for avian reovirus on chick embryo cells (Fig. 1; WINSHIP and MARCUS 1980). From the LAI and JOKLIK (1973) study we calculated that with mouse L-cells as hosts, the ratio of attached human reovirus type 3 physical particles: PFP: IFP was about 800: 16: 1. From the LONG and BURKE (1971) study using chick cells as hosts we calculated that same ratio as about 1,000: 20: 1, i.e., essentially the same.[1] From the good fit to the $r \geqq 1$ type of induction curve in these studies we conclude that about 999 of 1,000 physical particles never interact with the cell as IFP. However, with respect to the induction and production of interferon, it is clear that 1 IFP per 1,000 particles does interact with the cell in a functionally significant way. These considerations make it easy to appreciate use of the term "never" as it is often applied to the liberation of reovirus dsRNA into the cytoplasma of the cell (HENDERSON and JOKLIK 1978). However, we think that term requires modification so as to accommodate that rare particle (or event) which may contribute genomic dsRNA to the cell and function as an interferon inducer moiety.[2] With so many particles produced during reovirus infection, this rare event may assume biologic significance in natural infection.

If particles of human reovirus type 3 epitomize the inefficiency with which genomic dsRNA is presented to the cell's recognition system for interferon induction, then particles of the vaccine strain (S1133) of avian reovirus (VAN DER HEIDE and KALBAC 1975) epitomize the efficiency with which this process can function (WINSHIP and MARCUS 1980). For example, Fig. 1 shows that an average of 1 IFP avian reovirus S1133 per cell is reached only after the stock virus has been diluted to an infectious particle multiplicity of $m_{PFP} = 0.017$. This means that there is 60 times more IFP than PFP in this vaccine stock. The ratio IFP: PFP can be increased from 60: 1 to 197: 1 upon exposing the virus stock to 9.4 lethal hits of UV radiation (WINSHIP and MARCUS 1980). These data suggest that many of the physical particles are intrinsically capable of functioning as IFP in chick cells and that UV radiation may, in some systems, enhance that capability.[3]

---

1 The fact that these ratios are virtually the same in both a permissive (L-cell) and nonpermissive (chick cell) host strengthens the argument that the interferon-inducing moiety is associated with the input particle and not a replicative event. This argument will be developed further in the text

2 We also note the possibility that this low efficiency of expressing IFP may reflect the presence of naked dsRNA on the surface of some (possibly, damaged) (LONG et al. 1976) human reovirus particles (LENGYEL et al. 1980) and its delivery into the cell upon virion entry (BORSA et al. 1979)

3 Following UV radiation, the interferon-inducing capacity of human reovirus type 3 can be enhanced (HENDERSON and JOKLIK 1978) or reduced (LONG and BURKE 1971; LAI and JOKLIK 1973; WINSHIP and MARCUS 1980) and, in the case of bluetongue virus, can be unaffected (JAMESON and GROSSBERG 1979) or enhanced (JAMESON et al. 1980), and with Colorado tick fever virus can be enhanced (DUBOVI and AKERS 1972). Clearly, the efficacy with which reovirus particles induce interferon (present dsRNA to the cell) can vary widely, with the host cell playing a critical role in regulating the expression of IFP activity (WINSHIP and MARCUS 1981)

While lack of precise quantitation of the IFP activity of reoviridae makes it difficult to interpret the results of many interferon induction studies, the bulk of the evidence suggests that the virion-derived genome dsRNA segments constitute the interferon-inducing moiety of this family of viruses. Accepting that the dsRNA from the vast majority of entering human reovirus type 3 particles may never become free within the cell, there is nonetheless the possibility that, during each reovirus–cell interaction, at least one dsRNA segment of the virion is exposed, perhaps transiently, to the cell's recognition system for interferon induction. Possibly, primary transcription may help display the dsRNA (WINSHIP and MARCUS 1980). Apparently, the efficiency with which genomic dsRNA may be presented to the cell as a protein-free double helix may vary widely. In chick cells, virtually all physical particles of avian reovirus appear to function as IFP, whereas human reoviruses are intrinsically inefficient in expressing this function, even after UV irradiation. Furthermore, all of the *ts* mutants of human reovirus tested, representing nine of the ten complementation groups (CROSS and FIELDS 1977), induced interferon at a nonpermissive temperature, including *ts*447(C), a tight RNA^- mutant (WINSHIP and MARCUS 1980). Notably, reovirus particles lacking dsRNA fail to induce interferon (LAI and JOKLIK 1973). Taken in concert, these data provide strong evidence that the dsRNA intrinsic to the reovirion genome is the interferon-inducing moiety and that this dsRNA may be made available to the cell's recognition system for induction with widely differing efficiencies: low in the case of human reovirus on mouse L-cells or chick embryo cells, and high in the case of avian reovirus on chick embryo cells.

Finally, we note that the physiology of the host cell can be critical in regulating the expression of IFP activity of reoviruses. Thus, human reovirus type 3 and its *ts* mutants failed to function as IFP in mouse L(Y) cells until they had "aged" (CARVER and MARCUS 1967) appropriately in vitro (WINSHIP and MARCUS 1981). This critical dependence on cell "age" for the expression of IFP activity provides an explanation for the need to form progeny reovirus to induce interferon, as reported by LAI and JOKLIK (1973). For example, when inadequately "aged" mouse L(Y) cells (3-day-old) were infected with *ts* mutants at 39 °C they failed to function as IFP. However, when these same mutants were used to infect cells 1 day later (4-day-old cells), they induced high levels of interferon! Furthermore, when 3-day-old cells were infected with wild-type reovirus they did not begin to produce interferon until 1 day later, i.e., until the cells had become 4 days old. We interpret these results to mean that progeny virus synthesized during the first 24 h of infection were present to superinfect the cells when they became receptive hosts 1 day later. Proof that progeny virus, and not parental virus, was responsible for the appearance of interferon 48 h after the initial infection was obtained by demonstrating that anti-reovirus type 3 serum added during the first 24 h (immediately after virus entry) prevented interferon production 24 h later, i.e., prevented superinfection of the by then, 4-day-old cells. In this context, the failure of *ts* mutants to induce interferon in 3-day-old cells is seen as a failure to produce progeny virus at the nonpermissive temperature. Thus, new virus would not be available when the cells became physiologically receptive hosts for IFP expression 1 day later (WINSHIP and MARCUS 1981).

IV. Mengo Virus

Picornaviridae generally are not chosen for their propensity to induce interferon, and hence might not be considered a research object worthy for studies on interferon induction. However, under appropriate conditions many members of this family can induce significant levels of interferon (JOHNSON and MCLAREN 1965; GIRON et al. 1971; STEWART et al. 1971). In this regard, we have demonstrated recently that a mutant of Mengo virus, *is*-1, designated as "interferon sensitive" by SIMON et al. (1976), is an excellent inducer of interferon and is more accurately described phenotypically as *ifp* (MARCUS et al. 1981a). In an excellent fit to a type $r=1$ dose–response curve (cf. theoretical and observed curves in Fig. 4), mutant *is*-1 induced over 25,000 U interferon per 4×10^6 mouse L(Y) cells, thus providing an opportunity to characterize the requirements for IFP activity by this picornavirus. From Fig. 4 we note the ratio IFP : PFP ~ 1 : 1, suggesting that only infectious particles can function as IFP. Indeed, when Mengo virus mutant *is*-1 is UV irradiated, both IFP and PFP activities are lost at the same rate (MARCUS et al. 1981b). From this we infer that a single hit, i.e., uracil dimer formation (MILLER and PLAGEMANN 1974) suffices to prevent translation of the positive-strand genome (FULLER and MARCUS 1980c) and therefore synthesis of some gene product or products essential for interferon inducer formation.

While these results appear to implicate amplified viral RNA synthesis as a requisite event for inducer formation, we favor an alternative interpretation based on our model for dsRNA formation in another positive-strand virus, Sindbis (references cited in Sect. E.II). In the case of Sindbis virus the [−]RNA polymerase genes are located at the extreme 5′ end of the genome where translation is initiated. Thus, several UV hits can be sustained by the RNA genome without any adverse effect on the two negative-strand polymerase genes or their action to produce a dsRNA molecule at the 3′ end and hence IFP activity (FULLER and MARCUS 1980 a). However, and in marked contrast, the polymerase gene or genes of picornaviruses are located at the 3′ end of the genome, far distant from the initiation site, and thus a single UV hit would prevent its expression (translation). We postulate that as a result of this polymerase activity, a threshold amount of base pairing between positive-strand genome and its negative-strand complement produces a dsRNA molecule, the putative interferon-inducing moiety.

One puzzling aspect of interferon induction by Mengo virus mutant *is*-1 is its complete abrogation upon coinfection of cells with wild-type, *is*$^+$, virus (MARCUS et al. 1981), i.e., the *ifp*$^-$ phenotype of the wild-type virus is dominant to the *ifp*$^+$ phenotype of the mutant. Usually the rapid turnoff of cellular macromolecular synthesis by viruses is offered to explain the *ifp*$^-$ phenotype for poor inducers of interferon (reviewed in STEWART 1979, p 72–73). However, FOUT and SIMON (1981) provided evidence that wild-type and mutant virus were equally effective in suppressing host cell macromolecular synthesis. Consequently, we sought an alternative explanation for the dominant expression of the *ifp*$^-$ phenotype, based in concept on our model for the interferon-inducing moiety of VSV (MARCUS and SEKELLICK 1980). We postulate that in the presence of wild-type Mengo virus proteins there is minimal base pairing between the genome strand and its newly synthesized complement, not enough to trigger the interferon induction system. In contrast, we hypothesize that in the mutant virus a non-*ts* defect in one or more proteins permits a threshold length, and/or an extended time, of base pairing during replication – sufficient to trigger the cell's recognition system for interferon induction, but not sufficient to disrupt the replication process itself. In a mixedly infected cell, we postulate that expression of the wild-type viral protein or proteins dominates and base pairing and/or its duration are held below the threshold for induction. It will be of interest to determine the relationship between this postulated threshold for the base pairing length and the minimum of about 50 paired nucleotides required to activate the 2′,5′-oligo(A) synthetase associated with interferon action (NILSEN and BAGLIONI 1979).

Finally, we note the perceptive comments of STEWART (1979, p 35), who points out that the factors which affect interferon induction by viruses are so variable that the terms "good" or "poor" inducer are not particularly enlightening. We agree, and point out that Mengo virus mutant *is*-1 used at $m_{IFP} \sim 1$ would be scored as a "good" inducer, but when tested at $m_{IFP} \geqq 5$, a commonly used multiplicity, would rate as only a "poor" inducer (Fig. 4; MARCUS et al. 1981 a, b).[4] This underscores the necessity of carrying out interferon induction studies over a complete range of virus multiplicities.

V. Newcastle Disease Virus

Newcastle disease virus (NDV) perhaps has been studied more extensively than any other virus to discern the mechanism of interferon induction. Much of this effort has come from the laboratories of D.C. BURKE (reviewed in JOHNSTON and BURKE 1973), J. VILČEK (reviewed in VILČEK and KOHASE 1977), and J.S. YOUNGNER (reviewed in KOWAL and YOUNGNER 1978). Two aspects of the literature have been culled and information analyzed regarding the nature of the interferon-inducing moiety of this well-studied virus. These are discussed in Sects. E.V.1 and 2 in the context of the approach to this problem we have emphasized throughout the chapter.

1. Dose (Multiplicity)–Response (Interferon Yield) Curves

Table 1 records the studies which reported dose–response curve data for NDV on various host cells. By appropriately replotting the data we have been able to categorize the curves. It is evident that both $r=1$ and $r \geqq 1$ curves have been observed. No obvious explanation for the different responses is apparent. In the study by SLATTERY et al. (1980) the experimental fit to an $r=1$ curve was particularly good, and revealed that only 1 in 20 PFP registered as an IFP on the mouse Ehrlich

4 Accurate values of m_{IFP} can be obtained only if specific anti-Mengo virus serum is present after virus attachment and entry. This treatment prevents superinfection by newly released virus and hence maintains equivalence between the input and the effective multiplicity. Antiserum to Semliki Forest virus was used in a related manner by GOORHA and GIFFORD (1970) who cleverly implicated the role of priming in enhancing the induction/production of interferon at low multiplicities of infection

Table 1. Newcastle disease virus dose–response curves and IFP : PFP ratios

Reference	Data source[a]	NDV strain	Host cell	Type of dose–response curve[b]	Ratio IFP : PFP[c]
WHEELOCK (1966)	Fig. 1	Hickman	Human leukocytes	$r=1$	1 : 1
YOUNGER et al. (1966)	Fig. 4	Herts	Mouse L	$r \geqq 1$	1 : 1
FLEISCHMANN and SIMON (1974)	Fig. 1	Beaudette	Mouse L	$r \geqq 1$	1 : 2
Kohase and VILČek (1979)	Fig. 5	Hickman	Human FS-4	$r \geqq 1$	1 : 9
Slattery et al. (1980)	Fig. 3	Beaudette	Mouse EAT	$r=1$	1 : 20
MARCUS et al. (1982) (unpublished work)		Australia–Victoria, 1932	Mouse L(Y)	$r \geqq 1$	1 : 1

[a] Refers to figures in the cited reference
[b] Defined in Sects. C.I and C.II
[c] Values of m_{PFP} were obtained from the cited reference. Values of m_{IFP} were calculated according to the type of curve (discussed in Sects. C.I and C.II)

ascites tumor cells used as hosts. While the reported yield (quantum value) of interferon was extremely high in that study (0.4 U/cell; enhanced three fold by the presence of theophylline), the actual yield on a per cell basis was even higher, since at the optimal multiplicity for interferon yield ($m_{IFP}=1$, $m_{PFP}=20$) in an $r=1$ type of response only 63% ($=1-e^{-1}$) of the cells are actually infected with an IFP. Consequently, the real yield of interferon is calculated as 0.63 (0.40/0.63) U/cell. We note that the data of FLEISCHMANN and SIMON (1974) and of KOHASE and VILČEK (1979) show a good fit to an $r \geqq 1$ curve, i.e., show near congruence of experimental and theoretical curves, when one assumes that only 1 of 2 PFP and 9 PFP, respectively, register in a cell as an IFP.

2. Genome Integrity and Interferon Induction

Table 2 records several studies in which the interferon-inducing capacity of NDV was evaluated following UV irradiation of the virus. Initially, this determination appeared complicated because most of the studies were done under conditions (chick embryo cells as hosts and virus derived from chick eggs) where low doses of UV radiation enhanced rather than inactivated IFP activity. This effect was quantitated first by HO and BREINIG (1965) and has been substantiated by all sub-

Table 2. Newcastle disease virus: relative target sizes for inactivation of PFP and IFP activities by UV radiation

Reference	Data source[a]	UV targets for PFP and IFP activities	
		Relative rates of inactivation (PFP:IFP)[b]	Fraction of genome required for IFP activity[c]
Ho and Breinig (1965)	Fig. 1	1:50	0.02
Youngner et al. (1966)	Fig. 1	1:33	0.03
	Fig. 2	1:10	0.10
Kohno and Kohase (1969)	Fig. 1	1:14	0.07
	Fig. 2	1:14	0.07
Gandhi et al. (1970)	Table 1	1:66	0.02
Clavell and Bratt (1971)	Fig. 1	1:37	0.03
Meager and Burke (1972)	Fig. 1	1:33	0.03
Sheaff et al. (1972)	Fig. 7b	1:41	0.02
Kowal and Youngner (1978)	Fig. 4	1:50	0.02
P.I. Marcus et al. (1982) (unpublished work)		1:10	0.10
			Mean = 0.04

[a] Refers to figures or tables in the cited reference
[b] For IFP activity the rate of inactivation was calculated from the region of the curve (high doses of UV) showing an exponential decay
[c] The rate of loss of infectivity (PFP activity) is considered to reflect a hit (uracil dimer formation) to a target equivalent to the molecular weight of the entire NDV [−]RNA genome, $\sim 5.4 \times 10^6$ daltons (Collins et al. 1980). The target size for IFP activity, representing the fraction of the genome required for its expression, is calculated from the rate of inactivation of IFP relative to PFP. The mean value of 0.04 represents a target of about 2.2×10^5 daltons

sequent studies in which chick cells were used as hosts (references in Table 2), with one notable exception.[5]

When we analyzed the high UV dose region of the interferon induction curves, where the IFP capacity decreased exponentially with UV dose (after being enhanced at the lower doses), it became apparent that the curves extrapolated to a "hit" number approximating the multiplicity of infection. We interpret these results to mean that each virion of NDV contains one or more UV radiation-sensitive functions that, when expressed, prevent either formation of the interferon inducer moiety, or its action.[6] On this basis, only when that function has been inactivated

5 Kohno and Kohase (1969) reported that NDV propagated in primary chick embryo cells (rather than in eggs), was capable of inducing interferon in chick cells, even though unirradiated. Furthermore, they showed that following UV irradiation chick cell-derived NDV induced decreasing amounts of interferon

6 This concept in a similar form was first advanced by Kohno et al. (1969) and elaborated on by Sheaff et al. (1972) who recognized the need for limited polymerase activity in interferon induction by NDV. Furthermore, based on their data, they argued convincingly that a newly synthesized viral protein or proteins acted to inhibit interferon formation by NDV in chick embryo cells

in all of the virions in a multiply infected cell would interferon be produced. Thus, the action in chick embryo cells of a putative inhibitor protein or proteins confers an *ifp*$^-$ phenotype on NDV. The relatively slow rate of inactivation of IFP activity at high doses of UV radiation indicates there is only a small region of the viral genome which must remain intact for the expression of that activity. The size of that region (target) is deduced from the mean value of the ratio of the slopes of the survival curves for IFP and PFP activity. From the data compiled in Table 2, we estimate that target at about 4% of the NDV genome, i.e., $0.04 \times 5.4 \times 10^6 = 2.2 \times 10^5$ daltons RNA. Because the IFP activity of NDV is sensitive to heat, as is viron-associated transcriptase activity (SHEAFF et al. 1972), we conclude, in agreement with these workers, that limited transcription is required to produce an interferon-inducing moiety. Furthermore, since the NDV genome contains only one initiation (promoter) site for transcription (COLLINS et al. 1980) and a UV hit (uracil dimer) blocks traversal of the transcriptase, we conclude that this transcriptase activity is used to copy the 4% (2.2×10^5 daltons) of the genome required for IFP activity and that it must be located at the extreme 3′ end of the genome. Based on the gene order of transcription for NDV (COLLINS et al. 1980), this region encodes for NP (nucleoprotein) and represents about 45% of that cistron.

Drawing largely on a model developed to define the interferon-inducing moiety of another [−]RNA strand virus, VSV (MARCUS and SEKELLICK 1980), we propose that in chick embryo cells infected with NDV newly synthesized NP acts to prevent a threshold level of base pairing between the [−]RNA genome and its [+]RNA primary transcripts, and hence blocks formation of the dsRNA, which we suggest constitutes the interferon-inducing moiety of NDV.[7] However, when synthesis of NP is prevented, as for example by creating a uracil dimer in the NP cistron, any endogenous NP in the RNP complex which is lost during the transcription process cannot be replaced. We think the gradual loss of NP during each round of transcription increases the chances that a significant length of paired bases will be formed between the [−]RNA genome and a partially completed complementary transcript of NP mRNA. We argue that the target of 2.2×10^5 daltons represents the minimal length of RNA required to form base paired structures of adequate length and stability to produce a signal of sufficient magnitude to activate the cell's recognition system for interferon induction. We note, without understanding its significance, the similarity in lengths of the RNA required to express an *ifp*$^+$ phenotype for VSV ($\sim 4 \times 10^5$ daltons), NDV ($\sim 2 \times 10^5$ daltons) and the [±]RNA DI-011 particle ($8 \times 10^5/2 = 4 \times 10^5$ daltons).

In summary, we propose two requirements for interferon induction by particles of NDV: (1) virion-associated transcriptase activity is needed to transcribe about

7 By this model, NP would constitute the "inhibitor" which confers an *ifp*$^-$ phenotype on NDV in chick embryo cells. In cells mixedly infected with NDV containing a functional (unirradiated wild-type: *ifp*$^-$ phenotype) and a nonfunctional (UV-irradiated wild type: *ifp*$^+$ phenotype) NP gene, respectively, the NP synthesized by the unirradiated NDV would "dominate", prevent base pairing and hence produce an *ifp*$^-$ phenotype. These events provide an explanation for the observations of KOWAL and YOUNGNER (1978) that relate to mixedly infected cells. We also note that interferon pretreatment might act to lower the effective concentration of NP – or a comparable molecule in other virus systems, for example, in the conversion of an *ifp*$^-$ MM virus to an *ifp*$^+$ phenotype (STEWART et al. 1971) – and hence convert an *ifp*$^-$ to an *ifp*$^+$ phenotype

one-half of the NP gene; and (2) loss of NP from the transcribing NP complex must take place to facilitate a threshold amount of base pairing between the genome and its complementary transcript.[8] We suggest that the dsRNA thus formed constitutes the interferon induction signal.

VI. Sendai Virus

A recent investigation on interferon induction by Sendai virus deserves special consideration in that it reveals a new facet of complexity in the induction process, at last in one type of host cell. JOHNSTON (1981) has shown that the capacity of a stock of egg-grown Sendai virus to induce interferon in the human lymphoblastoid cell, Namalwa was dependent upon its content of defective interfering particles. JOHNSTON showed that Sendai virus alone, or Sendai defective interfering particles alone, induced little or no interferon. However, when cells were mixedly infected with both standard and defective interfering particles, large quantities of interferon were induced. Maximal levels of interferon were induced when every cell in the population was mixedly infected, a condition achieved when the multiplicity was about three or four particles of each type per cell. Although the nature of the interferon inducer moiety remains inknown, JOHNSTON points out that PORTNER and KINGSBURY (1972) found a partially double-stranded structure unique to cells mixedly infected with standard virus and defective interfering particles. He also suggests that the presence of the defective interfering particles may prevent production of an inhibitor of interferon synthesis. Assuming that NP is the inhibitor, as already proposed,[7] then the accumulation of detective interfering particle RNA may act to siphon off NP, thereby reducing the number of molecules available to coat the transcribing NP complex. This would enhance base pairing of the type suggested for VSV (Sect. E.I.) and NDV (Sect. E.V), and provide a mechanism for interference.

The cooperative effect for interferon induction discovered by JOHNSTON (1981) may be regulated by a host cell function, since Sendai defective interfering particles do not induce interferon in chick cells (PORTNER and KINGSBURY 1971), nor do they affect the IFP activity of standard Sendai virus upon mixed infection (M. J. SEKELLICK and P. I. MARCUS 1980, unpublished work). Clearly, the factors which affect interferon induction by viruses in vitro can be complex. Apparently, the situation is no less complex in vivo. For example, in mice the interferon inducer moiety of Sendai virus appears to be, at least in part, the virion-associated glycoproteins (ITO et al. 1978).

F. Summary

The selected studies reviewed in this article were chosen largely because they contained data amenable to quantitative analysis of interferon induction dose–re-

8 HUPPERT et al. (1969) first suggested that base pairing between the genome strand and its newly synthesized complement may constitute the interferon-inducing moiety for NDV, a suggestion which has gained credence with further experimentation (CLAVELL and BRATT 1971; SHEAFF et al. 1972)

sponse curves and the IFP activity they represented. The interpretation of the data in these studies was predicated on the assumption that a single molecule of dsRNA when properly introduced into a cell, either as a preformed entity or formed therein following some synthetic event or events, can induce a quantum yield of interferon. This novel view of interferon induction by viruses has provided an explanation for many seemingly discordant results reported for the interferon-inducing capacity of viruses, and offers a unifying hypothesis regarding the nature of the interferon-inducing moiety for viruses from widely different families.

We contend that for viruses, dsRNA is the common interferon-inducing molecule, while noting the reluctance of some to accept this view (McKIMM and RAPP 1977; KOWAL and YOUNGNER 1978; JOKLIK 1980), and that the threshold for activating the interferon induction system is one molecule of dsRNA per cell. In some cases of interferon induction (the $r=1$ type of dose–response curve) there is an extremely responsive modulation of interferon production when a second molecule of dsRNA is introduced into the cell. The experimental approach and concepts discussed herein offer a new perspective on the mechanism of interferon induction by viruses and its regulation, and point out the incredible biologic potency of a dsRNA molecule – a molecule bound to play a key role in viral infection, host defense (CARTER and DECLERCQ 1974), and perhaps some yet to be defined function in differentiation (KEAYS and GROSSBERG 1977) through its capacity to activate the interferon system.

Acknowledgments. The studies of interferon induction carried out in my laboratory over the past 5 years have been supported by grants from the National Institutes of Health (CA-20882 and AI-18381) and the National Science Foundation (PCM-77-24875 and PCM-80-21882), and benefited from the use of the Cell Culture Facility supported by NCI grant CA 14733. I thank Dr. MARGARET J. SEKELLICK for a critical reading of the manuscript, and my many colleagues who generously provided seed cultures of viruses and cells.

References

Ball LA, White CN (1978) Coupled transcription and translation in mammalian and avian cell-free systems. Virology 84:479–495

Baron S, Dianzani F (eds) (1977) The interferon system: a current review to 1978. Tex Rep Biol Med 35:1–573

Bay PHS, Reichmann ME (1979) UV inactivation of the biological activity of DI particles generated by VSV. J Virol 32:876–884

Borsa J, Morash BD, Sargent MD, Copps TP, Lievaart PA, Szekely JG (1979) Two modes of entry of reovirus particles into L cells. J Gen Virol 45:161–170

Carter WA, DeClercq E (1974) Viral infection and host defense. Science 186:1177–1178

Carver DH, Marcus PI (1967) Enhanced interferon production from chick embryo cells aged in vitro. Virology 32:247–257

Clavell LA, Bratt MA (1971) Relationship between the RNA-synthesizing capacity of UV-NDV and its ability to induce IFN. J Virol 8:500–508

Clewley JP, Kennedy SIT (1976) Purification and polypeptide composition of Semliki Forest Virus RNA polymerase. J Gen Virol 32:395–411

Colby C, Morgan MJ (1971) IFN induction and action. Annu Rev Microbiol 25:333–360

Collins PL, Hightower LE, Ball LA (1980) Transcriptional map for Newcastle disease virus. J Virol 35:682–693

Cross RK, Fields BN (1977) Genetics of reovirus. In: Fraenkel-Conrat H, Wagner RR (eds) Comprehensive virology, vol 9. Plenum, New York, chap 7, p 291

DeClercq E, Merigan TC (1970) Current concepts of IFN and IFN induction. Annu Rev Med 21:17–33

De Maeyer E, De Maeyer-Guignard J (1979) In: Fraenkel-Conrat H, Wagner RR (eds) Comprehensive virology, vol 15. Plenum, New York, pp 205–284
Desmyter J, Melnick JL, Rawls WE (1968) Defectiveness of interferon production and of Rubella virus interference in a line of African Green Monkey kidney cells (Vero). J Virol 2:955–961
Dubovi EJ, Akers TG (1972) Interferon induction by Colorado Tick Fever virus: a double-stranded RNA virus. Proc Soc Exp Biol Med 139:123–127
Emerson SU, Dierks PM, Parsons JT (1977) In vitro synthesis of a unique RNA species by a T particle of VSV. J Virol 23:708–716
Field AK, Tytell AA, Lampson GP, Hilleman MR (1967) Inducers of interferon and host resistance. II. Multistranded synthetic polynucleotide complexes. PNAS 58:1004–1009
Finter NB (ed) (1973) Interferons and interferon inducers. Elsevier, Amsterdam
Fleischmann WR Jr, Simon EH (1974) Mechanism of interferon induction by NDV: a monolayer and single cell study. J Gen Virol 25:337–349
Fout GS, Simon EH (1981) Studies on an interferon-sensitive mutant of Mengovirus: effects on host RNA and protein synthesis. J Gen Virol 52:391–394
Francoeur AM, Lam T, Stanners CP (1978) The role of interferon in persistent infection with T1026. J Supramol Struct Cell Biochem [Suppl 2], p 245
Frey TK, Strauss JH (1978) Replication of Sindbis virus. VI. Poly(A) and Poly(U) in virus-specific RNA species. Virology 86:494–506
Frey TK, Jones EV, Cardamone JJ, Youngner JS (1979) Induction of interferon in L cells by defective-interfering (DI) particles of Vesicular Stomatitis virus: lack of correlation with content of [$\pm$] snap back RNA. Virology 99:95–102
Frey TK, Frielle DW, Youngner JS (1980) Standard Vesicular Stomatitis virus is required for interferon induction in L cells by defective interfering particles. In: Bishop DHL, Compans RW (eds) Replication of negative strand viruses. Elsevier, Amsterdam
Fuller FJ, Marcus PI (1980a) Interferon induction by viruses. IV. Sindbis virus: early passage defective-interfering particles induce interferon. J Gen Virol 48:63–73
Fuller FJ, Marcus PI (1980b) Interferon induction by viruses. V. Sindbis virus: defective-interfering particles temperature-sensitive for interferon induction. J Gen Virol 48:391–394
Fuller FJ, Marcus PI (1980c) Sindbis virus. I. Gene order of translation in vivo. Virology 107:441–451
Gandhi SS, Burke DC, Scholtissek C (1970) Virus RNA synthesis by UV-irradiated NDV and interferon production. J Gen Virol 9:97–99
Giron DJ, Allen PT, Pinkad FF, Schmidt JP (1971) Interferon-inducing characteristics of MM virus. Appl. Microbiol 21:387–393
Goorha RM, Gifford GE (1970) An explanation for increased interferon production at low multiplicities of infection. Proc Soc Exp Biol Med 135:91–93
Gordon J, Minks MA (1981) The interferon renaissance: molecular aspects of induction and action. Microbiol Rev 45:244–266
Guild GM, Stollar V (1977) Defective-interfering particles of Sindbis virus. V. Sequence relationships between SV_{STO} RNA and intracellular defective viral RNAs. Virology 77:175–188
Henderson DR, Joklik WK (1978) The mechanism of interferon induction by UV-irradiated reovirus. Virology 91:389–406
Ho M, Breinig MK (1965) Metabolic determinants of interferon formation. Virology 25:331–339
Hughes JV, Johnson TC (1981) Alterations in peptide structure of Vesicular Stomatitis virus mutant and its central nervous system isolate. J Gen Virol 53:309–319
Huppert J, Hillova J, Gresland L (1969) Viral RNA synthesis in chicken cells infected with UV-irradiated NDV. Nature 223:1015–1017
Isaacs A, Lindenmann J (1957) Virus interference. I. The interferon. Proc R Soc Lond [Biol] 147:258–267
Isaacs A, Cox RA, Rotem Z (1963) Foreign nucleic acids as the stimulants to make interferon. Lancet II 7299:113–116

Ito Y, Nishiyama Y, Shimokata K, Takeyama H, Kunii A (1978) Active component of HVJ (Sendai virus) for interferon induction in mice. Nature 274:801–802

Jameson P, Grossberg SE (1979) Production of interferon by human tumor cell lines. Arch Virol 62:209–219

Jameson P, Taylor JL, Grossberg SE (1980) Blue tongue virus induction of interferon: potential for cancer therapy. In: Hersh EM (ed) Augmenting agents in cancer therapy. Raven, New York, pp 193–204

Jarvis AP, Colby C (1978) Regulation of the murine interferon system: isolation and characterization of a mutant 3T6 cell engaged in the semiconstitutive synthesis of interferon. Cell 14:355–364

Johnson TC, McLaren LC (1965) Plaque development and induction of interferon synthesis by RMC poliovirus. J Bacteriol 90:565–570

Johnston MD (1981) The characteristics required for a Sendai virus preparation to induce high levels of interferon in human lymphoblastoid cells. J Gen Virol 56:175–184

Johnston MD, Burke DC (1973) Interferon induction by viruses: molecular requirements. In: Carter WA (ed) Selective inhibitors of viral functions. CRC, Boca Raton, pp 123–148

Joklik WK (1980) Induction of interferon by reovirus. In: Schlessinger D (ed) Microbiology – 1980. Am Soc Microbiol, Washington DC, pp 200–203

Keays S, Grossberg SE (1980) Interferon inhibits the conversion of 3T3-L1 mouse fibroblasts into adipocytes. Proc Natl Acad Sci USA 77:4099–4103

Kohase M, Vilček J (1979) Interferon induction with NDV in FS-4 cells: effect of priming with interferon and of virus inactivating treatments. Jpn J Med Sci Biol 32:281–293

Kohno S, Kohase M (1969) Studies on interferon induction by NDV. I. Interferon induction by NDV grown in primary chick embryonic cells. Arch Ges Virusforsch 28:177–187

Kohno S, Kohase M, Shimizu Y (1969) Studies on interferon induction by NDV. II. Interferon inductions by heat- and acid-treated NDV. Arch Ges Virusforsch 28:188–196

Kowal KJ, Youngner JS (1978) Induction of interferon by temperature-sensitive mutants of Newcastle disease virus. Virology 90:90–102

Lai MT, Joklik WK (1973) The induction of interferon by temperature-sensitive mutants of reovirus, UV-irradiated reovirus, and subviral particles. Virology 51:191–204

Lazzarini RA, Weber GH, Johnson LD, Stamminger GM (1975) Covalently linked message and anti-message (genomic) RNA from a defective Vesicular Stomatitis virus particle. J Mol Biol 97:289–307

Lengyel P, Desrosiers R, Broeze R, Slattery E, Taira H, Dougherty J, Samanta H, Pichon J, Farrell P, Ratner L, Sen G (1980) Biochemistry of the interferon system. In: Schlessinger D (ed) Microbiology – 1980. Am Soc Microbiol, Washington DC, pp 219–226

Lockart RZ Jr (1970) Interferon induction by viruses. J Gen Physiol 56:3–12s

Long DG, Borsa J, Sargent MD (1976) A potential artifact generated by pelleting viral particles during preparative ultracentrifugation. Biochim Biophys Acta 451:639–642

Long WF, Burke DC (1971) Interferon production by double-stranded RNA; a comparison of induction by reovirus to that by a synthetic double-stranded polynucleotide. J Gen Virol 12:1–11

Luria SE (1940) Méthodes statistiques appliquees à l'étude du Mode d'action des ultravirus. Ann Inst Pasteur 64:415–436

Marcus PI (1959) Symposium on the biology of cells modified by viruses or antigens. IV. Single-cell techniques in tracing virus-host interactions. Bacteriol Rev 23:232–249

Marcus PI (1980) The interferon system and rhabdoviruses. In: Bishop DHL (ed) Rhabdoviruses, vol 3. CRC, Boca Raton, pp 1–12

Marcus PI (1981–1982) The interferon inducer moiety of viruses: a single molecule of dsRNA. Tex Rep Biol Med 41:70–75

Marcus PI, Fuller FJ (1979) Interferon induction by viruses. II. Sindbis virus: interferon induction requires one-quarter of the genome – Genes G and A. J Gen Virol 44:169–177

Marcus PI, Sekellick MJ (1974) Cell killing by viruses. I. Comparison of cell-killing, plaque-forming, and defective-interfering particles of Vesicular Stomatitis virus. Virology 57:321–338

Marcus PI, Sekellick MJ (1975) Cell killing by viruses. II. Cell killing by Vesicular Stomatitis virus: a requirement for virion-derived transcription. Virology 63:176–190

Marcus PI, Sekellick MJ (1976) Cell killing by viruses. III. The interferon system and inhibition of cell killing by Vesicular stomatitis virus. Virology 69:378–393

Marcus PI, Sekellick MJ (1977) Defective-interfering particles with covalently linked [±]RNA induce interferon. Nature 266:815–819

Marcus PI, Sekellick MJ (1980) Interferon induction by viruses. III. Vesicular Stomatitis virus: interferon-inducing particle activity requires partial transcription of gene N. J Gen Virol 47:89–96

Marcus PI, Guidon PT Jr, Sekellick MJ (1981 a) Interferon induction by viruses. VII. Mengovirus: "interferon-sensitive" mutant phenotype attributed to interferon-inducing particle activity. J Interferon Res 1:601–611

Marcus PI, Guidon PT Jr, Sekellick MJ (1981 b) Interferon induction by Mengovirus: "interferon-sensitive" mutant phenotype attributed to interferon-inducing particle activity. 5th International congress of virology, abstracts, Strasbourg, 2–7 August

Marvaldi JL, Lucas-Lenard J, Sekellick MJ, Marcus PI (1977) Cell killing by viruses. IV. Cell killing and protein synthesis inhibition by Vesicular Stomatitis virus require the same gene functions. Virology 79:267–280

Meager A, Burke DC (1972) Production of interferon by ultraviolet radiation inactivated Newcastle disease virus. Nature 235:280–282

Meurs E, Hovanessian AG, Montagnier L (1981) Interferon-mediated antiviral state in human MRC5 cells in the absence of detectable levels of 2–5A synthetase and protein kinase. J Interferon Res 1:219–232

Miller RL, Plagemann PGW (1974) Effect of ultraviolet light on Mengovirus. Formation of uracil dimers, instability and degradation of capsid and covalent linkage of protein to viral RNA. J Virol 13:729–739

McKimm J, Rapp F (1977) Variation in ability of measles virus plaque progeny to induce interferon. Proc Natl Acad Sci USA 74:3056–3059

Nilsen TW, Baglioni C (1979) Mechanism for discrimination between viral and host mRNA in interferon-treated cells. Proc Natl Acad Sci USA 76:2600–2604

Nilsen TW, Wood DL, Baglioni C (1981) Cross-linking of viral RNA by 4′-aminomethyl-4,5′,8-trimethylpsoralen in HeLa cells infected with encephalomyocarditis virus and the tsG114 mutant of Vesicular Stomatitis virus. Virology 109:82–93

Pfefferkorn ER, Burge BW (1967) Genetics and biochemistry of arbovirus temperature-sensitive mutants. In: Colter J (ed) The molecular biology of viruses. Academic, New York, pp 403–426

Portner A, Kingsbury DW (1971) Homologous interference by incomplete Sendai virus particles: changes in virus-specific RNA synthesis. J Virol 8:388–394

Portner A, Kingsbury DW (1972) Identification of transcriptive and replicative intermediates in Sendai virus infected cells. Virology 47:711–725

Sawicki DL, Sawicki SG (1980) Short-lived minus-strand polymerase for Semliki forest virus. J Virol 34:108–118

Schnitzlein WM, Reichmann ME (1977) A possible effect of viral proteins on the specificity of interference by defective Vesicular Stomatitis virus particles. Virology 80:275–288

Schubert M, Lazzarini RA (1981) Structure and origin of a snapback defective interfering particle RNA of Vesicular Stomatitis virus. J Virol 37:661–672

Sekellick MJ, Marcus PI (1978) Persistent infection. I. Interferon-inducing defective-interfering particles as mediators of cell sparing: Possible role in persistent infection by Vesicular Stomatitis virus. Virology 85:175–186

Sekellick MJ, Marcus PI (1979) Persistent infection. II. Interferon-inducing temperature-sensitive mutants as mediators of cell sparing: possible role in persistent infection by Vesicular Stomatitis virus. Virology 95:36–47

Sekellick MJ, Marcus PI (1980 a) Persistent infections of rhabdoviruses. In: Bishop DHL (ed) Rhabdoviruses, vol 3. CRC, Boca Raton, pp 67–97

Sekellick MJ, Marcus PI (1980 b) Viral interference by defective particles of vesicular stomatitis virus measured in individual cells. Virology 104:247–252

Sekellick MJ, Marcus PI (to be published) Requirements for expression of defective-interfering particle-mediated interference. 5th International congress of virology, abstracts, Strasbourg, 2–7 August
Sekellick MJ, Marcus PI (1982) Interferon induction by viruses. VIII. Vesicular stomatitis virus: [±]DI-011 particles induce interferon in the absence of standard virions. Virology 117:280–285
Sheaff ET, Meager A, Burke DC (1972) Factors involved in the production of interferon by inactivated NDV. J Gen Virol 17:163–175
Silverstein SC, Dales S (1968) The penetration of reovirus RNA and initiation of its genetic function in L-strain fibroblasts. J Cell Biol 36:197–230
Simon EH, Kung S, Koh TT, Brandman P (1976) Interferon-sensitive mutants of Mengovirus. I. Isolation and biological characterization. Virology 69:727–736
Slattery E, Taira H, Broeze R, Lengyel P (1980) Mouse interferons: production by Ehrlich ascites tumor cells infected with Newcastle disease virus and its enhancement by theophylline. J Gen Virol 49:91–96
Solov'ev VD, Bektemirov TA (1973) Interferon, theory and applications. Plenum, New York
Stark C, Kennedy SIT (1978) The generation and propagation of defective-interfering particles of Semliki forest virus in different cell types. Virology 89:285–299
Stewart WE II (1979) The interferon system. Springer, Wien New York
Stewart WE II, Gosser LB, Lockart RZ Jr (1971) Priming: a nonantiviral function of interferon. J Virol 7:792–801
Strauss EG, Lenches EM, Strauss JH (1976) Mutants of Sindbis virus. I. Isolation and partial characterization of 89 new temperature-sensitive mutants. Virology 74:154–168
Stringfellow DA (ed) (1980) Interferon and interferon inducers: clinical applications. In: Modern pharmacology-toxicology, vol 17. Dekker, New York, chap 6, pp 145–165
Szilágyi JF, Pringle CR (1972) Effect of temperature-sensitive mutations on the virion-associated RNA transcriptase of Vesicular Stomatitis virus. J Mol Biol 71:281–291
Thang MN, DeMaeyer-Guignard J, DeMaeyer E (1977) Interaction of interferon with tRNA. FEBS Lett 80:365–370
Van Der Heide L, Kalbac M (1975) Infectious tenosynovitis (viral arthritis): characterization of a Connecticut viral isolate as a reovirus and evidence of viral egg transmission by reovirus-infected broiler breeders. J Avian Dis 19:683–688
Vilček J (1970) Cellular mechanisms of interferon production. J Gen Physiol 56:76–89
Vilček J, Kohase M (1977) Regulation of interferon production: cell culture studies. Tex Rep Biol Med 35:57–62
Wagner RR, Schnaitman TC, Snyder RM (1969) Structural proteins of Vesicular Stomatitis viruses. J Virol 3:395–403
Wertz GW, Youngner JS (1970) Interferon production and inhibition of host synthesis in cells infected with VSV. J Virol 6:476–484
Wheelock EF (1966) Virus replication and high-titered interferon production in human leukocyte cultures inoculated with NDV. J Bacteriol 92:1415–1421
Winship TR, Marcus PI (1980) Interferon induction by viruses. VI. Reovirus: virion genome dsRNA as the interferon inducer in aged chick embryo cells. J Interferon Res 1:155–167
Winship TR, Marcus PI (1981) Interferon-inducing particle activity of reoviruses: regulation by the host cell. 81st Annual Meeting, Am Soc Microbiol, abstracts, p 242
Yabrov AA (1980) Interferon and nonspecific resistance. Human Sciences, New York
Youngner JS, Scott AW, Hallum JV, Stinebring WR (1966) Interferon production by inactivated NDV in cell cultures and in mice. J Bacteriol 92:862–868

CHAPTER 11

Interferon Induction by Nucleic Acids: Structure-Activity Relationships

P. F. TORRENCE and E. DE CLERCQ

A. General Considerations

The first report of a nucleic acid as an interferon inducer was that of ISAACS et al. (1963) who suggested that "foreign" nucleic acids, i.e., those heterologous to the cell in question, were interferon inducers. This concept was abandoned when the supporting experiments could not be reproduced either by ISAACS' group or by others. In 1967, nucleic acids regained favor as interferon inducers when workers at Merck and Company demonstrated highly efficient induction of interferon in vitro and in vivo by the synthetic double-stranded (ds) polynucleotide, poly(I)·poly(C) (FIELD et al. 1967). In the meantime, the interferon-inducing agent of the fungal products, helenine and statolon had also been shown to be dsRNA in nature (LAMPSON et al. 1967; KLEINSCHMIDT et al. 1968). While nucleic acids are by no means the only class of interferon inducers, they are the most potent, least toxic, hence the most specific. They also possess that widest host cell spectrum of interferon-inducing activity. The superiority of dsRNAs as interferon inducers may be related to the possibility that dsRNA is the actual molecular signal for interferon induction during virus infection.

Quite a variety of dsRNAs of phage or viral origin have been found to induce interferon (as reviewed by TORRENCE and DE CLERCQ 1977b). This includes viral replicative forms, for instance, those of vaccinia virus, influenza virus, and Mengo virus (FALCOFF et al. 1973; COLBY and DUESBERG 1969). DsRNAs from nonviral sources have also been shown to induce interferon. BEVAN et al. (1973) found that the dsRNA of "killer" strains of *Saccharomyces cerevisiae* could induce interferon in mouse L-cells. dsRNAs isolated from apparently uninfected cells have also been reported to induce interferon (STERN and FRIEDMAN 1970; KIMBALL and DUESBERG 1971; DE MAEYER et al. 1971). Incidentally, DE MAEYER et al. (1971) showed that this latter DsRNA could provide protection against viral infection in cells from which it was derived, in direct contradiction to the hypothesis that interferon induction is the cell's response to "foreign" nucleic acids.

The relationship between the structure of a nucleic acid and its ability to induce interferon has been the subject of considerable investigation since such studies might yield information that would be valuable in constructing the ideal interferon inducer. Interferon induction also provides the opportunity to study the role of dsRNAs in the biologic responsiveness of the cell; dsRNAs may, indeed, be considered as modifiers of these biologic responses (Sect. F). The critical role of *endogenous* nucleic acids in the replication, maintenance, and functioning of the cell has long been recognized. During virus infection, the dsRNA replicative intermediate may contribute to both the pathogenesis and recovery from the disease (CARTER and DE CLERCQ 1974). Interferon induction by dsRNA provides a firsthand view of the biochemistry of *exogenous* nucleic acids and essentially opens a new field of study; that is, the medicinal chemistry of nucleic acids. Finally, the phenomenon of interferon induction points to an important role for dsRNA in the regulation of gene expression.

Structure–activity studies with nucleic acid interferon inducers assume, quite literally, some added dimensions compared with the study of more classical agonists. Nucleic acids consist of monomeric units which themselves can be chemically modified. These monomers (nucleotides) are then arranged via phosphodiester bonds in some specific sequence (polynucleotide), except for the case when all the monomers are the same as in a homopolynucleotide. This polynucleotide can assume a variety of different conformations, whether or not it is complexed with a complementary polynucleotide. The conformation assumed depends on the environment of the nucleic acid, but also, more fundamentally, on the chemical nature of the monomeric constituents of the nucleic acid. Thus, any single structural variation in the nucleotide building block of the polynucleotide will affect the higher order structure of the polynucleotide as well. In studies on DNA–protein interaction, as particularly exemplified by the restriction endonucleases, considerable emphasis has been placed on specific base sequences as recognition elements. The the case of interferon induction, we will see that nucleic acid conformation, rather than base sequence, is a recognition element of crucial importance.

B. Nucleic Acid Strandedness and Its Consequences for Interferon Induction

One of the simplest classifications of the higher order structure of nucleic acids in based on the strandedness of the polymer. Strictly speaking, the strandedness of a nucleic acid refers to the number of independent polynucleotide chains that associate in the formation of a higher order structure. A nucleic acid may, however, be nominally single-stranded, but possess considerable secondary structure consisting of double-stranded regions generated by a folding back of the single strand. In fact, quite a few nominally single-stranded nucleic acids have varying degrees of multistrandedness. This consideration is the more important, since single-stranded nucleic acids are usually assumed to be inactive as interferon inducers

I. Double-Strandedness is an Absolute Prerequisite for the Interferon-Inducing Ability of Polynucleotides

Aside from base stacking, poly(U) shows little, if any, hydrogen-bonded secondary structure at room temperature or above (GUSCHLBAUER 1976; BLOOMFIELD et al. 1974); poly(U) is completely inactive as an interferon inducer (DE CLERCQ and MERIGAN 1969). On the other hand, the homopolynucleotide poly (G) possesses a highly ordered structure, existing as a four-stranded helix (ZIMMERMAN et al. 1975). Nonetheless, poly(G) does not induce interferon (DE CLERCQ and MERIGAN 1969).

In general, homopolynucleotides and single-stranded nucleic acids are very poor inducers of interferon. However, at least one exception to this generalization has been reported. Poly(I), like poly(G), can, depending on environmental conditions, assume a four-stranded structure (THIELE and GUSCHLBAUER 1973); in fact, very low potassium ion concentration can provoke considerable multistrandedness in poly(I) (MILES and FRAZIER 1978). Some preparations of poly(I) have been reported to induce interferon in vitro and in vivo, and these poly(I) preparations were only slightly less effective than poly(I)·poly(C) itself (THANG et al. 1977; DE CLERCQ et al. 1978a). The characteristics of these active poly(I) preparations were: (1) in contrast to most polynucleotides prepared with the aid of soluble polynucleotide phosphorylase, these preparations were synthesized with an insolubilized matrix-bound enzyme; (2) reproducibly active material could not be made; (3) poly(I) preparations that were effective interferon inducers reacted poorly with antibody prepared against poly(I) that did not induce interferon; and (4) to some extent these interferon-inducing poly(I) preparations reacted with antibody specific for dsRNA (STOLLAR et al. 1978). Thus, it appeared that the interferon-inducing poly(I) molecules contained local regions of double-helical conformation. Furthermore, these results suggested that a continuous high molecular weight base paired structure is not an absolute requirement for a polynucleotide inducer interferon (THANG et al. 1977).

Triple-helical nucleic acids are notoriously poor, if not totally ineffective, interferon inducers (COLBY and CHAMBERLIN 1969; DE CLERCQ et al. 1970a, 1974b, 1975d, 1976b, 1979; TORRENCE et al. 1976; TORRENCE and DE CLERCQ 1977a). This characteristic lack of interferon-inducing capacity has led to the identification of several previously unrecognized polynucleotide triplexes (DE CLERCQ et al. 1975d; TORRENCE et al. 1976; TORRENCE and DE CLERCQ 1977a). For instance, when poly(I) was added to cell cultures 1 h prior to, simultaneously with, or 1 h after the active interferon inducers poly(A)·poly(U) or poly(A)·poly(rT), dramatic reductions in interferon production resulted. Based on experiments involving sucrose gradient ultracentrifugation, pancreatic ribonuclease A resistance, ultraviolet absorbance–mixing curves, and ultraviolet absorbance–temperature profiles, the explanation of these phenomena was determined to be the formation of polynucleotide triplexes according to the following equations (DE CLERCQ et al. 1975d):

$$\text{poly(A)}\cdot\text{poly(U)}+\text{poly(I)} \rightarrow \text{poly(A)}\cdot\text{poly(U)}\cdot\text{poly(I)}$$
$$\text{poly(A)}\cdot\text{poly(rT)}+\text{poly(I)} \rightarrow \text{poly(A)}\cdot\text{poly(rT)}\cdot\text{poly(I)}\,.$$

Besides poly(U)·poly(A)·poly(I), poly(rT)·poly(A)·poly(I), several other triple-helical polynucleotides were established with the aid of interferon induction assays, i.e., poly(dUz)·poly(A)·poly(U), poly(rT)·poly(A)·poly(dUz) (TORRENCE et al. 1976), poly(dUfl)·poly(A)·poly(U) (DE CLERCQ et al. 1976b), poly(X)·poly(A)·poly(U) (TORRENCE and DE CLERCQ 1977a), and poly(U)·poly(A)·poly(I_x,U) ($0.1>x>10$) (DE CLERCQ et al. 1979) [in these complexes the homopolynucleotide written to the left of poly(A) would be involved in Watson–Crick hydrogen bonding, whereas the homopolynucleotide written to the right of poly(A) would be involved in Hoogsteen hydrogen bonding].

To induce interferon, a nucleic acid need not necessarily be double-helical over its whole length, as originally suggested by the studies of THANG et al. (1977) and DE CLERCQ et al. (1978). Imperfectly matched duplexes such as poly(I_x,U) · poly(C) are still effective as inducers of interferon if $x \geqq 10$ (DE CLERCQ et al. 1979), indicating that intact double-helical RNA segments of at least ten base pairs long (on the average) may suffice to trigger the interferon response. This latter concept is in harmony with the hypothesis of GREENE et al. (1978) that interaction of poly(I) · poly(C) with the cell may occur in a biphasic manner, involving first the recognition of a large portion of the dsRNA to permit proper binding to the (putative) cellular receptor, followed by recognition of a smaller region of the dsRNA (6–12 consecutive base pairs or 0.5–1 double-helical turn). The second interaction would be responsible for the triggering of the interferon-inducing process.

II. To Act as an Interferon Inducer, the Double-Helical Complex Should be Sufficiently Thermostable

Another expression of the requirement for double-strandedness is the dependence of interferon-inducing ability on the T_m (the temperature at which one-half of the base pairs of the helix have been disrupted) of the double-stranded complex. This means that the double helix must be intact under conditions of the interferon induction assay. Generally speaking, polynucleotide duplexes with $T_m < 40$ °C are unable to induce interferon at all,[1] those with T_m of intermediate range (~40 °–60 °C) can induce interferon, but they are less effective than polynucleotide complexes with $T_m > 60$ °C. On occasion, nucleic acid duplexes do not melt directly to single strands, but may rearrange first to triple-helical complexes which are themselves inactive as interferon inducers. The temperature at which this double–triple-helical rearrangement occurs is termed the $T_{m(2\to3)}$, as opposed to direct melting out of a double helix to its constituent strands [$T_{m(2\to1)}$]. This rearrangement has been extensively studied in the case of poly(A) · poly(U) (STEVENS and FELSENFELD 1964; MILES and FRAZIER 1964; BLAKE et al. 1967):

$$2\text{poly(A)} \cdot \text{poly(U)} \xrightarrow{T_m(2\to1)} \text{poly(A)} \cdot 2\text{poly(U)} + \text{poly(A)}.$$

The temperature at which this rearrangement occurs is quite sensitive to environmental conditions (e.g., divalent cations, ionic strength, pH). DE CLERCQ et al. (1974b) have related the $T_{m(2\to3)}$ to the ability of several complexes to induce interferon: poly(A) · poly(br^5U) [$T_{m(2\to3)} = 45$ °C] did not induce interferon, poly(A) · poly(U) [$T_{m(2\to3)} = 49$ °C] was intermediate in activity and poly(A) · poly(rT) [$T_{m(2\to3)} = 53$ °C] was nearly as active as poly(I) · poly(C), a duplex that cannot rearrange to a triple helix.

Still another restatement of the importance of the $T_{m(2\to1)}$ and double-strandedness is illustrated by the following experiment. The polynucleotide complex, poly(L) · poly(br^5C) is completely inactive as an interferon inducer (TORRENCE et al. 1975). When, however, an equimolar amount of the inactive single-stranded

1 T_m determined under physiologic conditions (0.15 M Na^+, pH 7.0–7.5)

poly(c^7I) is added to it, the resulting mixture is able to induce high titers of interferon. This phenomenon is due to the following displacement reaction:

poly(L) · poly(br^5C) + poly(c^7I)	→	poly(c^7I) · poly(br^5C) + poly(L)
$T_{m(2\to1)} = 72\ °C$		$T_{m(2\to1)} = 83\ °C$ (0.15 *M* NaCl)
IFN titer < 10 U/ml		IFN titer = 3,000 U/ml.

A large number of such polynucleotide displacement reactions has been demonstrated with the aid of interferon induction assays, e.g.,

poly(A) · 2poly(I) + 2poly(C)	→	2poly(I) · poly(C) + poly(A)
poly(A) · 2poly(I) + 2poly(br^5C)	→	2poly(I) · poly(br^5C) + poly(A)
poly(I) · poly(C) + poly(br^5C)	→	poly(I) · poly(br^5C) + poly(C)
poly(c^7I) · poly(C) + poly(I)	→	poly(I) · poly(C) + poly(c^7I)
poly(c^7I) · poly(C) + poly(br^5C)	→	poly(c^7I) · poly(br^5C) + poly(C),

(DE CLERCQ et al. 1976d). The reaction proceeded uniformly in the direction of the helix with the higher $T_{m(2\to1)}$ and greater interferon-inducing activity.

III. The Polynucleotide Should not be Degraded by Nucleases Before it Reaches Its Destination

As a rule, effective polynucleotide interferon inducers are relatively resistant to the action of nucleases. Since the double helix must survive the attack of extracellular and intracellular nucleases to reach its receptor site, and since double-helical nucleic acids are usually more resistant to nucleases than single-stranded forms, the double-strandedness helps insure delivery of the nucleic acid. Nucleic acids with low $T_{m(2\to1)}$ values "breathe" extensively; that is, single-stranded regions are being continually exposed and would serve as likely targets for the abundance of nucleases found in biologic fluids and organs. The relationship between interferon-inducing ability [$T_{m(2\to1)}$] and nuclease resistance is not easy to generalize, however. Some duplexes, like poly(dAz) · poly(dUz) (DE CLERCQ et al. 1978b) and poly(AM) · (poly(Um) (TORRENCE and FRIEDMAN 1979), are completely resistant to most nucleases, but they are also totally inactive as inducers of interferon. Mismatched complexes, like poly(I) · poly(C_{12},U), show enhanced sensitivity to nucleases like pancreatic ribonuclease A, but they are potent interferon inducers (TS'O et al. 1976; CARTER et al. 1976).

Resistance to nuclease degradation may become of critical importance when polynucleotide inducers of interferon are administered to humans, since human serum contains a nuclease activity that quickly hydrolyzes and inactivates poly(I) · poly(C) (STERN 1970; NORDLUND et al. 1970). This inactivation is apparently due to a specific degradation of the poly(C) strand (DE CLERCQ 1979). Poly(I) · poly(C) analogs in which the poly(C) strand has been replaced by either poly(br^5C) or poly(s^2C) (DE CLERCQ 1979), or mixtures of poly(I) · poly(C) with poly-L-lysine and carboxymethylcellulose (referred to as PICLC) are much more resistant to the action of human serum nucleases, and, in contrast to poly(I) · poly(C) itself, PICLC is an effective inducer of interferon in primates (LEVY 1977).

Table 1. Interferon induction by synthetic double-helical polynucleotides: structure–activity relationship

General structural formula[a]

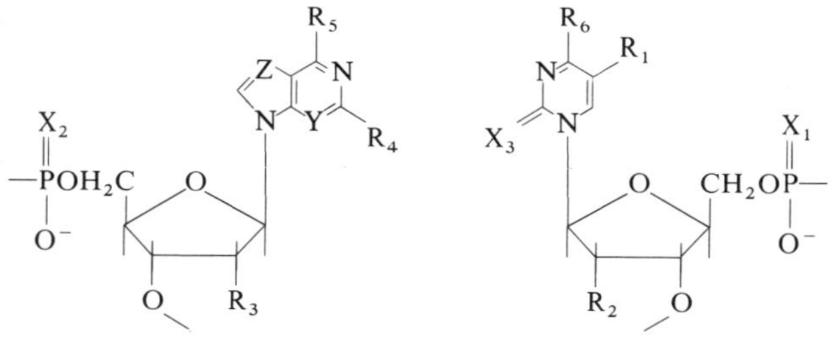

Polynucleotide	Structure[b]											IFN induction		References[c]
	R_1	R_2	R_3	R_4	R_5	R_6	X_1	X_2	X_3	Y	Z	In vitro	In vivo	
Homopolymer · homopolymer duplexes														
poly(I) · poly(C)	H	OH	OH	H	OH	NH_2	O	O	O	N	N	+	+	[1, 2]
poly(I) · poly(br^{5}C)	**BR**	OH	OH	H	OH	NH_2	O	O	O	N	N	+	+	[3, 4]
poly(I) · poly(io^{5}C)	**I**	OH	OH	H	OH	NH_2	O	O	O	N	N	N.D.	+	[5]
poly(I) · poly(fl^{5}C)	**F**	OH	OH	H	OH	NH_2	O	O	O	N	N	+	N.D.	[6]
poly(I) · poly(m^{5}C)	**CH_3**	OH	OH	H	OH	NH_2	O	O	O	N	N	+	N.D.	[7]
poly(I) · poly(s^{2}C)	H	OH	OH	H	OH	NH_2	O	O	**S**	N	N	+	+	[8]
poly(I) · poly($_s$C)	H	OH	OH	H	OH	NH_2	**S**	O	O	N	N	+	+	[9, 10]
poly($_s$I) · poly(C)	H	OH	OH	H	OH	NH_2	O	**S**	O	N	N	+	+	[10]
poly($_s$I) · poly($_s$C)	H	OH	OH	H	OH	NH_2	**S**	**S**	O	N	N	+	+	[10]
poly(c^{7}I) · poly(C)	H	OH	OH	H	OH	NH_2	O	O	O	N	**CH**	+	+	[3, 4]
poly(c^{7}I) · poly(br^{5}C)	**Br**	OH	OH	H	OH	NH_2	O	O	O	N	**CH**	+	+	[3, 4]
poly(c^{3}I) · poly(br^{5}C)	**Br**	OH	OH	H	OH	NH_2	O	O	O	**CH**	N	–	N.D.	[11]
poly(m^{7}I) · poly(C)	H	OH	OH	H	OH	NH_2	O	O	O	N	**N^+CH_3**	N.D.	–	[5]
poly(m^{7}I) · poly(br^{5}C)	**Br**	OH	OH	H	OH	NH_2	O	O	O	N	**N^+CH_3**	N.D.	–	[5]
poly(X) · poly(U)	H	OH	OH	**OH**	OH	**OH**	O	O	O	N	N	–	N.D.	[12]
poly(X) · poly(rT)	**CH_3**	OH	OH	**OH**	OH	**OH**	O	O	O	N	N	–	N.D.	[13]
poly(X) · poly(br^{5}U)	**Br**	OH	OH	**OH**	OH	**OH**	O	O	O	N	N	–	N.D.	[13]
poly(G) · poly(C)[d]	H	OH	OH	**NH_2**	OH	NH_2	O	O	O	N	N	+?	+?	[14–16]
poly(dI) · poly(C)	H	OH	**H**	H	OH	NH_2	O	O	O	N	N	–	N.D.	[17]
poly(I) · poly(dC)	H	**H**	OH	H	OH	NH_2	O	O	O	N	N	–	N.D.	[17, 18]
poly(dI) · poly(dC)	H	**H**	**H**	H	OH	NH_2	O	O	O	N	N	–	N.D.	[17, 18]
poly(dI) · poly(cl^{5}C)	**Cl**	OH	**H**	H	OH	NH_2	O	O	O	N	N	–	N.D.	[19]
poly(dI) · poly(br^{5}C)	**Br**	OH	**H**	H	OH	NH_2	O	O	O	N	N	–	N.D.	[19]

poly(dI) · poly(io^{5}C)	**I**	OH	**H**	H	OH	NH_2	O	O	O	N	N	–	N.D.	[19]
poly(Im) · poly(C)	H	OH	**OCH_3**	H	OH	NH_2	O	O	O	N	N	–	N.D.	[20]
poly(I) · poly(Cm)	H	**OCH_3**	OH	H	OH	NH_2	O	O	O	N	N	–	N.D.	[7, 20]
poly(Im) · poly(Cm)	H	**OCH_3**	**OCH_3**	H	OH	NH_2	O	O	O	N	N	–	–	[20]
poly(dIz) · poly(C)	H	**N_3**	OH	H	OH	NH_2	O	O	O	N	N	+	+	[21]
poly(dIz) · poly(br^{5}C)	**Br**	**N_3**	OH	H	OH	NH_2	O	O	O	N	N	–	N.D.	[21]
poly(I) · poly(dCc1)	H	**Cl**	OH	H	OH	NH_2	O	O	O	N	N	–	N.D.	[9]
poly(I) · poly(dCz)	H	**N_3**	OH	H	OH	NH_2	O	O	O	N	N	–	N.D.	[21]
poly(dIc1) · poly(C)	H	OH	**Cl**	H	OH	NH_2	O	O	O	N	N	+	+	[22]
poly(dIf1) · poly(C)	H	OH	**F**	H	OH	NH_2	O	O	O	N	N	+	+	[22]
poly(dIf1) · poly(br^{5}C)	**Br**	OH	**F**	H	OH	NH_2	O	O	O	N	N	+	N.D.	[22]
poly(dG) · poly(dC)	H	**H**	**H**	**NH_2**	OH	NH_2	O	O	O	N	N	–	N.D.	[13, 17]
poly(A) · poly(U)	H	OH	OH	H	**NH_2**	**OH**	O	O	O	N	N	+	+	[1, 23]
poly(A) · poly(rT)	**CH_3**	OH	OH	H	**NH_2**	**OH**	O	O	O	N	N	+	N.D.	[23]
poly(A) · poly(fl^{5}U)	**F**	OH	OH	H	**NH_2**	**OH**	O	O	O	N	N	–	N.D.	[13]
poly(A) · poly(cl^{5}U)	**Cl**	OH	OH	H	**NH_2**	**OH**	O	O	O	N	N	–	N.D.	[13]
poly(A) · poly(br^{5}U)	**Br**	OH	OH	H	**NH_2**	**OH**	O	O	O	N	N	–	N.D.	[13, 23]
poly(c^{7}A) · poly(U)	H	OH	OH	H	**NH_2**	**OH**	O	O	O	N	**CH**	–	N.D.	[23]
poly(c^{7}A) · poly(rT)	**CH_3**	OH	OH	H	**NH_2**	**OH**	O	O	O	N	**CH**	–	N.D.	[23]
poly(c^{7}A) · poly(br^{5}U)	**Br**	OH	OH	H	**NH_2**	**OH**	O	O	O	N	**CH**	–	N.D.	[23]
poly(A) · poly(Um)	H	**OCH_3**	OH	H	**NH_2**	**OH**	O	O	O	N	N	–	N.D.	[7, 13]
poly(Am) · poly(U)	H	OH	**OCH_3**	H	**NH_2**	**OH**	O	O	O	N	N	–	N.D.	[13]
poly(Am) · poly(Um)	H	**OCH_3**	**OCH_3**	H	**NH_2**	**OH**	O	O	O	N	N	–	N.D.	[13]
poly(A) · poly(dU)	H	**H**	OH	H	**NH_2**	**OH**	O	O	O	N	N	–	N.D.	[17]
poly(dA) · poly(dT)	**CH_3**	**H**	**H**	H	**NH_2**	**OH**	O	O	O	N	N	–	N.D.	[13]
poly(A) · poly(dUz)	H	**N_3**	OH	H	**NH_2**	**OH**	O	O	O	N	N	–	N.D.	[24, 25]
poly(A) · poly(dUfl)	H	**F**	OH	H	**NH_2**	**OH**	O	O	O	N	N	–	N.D.	[26, 27]
poly(Ae) · poly(U)	H	OH	**OEt**	H	**NH_2**	**OH**	O	O	O	N	N	–	N.D.	[28]
poly(A) · poly(Ue)	H	**OEt**	OH	H	**NH_2**	**OH**	O	O	O	N	N	–	N.D.	[28]
poly(A) · poly(dUc1)	H	**Cl**	OH	H	**NH_2**	**OH**	O	O	O	N	N	–	N.D.	[9]
poly(dAf1) · poly(U)	H	OH	**F**	H	**NH_2**	**OH**	O	O	O	N	N	–	N.D.	[22]
poly(dAc1) · poly(U)	H	OH	**Cl**	H	**NH_2**	**OH**	O	O	O	N	N	–	N.D.	[22]
poly(dAz) · poly(U)	H	OH	**N_3**	H	**NH_2**	**OH**	O	O	O	N	N	–	N.D.	[21]
poly(dAz) · poly(rT)	**CH_3**	OH	**N_3**	H	**NH_2**	**OH**	O	O	O	N	N	–	N.D.	[21]
poly(dAz) · poly(dUz)	H	**N_3**	**N_3**	H	**NH_2**	**OH**	O	O	O	N	N	–	N.D.	[21]
poly(dAf1) · poly(rT)	**CH_3**	OH	**F**	H	**NH_2**	**OH**	O	O	O	N	N	–	N.D.	[22]
poly(dAf1) · poly(br^{5}U)	**Br**	OH	**F**	H	**NH_2**	**OH**	O	O	O	N	N	–	N.D.	[22]
Random copolymer · homopolymer complexes[e, f]														
poly(I) · poly((ac^{4}C)$_3$, C$_7$)	H	OH	OH	H	OH	**NHAc**	O	O	O	N	N	+	N.D.	[29]
poly(I$_x$, (m$_2{}^2$G)$_y$) · poly(C)	H	OH	OH	**$(CH_3)_2N$**	OH	NH_2	O	O	O	N	N	+ (if $x/y \geqq 5$)	N.D.	[30]

Table 1 (continued)

Polynucleotide	Structure[b]											IFN induction		References[c]
	R_1	R_2	R_3	R_4	R_5	R_6	X_1	X_2	X_3	Y	Z	In vitro	In vivo	
poly(I_x, $(ms^2I)_y$) · poly(C)	H	OH	OH	**CH_3S**	OH	NH_2	O	O	O	N	N	+ (if $x/y \geqq 4$)	N.D.	[30]
poly(I_x, $(Im)_y$) · poly(C)	H	OH	**OCH_3**	H	OH	NH_2	O	O	O	N	N	+ (if $x/y \geqq 0.25$)	N.D.	[20, 31]
poly(I) · poly(C_x, $(Cm)_y$)	H	**OCH_3**	OH	H	OH	NH_2	O	O	O	N	N	+ (if $x/y \geqq 1$)	N.D.	[20, 31]
poly(I) · poly(C_x, $(s^5C)_y$)	**SH**	OH	OH	H	OH	NH_2	O	O	O	N	N	+ (if $x/y > 50$)	N.D.	[32]
poly(A_x, $(Aac)_y$) · poly(U)	H	OH	**OAc**	H	**NH_2**	**OH**	O	O	O	N	N	+ (if $x/y \geqq 2.3$)	N.D.	[33]
poly(I_x, $(Iac)_y$) · poly(C)	H	OH	**OAc**	H	OH	NH_2	O	O	O	N	N	+ (if $x/y \sim 15$)	N.D.	[33]
poly(I) · poly(C_x, $(Cac)_y$)	H	**OAc**	OH	H	OH	NH_2	O	O	O	N	N	+ (if $x/y \gg 0.3$)	N.D.	[33]
poly(I) · poly(C_x, U_y)	H	OH	OH	H	OH	**OH**	O	O	O	N	N	+ (if $x/y \geqq 12$)	+ (if $x/y \geqq 12$)	[34–36]
poly(I) · poly(C_x, G_y)												+ (if $x/y \geqq 20$)	+ (if $x/y \geqq 20$)	[34–36]
poly(I_x, U_y) · poly(C)												+ (if $x/y \geqq 10$)	+ (if $x/y \geqq 10$)	[37]
poly(I_x, G_y) · poly(C)	H	OH	OH	**NH_2**	OH	NH_2	O	O	O	N	N	N.D.	+ (if $x/y \geqq 0.3$)	[38]
Alternating copolymers[g]														
poly(G–C)												±	N.D.	[39]
poly(A–U)												+	–	[39–40]
poly(I–C)												+	–	[39–41]
poly($_s$I–$_s$C)												+	+	[41, 42]
poly($_s$A–$_s$U)												+	+	[40–42]
poly(A–$_s$U)												+	N.D.	[41, 42]
poly($_s$I–C)												+	+	[41, 42]
poly(A–br^5U)												+	N.D.	[17]
poly(I–br^5C)												+	N.D.	[17]
poly(dA–dT)												–	N.D.	[13, 17]
poly(A–s^2U)												+	N.D.	[8]
Miscellaneous[h]														
poly(A) · poly(X)												–	N.D.	[13, 43]
poly(isoA) · poly(I)												N.D.	–	[44]

poly(isoA) · poly(U)	N.D.	–	[44]
poly(L) · poly(C)	–	N.D.	[45]
poly(L) · poly(br^5C)	–	N.D.	[45]
poly(aza^2I) · poly(C)	–	N.D.	[46]
poly(aza^2I) · poly(br^5C)	–	N.D.	[46]
poly(aza^2A) · poly(U)	–	N.D.	[46]
poly(aza^2A) · poly(br^5U)	–	N.D.	[46]
poly(A) · poly(U_x, $(m^3U)_y$)	–	N.D.	[24]

[1] FIELD et al. (1967); [2] FIELD et al. (1968); [3] TORRENCE et al. (1974); [4] DE CLERCQ et al. (1976a); [5] DE CLERCQ et al. (1970a); [6] FOLAYAN and HUTCHINSON (1974); [7] DE CLERCQ et al. (1972); [8] REUSS et al. (1976); [9] BLACK et al. (1972); [10] BLACK et al. (1973); [11] DE CLERCQ et al. 1976c); [12] DE CLERCQ and MERIGAN (1969); [13] TORRENCE and FRIEDMAN (1979); [14] AKSENOV et al. (1973); [15] TIMKOVSKY et al. (1973); [16] NOVOHATSKY et al. (1975); [17] COLBY and CHAMBERLIN (1969); [18] VILCEK et al. (1968); [19] HUTCHINSON et al. (1974); [20] MERRIGAN and ROTTMAN (1974); [21] DE CLERCQ et al. (1978); [22] DE CLERCQ et al. (1980); [23] DE CLERCQ et al. (1974b); [24] TORRENCE et al. (1973); [25] TORRENCE et al. (1976); [26] DE CLERCQ and JANIK (1973); [27] DE CLERCQ et al. (1976b); [28] DE CLERCQ et al. (1974a); [29] PITHA and PITHA (1971); [30] DE CLERCQ et al. (1975c); [31] GREENE et al. (1978); [32] O'MALLEY et al. (1975); [33] STEWARD et al. (1972); [34] CARTER et al. (1972); [35] CARTER et al. (1976); [36] Ts'o et al. (1976); [37] DE CLERCQ et al. (1979); [38] MATSUDA et al. (1971); [39] CONTENT et al. (1978); [40] DE CLERCQ et al. (1969); [41] DE CLERCQ et al. (1970b); [42] DE CLERCQ et al. (1970c); [43] TORRENCE et al. (1977); [44] UCHIC (1975); [45] TORRENCE et al. 1975); [46] DE CLERCQ et al. (1977).

N.D. not determined

[a] The predominant tautomer is not to be inferred from the representation which only serves as a general structural formula for duplexes belonging to the G · C, A · U, and I · C families

[b] **Boxed-in** are those substituents that are modified compared with the parent complex, poly(I) · poly(C)

[c] This is not an exhaustive listing of each instance in which the interferon-inducing ability of the relevant complex was determined; but rather represents those references in which determination of the relevant polynucleotide's interferon-inducing activity was a significant aspect of the work

[d] There is substantial disagreement in the literature regarding the interferon-inducing ability of poly(G) · poly(C); thus COLBY and CHAMBERLIN (1969), AKSENOV et al. (1973), TIMKOVSKY et al. (1973), and NOVOKHATSKY et al. (1975) found poly(G) · poly(C) to be an active interferon inducer, whereas MATSUDA et al. (1971), DE CLERCQ et al. (1970a) and DE CLERCQ and TORRENCE (1977) found poly(G) · poly(C) to be devoid of significant interferon-inducing capacity

[e] For random copolymer · homopolymer duplexes, the interferon-inducing activity, if any, is critically dependent on the proportion of modified nucleotide in the copolymer

[f] For these duplexes, only the structure of the modified or "fraudulent" nucleotide in the copolymer is represented

[g] The detailed structure of these alternating copolymers may be obtained by consulting the homopolymer ·homopolymer complex section of the table since these structures are represented there

[h] The structure of a number of the constituent homopolymers may be determined by consultation of earlier sections of this table. Previously unintroduced structures are given here since they could not be incorporated conveniently into the general structural formula of the table

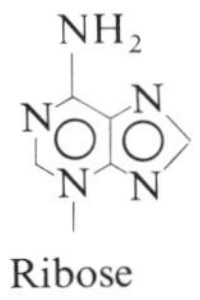

isoA
(isoadenosine)

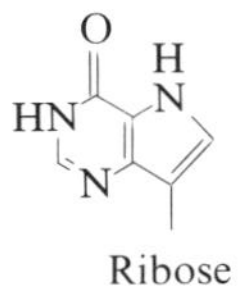

L
(laurusin, formycin B)

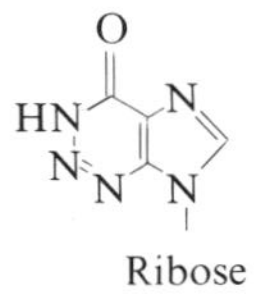

aza^2I
(2-azainosine)

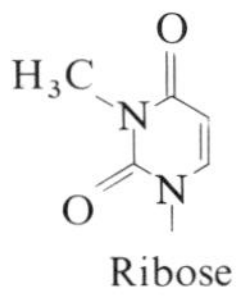

m^3U
(3-methyluridine)

The relationship between nuclease resistance, T_m, and interferon induction becomes complicated when complexes with built-in chemical resistance to nuclease action are examined. Poly(I) · poly(s^2C) is resistant to the action of nucleases and is an excellent interferon inducer in several systems (REUSS et al. 1976; DE CLERCQ and TORRENCE 1977), but since its $T_{m(2\rightarrow 1)}$ is also raised by the substitution of sulfur of oxygen at the C-2 position of the cytosine ring, it is difficult to determine the relative contributions of T_m and nuclease resistance in the interferon-inducing ability of the compound. As will be discussed later, substitutions such as those leading from poly(I) · poly(C) to poly(I) · poly(s^2C) may also affect the conformation of the nucleic acid, thereby altering its interaction with the putative receptor for interferon induction.

C. The Effectiveness of a Nucleic Acid Complex as an Interferon Inducer Depends on the Molecular Size of the Complex and/or Its Constituent Homopolymer Strands

Experiments in which the molecular size of the whole complex [i.e., poly(I) · poly(C)] was varied by simultaneously reducing the molecular size of the individual homopolymer constituents have indicated that, as the size of the nucleic acid complex falls below a critical level (about 4–5 *S*), the interferon-inducing ability of the complex rapidly diminishes (LAMPSON et al. 1970; NIBLACK and MCCREARY 1971; MORAHAN et al. 1972; SHIOKAWA and YAOI 1972; BLACK et al. 1973; STEWART and DE CLERCQ 1974; MACHIDA et al. 1976). Experiments in which the molecular size of one constituent homopolymer was held constant while the molecular size of the complementary homopolymer was varied revealed that there is a critical range (2–5 *S*) where the interferon-inducing ability of the nucleic acid complex decreases almost linearly with decreasing molecular size of either component of poly(I) · poly(C) (TYTELL et al. 1970; CARTER et al. 1972; MOHR et al. 1972; STEWART and DE CLERCQ 1974). These investigations have also ascertained that the interferon-inducing potency of poly(I) · poly(C) is more dependent on maintaining a high molecular size of the poly(I) strand than of the poly(C) strand. The threshold molecular size that a polynucleotide inducer of interferon must exceed to trigger the interferon response may differ considerably from one induction system to another. In a highly optimized interferon production system, such as human diploid fibroblasts "primed" with interferon and "superinduced" with metabolic inhibitors (cycloheximide, actinomycin D), the threshold molecular size may be rather small. In this system, poly(I) · poly(C) preparations composed of a low molecular size (2.5 *S*) poly(I) and low molecular size (3.1 *S*) poly(C) proved nearly as effective in inducing interferon as poly(I) · poly(C) preparations composed of a high molecular size (12.5 *S*) poly(I) and a high molecular size (13.2 *S*) poly(C) (DE CLERCQ and TORRENCE 1977).

D. Interferon Induction by Synthetic Polynucleotides Depends on the Structure of the Nucleotide Building Block

More than 80 synthetic nucleic acid duplexes have been evaluated for interferon-inducing ability (Table 1). Most, if not all, of these complexes fulfilled the minimum requirements for an interferon inducer: they were shown to be double-stranded and to be endowed with a T_m that would insure double-strandedness under assay conditions. Usually, these duplexes were also shown to possess the minimum requirements of molecular size and nuclease resistance to insure their interferon-inducing potentials. Although the minimum requirements for interferon induction were met, many synthetic polynucleotides failed to induce interferon (Table 1). From the data presented in Table 1, it becomes clear that the interferon-inducing ability of polynucleotides depends to a large extent on the chemical constitution of their monomeric nucleotide unit.

I. Interferon Induction by Synthetic Polynucleotides is Critically Dependent on the Nature of the Ribose-Phosphate Backbone

The nature of the substituent at ribose C2′ position is of strategic importance in determining the interferon-inducing ability of a nucleic acid (TORRENCE and DE CLERCQ 1977b). As presented in Table 1, duplexes such as poly(Am) · poly(Um), poly(dAfl) · poly(U), poly(A) · poly(dUz), poly(dI) · poly(br^5C), poly(Im) · poly(C), or poly(I) · poly(dCcl) are all devoid of interferon-inducing ability. This apparent requirement for the presence of a 2′-hydroxyl group on both strands of the double helix is, however, not an absolute one, since poly(dIz) · poly(C), poly(dIcl) · poly(C), and poly(dIfl) · poly(C) are excellent interferon inducers, both in vitro and in vivo (DE CLERCQ et al. 1978b, 1980). While substitution of phosphorothioate for phosphate in the poly(I) and/or poly(C) strand of poly(I) · poly(C) does not enhance its interferon-inducing ability (BLACK et al. 1972, 1973), the same substitution in the alternating copolymers, poly(A-U) and poly(I-C), does lead to a significant increase in interferon-inducing ability (DE CLERCQ et al. 1969, 1970b, c).

II. Interferon Induction by Synthetic Polynucleotides is Critically Dependent on the Nature of the Heterocyclic Bases in the Interior of the Double Helix

The critical importance of the nature of the base pairs in the interior of the double helix (TORRENCE and DE CLERCQ 1977b) was first demonstrated by the observation (DE CLERCQ et al. 1974b) that a series of poly(7-deazaadenylic acid) [poly(c^7A)]-derived duplexes (TORRENCE and WITKOP 1975), even though satisfying all previously recognized requirements for interferon induction, proved completely inactive as interferon inducers. In marked contrast with the poly(c^7A)-derived duplexes, the duplexes based on poly(7-deazainosinic acid) [poly(c^7I)], i.e., poly(c^7I) · poly(C) and poly(c^7I) · poly(br^5C), were quite effective as interferon inducers (TORRENCE et al. 1974; DE CLERCQ et al. 1976a). Complexes derived from polylaurusin [poly(L)] (TORRENCE et al. 1975), polyxanthylic acid [poly(X)] (TORRENCE et al. 1977), polyisoadenylic acid [poly(isoA)] (UCHIC 1975), poly(3-deazainosinic acid) [poly (c^3I)] (DE CLERCQ et al. 1976c), and poly(2-azainosinic acid) [poly(aza^2I)] (DE CLERCQ et al. 1977) are also inactive as interferon inducers, although in the case of the complexes arising from the latter two polynucleotides, low thermal stability may preclude an accurate assessment of their interferon-inducing abilities.

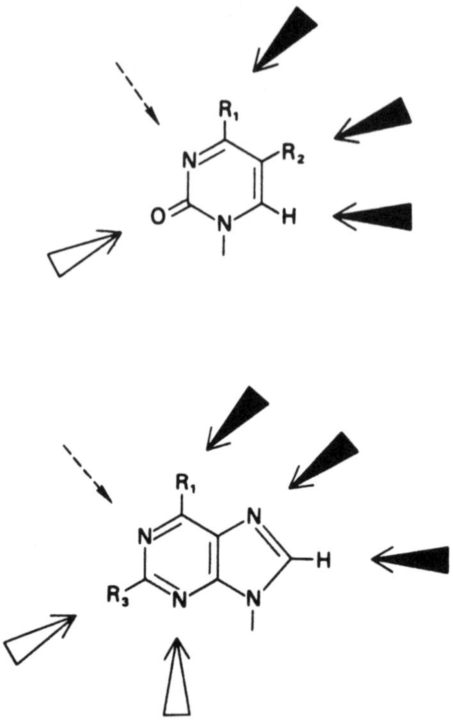

Fig. 1. Potential recognition sites on purine or pyrimidine bases. *Full arrows* denote those positions accessible from the major groove of a double-helical nucleic acid; *open arrows* denote accessiblity from the minor groove of a double-helical nucleic acid; *broken arrows* signify those sites that would be inaccessible from either groove unless the nucleic acid were at least partially denatured, in which case all sites would be available for recognition. For purpose of illustration, the rare tautomeric forms of the bases uracil (thymine), guanine, or hypoxanthine are indicated. Torrence and De Clercq (1977)

E. Role of Polynucleotide Conformation in the Interferon Induction Process

On the basis of these structure–function considerations and several experiments to be described this section, the hypothesis has been advanced that the interferon-inducing ability of a nucleic acid depends on the recognition of a particular conformation (i.e., the spatial and steric configuration) of the nucleic acid (Torrence et al. 1974; De Clercq et al. 1974b; Torrence et al. 1975; Johnston et al. 1975; Bobst et al. 1976; Torrence and De Clercq 1977b). There is no evidence to lead one to believe that interferon induction depends on the recognition of a particular base or base sequence in the nucleic acid; many, if not all, of the purine and pyrimidine base recognition sites that would be available through the major or minor grooves of the double helix (Fig. 1) can be excluded as potential recognition elements by the data of Table 1. Insofar as poly(I)·poly(C), poly(A)·poly(U), poly(A-U)·poly(I-C), poly(c^7I)·poly(br^5C), poly(I)·poly(s^2C), poly(I)·poly(br^5C), and poly(A)·poly(rT) have been established as active interferon inducers, pyrimidine sites O-4, HN-4, C-5, and O-2 as well as purine sites N-7, HN-6, O-6, and HN-2 can be reasonably eliminated as potential recognition sites. Purine N-1 and pyrimidine N-3 would become available only after the unlikely event of helix denaturation (TORRENCE and DE CLERCQ 1977b). Likewise, purine N-3 and C-8 and pyrimidine C-6 would seem insufficient to specify recognition, since this would require poly(c^7A)- and poly(m^7I)-derived complexes to be active inducers. Yet, the latter are inactive as interferon inducers (Table 1).

The data presented in Table 1 show that the putative interferon inducer receptor can discriminate between double-helical nucleic acids which differ in nucleotide composition and, as alrealy discussed, this discrimination does not seem to be based on a recognition of specific functional groups or sites of the nucleic acid bases. Using experimentally induced antibodies to dsRNA as a probe, JOHNSTON et al. (1975) addressed the question: can any other receptor of nucleic acids recognize the apparent differences among double-stranded nucleic acids in a manner similar to the interferon inducer receptor? It was found that the same structural features that determined the recognition of the polynucleotide by antibody also specified the interferon-inducing capacity of the polynucleotide. For instance, substitution of one or both hydroxyl groups of one or both strands of the double-helical nucleic acid, as in poly(I)·poly(dCcl), poly(A)·poly(dUfl), poly(Am)·poly(U), or poly(Am)·poly(Um), led to a dramatic decrease in reactivity of those duplexes with antibody to poly(A)·poly(U). The only exception to this generalization were those 2′-modified helices, poly(dIz)·poly(C), poly(dIcl)·poly(C), and poly(dIfl)·poly(C), that were found to be effective interferon inducers (DE CLERCQ et al. 1978 b, 1980). These latter helices reacted much more like unmodified poly(I)·poly(C) than any other 2′-modified duplexes. Alterations of the bases of the polynucleotide complexes also led to changes in their reactivity towards poly(A)·poly(U) antisera, just as had been observed for interferon induction. Poly(L)-derived complexes, for instance, showed a large decrease in reactivity with anti-poly(A)·poly(U) sera [as compared with poly(I)·poly(C)], concomitantly with an almost total loss of interferon-inducing potency (TORRENCE et al. 1975). Finally, both interferon induction and serologic reactivity would require the recognition of a small segment of the double helix, encompassing no more than four base pairs (serologic reactivity: JOHNSTON and STOLLAR 1978) to 6–12 base pairs (interferon induction: GREENE et al. 1978; DE CLERCQ et al. 1979).

The similarities between two independent nucleic acid receptor systems (interferon induction and immunoreactivity) provide strong circumstantial evidence for the hypothesis that, as first suggested by COLBY and CHAMBERLIN (1969), the putative interferon inducer receptor may be protein in nature; moreover, the results of the structure–function analysis indicated that interferon induction, like reactivity with dsRNA antibody, might depend on the recognition of a particular spatial and steric configuration of the nucleic acid double helix.

BOBST et al. (1976) related the interferon-inducing ability of a polynucleotide double helix to base tilt, a measure of the displacement of the base pairs with respect to a perpendicular to the helix axis (Fig. 2). Using ultraviolet and circular dichroism spectroscopy, BOBST et al. (1976) found that substitution of CH for pu-

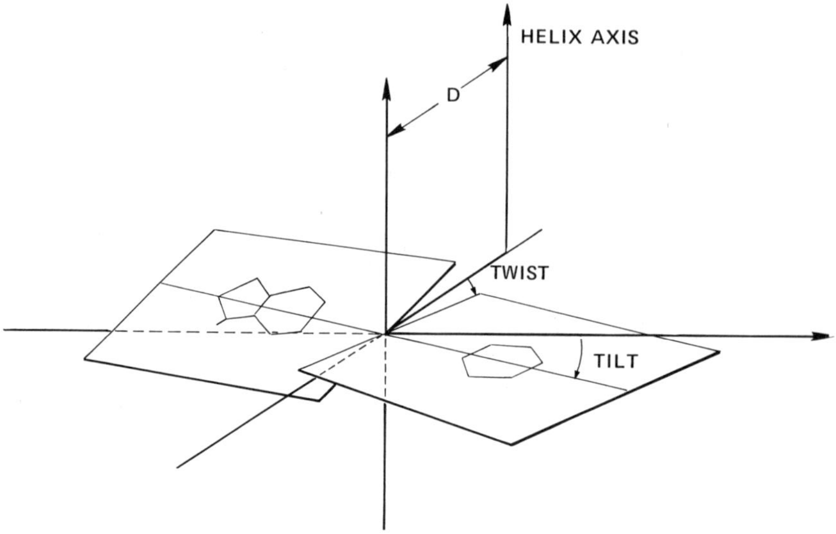

Fig. 2. Definition of the base parameters of a helical nucleic acid such as dsRNA; specifically, tilt (a measure of the displacement of the base pairs with respect to a perpendicular to the helix axis, twist (a measure of the relation of the plane of one base to the plane of the other member of the base pair), and *D* (a measure of the displacement of the base pair from the helix axis). After ARNOTT (1970), Fig. 7

rine N-7 of poly(A) or poly(I) differentially affected the conformation of the duplexes derived from these two polymers. The modification poly(A)→poly(c^7A) effected an increase of the positive base tilt of poly(c^7A) · poly(U) relative to poly(A) · poly(U). This modification also resulted in a loss of interferon-inducing ability (DE CLERCQ et al. 1974b). Conversely, the change poly(I)→poly(c^7I) brought about a decrease in positive base tilt of poly(c^7I) · poly(C), relative to poly(I) · poly(C); like poly(I) · poly(C), poly(c^7I) · poly(C) was also found to be an effective interferon inducer (DE CLERCQ et al. 1976a). Thus, duplexes derived from poly (c^7A) and poly(c^7I) undergo conformation changes in different directions as compared with their parent compounds, and these conformational changes are reflected by the interferon-inducing properties of the corresponding complexes. This study, therefore, links the interferon-inducing ability of a nucleic acid to a defined physical parameter of the double helix, base tilt.

Theoretical calculations (MILES et al. 1979) have suggested that the existence of certain stable glycosidic orientations may determine whether or not a polynucleotide duplex will be an active interferon inducer. In particular, it is proposed that stability of glycosidic orientations near 20°, 80°, and 160° (Fig. 3) may be necessary to endow polynucleotide duplexes with interferon-inducing activity. Inosine and 7-deazainosine (c^7I) possess nearly the same conformational stability in the regions near 20°, 80°, and 160°; however, the glycosidic orientation of 7-deazaadenosine (c^7A) is markedly destabilized in the 60°–80° region, as compared with adenosine. Finally, removal of the 2-OH group can destabilize the high *anti*

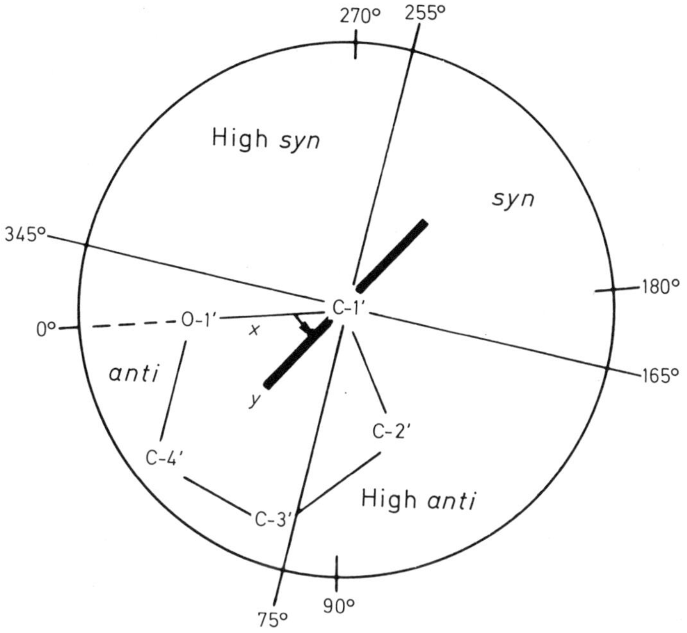

Fig. 3. Definition of glycosidic conformational ranges. A *cis* planar arrangement of the O-1′–C-1′–N-9–C-8 atoms of purine nucleosides in defined as a dehedral angle of 0°. The *heavy line* represents the purine base viewed edgewise. When viewed down the C-1′–N-9 bond, a positive rotation about the C-1′–N-9 bond is defined as a clockwise rotation of the C-1′–0-1′ of the ribose MILES et al. (1979)

conformation near 160°. Thus, different interferon-inducing abilities at the polynucleotide level may originate from different conformational stabilities at the nucleoside level.

It has been abundantly demonstrated that nucleic acids, depending on their composition, sequence, and environment, may belong to different conformational families, each of which is defined by a set of characteristic conformational parameters (Table 2). When the 2′-OH groups of a dsRNA, such as poly(A)·poly(U), are replaced by hydrogen to give a dsRNA, there is an accompanying change in conformation from the A RNA family to the B RNA family. These helical families differ considerably in conformational parameters such as base tilt, axial rise per residue, and sugar conformation (Table 2, Figs. 2 and 4). If, as in the simplest possible case, a nucleic acid receptor existed that specifically recognized the A family of nucleic acids, based on the electrostatic interaction of two lysine residues with two phosphate residues of the double helix, a significant change in the distribution of the phosphate residues (as occurs during the transition from the A family to the B family) would substantially decrease the affinity of the nucleic acid for the receptor. Thus, a conformational change (from A to B, or Z) could by itself suffice to explain the lack of interferon-inducing ability of dsRNA's.

In other instances the conformation of the nucleic acid may remain the same, but a modification of the 2′-OH groups might abolish effective binding to the puta-

Table 2. Conformational parameters[a] of nuclei acid double helices

Family	Helix sense	Helix pitch Å	Axial rise per residue Å	Base pairs per helical turn	Base tilt (°)	Glycosyl bond	Sugar conformation
A	Right	30.9	2.8	11	16–19	*anti*	C-3′-*endo*
A′	Right	36	3.0	12	10	*anti*	C-3′-*endo*
B	Right	33.8	3.38	10–10.4	− 6	*anti*	C-3′-*exo* (or C-2′-*endo*)
C	Right	31	3.31	9.33	− 8	*anti*	C-3′-*exo* (or C-2′-*endo*)
Z[c]	Left	44.6	7.43/2[b]	12	− 7	*syn* (dG) *anti* (dG)	C-3′-*endo* (dG) C-2′-*endo* (dG)
Z′[c]	Left	45.7	7.61/2[b]	12	9	*syn* (dG) *anti* (dG)	C-3′-*endo* (dG) C-2′-*endo* (dG)

[a] The definitions of base tilt, glycosyl bond angle, and sugar conformation are presented in Figs. 2, 3, 4
[b] The Z family has two nucleotides in the asymmetric unit
[c] These families have been described so far only for poly(dG-dC)

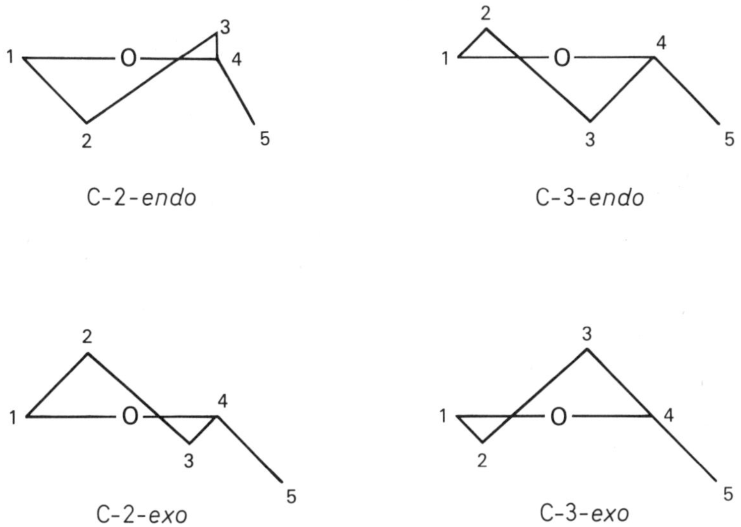

Fig. 4. Projections parallel to C-1–O-5–C-4 showing the four modes of ribose puckering

tive receptor. Such a situation may occur with poly(A_m) · poly(U), poly(Im) · poly(C), poly(I) · poly(Cm), and poly(Im) · poly(Cm), all of which have conformations similar to poly(A) · poly(U) or poly(I) · poly(C) (BOBST et al. 1969; GREENE et al. 1978). To explain the lack of interferon-inducing ability of these 2′-modified polynucleotides, one may assume the existence within the putative interferon inducer receptor of a specific site that accomodates the 2′-OH groups of the ribose–phosphate backbone. Owing to steric hindrance, the bulky *O*-methyl group may not be able to fit this binding site, even though the relative conformational disposition of the *O*-methyl group is the same as that of the hydroxyl group in the unmodified nucleic acid. Following this lead, one may also assume that poly(dIz) · poly(C), poly(dIfl) · poly(C), and poly(dIcl) · poly(C) owe their interferon-inducing potency to the fact that the azido, fluoro, and chloro groups do not significantly alter the conformation of the duplex and also are able to replace the hydroxyl groups in binding to the specific site within the interferon inducer receptor. According to their circular dichroism spectra, poly(dIz) · poly(C) and poly(dIfl) · poly(C) bear a close conformational resemblance to poly(I) · poly(C) (FUKUI et al. 1977; KAKIUCHU et al. (1980). As for serologic reactivity poly(dIz) · poly(C), poly (dIfl) · poly(C), and poly(dIcl) · poly(C) also exhibit a much greater resemblence to poly(I) · poly(C) or poly(A) · poly(U) than do any other 2′-modified double-helical nucleic acids (DE CLERCQ et al. 1978 b, 1980). Furthermore, the purine strand of poly(I) · poly(C) is much more tolerant to 2′-substitutions since poly(I) · poly(dCz) and poly(I) · poly(dCcl) are, in marked contrast with poly(dIz) · poly(C) and poly(dIcl) · poly(C), totally inactive as interferon inducers (BLACK et al. 1972; DE CLERCQ et al. 1978, 1980). Likewise, introduction of 2′-*O*-methyl groups in the poly(I) strand appears to cause a relatively smaller reduction in interferon-inducing capacity than a similar modification of the poly(C) strand (MERIGAN and ROTTMAN 1974; GREENE et al. 1978). To unravel the differential conformational effects imposed by 2′-substitutions on the purine and pyrimidine strand of poly(I)·poly(C), it may seem necessary to apply more sophisticated approaches than those applied thus far.

In an attempt to gain better insight in the mode of action of the polynucleotide interferon inducers and noninducers at the cellular level, competition experiments have been carried out, in which single-stranded, triple-stranded, or inactive double-stranded polymers were investigated for their effects on the interferon-inducing ability of active inducers (DE CLERCQ et al. 1974b, 1975f; O'MALLEY et al. 1975; JOHNSTON et al. 1976; GREENE et al. 1978). Single-stranded polynucleotides did not reduce the interferon response to the active inducers (DE CLERCQ et al. 1974b, 1975f; O'MALLEY et al. 1975), unless they were applied to the cell at 4 °C or could be metabolized to a cytotoxic nucleoside (DE CLERCQ et al. 1975f). Some triple-helical nucleic acids [i.e., poly(A)·poly(U)] and inactive double-helical nucleic acids [i.e., poly(Im)·poly(Cm)] were found to inhibit interferon induction by active inducers (DE CLERCQ et al. 1974b, 1975f; GREENE et al. 1978). These data have been interpreted to suggest that single-stranded nucleic acids cannot bind to the putative interferon inducer receptor, while triple-helical complexes and (some) inactive duplexes may bind to the receptor site, but not to such an extent that an interferon response ensues (DE CLERCQ et al. 1974b, 1975f; GREENE et al. 1978). GREENE et al. (1978) further observed that the interferon-inducing ability of copolymer duplexes [poly(Im,I)·poly(Cm,C)] of varying degrees of methylation and residue clustering correlated with the presence of clusters containing 6–12 consecutive unmodified ribosyl base pairs. This result suggested that the triggering of interferon required the recognition of a dsRNA region comprising only 0.5–1 helical turn. As already mentioned, DE CLERCQ et al. (1979) reached a similar conclusion from their studies with a series of mismatched poly(Ix,U)·poly(C) duplexes.

F. The Spectrum of Biologic Activity of Exogenous Nucleic Acids

Exposure of the cells to a dsRNA of the proper structure and conformation results in the production of interferon, a biologic response modifier which itself has a wide variety of effects. In addition to its well-known antiviral and antitumor activity (GRESSER and TOVEY 1978), interferon also blocks the replication of intracellular parasites (DE CLERCQ and STEWART 1973), primes cells for interferon production (ISAACS and BURKE 1958), inhibits cell proliferation (PAUCKER et al. 1962), stimulates the synthesis of certain induced or noninduced cellular enzymes (NEBERT and FRIEDMAN 1973), enhances the toxicity of dsRNA (STEWART et al. 1972), alters the cell membranes (KOHN et al. 1976), modulates the immune system (HERBERMAN et al. 1979), regulates differentiation (KEAY and GROSSBERG 1980), stimulates prostaglandin production (FITZPATRICK and STRINGFELLOW 1980), and abolishes the mitogenic effect of epidermal growth factor (LIN et al. 1980).

In addition to these effects, which are all mediated by interferon, dsRNA possesses various other biologic activities that may be independent of the dsRNAs' ability to induce interferon. Poly(I)·poly(C) induces, in addition to interferon, a number of polypeptides that are not synthesized in response to interferon itself (RAJ and PITHA 1980). Poly(A)·poly(U) and poly(I)·poly(C) are effective adjuvants of humoral and cellular immunity (JOHNSON 1979). In extracts of interferon-treated cells, poly(I)·poly(C) causes an activation of the 2′,5′-oligoadenylate synthetase (ROBERTS et al. 1976; HOVANESSIAN et al. 1977) and an activation of a 67,000 daltons (protein P_1) kinase (ROBERTS et al. 1976; BROWN et al. 1976), and, thereby switches on two enzymatic pathways which will ultimately lead to an inhibition of protein synthesis (KERR et al. 1974). The existence of these additional activities of dsRNAs coupled with the possible role of these phenomena in the mechanism of interferon action (as reviewed by BAGLIONI 1979; HOVANESSIAN 1979; TORRENCE 1982) have provided an entirely new forum for the use of modified polynucleotides and the relation of nucleic acid structure to biologic activity. The structure–activity approach has been used to address the question whether the other biologic activities of dsRNA (i.e., inhibition of protein synthesis) might be related to interferon induction (CONTENT et al. 1978; TORRENCE and FRIEDMAN 1979; MINKS et al. 1979). In some respects, i.e., molecular size of the homopolymer components, double-strandedness versus single-strandedness, nature of the 2′-substituent, there are definite similarities between the structural requirements for interferon induction and those for protein synthesis inhibition (CONTENT et al. 1978; TORRENCE and FRIEDMAN 1979). However, inhibition of protein synthesis proves much more sensitive to the nature of the heterocyclic bases and their substituents, since poly(I)·poly(br^{5}C) and poly(I)·poly(s^{2}C), while effective interferon inducers, are completely inactive as inhibitors of protein synthesis. Conversely, triple-helical nucleic acids such as poly(U)·poly(A)·poly(I) and poly(X)·poly(A)·poly(U), while lacking interferon-inducing ability, are potent inhibitors of protein synthesis (TORRENCE and FRIEDMAN 1979).

In Table 3, the structural requirements for interferon induction are compared with those required for the other biologic activities, using just a few key polymers. Two other significant biologic activities of nucleic acids are anticomplement activity and inhibition of reverse transcriptase. However, as pointed out by DE CLERCQ (1977), the structural features that provide significant anticomplement activity or reverse transcriptase inhibitory activity are often antagonistic to those needed for interferon induction. Single-stranded polynucleotides are invariably inactive as interferon inducers. They also fail to inhibit protein synthesis or to activate any of the enzymatic pathways that lead to an inhibition of protein synthesis. However, several single-stranded polynucleotides [i.e., poly(X), poly(dUz), poly(dCcl)] are potent inhibitors of complement or reverse transcriptase activity, and those that inhibit complement cause a concomitant inhibition of reverse transcriptase activity. Double-stranded polynucleotides can act as interferon inducers if they comply with the structural and conformational requirements outlined in Sects. D and E. Some of these dsRNA molecules can also act as inhibitors of protein synthesis. However, none of the dsRNAs is capable of inhibiting either complement or reverse transcriptase activity. Comparison of the systems (Table 3) than can be activated by dsRNA reveals that there is some discrimination among the structures required for inhibition of cell-free protein synthesis, 2′,5′-oligoadenylate synthetase activation and protein P_1, kinase activation. Finally, triple-stranded RNA complexes are inactive as interferon inducers, complement inhibitors, and reverse transcriptase inhibitors. Yet, some triple-stranded RNA complexes have been found to be potent inhibitors of protein synthesis and this inhibition presumably depends on an activation of the protein P_1, kinase pathway (Table 3).

Table 3. Relative biologic activities of some representative synthetic polynucleotides

Polynucleotide	Reverse transcriptase inhibition	Anti-complement activity	Interferon induction[a]	Inhibition of cell-free protein synthesis	Activation of 2′,5′-oligo(A) synthetase	Activation of protein P_1 kinase	References
Single-stranded							
poly(A)	–	–	–	–	–	–	[1–8]
poly(I)	+	+	–	–	–	–	[1–9]
poly(dT)	–	–	–	–	–	–	[1, 4, 8, 10]
poly(Cm)	–	–	–	–	–	–	[4, 8, 11]
poly(dUz)	+	+	–	–	–	–	[1, 4, 8, 12]
Double-stranded							
poly(I) · poly(C)	–	–	+	+	+	+	[1, 2, 4–8, 13, 14]
poly(I) · poly(br^5C)	–	–	+	–	+[b]	+	[1, 4, 5, 8, 14, 15]
poly(c^7I) · poly(C)	–	–	+	–	+[b]		[1, 2, 4, 8]
poly(dIz) · poly(C)	–	–	+	–	–	–	[15]
poly(A) · poly(U)	–	–	+	+	+[b]	+	[1, 2, 4–8]
poly(A) · poly(dUfl)	–	–	–	–	–	+[b]	[4, 8, 10, 16, 17]
poly(A) · poly(dUz)	–	–	–	–	–	–	[1, 4, 8, 12]
Triple-stranded							
poly(A) · 2poly(U)	–	–	–	+[b]	–	+	[1, 4–8]
poly(A) · 2poly(I)	–	–	–	–	–	–	[1, 4, 8]
poly(A) · poly(U) · poly(I)	–	–	–	+	–	+	[1, 4, 8]

[1] DE CLERCQ et al. (1975e); [2] DE CLERCQ et al. (1975b); [3] DE CLERCQ et al. (1976c); [4] TORRENCE and FRIEDMAN (1979); [5] CONTENT et al. (1978); [6] HUNTER et al. (1975); [7] MINKS et al. (1979); [8] TORRENCE et al. (1981); [9] ARYA et al. (1974); [10] ERICKSON and GROSCH (1974); [11] ARYA et al. (1975); [12] DE CLERCQ et al. (1975a); [13] HOVANESSIAN et al. (1977); [14] EPSTEIN et al. (1980); [15] TORRENCE PF, DE CLERCQ E, IKEHARA M (1981, UNPUBLISHED WORK); [16] BAGLIONI et al. (1981); [17] JACOBSON et al. (1983)

[a] See Table 1 for references on interferon induction
[b] Definitely active, but not as potent as poly(I) · poly(C)

By virtue of the myriad nature of biochemical and biologic effects they exert, dsRNA molecules should play a fundamental role in the functioning of a cell. In an optimistic vein, one may hope that a systemic exploration of the structure-activity relationship of the various biologic effects of dsRNA will aid in the development of a biologic response modifier that would be useful clinically. At the very least, such studies should contribute to a better understanding of the mechanisms by which dsRNA regulates the cell's responsiveness to various endogenous and exogenous stimuli.

References

Aksenov OA, Timkowsky AL, Ageeva ON, Kogan EM, Bresler SE, Smorodinstev AA, Tikhomirova-Sidorova NS (1973) Interferon-inducing and antiviral activities of the double-stranded polyriboguanylic acid-polyribocytidylic acid complex. Vopr Virusol 18:345–349

Arnott S (1970) The geometry of nucleic acids. Progr Biophys Mol Biol 21:267–319

Arya SK, Carter WA, Alderfer JL, Ts'o POP (1974) Inhibition of RNA-directed DNA polymerase of murine leukemia virus by 2′-O-alkylated polyadenylic acids. Biochem Biophys Res Commun 59:608–615

Arya SK, Carter WA, Alderfer JL, Ts'o POP (1975) Inhibition of ribonucleic acid-directed deoxyribonucleic acid polymerase of murine leukemia virus by polynucleotides and their 2′-*O*-methylated derivatives. Mol Pharmacol 11:421–426

Baglioni C (1979) Interferon-induced enzymatic activities and their role in the antiviral state. Cell 17:255–264

Baglioni C, Minks MA, De Clercq E (1981) Structural requirements of polynucleotides for the activation of (2′–5′)A_n polymerase and protein kinase. Nucleic Acids Res 9:4939–4950

Beck G, Poindron P, Illinger D, Beck JP, Ebel JP, Falcoff R (1974) Inhibition of steroid inducible tyrosine aminotransferase by mouse and rat interferon in hepatoma tissue culture cells. FEBS Lett 49:297–299

Bevan EA, Herring AJ, Mitchell DJ (1973) Preliminary characterization of two species of dsRNA in yeast and their relation to the "killer" character. Nature 245:81–86

Black DR, Eckstein F, Hobbs JB, Sternbach H, Merigan TC (1972) The antiviral activity of certain thiophosphate and 2′-chloro substituted homopolymer duplexes. Virology 48:537–545

Black DR, Eckstein F, De Clercq E, Merigan TC (1973) Studies on the toxicity and antiviral activity of various polynucleotides. Antimicrob Agents Chemother 3:198–206

Blake RD, Massoulie' J, Fresco JR (1967) Polynucleotides VIII. A spectral approach to the equilibria between poly(A) and poly(U) and their complexes. J Mol Biol 30:291–308

Bloomfield VA, Crothers DM, Tinoco IM (1974) Physical chemistry of nucleic acids. Harper and Row, New York

Bobst AM, Rottman F, Ceratti PA (1969) Effect of the methylation of the 2′-hydroxyl groups in polyadenylic acid on its structure in weakly acidic and neutral solutions and on its capacity to form ordered complexes with polyuridylic acid. J Mol Biol 46:221–234

Bobst AM, Torrence PF, Kouidou S, Witkop B (1976) Dependence of interferon induction on nucleic acid conformation. Proc Natl Acad Sci USA 73:3788–3792

Brown GE, Lebleu B, Kawakita M, Shaila S, Sen GC, Lengyel P (1976) Increased endonuclease activity in an extract from mouse Ehrlich ascites tumor cells which had been treated with a partially purified interferon preparation: dependence on double-stranded RNA. Biochem Biophys Res Commun 69:114–122

Carter WA, De Clercq E (1974) Viral infection and host defense. Science 186:1172–1178

Carter WA, Pitha PM, Marshall LW, Tazawa I, Tazawa S, Ts'o POP (1972) Structural requirements of the $rI_n \cdot rC_n$ complex for induction of human interferon. J Mol Biol 70:567–587

Carter WA, O'Malley J, Beeson M, Cunnington P, Kelvin A, Vere-Hodge A, Alderfer JL, Ts'o POP (1976) An integrated and comparative study of the antiviral effects and other biological properties of the polyinosinic · polycytidylic acid duplex and its mismatched analogues. III. Chronic effects and immunological features. Mol Pharmacol 12:440–453
Colby C, Chamberlin MJ (1969) The specificity of interferon induction in chich embryo cells by helical RNA. Proc Natl Acad Sci USA 63:160–167
Colby C, Duesberg PH (1969) Double-stranded RNA in vaccinia virus infected cells. Nature 222:940–944
Content J, Lebleu B, De Clercq E (1978) Differential effects of various double-stranded RNAs on protein synthesis in rabbit reticulocyte lysates. Biochemistry 17:88–94
De Clercq E (1977) Interferon induction by polynucleotides: structure-function relationship. Tex Rep Biol Med 35:29–38
De Clercq E (1979) Degradation of poly(inosinic acid) · poly(cytidylic acid) $[(I)_n \cdot (C)_n]$ by human plasma. Eur J Biochem 93:165–172
De Clercq E, Janik B (1973) Antiviral activity of polynucleotides: poly-(2′-fluoro-2′-deoxyuridylic acid). Biochim Biophys Acta 324:50–56
De Clercq E, Merigan TC (1969) Requirement of a stable secondary structure for the antiviral activity of polynucleotides. Nature 222:1148–1152
De Clercq E, Stewart WE II (1973) The breadth of interferon action. In: Carter WA (ed) Selective inhibitors of viral functions. CRC, Cleveland, pp 81–106
De Clercq E, Eckstein F, Merigan TC (1969) Interferon induction increased through chemical modification of a synthetic polynucleotide. Science 165:1137–1139
De Clercq E, Eckstein F, Merigan TC (1970a) Structural requirements for synthetic polyanions to act as interferon inducers. Ann NY Acad Sci 173:444–461
De Clercq E, Eckstein F, Sternbach H, Merigan TC (1970b) The antiviral activity of thiophosphate-substituted polyribonucleotides in vitro and in vivo. Virology 42:421–428
De Clercq E, Eckstein F, Sternbach H, Merigan TC (1970c) Interferon induction by, and ribonuclease sensitivity of thiophosphate-substituted polyribonucleotides. Antimicrob Agents Chemother 1969:187–191
De Clercq E, Zmudzka B, Shugar D (1972) Antiviral activity of polynucleotides: role of the 2′-hydroxyl and a pyrimidine 5-methyl. FEBS Lett 24:137–140
De Clercq E, Torrence PF, Witkop B (1974) Interferon induction by synthetic polynucleotides: importance of purine N-7 and strandwise rearrangement. Proc Natl Acad Sci USA 71:182–186
De Clercq E, Billiau A, Hobbs J, Torrence PF, Witkop B (1975a) Inhibition of oncornavirus functions by 2′-azido polynucleotides. Proc Natl Acad Sci USA 72:284–288
De Clercq E, Billiau A, Torrence PF, Waters JA, Witkop B (1975b) Antiviral and antimetabolic activities of poly(7-deazaadenylic acid) and poly(7-deazainosinic acid). Biochem Pharmacol 24:2233–2238
De Clercq E, Hattori M, Ikehara M (1975c) Antiviral activity of polynucleotides: copolymers of inosinic acid and N2-dimethylguanylic or 2-methylthioinosinic acid. Nucleic Acids Res 2:121–129
De Clercq E, Torrence PF, De Somer P, Witkop B (1975d) Biological, biochemical and physicochemical evidence for the existence of the polyadenylic · polyuridylic · polyinosinic acid triplex. J Biol Chem 250:2521–2531
De Clercq E, Torrence PF, Hobbs J, Janik B, De Somer P, Witkop B (1975e) Anticomplement activity of polynucleotides. Biochem Biophys Res Commun 67:255–263
De Clercq E, Torrence PF, Witkop B, De Somer P (1975f) Interferon induction by synthetic polynucleotides. Competition between inactive and active polymers. In: Geraldes A (ed) Effects of interferon on cells, viruses and the immune system. Academic, New York, pp 215–236
De Clercq E, Edy VG, Torrence PF, Waters JA, Witkop B (1976a) In vitro and in vivo antiviral activity of poly(7-deazainosinic acid)derived complexes. Mol Pharmacol 12:1045–1051
De Clercq E, Janik B, Sommer RG (1976b) Biological, biochemical and physicochemical evidence for the existence of the polyadenylate · polyuridylate · poly2′-fluoro-2′-deoxyuridylate triple stranded complex. Chem Biol Interactions 4:113–125

De Clercq E, Torrence PF, Fukui T, Ikehara M (1976c) Role of purine N-3 in the biologic activities of poly(A) and poly(I). Nucleic Acids Res 3:1591–1601

De Clercq E, Torrence PF, Witkop B (1976d) Polynucleotide displacement reactions: detection by interferon induction. Biochemistry 15:717–724

De Clercq E, Huang GF, Torrence PF, Fukui T, Kakiuchi N, Ikehara M (1977a) Biologic activities of poly(2-azaadenylic acid) and poly(2-azainosinic acid). Nucleic Acids Res 4:3643–3654

De Clercq E, Torrence PF (1977b) Comparative study of various double-stranded RNAs as inducers of human interferon. J Gen Virol 37:619–623

De Clercq E, Stollar BD, Thang MN (1978a) Interferon inducing activity of polyinosinic acid. J Gen Virol 40:203–212

De Clercq E, Torrence PF, Stollar BD, Hobbs J, Fukui T, Kakiuchi N, Ikehara M (1978b) Interferon induction by a 2′-modified double-helical RNA, poly(2′-azido-2′-deoxyinosinic acid) · polycytidylic acid. Eur J Biochem 88:341–349

De Clercq E, Huang GF, Booshan B, Ledley G, Torrence PF (1979) Interferon induction by mismatched analogues of polyinosinic acid · polycytidylic acid $[(I_x,U)_n \cdot (C)_n]$. Nucleic Acids Res 7:2003–2014

De Clercq E, Stollar BD, Hobbs J, Fukui T, Kakiuchi N, Ikehara M (1980) Interferon induction by two 2′-modified double-helical RNA's, poly(2′-fluoro-2′-deoxyinosinic acid) · poly(cytidylic acid) and poly(2′-chloro-2′-deoxyinosinic acid) · poly(cytidylic acid). Eur J Biochem 107:279–288

De Maeyer E, De Maeyer-Guignard J, Montagnier L (1971) Double-stranded RNA from rat liver induces interferon in rat cells. Nature 229:109–110

Epstein DA, Torrence PF, Friedman RM (1980) Double-stranded RNA inhibits a phosphoprotein phosphatase present in interferon-treated cells. Proc Natl Acad Sci USA 77:107–111

Erickson RJ, Grosch JC (1974) The inhibition of avian myeloblastosis virus deoxyribonucleic acid polymerase by synthetic polynucleotides. Biochemistry 13:1987–1993

Falcoff E, Falcoff R, Cherby J, Florent J, Lunel J, Ninet L, De Ratuld Y, Tissier R, Vuillemin B, Werner GH (1973) Double-stranded ribonucleic acid from mengo virus: production, characterization, and interferon-inducing and antiviral activities in comparison with polyriboinosinic · polyribocytidylic acid. Antimicrob Agents Chemother 3:590–598

Field AK, Tytell AA, Lampson GP, Hilleman MR (1967) Inducers of interferon and host resistance. II. Multistranded synthetic polynucleotide complexes. Proc Natl Acad Sci USA 58:1004–1009

Field AK, Tytell AA, Lampson GP, Hilleman MR (1968) Inducers of interferon and host resistance. V. In vitro studies. Proc Natl Acad Sci USA 61:340–346

Fitzpatrick FA, Stringfellow DA (1980) Virus and interferon effects on cellular prostaglandin biosynthesis. J Immunol 125:431–437

Folayan JO, Hutchinson DW (1974) Poly(5-fluorocytidylic acid). Biochim Biophys Acta 340:194–198

Fukui T, Kakiuchi N, Ikehara M (1977) Polynucleotides. XLV. Synthesis and properties of poly(2′-azido-2′-deoxyinosinic acid). Nucleic Acids Res 4:2629–2639

Greene JJ, Alderfer JL, Tazawa I, Tazawa S, Ts'o POP, O'Malley JA, Carter WA (1978) Interferon induction and its dependence on the primary and secondary structure of poly(inosinic acid) · poly(cytidylic acid). Biochemistry 17:4214–4220

Gresser I, Tovey MG (1978) Antitumor effects of interferon. Biochim Biophys Acta 516:231–247

Guschlbauer W (1976) Nucleic acid structure. Springer, Berlin Heidelberg New York

Herberman RB, Ortaldo J, Bonnard G (1979) Augmentation by interferon of human natural and antibody dependent cell-mediated cytotoxicity. Nature 277:221–223

Hovanessian AG (1979) Intracellular events in interferon-treated cells. Differentiation 15:139–151

Hovanessian AG, Brown RE, Kerr IM (1977) Synthesis of low molecular weight inhibitor of protein synthesis with enzyme from interferon-treated cells. Nature 268:537–540

Hunter T, Hunt T, Jackson RJ, Robertson HD (1975) The characteristics of inhibition of protein synthesis by double-stranded ribonucleic acid in reticulocyte lysates. J Biol Chem 250:409–417

Hutchinson DW, Johnston MD, Eaton MAW (1974) Necessity for the 2′-hydroxyl group for the antiviral activity of synthetic polynucleotides. J Gen Virol 23:331–333

Isaacs A, Burke DC (1958) Mode of action of interferon. Nature 182:1073–1074

Isaacs A, Cox RA, Rotem A (1963) Foreign nucleic acids as the stimulants to make interferon. Lancet 2:113–116

Jacobsen H, Epstein DA, Friedman RM, Safer B, Torrence PF (1983) Double-stranded RNA-dependent phosphorylation of protein P1 and eukaryotic initiation factor 2α does not correlate with protein synthesis inhibition in a cell-free system from interferon-treated mouse L cells. Proc Natl Acad Sci USA 80:41–45

Johnson AG (1979) Modulation of the immune system by synthetic polynucleotides. Springer Semin Immunopathol 2:149–168

Johnston MD, Atherton KT, Hutchinson DW, Burke DC (1976) The binding of poly(rI) · poly(rC) to human fibroblasts and the induction of interferon. Biochim Biophys Acta 435:69–75

Johnston MI, Stollar BD (1978) Antigenic structure of double-stranded RNA analogues having varying activity in interferon induction. Biochemistry 17:1959–1964

Johnston MI, Stollar BD, Torrence PF, Witkop B (1975) Structural features of double-stranded polyribonucleotides required for immunological specificity and interferon induction. Proc Natl Acad Sci USA 72:4564–4568

Kakiuchi N, Marck C, Guschlbauer W (1980) New polynucleotide complexes: an attempt to understand the influence of sugar conformation and strand contributions on polynucleotide duplex stability and geometry. 4th CMEA symposium on Biophysics of nucleic acids and proteins, Schloss Reinhardsbrunn, GDR, March 1980

Keay A, Grossberg SE (1980) Interferon inhibits the conversion of 3T3-L1 mouse fibroblasts into adipocytes. Proc Natl Acad Sci USA 77:4099–4103

Kerr IM, Brown RE, Ball LA (1974) Increased sensitivity of cell-free protein synthesis to double-stranded RNA after interferon treatment. Nature 250:57–59

Kimball PC, Duesberg PH (1971) Virus interference by cellular double-stranded ribonucleic acid. J Virol 7:697–706

Kleinschmidt WJ, Ellis LF, Van Frank RM, Murphy EB (1968) Interferon stimulation by a double-stranded RNA of a mycophage in statolon preparations. Nature 220:167–168

Kohn LD, Friedman RM, Holmes JM, Lee G (1976) Use of thyrotropin and cholera toxin to probe the mechanism by which interferon initiates its antiviral activity. Proc Natl Acad Sci USA 73:3695–3699

Lampson GP, Tytell AA, Field AK, Nemes MM, Hilleman MR (1967) Inducers of interferon and host resistance. I. Double-stranded RNA from extracts of *Penicillium funiculosum*. Proc Natl Acad Sci USA 58:782–789

Lampson GP, Field AK, Tytell AA, Nemes MM, Hilleman MR (1970) Relationship of molecular size of rI_n:rC_n (PolyI:C) to induction of interferon and host resistance. Proc Soc Exp Biol Med 135:911–916

Levy HB (1977) Induction of interferon in vivo by polynucleotides. Tex Rep Biol Med 35:91–95

Lin SL, Ts'o POP, Hollenberg MD (1980) The effects of interferon on epidermal growth factor action. Biochem Biophys Res Commun 97:168–174

Machida H, Kuninaka A, Yoshino H (1976) Relationship between the molecular size of polyI · polyC and its biological activity. Jpn J Microbiol 20:71–76

Matsuda S, Kida M, Shirafuji H, Yoneda M, Yaoi H (1971) Induction of interferon and host resistance in vivo by double-stranded complexes of copolyribonucleotide of inosinic and guanylic acids with polyribocytidylic acid. Arch Ges Virusforsch 34:105–118

Merigan TC, Rottman F (1974) Influence of increasing 2′-*O*-methylation on the interferon stimulating capacity of poly(rI) · poly(rC). Virology 60:297–301

Miles HT, Frazier J (1964) A strand disproportionation reaction in a helical polynucleotide system. Biochem Biophys Res Commun 14:21–28

Miles HT, Frazier J (1978) Poly(I) helix formation dependence on size-specific complexing to alkali metal ions. J Am Chem Soc 100:8037-8038

Miles DL, Miles DW, Eyring H (1979) Interferon induction: a conformational hypothesis. Proc Natl Acad Sci USA 76:1018–1021

Minks MA, Benvin S, Maroney PA, Baglioni C (1979) Synthesis of 2′,5′-oligo(A) in extracts of interferon-treated HeLa cells. J Biol Chem 254:5058–5064

Mohr SJ, Brown DG, Coffey DS (1972) Size requirement of polyinosinic acid for DNA synthesis, viral resistance and increased survival of leukaemic mice. Nature 240:250–252

Morahan PS, Munson AE, Regelson W, Commerford SL, Hamilton LD (1972) Antiviral activity and side effects of polyriboinosiniccytidylic acid complexes as affected by molecular size. Proc Natl Acad Sci USA 69:842–846

Nebert DW, Friedman RM (1973) Stimulation of aryl hydrocarbon hydroxylase induction in cell cultures by interferon. J Virol 11:193–197

Niblack JF, McCreary MB (1971) Relationship of biological activities of poly(I)·poly(C) to homopolymer molecular weights. Nature 233:52–53

Nordlund JJ, Wolff SM, Levy HB (1970) Inhibition of biologic activity of polyI:polyC by human plasma. Proc Soc Exp Biol Med 133:439–444

Novokhatsky AS, Ershov FI, Timkovsky AL, Bresler SE, Kogan EM, Tikhomirova-Sidorova NS (1975) Double-stranded complex of polyguanylic and polycytidylic acids and its antiviral activity in tissue culture. Acta Virol 19:121–129

O'Malley JA, Ho YK, Chakrabarti D, DiBerardino L, Chandra P, Orinda DAO, Byrd DM, Bardos TJ, Carter WA (1975) Antiviral activity of partially thiolated polynucleotides. Mol Pharmacol 11:61–69

Paucker K, Cantell K, Henle W (1962) Quantitative studies on viral interference in suspended L-cells. III. Effect of interfering viruses and interferon on the growth rate of cells. Virology 17:324–334

Pitha J, Pitha PM (1971) Antiviral resistance by the polyinosinic acidpoly(1-vinylcytosine) complex. Science 172:1146–1148

Raj NBK, Pitha PM (1980) Synthesis of new proteins associated with the induction of interferon in human fibroblast cells. Proc Natl Acad Sci USA 77:4918–4922

Reuss K, Scheit KH, Saiko O (1976) Induction of interferon by polyribonucleotides containing thiopyrimidines. Nucleic Acids Res 3:2861–2875

Roberts WK, Clemens MJ, Kerr IM (1976) Interferon-induced inhibition of protein synthesis in L-cell extracts: an ATP-dependent step in the activation of an inhibitor by double-stranded RNA. Proc Natl Acad Sci USA 73:3136–3140

Sen GC, Lebleu B, Brown GE, Kawakita M, Slattery E, Lengyel P (1976) Interferon, double-stranded RNA and mRNA degradation. Nature 264:370–373

Shiokawa L, Yaoi H (1972) Effects of sonication on physicochemical and biological properties of synthetic double-stranded polyribonucleotides as interferon inducer. Arch Ges Virusforsch 38:109–124

Stern R (1970) A nuclease from animal serum which hydrolyzes double-stranded RNA. Biochem Biophys Res Commun 41:608–614

Stern R, Friedman RM (1970) Double-stranded RNA synthesized in animal cells in the presence of actinomycin D. Nature 226:612–616

Stevens G, Felsenfeld G (1964) The conversion of two-stranded poly(A+U) to three-stranded poly(A+2U) and poly(A) by heat. Biopolymers 2:293–314

Steward DL, Herndon WC, Schell KR (1972) Influence of 2′-*O*-acetylation on the antiviral activity of polynucleotides. Biochim Biophys Acta 262:227–232

Stewart WE II, De Clercq E (1974) Relationship of cytotoxicity and interferon-inducing activity of polyriboinosinic acid·polyribocytidylic acid to the molecular weights of the homopolymers. J Gen Virol 23:83–89

Stewart WE II, De Clercq E, Billiau A, Desmyter J, De Somer P (1972) Increased susceptibility of cells treated with interferon to the toxicity of polyriboinosinic-polyribocytidylic acid. Proc Natl Acad Sci USA 69:1851–1854

Stollar BD, De Clercq E, Drocourt JL, Thang MN (1978) Immunochemical measurement of conformational heterogeneity of poly(inosinic) acid. Eur J Biochem 82:339–346

Thang MN, Bachner L, De Clercq E, Stollar BD (1977) A continous high molecular weight base-paired structure is not an absolute requirement for a potential polynucleotide inducer of interferon. FEBS Lett 76:159–165
Thiele D, Guschlbauer W (1973) The structure of polyinosinic acid. Biophysik 9:261–277
Timkovsky AL, Aksenov OA, Bresler SE, Kogan EM, Smorodintsev AA, Tikhomirova-Sidorova NS (1973) Molecular weight characteristics of the poly(G) · poly(C) complex and their relationship to the interferon-inducing and antiviral activities. Vopr Virusol 18:350–355
Torrence PF (1982) Molecular foundations of interferon action. Md Aspects Med 5:129–171
Torrence PF, De Clercq E (1977 b) Inducers and induction of interferons. Pharmacol Ther A 2:1–88
Torrence PF, De Clercq E (1977 a) The polyadenylic-polyxanthylic-polyuridylic acid triple-helix. Biochemistry 16:1039–1043
Torrence PF, Friedman RM (1979) Are double-stranded RNA-directed inhibition of protein synthesis in interferon-treated cells and interferon induction related phenomena? J Biol Chem 254:1259–1267
Torrence PF, Witkop B (1975) Polynucleotide duplexes based an poly(7-deazaadenylic acid). Biochim Biophys Acta 395:56–66
Torrence PF, Waters JA, Buckler CE, Witkop B (1973) Effect of pyrimidine and ribose modifications on the antiviral activity of synthetic polynucleotides. Biochem Biophys Res Commun 52:890–898
Torrence PF, De Clercq E, Waters JA, Witkop B (1974) A potent inducer of interferon derived from poly(7-deazainosinic acid). Biochemistry 13:4400–4408
Torrence PF, De Clercq E, Waters JA, Witkop B (1975) Failure of duplexes based on polylaurusin [poly(L), 'polyformycin B'] to induce interferon. Biochem Biophys Res Commun 62:658–664
Torrence PF, De Clercq E, Witkop B (1976) Triple-helical polynucleotides. Mixed triplexes of the poly(uridylic acid) · poly(adenylic acid) · poly(uridylic acid) class. Biochemistry 15:724–734
Torrence PF, De Clercq E, Witkop B (1977) The interaction of polyadenylic acid with polyxanthylic acid. Biochim Biophys Acta 475:1–6
Torrence PF, Johnston MI, Epstein DA, Jacobsen H, Friedman RM (1981) Activation of human and mouse 2-5A synthetases and mouse protein P_1 kinase by nucleic acids. FEBS Lett 136:291–296
Ts'o POP, Alderfer JL, Levy J, Marshall LW, O'Malley J, Horoszewicz JS, Carter WA (1976) An integrated and comparative study of the antiviral effects and other biological properties of polyinosinic acid · polycytidylic acid and its mismatched analogues. Mol Pharmacol 12:299–312
Tytell AA, Lampson GP, Field AK, Nemes MM, Hilleman MR (1970) Influence of size of individual homopolynucleotides on the physical and biological properties of rI_n:rC_n (polyI:C). Proc Soc Exp Biol Med 135:917–921
Uchic JT (1975) Potential interferon-inducers. Complexes of poly(3-isoadenylic acid). Abstracts of the 170th national meeting of the American Chemical Society, abstract no. MEDI 43
Vilcek J, Ng MH, Friedman-Kien AE, Krawciw T (1968) Induction of interferon synthetic double-stranded polynucleotides. J Virol 2:648–650
Zilberstein A, Kimchi A, Schmidt A, Revel M (1978) Isolation of two interferon-induced translational inhibitors: a protein kinase and an oligo-isoadenylate synthetase. Proc Natl Acad Sci USA 75:4734–4738
Zimmerman SB, Cohen GH, Davies DR (1975) X-ray fiber diffraction and model-building study of polyguanylic acid and polyinosinic acid. J Mol Biol 92:181–192

CHAPTER 12

Production and Characterization of Human Leukocyte Interferon

N. O. HILL

A. Introduction

The development of production methods for human leukocyte interferon (IFN-α) is significant not only for basic and clinical needs, but also as a model for production of many other biologically interesting leukocyte products. The therapeutic potential of interferon was well appreciated early. After its discovery by ISAACS and LINDENMANN (1957), further recognition of its action in vitro and in vivo (LINDENMANN et al. 1957; ISAACS and BURKE 1958; CANTELL and TOMMILA 1960), of factors affecting in vitro production (BURKE and ISAACS 1958; ISAACS and BURKE 1958), and of pharmaceutical possibilities for human IFN-α (ISAACS 1959, 1961) soon followed. However, many years passed before amounts sufficient for clinical trials were produced. Progress toward IFN-α production began with the observation in 1961 that leukocyte cultures were capable of producing interferon (GRESSER 1961). Soon thereafter, CANTELL and his associates reported progress in the development of IFN-α production from Sendai virus-stimulated leukocyte suspension cultures (STRANDER and CANTELL 1966; STRANDER and CANTELL 1967; TOVELL and CANTELL 1971; CANTELL et al. 1974; KAUPPINEN et al. 1978). In this chapter, our procedures adopted from CANTELL will be described to emphasize what has been most suitable in our hands. The importance of certain steps will be discussed as they are presented, as will pertinent variations from CANTELL's methods.

B. Production

I. Leukocyte Preparation

Leukocytes are obtained as a by-product of conventional blood donation. Whole blood, 450 ml, is collected into blood bags containing 63 ml citrate–phosphate–dextrose (CPD) or CPD–adenine anticoagulant. Up to four attached satellite bags enable subsequent preparation of packed red cells, platelet concentrate, cryoprecipitated antihemophilic factor, and/or cryoprecipitate–poor fresh frozen plasma for transfusion therapy. In addition, it enables preparation of source leukocytes for subsequent suspension cultures.

After collection, the blood is cooled to room temperature and centrifuged within 4 h at 4,132 *g* for 2.5 min at 18 °–20 °C. The primary bag and satellites are removed from the centrifuge and carefully placed in a plasma expressor to avoid agitation of the red cells. A hemostat is placed on the tubing of the white cell concentrate bag. This bag is always the satellite bag closest to the primary blood bag. The supernatant platelet-rich plasma is expressed into a second satellite bag until the buffy coat reaches the top of the primary bag. A clamp is then placed on the tubing just above the Y joint which separates the lower satellite bags from the primary blood bag and white cell concentrate bag. The hemostat on the tubing to the white cell concentrate bag is released. The lateral corners of the bag are immediately pushed from the outside towards the center of the bag to facilitate removal of the buffy coat with the least amount of red cell contamination. This should result in the collection of a 25–35 ml volume in the leukocyte bag. A clamp is placed on the tubing as close as possible to the blood bag which is then removed from the expressor. With another hemostat, the tubing is stripped from the red cell bag toward the white cell bag to capture the remaining white cells. A dielectric heat sealer is used on the tubing in three places above the white cell bag. The tubing is separated at the middle seal, and the leukocyte bag removed. The remaining red cell bag and satellites can be processed into the conventional components. The white cell concentrate is then stored in an expanded polystyrene container slightly chilled with a bag of ice separated at the opposite end of the container.

White cell concentrates prepared by this method in other United States blood centers are shipped by air in the insulated containers such that they arrive in the interferon production laboratory early on the morning following their collection and preparation. U. S. Food and Drug Administration regulations require that the source leukocytes come from donor blood which is hepatitis B surface antigen (HB_sAg) negative. Sometimes it is not possible to complete testing prior to shipment because of the testing and flight schedules involved. Therefore, it is necessary either to complete the testing to exclude potentially dangerous units prior to shipment of the blood or to have an approved communication procedure, in the event that the white cells must be shipped prior to completion of tests, which assures that positive units will be removed and destroyed prior to the leukocyte pooling procedure.

The temperatures of white cell concentrates are generally 12 °–15 °C upon arrival the following morning. In our experience, pooling of individual leukocyte concentrates which have first reached temperatures below 10 °C is more likely to be associated with clumping problems in the final suspension culture. This is in contrast to CANTELL's preparation procedure where the buffy coats are pooled on the day of collection by expressing them from a primary bag into a graduated cylinder which contains a total of 10–15 pooled buffy coats. This pool is then stored overnight at 4 °–8 °C while test results of HB_sAg are awaited. In the event of a positive unit, the small pool is discarded by CANTELL prior to forming a larger pool from multiple graduated cylinders. Owing to an extraordinarily low incidence of HB_sAg positive subjects studied by CANTELL in Finland, unusable pools are highly unlikely to result.

The buffy coat preparations are then pooled into 2-l vacuum pooling bottles. This is accomplished by cutting across the stub of tubing originally directed towards the satellite bags. A multispiked collector (Fig. 1) is inserted into the tubing of 20 bags. The collector is connected to the vacuum pooling bottle and the connecting tubing unclamped allowing the pool to enter the bottle. Each pool then contains only cells from individual source blood banks so that determination of buffy coat volume, leukocyte count, and average leukocyte collection per donation

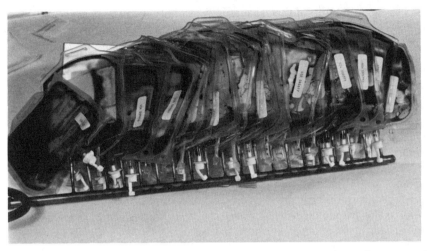

Fig. 1. Multispiked buffy coat satellite bag aspiration device. The aspirator is connected by rubber tubing to a 2-l vacuum pooling bottle

can be estimated as a quality control check on the procedures of the shipping blood center.

The leukocyte pools are then added to 3 volumes 0.83% NH_4Cl which has been previously cooled to 4 °–8 °C. After mixing, lysis is allowed to take place for 15 min. The lysate is then spun at 600 *g* for 15 min at 5 °–10 °C. It is important that the lysing procedure and centrifugation be carried out expeditiously to avoid excessive lysis and therefore leukocyte damage. Next, the cells are washed by suspension in 1 l phosphate-buffered saline (PBS) at 4 °C for every 250 buffy coats in the original pools. They are then centrifuged at 600 *g* for 15 min at 5 °–10 °C and the PBS is decanted. The cells of each 250 original buffy coats are then contained as a pellet in 1 l centrifuge bottles. To this cell pellet is added 1 l 0.83% NH_4Cl at 4 °C for each 250 original buffy coats. After 5 min of mixing, the cells are spun at 600 *g* for 15 min at 4 °C. The supernatant NH_4Cl is removed by decanting. The cells are then resuspended in 1 l tissue culture fluid at 4 °–8 °C. They are left stirring at room temperature while the leukocytes are counted and the total cell yield calculated. Immediately after this prodedure they are put into the final tissue culture vessel with media sufficient to achieve the appropriate cell concentration.

II. Propagation of Inducing Virus

CANTELL's strain of Sendai virus is passed into 10-day-old chick embryos by inoculation with 0.2 ml 1:10,000 dilution of virus-containing chorioallantoic fluid. Biologically tested utility grade embryonated eggs are utilized (Spafas, Inc., Norwich, Connecticut). After inoculation into the chorioallantoic space, the eggs are incubated for 65 h in a 37.5 °C, 50% wet bulb humidity incubator which autmatically turns the eggs every 2 h. They are then placed in a 4 °C cold room overnight.

In a clean room the following morning, egg tops are swabbed with 70% ethanol. Then an egg puncher (Tri R Instruments, Rockville Center, New York, is used to break the top of the egg circumferentially, and the top is removed. With sterile tweezers, the chorioallantoic membrane is lifted off, the embryo gently pushed aside, and the clear fluid removed with a fresh, sterile syringe. Bloody fluid, or that from obviously damaged or contaminated embryos, is discarded. Nine of ten embryos are generally satisfactory for fluid harvest. The fluid is pooled into sterile 1-l plastic bottles kept on ice. Pooled fluid is clarified by centrifugation at 1,100 *g* for 30 min at 4 °C. The supernatant is transferred to fresh 500-ml vaccum bottles by aspiration. The fluid is usually refrigerated for up to 1 week until used. For stock virus, human agamma serum is added to a concentration of 4% and the bottle frozen at −70 °C. The fluid is cultured on tryptic soy broth and blood agar, then observed for up to 48 h for contamination. It should be noted that the chorioallantoic fluid may on occasion have low level bacterial contamination, as evidenced by a noticeable growth in broth, but little or no growth on agar plates. As long as the growth on plates is not substantial, the virus may be used. However, complete sterility is desirable for best results.

Viral yield is assayed by hemagglutination. A 0.2-ml sample of a 5% chick red cell suspension is added to wells of chorioallantoic fluid diluted with PBS containing 8 m*M*$CaCl_2$ and 8 m*M* $MgCl_2$. After incubation at room temperature for 20 min or until the control samples pellets, the titer is read as the last dilution which pellets. Titers usually range between 3,000 and 10,000 U/ml. We have made a practice of freezing aliquots of 100 ml from batches which have a titer of 8,000–12,000 U/ml. If the refrigerated fluid from that batch, used within 1 week after harvest, was found to produce titers of interferon in the range 30,000–60,000 U/ml, we have considered this to be a good seed stock for production of batches of inducing virus. For induction, titers of 8,000–10,000 U/ml are of more practical volume than are lower titers.

III. Preparation of Agamma Serum and Media

1. Agamma Serum

To prepare agamma serum, cryoprecipitate-poor fresh plasma is obtained from the blood bank and pooled into 6-l Florence flasks. Powdered $(NH_4)_2SO_4$ is added to 37.5% saturation at 4 °C and stirred for 2 h. After centrifugation at 4,132 *g* for 1 h at 4 °C, the supernatant is decanted into 2-l sterile bottles. It is then applied in 8-l batches directly to a 25 × 120-cm column containing Sephadex G-25 (coarse) and eluted with triply deionized water. Fractions of 1 l are collected and assayed for protein and ammonia. The ammonia-free protein fractions which elute first are collected. These are pooled and sterilized by double filtration, first through a coarse Millipore filter, then through an 0.22-μm Millipore filtration membrane. The agamma serum is stored in 2-l pooling bottles at 4 °C until use after characterization by protein assay and electrophoresis.

2. Media Preparation

Powdered minimal essential medium (MEM) without phosphate, but with 265 mg/l $CaCl_2$ and 200 mg/l $MgCl_2$ are mixed with triply deionized, reverse osmosis-treated, water in a 100-l tank. This is doubly filtered through 0.22 μm Millipore filters

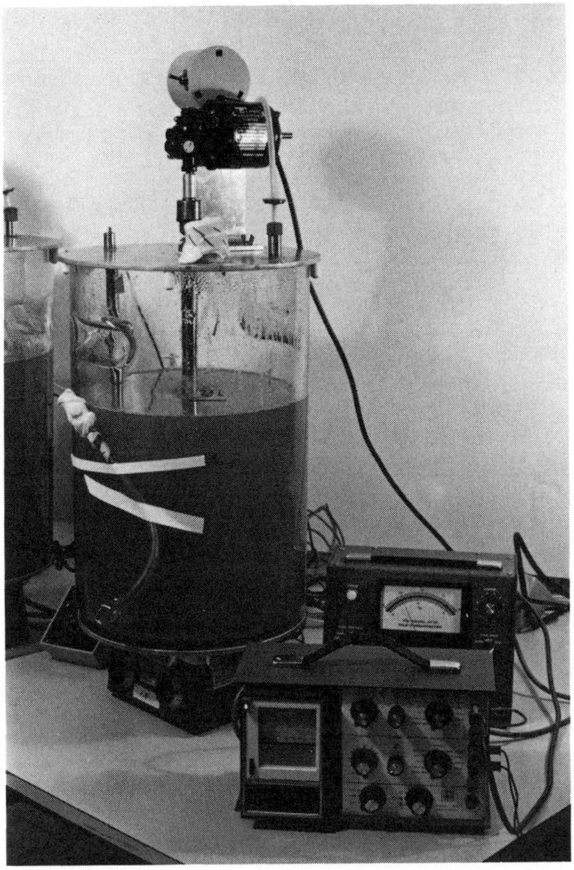

Fig. 2. Vessel (30-l) used for culture of leukocytes during interferon production. An electric heating unit, top drive stirring device, and temperature monitor are utilized for each vessel to maintain desired temperature. Filtered air flow is introduced by needle through the rubber portal cap

and stored in sterile 50-l bottles at 4 °C. Each bottle is cultured in tryptic soy broth and on blood agar plates with observation for up to 48 h. Only bottles free of bacterial contamination are utilized.

IV. Interferon Induction in Leukocyte Cultures

As shown in Fig. 2, 30-l cylindrical vessels are filled to 20 l with a solution containing MEM with 4% agamma serum and 100 U/ml IFN-α. An aluminum plate covers the vessel and anchors a top drive apparatus. The vessels are placed on electrical heating units and the temperature monitored by a thermistor probe placed in a metal well extending well into the fluid. After the temperature has reached 37 °C, cells are added to a concentration of 5–10 $\times$ 10^6 leukocytes/ml in the 20-l final volume. At 2 h, 100–200 hemagglutinating units of Sendai virus per milliliter are added to induce interferon production. An electrical timer is attached to the heating unit which turns the heater off at 12 h after induction. This allows the fluid to begin cooling before harvest the following morning. To harvest the crude IFN-α, the fluid is spun in 1-l centrifuge bottles at 1,100 *g* for 15 min. The fluid is then stored in 20-l batches at 4 °C until completion of the crude titers before beginning purification. As a quality control measure, samples of each vessel are taken for culture in tryptic soy broth and on blood agar plates. Assay of IFN-α is by vesicular stomatis virus plaque reduction in U amnion cells. A laboratory standard, frequently compared with the National Institutes of Health Standard G-023-901-527, is used in each assay run. Expected titers for crude IFN-α may be from 10,000 to 80,000 U/ml with an average of 40,000 U/ml.

C. Purification

I. Cantell Method

The harvested crude IFN-α is stored pending completion of the interferon assays. For purification, the crude IFN-α is then transferred to several round-bottom flasks, each holding 10 l. All purification steps are carried out at 4 °C. First, 5 *M* KSCN is poured in to a final concentration of 0.5 *M*. Then 2 *N* HCl is added dropwise over approximately 15 min until the pH reaches 3.8. The mixture is stirred for 15 min. It is then centrifuged in 1-l centrifuge bottles for 20 min at 1,030 *g*. The supernatant is decanted and discarded. Between 40 and 50 ml 95% ethanol previously cooled to −20 °C is poured into each of the 1-l bottles sufficient to wash the precipitate out into a Waring blender. Then each bottle is rinsed with ethanol so that 250 ml ethanol is used for every four bottles. This fills the Waring blender approximately one-third full. The blender is then turned on for 5 s and off for 5 s. This cycle is repeated five times. Then the material is decanted from the blender into a round-bottom flask. When all of the material from the centrifuge bottles has been processed in the blender and added to the pooling flask, the total alcohol volume is brought to one-fifth of that contained in the original crude interferon and allowed to stir for 15 min. It is then centrifuged for 15 min at 1,100 *g* and decanted into a clean round-bottom flask. The solid is discarded.

Next, 0.1 *N* NaOH is added dropwise over about 1 h to raise the pH to 5.3. This is centrifuged as before and the supernatant decanted to a clean bottle. The solid is saved and frozen for further research. Continued addition of 0.1 *N* NaOH over the next 30–60 min raises the pH to 5.6. The fluid is centrifuged at 600 *g* for 15 min. The supernatant is decanted into another clean round-bottom flask, and the precipitate saved and frozen for further research. Finally, the pH is raised to 8.0 with further addition of 0.1 *N* NaOH. After centrifugation of 1,100 *g* for 15 min, the supernatant is decanted and discarded. The precipitate containing IFN-α is saved. The precipitate is promptly dissolved in phosphate buffer containing 0.5 *M* KSCN at 1/50 the volume of the original crude. This is stirred for 3 h until completely dissolved, centrifuged at 2,500 *g* for 30 min and the supernatant transferred to a clean beaker. Then, 2 *N* HCI is slowly added over a 15-min period until pH 5.0 is reached

Table 1. IFN-α production January 1 through April 30, 1981 at Wadley Institutes of Molecular Medicine, Dallas, Texas

White cell concentrates	26,200
Volume of culture (l)	3,633
Crude interferon (U)	96.7×10^9
Purified interferon (U)	45×10^9
Recovery (%)	47

or heavy turbidity starts. In no case should the pH go below 4.8. This is mixed for 5 min, then spun at 260 *g* for 30 min. The precipitate is purified interferon B (PIFB) which is resuspended in 50–100 ml saline and dialyzed as described in the next paragraph for PIFA before bottling.

The supernatant is then brought to pH 3.5 and centrifuged as for PIFB. The precipitate (PIFA) is saved and dissolved in 100–500 ml sterile saline, depending on yield estimates based on total crude IFN-α processed. This is dialyzed against PBS pH 7.4 for 8 h per change with four changes occurring in 32 h. The PIFA is then clarified by centrifugation at 20,000 *g* in a refrigerated centrifuge for 30 min. The supernatant is decanted directly onto an 0.22 μm Falcon disposable filter for sterilization. The membrane had previously been wetted with saline to minimize IFN-α absorption. Only a slight vacuum is applied to prevent foaming. The membrane is rinsed with 10 ml saline at the end to assure passage of residual IFN-α. Prior to bottling, samples of the filtrate are assayed for IFN-α and cultured, as well as tested in animals for safety and pyrogenicity.

Table 1 presents interferon production data for January 1 through April 30, 1981 at the Wadley Institutes of Molecular Medicine, Dallas, Texas.

Alternate methods of purifying interferon have not been performed on the scale of the Cantell method. However, interferon can be purified by alternate methods of precipitation and gel filtration (Matsuo et al. 1974; Torma and Pauker 1976; Reuveni et al. 1979; S. Grossberg 1980, personal communication) however, these have not been applied on a large scale basis for IFN-α production from buffy coats.

II. High Pressure Liquid Chromatography

Conventional column chromatography using a number of affinity ligands has been performed in an attempt to attain highly purified interferon. These include polynucleotides and lectins (Matsuo 1978), hydrophobic groups (Jankowski et al. 1976; Sulkowski et al. 1976), and copper chelate chromatography (Berg et al. 1979), among others. More recently IFN-α has been purified to apparent homogeneity through the use of high pressure liquid chromatography (Rubenstein et al. 1978, 1979). Furthermore, these workers demonstrated activity in at least three distinct eluted peaks.

III. Antibody Affinity Chromatography

Conventional antibody affinity chromatography utilizing antisera from sheep hyperimmunized with partially purified IFN-α has shown promise as an additional method of purification (BERG 1977; BERG et al. 1978). Indeed, conventional antibody affinity columns of sufficient specificity have been developed such that partially purified human IFN-α has been brought to apparent homogeneity (BERG et al. 1979). More recently, an interesting monoclonal antibody holding promise for large scale purification of IFN-α from the crude state has been developed (SECHER and BURKE 1980). Their report describes utilization of this antibody against lymphoblastoid interferon to achieve a 5,300-fold purification and 97% yield. Purity estimated at 180×10^6 U per milligram protein shows near homogeneity on sodium dodecylsulfate polyacrylamide gel electrophoresis (SDS PAGE). A second pass through this column results in a homogeneous band on SDS PAGE.

D. Characterization

Leukocyte interferons of partial purity have, in the past, been characterized as to a variety of chemical properties. Size and charge heterogeneity with molecular weights ranging from 16,000 to 26,000 (STEWART and DESMYTER 1975; DESMYTER and STEWART 1976; TORMA and PAUKER 1976; BERG 1977; BERG et al. 1979; VILCEK et al. 1978), and isoelectric points ranging from pH 5.2 to 6.1 have been reported (FANTES 1974; CHADA et al. 1979). A possible explanation for this heterogeneity has been variable glycosylation of leukocyte interferons. Indeed, STEWART et al. (1977, 1978) and CHADA et al. (1979) demonstrated disappearance of certain charge and size peaks after chemical treatment or culture conditions intended to free interferons of carbohydrate.

However, recombinant DNA methods which utilize gene isolation, cloning, and sequencing, demonstrate multiple interferons genes of the same length, but which vary in 5%–15% of sequences (SHIGEKAZU et al. 1980; STREULI et al. 1980; GOEDDEL et al. 1981). Thus, heterogeneity in molecular weight, charge, and other properties, is expected. As to glycosylation, chemically mild purification methods such as specific antibody affinity chromatography should be of value. The presence or absence of carbohydrate on native species of IFN-α should be determined using such materials when samples thereof appear homogeneous by high resolution gel separation methods.

Recombinant DNA methods and/or anti-IFN-α monoclonal antibodies hold promise to help in defining the active site (or sites) on the different IFN-α species. For example, to the extent that monoclonal antibodies can be raised against different sites on the interferon molecule, commonality of these configurations may be determinable and related to activity. Using recombinant DNA information, WETZEL (1981) has presented evidence for highly conserved and distinct disulfide binding in IFN-α species. Tryptic digests matched to genetically determined amino acid sequences resulted in assignment of two disulfide bonds between Cys-1 and Cys-98, as well as between Cys-29 and Cys-138 for the seven leukocyte interferons so far genetically sequenced (GOEDDEL et al. 1981), cloned in bacterial plasmids, and produced in cultures of *Escherichia coli*. Since the fibroblast interferon (IFN-β) gene sequence indicates only one possible disulfide bond, this appears to be a distinct difference between IFN-α and IFN-β which may well be reflected in equally distinct configurational properties.

Because a number of interferon species appear to exist, biologic characterization of each, when highly purified, will be desirable. Although such characterization of interferon produced directly from leukocytes is limited, information assigning variable antiviral, anticellular, and cross-species activities to interferons produced by bacteria has been reported (STEBBING 1980; WECK 1980). For the less purified native interferons, biologic characterization has included, in addition to their antiviral activity, their activity in inhibiting the proliferation of standard cell lines, activation of natural killer cells, and the ability to inhibit growth of certain tumor lines as compared with other interferons. These studies have indicated differences between IFN-α and IFN-β. Although there are probably distinctive biologic differences, part of the differences observed may be due to other substances present in the more impure preparations used for most studies. An example of the type of differences which need to be unraveled with highly purified material is the report of BRADLEY and RUSCETTI (1981) who observed that myeloblastoid, lymphoblastoid, and fibroblast interferons had variable effects when utilized in the human tumor stem cell assay (HAMBURGER and SALMON 1977) to detect the direct anticellular effects of interferon. Of interest was the fact that, in a small proportion of the patient samples studied, interferon actually stimulated growth of the malignant cells although a majority of cell samples were suppressed. By extension of these studies to include highly purified interferon species, it should now be possible to characterize their biologic activities more thoroughly.

E. Discussion

Human leukocyte interferon production methods have served quite well in providing the necessary material for initial laboratory and clinical investigation of potential usefulness. These production methods may soon be supplanted entirely by production from bacteria which have been genetically engineered through recombinant DNA methods to enable their production of selected IFN-α species. However, the leukocyte culture method remains useful as a model for studying the whole question of interferon induction and production, evaluating the response capability of patient leukocytes, and especially as a model sytem for the production of biologically active leukocyte products. An example has been the observation that crude leukocyte interferon preparations contain chemotactic factor and migration-inhibitory factor (KHAN et al. 1980; KHAN and K. SINGH 1981, personal communication). Each of these substances, as well as a considerable list of lymphokines, are of interest either as therapeutic tools or for the value of studying their role in immunity.

It is also conceivable that the production of buffy coat interferon could remain as a competitive method to the recombinant DNA methods if the multiple products induced along with interferon can be successfully and efficiently captured from the same culture media. In addition, discovery of methods of substantially increasing the yield of interferon cultures or obtaining proof of glycosylated leukocyte interferon species could make continued preparation from buffy coat cultures desirable or necessary.

It is clear that many additional lymphokines can be produced from leukocytes derived from buffy coats. It is also likely that the large scale production methods presently used in a number of interferon laboratories around the world may be quite adaptable to the production of substances induced under a variety of other culture conditions. It is for these reasons that IFN-α production methods remain significant and are likely to be continued for a period of time.

References

Berg K (1977) Sequential antibody affinity chromatography of human leukocyte interferon. Scand J Immunol 6:77

Berg K, Heron I, Hamilton R (1978) Purification of human interferon by antibody affinity chromatography, using highly absorbed anti-interferon. Scand J Immunol 8:429

Berg K, Osther K, Heron I (1980) The complete purification of human leukocyte interferon by tandem affinity chromatography. In: Khan A et al. (eds) properties and clinical uses. Wadley Institutes of Molecular Medicine, Dallas p 33

Bradley E, Ruscetti F (1981) Effect of fibroblast, lymphoid, and myeloid interferons on human tumor colony formation in vitro. Cancer Res 41:244

Burke D, Isaacs A (1958) Some factors affecting the production of interferon. Br J Exp Path 452

Cantell K, Tommila V (1960) Effect of interferon on experimental vaccinia and herpes-simplex virus infections in rabbits eyes. Lancet 682

Cantell K, Hirvonen S, Mogensen K, Phala L (1974) Human leukocyte interferon: production, purification, stability and animal experiments. In: In Vitro [Monograph 3]: 35, 38

Chada K, Grob P, Hamill R, Sulkowski E (1979) Effects of tunicamycin on properties of human leukocyte interferon. In: Khan A et al. (eds) Interferon: properties and clinical uses. Wadley Institutes of Molecular Medicine, Dallas, pp 21–32

Desmyter J, Stewart II W (1976) Molecular modification of interferon. Attainment of human interferon in a conformation active on cat cells but inactive on human cells. Virology 70:451

Fantes KH (1974) Human leukocyte interferon: properties and purification. In Vitro [Monograph 3]: 48

Goeddel D, Leung D, Dull T, Gross M, Lawn R, McCandliss R, Seeburg P, Ullrich A, Yelverton E, Gray P (1981) The structure of eight distinct cloned human leukocyte cDNAs. Nature 290:20

Gresser I (1961) Production of interferon by suspensions of human leukocytes. Proc Soc Exp Biol Med 108:799

Hamburger A, Salmon S (1977) Primary bioassay of human myeloma stem cells. J Clin Invest 60:846

Isaacs A (1959) Interferon: The prospects. Practitioner 183:601

Isaacs A (1961) Interferon. Sci Am 204:51

Isaacs A, Burke D (1958) Mode of action of interferon. Nature 1073:4642

Isaacs A, Lindenmann J (1957) Virus interference. I. The Interferon. Proc R Soc Lond [Biol] 147:258

Jankowski W, Von Muenchenhausen W, Sulkowski E, Carter W (1976) Binding of human interferons to immobilized Cibacron Blue F3GA: The nature of molecular interaction. Biochemistry 15:5182

Kauppinen H, Myllyla G, Cantell K (1978) Large scale production and properties of human leukocyte interferon used in clinical trials. Human interferon. Adv Exp Med Biol 110:75

Khan A, Kiker C, Schpok S, Hill N, Hill J (1980) Monocyte chemotactic factor (human) as a by-product of large scale interferon production. Fed Proc II 39 (3):1156

Lindenmann J, Burke D, Isaacs A (1957) Studies on the production mode of action and properties of interferon. Br J Exp Path 38:551

Matsuo A (1978) Molecular heterogeneity of human leukocyte interferon. Differing properties in affinity chromatography on poly U and con A sepharose. Kyoto-furitsu Ika Daigaku Zasshi 87 (12):1115 (in Japanese with English abstract)
Matsuo A, Hayoshi S, Kishida T (1974) Production and purification of human leukocyte interferon. Jpn J Microbiol 18(1):21
Reuveni S, Bino T, Hagai R, Traub A, Mizrahi A (1979) Pilot plant scale production of human lymphoblastoid interferon. In: Khan A et al. (eds) Interferon: properties and clinical use. Wadley Institutes of Molecular Medicine, Dallas, p 75
Rubenstein M, Rubenstein S, Familletti P, Gross M, Miller R, Waldman A, Pestke S (1978) Human leukocyte interferon purified to homogeneity. Science 202:1289
Rubenstein M, Rubenstein S, Familletti P, Miller R, Waldman A, Pestka S (1979) Human leukocyte interferon: Production purification to homogeneity, and initial characterization. Proc Natl Acad Sci USA 76:640
Secher D, Burke D (1980) A monoclonal antibody for large-scale purification of human leukocyte interferon. Nature 285:446
Shigekazu N, Mantei N, Weissman C (1980) The structure of one of the eight or more distinct chromosomal genes for human interferon alpha. Nature 284:401
Stebbings N (1980) Protective effects of cloned human interferons in various animal models. 1st Annual international congress for interferon research, Washington, DC
Stewart W II, Desmyter J (1975) Molecular heterogeneity of human leukocyte interferon; two populations differing in molecular weights, requirements for renaturation, and cross-species antiviral activity. Virology 67:68
Stewart W II, Lin L, Chudzio T, Wiranowska-Stewart M (1977) Molecular alterations of interferons. Tex Rep Biol Med 35:193
Stewart W II, Chudzio T, Lin L, Wiranowska-Stewart M (1978) Interoids: in vitro and in vivo conversion of native forms. Proc Natl Acad Sci USA 75:48
Strander H, Cantell K (1966) Production of interferon by human leukocytes in vitro. Ann Med Exp Fenn 44:265
Strander H, Cantell K (1967) Further studies on the production of interferon by human leukocytes in vitro. Ann Med Exp Fenn 45:20
Streuli M, Nagota S, Weissman C (1980) At least three human type alpha interferons: structure of alpha 2. Science: 209:1343
Sulkowski E, Davey M, Carter W (1976) Interaction of human interferons with immobilized hydrophobic amino acids and dipeptides. J Biol Chem 251:5381
Torma E, Pauker K (1976) Purification and characterization of human leukocyte interferon components. J Biol Chem 251:4810
Tovell D, Cantell K (1971) Kinetics of interferon production in human leukocyte suspensions. J Gen Virol 13:485
Vilcek J, Havell E, Yamazake S (1977) Antigenic, physicochemical and biologic characterization of human interferons. Ann NY Acad Sci 284:703
Weck P (1980) Properties of cloned human interferons in various cell cultures. 1st Annual international congress for interferon research, Washington, DC
Wetzel R (1981) Assignment of the disulfide bonds of leukocyte interferon. Nature 289:606

CHAPTER 13

Lymphoblastoid Interferon: Production and Characterization

N. B. FINTER and K. H. FANTES

A. Introduction

The results of animal studies have long suggested that human interferons should be studied as antiviral and antitumour agents in medicine (see reviews by FINTER 1973; OXMAN 1973), but clinical trials have been hindered by the shortage of suitable material. Primary human leukocytes obtained from transfusion blood and processed as described by STRANDER and CANTELL (1966, 1967) have until recently provided nearly all the interferon used in humans. In 1976, Finnish workers made 10^{11} IU crude interferon from this source (CANTELL and HIRVONEN 1977), and have since increased their output severalfold (K. CANTELL, personal communication). Such preparations have played a key role in the development of clinical studies. Nevertheless, it is obvious that human blood could not provide enough cells to make interferon in really large amounts. Furthermore, only limited quality control procedures can be applied to individual white blood cell lots, and for example there are few countries where the incidence of hepatitis in blood donors is as low as in Finland.

FINTER (1966) – and perhaps others before – suggested that human cell lines might be used to provide interferon for clinical use. At that time, many scientists found this idea unacceptable: on theoretical grounds, they believed that a product made from transformed human cells might cause cancer in the recipient, or else be contaminated with a slow virus or other noxious replicating agent. Over the years attitudes have changes and, for example, WI-38 diploid human fibroblasts, which 15 years ago were regarded with some suspicion, are now a preferred substrate for making live virus vaccines. Similarly, transformed human cells can now be considered as substrates for the production of interferons and other substances, provided that the product is suitably processed and purified, and that there is due consideration of the ratio of possible risk to possible benefit (PETRICIANNI et al. 1982). STRANDER et al. (1975) showed that some lymphoblastoid cell lines produce large amounts of interferon, and this led to the study of these possible sources of interferon for clinical use.

Most human lymphoblastoid cell lines consist of transformed B-lymphocytes, which form immunoglobulin, are polyploid, and contain at least part of the genome of Epstein–Barr virus (EBV). If the whole genome is present, infectious EBV may be produced. Such lines can be derived by spontaneous transformation in vitro of white blood cells from donors who have been infected at some time in their life with EBV. The leukocytes transform more rapidly and consistently on superinfection with added EBV, and lines can usually only be derived in this way from cord blood (EBV does not cross the placenta) and from those who have never been infected with EBV. Lines are also readily derived from the white cells of patients with an active EBV infection, or EBV-related malignancy, and from biopsy samples of Burkitt's lymphoma tissue. There are in addition some B-cell lines which do not apparently contain EBV, and other lines which consist of T-cells, or non-B-, non-T-cells. NILSSON and PONTÉN (1975) have reviewed the different classes of lymphoblastoid cell and suggested a terminology.

Conventionally, interferon preparations derived from lymphoblastoid cells have been regarded as forming a separate category, and in relation to their production and safety, this has some merit. However, just as the interferon genes present in lymphoblastoid cell lines are the same as in the circulating B-lymphocytes from which they are derived, so their products are interferons of the appropriate type (i.e. IFN-α or -β) and subtype, and independent of the particular cell of origin. In this chapter, some of the chemical and biological properties specifically demonstrated with lymphoblastoid (and mainly with Namalwa) interferons will be described. It is likely that in due course all those other effects shown so far only with preparations of IFN-α from primary leukocytes will also be demonstrated. Conceivably, such expectations will not always be realised, if for example a particular molecular species of IFN-α has a predominant role in certain circumstances, and the number or proportion of the different interferons in preparations from the two sources differs very markedly. This chapter will deal only with interferons derived from human lymphoblastoid lines of B-cell origin. From this point of view, Namalwa cells have been very much the most extensively studied, and are currently the largest single source of interferon for clinical use. Their interferons will therefore be considered separately, after the relatively scanty information about those derived from other lymphoblastoid lines has been discussed.

B. Spontaneous Formation of Interferon by Lymphoblastoid Cells

In a study of a line EB2, derived from a Burkitt's lymphoma and latently infected with a herpesvirus (now identified as EBV), HENLE and HENLE (1965) found low concentrations of an interferon in the culture medium. In extension of this work, many lymphoblastoid cell lines of diverse origin were studied. ZAJAC et al. (1969) and HAASE et al. (1970) found that, respectively, 11 of 16 and 17 of 21 lines studied formed interferon spontaneously. There was no apparent correlation with the nature of the disease, or demonstrable EBV infection, and some were derived from healthy donors.

The reasons for this spontaneous production of interferon have been much discussed. HENLE and HENLE (1967) concluded that latent EBV infection of Burkitt's lymphoma lines stimulated production of interferon, which in turn played a role in controlling the expression of the EBV infection. The hypothesis proved difficult to sustain in the face of evidence suggesting that several of the lines forming interferon spontaneously were apparently not infected with EBV. Also, some lymphoblastoid cell lines derived from Burkitt's lymphoma patients did not form detectable amounts of interferon, although they were infected with EBV (reviewed by OXMAN 1973). HAASE et al. (1970) concluded that the spontaneous production of interferon was not related to EBV infection, and suggested instead that it resulted from a derepression of gene expression, associated with the transformed state of lymphoblastoid cells. It should however be noted that some of the more sophisticated techniques for detecting latent EBV infection, such as nucleic acid hybridisation, had not been developed at that time; for example Raji cells, which HAASE et al. (1970) considered EBV-negative, have since been shown to be infected with this virus.

ADAMS et al. (1975) studied three lymphoblastoid cell lines which formed no interferon spontaneously. These could all readily be superinfected with EBV, and could be induced to form early antigen (EA), i.e. to express the function of the EBV genes present, by treatment with 5′-iodo-2′-deoxyuridine (IdUrd). In contrast, Namalwa cells and cells of two other lines formed interferon spontaneously, could only be superinfected if at least 100 times more EBV was used, and did not form EA after treatment with IdUrd. They concluded that interferon may indeed be important in the regulation of EBV gene expression, and that IdUrd failed to induce EA formation because interferon suppressed the lytic function of EBV in the cells concerned. Later work in many laboratories has shown that Namalwa cells never form EA (for example PRITCHETT et al. 1976; KLEIN and VILCEK 1980), but the mechanism is uncertain. TOVEY et al. (1977) showed that Namalwa, Raji and BJAB cells treated with 5′-bromo-2′-deoxyuridine (BdUrd) at 25 μg/ml produced larger amounts of interferon spontaneously, whether or not EA formation was induced. KLEIN and VILCEK (1980) treated cells from a number of lymphoblastoid lines, including Namalwa, with various inducers of the EBV cycle [IdUrd; the tumour promotor, phorbol myristate acetate (TPA); sodium butyrate], or superinfected them with strains of EBV. They confirmed that induction of EA and formation of interferon in response to these agents were independent phenomena.

Several groups have characterised the interferons produced spontaneously by lymphoblastoid cells. PICKERING et al. (1980) studied three lines producing interferon spontaneously in amounts of 10–600 U/ml. Their interferon had significant antiviral activity on bovine cells and was neutralised by an anti-IFN-α serum; in contrast to IFN-α from leukocytes or Namalwa cells (after induction with Sendai virus), it was also neutralised by antisera to mouse interferon. It migrated in sodium dodecylsulphate polyacrylamide gel electrophoresis (SDS PAGE) as a homogeneous band of activity with a peak at 20,000 daltons, whereas IFN-α from leukocytes or Namalwa cells appeared much more disperse, with peaks at 21,000 and 15,000 daltons (see Sect. D.V.1).

YAMANE et al. (1982) studied 14 lymphoblastoid cell lines derived by infecting umbilical cord blood cells with EBV. All produced considerable amounts of interferon spontaneously. That from one such line was partially purified: it eluted from a gel permeation chromatography column as a single peak with antiviral activity and molecular mass of 23,000 daltons. It is interesting that both groups found that the interferon formed spontaneously was relatively homogenous. Presumably only a few of the many IFN-α genes are activated in the absence of an inducer. KLEIN and VILECK (1980) showed that Namalwa cells form IFN-α spontaneously but no IFN-β.

C. Interferon Formed by Lymphoblastoid Cells After Induction

Many lymphoblastoid cell lines form interferons when treated with a suitable virus. Newcastle disease virus (NDV) and Sendai virus have predominantly been used, probably because STRANDER and CANTELL (1966) found these the best for making primary leukocyte interferon. To generalise, some lines which form interferon spontaneously, form larger amounts if induced with a virus; of those which spontaneously form no detectable interferon, some respond when induced, but others still yield none (ZAJAC et al. 1969; PICKERING et al. 1980; YAMANE et al. 1982). No particular pattern relating the behaviour of a line to its origin emerges from these data, which also require some qualifications. First, failure to detect interferon could reflect the use of a very insensitive assay system, or its production in concentrations below the threshold of detection, and for example in the first study of spontaneously produced interferon, it was sometimes detected only after concentration of the culture fluid (HENLE and HENLE 1965). Second, suboptimal induction conditions may have been used by some working with viruses. Finally, different virus input multiplicities (ZAJAC et al. 1969), or other conditions, may be required for optimum production with different cells, and the arbitrary choice of particular conditions may affect the pattern of the results obtained.

Numerous lymphoblastoid cell lines have been screened for their capacity to form interferon after virus induction. STRANDER et al. (1975) tested 21 lines: Namalwa cells produced the most. CHRISTOFINIS and FINTER (1977) found that Namalwa was the best producer of 124 lines tested, and it also grew well in suspension culture. CHRISTOFINIS et al. (1981) studied 150 lines, of which 22 (14%) produced relatively large amounts of interferon after induction with Sendai virus. Of the cell lines which had developed spontaneously in culture and were mainly derived from adult donors, 61% were poor interferon producers. Some cell lines had been transformed by the addition of EBV, and 65% of these were relatively good producers [this could reflect the fact that most were derived from fetal or neonatal cells: YAMANE et al. (1982) found that such lines spontaneously produced much more interferon than those derived from adult peripheral blood]. Of 13 lines originating from patients with infectious mononucleosis, 10 were good interferon producers, but 29 of 34 lines established spontaneously from leukaemic donors were poor producers. There was some indication that the particular strain of EBV used to transform cells influenced the yield of interferon from the established lymphoblastoid cell line. Finally, when two or more lines were derived from the cells of a single donor, these sometimes yielded very different amounts of interferon. Thus the genetic make-up of the donor did not play a major role in determining yields.

D. Interferons Made by Namalwa Cells

I. Factors Influencing Production

1. Production Conditions

Namalwa cells readily grow in culture on a scale from a few millilitres up to many thousands of litres. JOHNSTON et al. (1978) described conditions for making interferon in 10–20-ml stationary cultures. Yields of 100,000 IU/ml or more can be obtained, especially if the cells are treated with sodium butyrate for 48 h before induction (see Sect. D.I.4). Yields are comparable from 100-ml volumes of cell suspension in Roux bottles, but somewhat lower from roller tube or spinner flask (1–5-l capacity) cultures. Some workers have reported yields of 1,000 U/ml or even less from their Namalwa cell cultures. Possible explanations are that perhaps:

a. the cells used were derived from a low-producing clone;
b. the cells were infected with a mycoplasma or other latent agent which impaired interferon production;
c. the inducing virus preparation was unsatisfactory (see Sect. D.I.3),
d. the medium contained high concentrations of inhibitors to the inducing virus, e.g. derived from the serum, so that, effectively, insufficient virus was used;
e. if induced in stationary culture, the cell suspension was in too deep a layer, or was cultured with too small an air space, so that, effectively, the cells were inadequately aerated.

Growth of lymphoblastoid cell lines in large tanks was pioneered at the Roswell Park Memorial Institute, Buffalo, New York (MOORE et al. 1967). TOVEY et al. (1974) described the production of interferon from small fermenter cultures or mouse L-cells, and they used the same system to make Namalwa interferon (I. GRESSER and M. TOVEY 1975, personal communication). Very large cultures of Namalwa cells are now used to make interferon on an industrial scale, as discussed in Sect. D.III.

2. Medium and Serum

Almost all workers have used the RPMI 1640 medium developed by MOORE et al. (1967) for the culture of lymphoblastoid cell lines, sometimes with minor modifications such as supplementation with 25 m*M* Hepes buffer. In laboratory scale cultures, animal serum, and commonly fetal calf serum, has been added to the medium at 5%–10%. ZOON and BUCKLER (1977) used 10% fetal serum in their 100-l cultures, but this is costly and could not be obtained in sufficient quantity for use in much bigger cultures. At the Wellcome laboratories, we have readily adapted Namalwa cells to grow with human, horse, pig or calf serum at 5%–10%, and have grown them for long periods with 2% serum supplemented with protein hydrolysates. MIZRAHI et al. (1980) grew 50-l volumes of Namalwa cells with RMPI 1640 medium supplemented with 3.5% (v/v) heat-inactivated and polyethylene glycol-treated bovine serum and various other additives. Cell growth and interferon yields were the same as when the medium was supplemented with 5% fetal calf serum. For cost reasons, media have been supplemented with 0.5%–1% bovine albumin and other additives in place of fetal calf serum (YAMANE et al. 1982; ZOON et al. 1979) and given comparable cell growth and interferon yields.

3. Inducers

Most workers have used NDV or Sendai virus. With the latter, different strains have given very different maximum yields of interferon, the Cantell strain usually giving the best results. Even with this, the results with different production batches of virus have not always been uniform. Recent work (JOHNSTON 1981) has thrown light on the reason. Passage of Cantell strain virus at high dilution gives highly infectious virus preparations (standard virus) which are poor inducers. Serial passage of the virus without dilution gives much better inducing preparations which contain large numbers of defective interfering (DI) particles. Although by themselves DI particles do not stimulate interferon production, they greatly potentiate its production by standard virus. Optimal virus preparations are those with the right mixture of standard virus and DI particles. Similar mixtures of other strains of Sendai virus or of NDV are equally effective as inducers (M. D. JOHNSTON 1981, personal communication).

Measles virus is another useful inducer (VOLCKAERT-VERVLIET and BILLIAU 1977). DE LEY et al. (1978) infected roller bottle cultures of Namalwa cells at 10^6/ml with the Enders–Edmonston strain of measles virus at a low input multiplicity (0.001 TCD_{50}/cell). When the number of living cells dropped below 50%, the medium was removed and assayed for interferon and an equal volume of fresh uninfected Namalwa cells was added. After the fourth passage, amounts of interferon in the harvests increased to about 10^4 U/ml, and this level was maintained in the next seven harvests over 25 days. There was an associated increase in the amount of haemagglutinin in the harvests, but not of infectious virus: it was suggested that this might reflect the presence of DI particles (cf. JOHNSTON 1981). To use measles virus in this way obviates the need to make an inducing virus in fertile eggs, and with two fermenters suitably linked, one growing Namalwa cells and the other containing measles-infected cells, a continuous fully automated interferon production system might be possible. When similarly tested, human parainfluenza II virus, NDV, vesicular stomatitis virus, parainfluenza III virus and Semliki Forest virus all induced less interferon than measles virus (HEREMANS et al. 1980).

Namalwa cells, especially if treated with sodium butyrate, produce small amounts of interferon when stimulated with the synthetic double-stranded RNA, poly(rI)·poly(rC) (JOHNSTON 1980), although some workers have not found any (VOLCKAERT-VERVLIET et al. 1980). H. WEIDELI (1980, personal communication) showed that DEAE-dextran at 200 µg/ml was needed in addition to this RNA for maximum yields (400 U/ml), and that the interferon was produced later than after induction of the cells with Sendai virus.

4. Enhancers

In spite of considerable attention to detail, such as the use of the same medium ingredients, serum and inducing virus, and standardised cultural and induction conditions, we have found that the yields of interferon per Namalwa cell have varied quite considerably from one occasion to another. Good yields can be obtained more consistently if Namalwa cells are treated with various chemicals, but in our experience, these substances do not raise the yield beyond what can on occasion be obtained without their use.

JOHNSTON (1979, 1980) and ADOLF and SWETLY (1979a) independently found that pretreatment of Namalwa cells with various straight chain carboxylic acids or their sodium salts improved interferon yields. Butyric acid was the best member of the series. JOHNSTON (1980) pretreated Namalwa cells with this at 1 m*M* for 48 h before induction with Sendai virus. Maximum interferon titres were obtained after about 16 h. Butyrate did not need to be present during the induction stage, and its enhancing effect was reversed if the cells were further incubated for 48 h in fresh butyrate-free medium before induction. Interferon production was also enhanced in Namalwa cells pretreated with butyrate and induced with NDV or poly(rI)·poly(rC), and in vervet monkey cells (V3 line) stimulated with Sendai virus, but there was no effect in MRC-5 human fibroblasts induced with NDV. Sodium butyrate inhibited the growth of Namalwa cells and their synthesis of DNA (ADOLF and SWETLY 1979a; BAKER et al. 1980), and led to a number of biochemical changes, most of which occurred quickly and well before there was any effect on interferon production (BAKER et al. 1980). However, the reduction in cellular RNA and protein synthesis was maximum at 36–48 h, the time when stimulation of interferon was also greatest. In butyrate-treated Namalwa cells, there was increased production of interferon messenger RNA (MORSER et al. 1980), but no formation of EA (KLEIN and VILCEK 1980). BAKER et al. (1979) found that BdUrd augmented interferon formation by Namalwa cells and human fibroblasts and inhibited their growth: again, these phenomena were not connected. Incorporation of the drug into cellular DNA seemed necessary for stimulation of interferon production, but was not by itself sufficient.

Since sodium butyrate induces erythropoietic differentiation of Friend leukaemia cells, ADOLF and SWETLY (1979b) tested other substances with similar effects. Only dimethylsulphoxide at 280 m*M* had effects on interferon production which approached the activity of butyrate. ADOLF and SWETLY (1279b, 1980) found that glucocorticoid hormones, particularly dexamethasone, and TPA inhibited DNA synthesis in Namalwa cells and enhanced formation of interferon in response to Sendai virus. Treatment with TPA for even 1 h increased interferon production 20 times; simultaneous treatment with TPA and butyrate gave a further 2- to 3-fold increase. TPA did not increase interferon production in three other lymphoblastoid cell lines. ADOLF and SWETLY (1980) reported that retinoic acid (*trans* isomer, 10^{-5} *M*) had no effect on interferon formation by Namalwa cells, but L. MONTAGNIER (1981, personal communication) claim that this substance has a profound effect.

5. Other Factors

P. TALBOT and M. KEEN (1980, personal communication) grew Namalwa cells in a cytostat. The conditions were varied so that the doubling time of the cells in the steady state ranged from 27 to about 47 h: the cells nevertheless produced the same amounts of interferon per cell when induced with Sendai virus, whether pretreated with sodium butyrate or not. BAKER et al. (1980) reported that butyrate-treated cells were blocked in the G1 phase of the cell cycle. However, this did not explain the stimulating effect of butyrate on interferon production, since a high proportion of the cells was already in the G1 phase in untreated cultures. The fact that changes in the doubling time of cells had no effect on interferon production also argues against this hypothesis.

II. Kinetics of Production

Namalwa cells produce interferon at a rate which depends on such conditions as the virus used for induction, the cell density, and whether sodium butyrate or some other substance is used to treat the cells. With Sendai virus, cumulative yields of interferon from cells stirred at a concentration of 10^7 cells/ml were maximum by about 10 h after induction (ZOON et al. 1978). JOHNSTON (1980) reported that stationary cultures at 3×10^6 cells/ml gave maximum yields at about 16 h. If cells were butyrate treated, the course of interferon production was not changed. With NDV, interferon production was complete in 22 h from stirred saturation density cultures ($1.5–3.5 \times 10^6$/ml), but not until about 27 h if the cells were diluted to $1–4 \times 10^5$/ml: under the latter conditions, interferon yields per cell were 2- to 4-fold greater (ZOON et al. 1978).

III. Large Scale Production

Namalwa cells can provide large amounts of interferon. At the Wellcome laboratories (FINTER 1982), the cells are grown in stainless steel tanks of up to 4,000-l capacity (even these are quite small compared with those used routinely to produce penicillin, tetracycline, etc). Sendai virus is used for induction, and the crude interferon is processed in line to a final purity of 80% or greater. Although considerable expertise is required for such large cultures, no new scientific principles are involved. Routinely, RPMI 1640 medium is used, supplemented with 7% γ-irradiated (2.5 Mrad) adult bovine serum.

KLEIN et al. (1979) and WHITE and KLEIN (1980) have outlined the procedures used at the Frederick Cancer Research Center, Frederick, Maryland, to produce interferon from 20-l cultures of Namalwa cells in 50-l fermenters. MIZRAHI et al. (1980) have produced $100–500 \times 10^6$ U crude interferon each week from Namalwa cells in a 130-l fermenter. Other groups in Austria, Denmark, and Sweden are making Namalwa interferon for clinical use, but they have not described their procedures.

IV. Clinical Use

1. Safety Aspects

Whether interferon derived from Namalwa cells should be used in patients has been the subject of much discussion. As outlined in Sect. A, the idea of using transformed human cells as the substrate for biological production raises problems which are not unique to Namalwa cells and interferon. Objections have stemmed from concern that such cells might contain an oncogenic agent, which could still contaminate a product derived from them, even after purification. However, although intact Namalwa cells can give rise to tumours when injected into hairless mice (NILSSON et al. 1977), no tumours result if the cells are first disrupted (J. GARRETT 1980, personal communication). Namalwa cells contain EBV, but the virus genome is present in about two copies per cell (PRITCHETT et al. 1976), and no infectious virus is ever formed. Less than 3 pg EBV DNA per 10^6 U biological activity could be detected in preparations of crude Namalwa interferon prepared at the Wellcome Research Laboratories and examined by a sensitive hybridisation technique (N. RAAB-TRAUB 1982, personal communication), but such tests cannot exclude contamination at a very low level. Equally, in the absence of appropriate tests, it is not possible to rule out the presence of any other human tumour virus or oncogene in the crude interferon. The case for the safety of a particular preparation of Namalwa interferon therefore rests on the final degree of purification, on the particular purification steps used and on the evidence that these are likely to eliminate or destroy those agents which on theoretical grounds could conceivably be present in the crude product. With Wellcome interferon, this has been done by deliberately adding marker substances to crude interferon batches, and showing that in every case, none was present in the purified product. The markers included: a range of animal and bacterial viruses representing all the known virus classes; radiolabelled DNA from EBV and from human cells; various bacteria and mycoplasmas; bacterial endotoxin; and scrapie agent (a slow virus infecting sheep, taken as a representative of this type of virus) (FINTER and FANTES 1980). In particular, from the elimination of DNA during purification, it can be calculated that there are likely to be less than 0.05 molecules EBV DNA and less than 10^{-8} oncogenes in 10^6 U interferon preparation. The detailed evidence has been provided to the authorities concerned with clinical trials in the United Kingdom, the United States, Japan, and Canada. Similar evidence is likely to be required for Namalwa interferon preparations purified by other methods (J.C. PETRICCIANI 1980, personal communication).

2. Clinical Trials

Namalwa interferon has only quite recently been available in any quantity, and there are as yet few results from clinical studies. Wellcome interferon was given by the intramuscular route in a phase I study (PRIESTMAN 1980). The results matched what has been seen with much cruder preparations of IFN-α derived from blood leukocytes, but there were somewhat fewer side effects, and in particular, no pain at the site of injection. Phase II trials are in progress in melanoma; multiple myeloma; non-Hodgkin's lymphoma; carcinoma of the breast, lung, ovary, and colon; various forms of leukaemia; juvenile laryngeal papilloma; and chronic hepatitis virus B infections. These studies will involve in total some hundreds of patients, and because of the nature of the diseases, final results will not be available for some years.

Although current evidence suggests that interferons may not be more active than other single anticancer agents already in routine clinical use, there is still much to be done to define the best route, dose and treatment schedule. Thus, for example, by continuous intravenous infusions of large amounts ($50–100 \times 10^6$ U per square metre body surface per day) of Namalwa interferon, it is possible to achieve and maintain high blood levels of interferon, which are high and exceed those shown to inhibit the growth in vitro of some tumour cells (ROHATINER et al. 1982). The effects of such regimens are now being explored in patients with various cancers and other diseases.

V. Characterization

In the first publication dealing with Namalwa interferon, STRANDER et al. (1975) showed that this resembled IFN-α (i.e. leukocyte interferon), but differed from IFN-β (i.e. fibroblast interferon) in its stability to heat and acid and in its antigenic behaviour. Later publications from various laboratories have all confirmed the great similarities between primary leukocyte and Namalwa cell interferons (e.g.

HAVELL et al. 1978). However, since both are complex multicomponent products (e.g. NAGATA et al. 1980; ALLEN and FANTES 1980) one cannot say whether they are identical, and indeed laboratory studies have shown that the composition of both can vary from batch to batch (HAVELL et al. 1978; RUBINSTEIN et al. 1979).

1. Heterogeneity and Carbohydrate Content

It was recognised early on that leukocyte and Namalwa interferons were heterogeneous in charge (FANTES 1970; HAVELL et al. 1978) and size (STEWART and DESMYTER 1975; BRIDGEN et al. 1977). It was assumed by many that the heterogeneity was mainly or entirely due to differences in the carbohydrate content of a single common peptide (15–18,000 daltons), and that removal of the carbohydrate from a glycosylated peptide (21–23,000 daltons) led to a single biologically active and homogeneous molecule. Thus, BOSE et al. (1976, 1977) reduced the charge and size heterogeneity of leukocyte interferon and changed the half-life of Namalwa interferon injected into the blood of rats by treating them with a mixture of carbohydrases; STEWART et al. (1977) claimed to have converted the 21,000 daltons component of leukocyte interferon to the 15,000 daltons component by treatment with periodate, which they attributed to removal of carbohydrate; BESANÇON and BOURGEADE (1974) and GROB and CHADHA (1979) concluded from the behaviour of leukocyte interferon towards concanavalin A that at least part of it was glycosylated; the latter authors (GROB and CHADHA 1979) also found that tunicamycin (or 2-deoxyglucose) prevented the biosynthesis of the 21,000 daltons fraction of leukocyte interferon, and similar results were obtained by STEWART et al. (1979) with 2-deoxyglucose or D-glucosamine; CUNDLIFFE and MORSER (1979) suggested that the presence of D-glucosamine or 2-deoxyglucose during the biosynthesis of Namalwa interferon might lead to its incorrect glycosylation and hence to reduced yields.

It should be emphasised that all this evidence that leukocyte and Namalwa IFN-α are glycoproteins is circumstantial, and that nobody as yet has actually shown by direct staining that a sugar is an integral part of any of these interferon molecules, as KNIGHT (1976) has shown for human IFN-β. The results from analysing and sequencing pure leukocyte and Namalwa interferons make it unlikely that these are indeed glycoproteins (RUBINSTEIN et al. 1979; ALLEN and FANTES 1980). Although the results do not with certainty exclude the presence of very small amounts of sugar or of unusual sugars, or the possibility that minor sugar-containing components were eliminated by the purification procedures, it now seems more likely that the observed heterogeneity is due to the different primary structures of the multiple components present, and not to differences in their carbohydrate content. Even the two main molecular classes, long accepted as having masses of approximately 18,000 and 22,000 daltons, probably do not differ by 4000 daltons or in their sugar content, but merely in the composition and arrangement of their 166 amino acids.

If IFN-α species do not contain sugar, one has to explain these effects ascribed to glycosidases, tunicamycin, glycosylation inhibitors and to periodate, and also the affinity for concanavalin A. It is possible that the rather impure glycosidases that were used could have been contaminated with proteases; glycosylation inhibitors could interfere with the biosynthesis per se of the "larger" molecular weight peptides, and periodate is known to act very readily on certain amino acids as well as on sugars (SKLARZ 1967). The affinity for concanavalin A could perhaps be nonspecific and was, in any case, not observed by JANKOWSKI et al. (1975). It is also worth mentioning that MOGENSEN et al. (1974) already believed that leukocyte interferon was not a glycoprotein.

Recently more has become known about the multiple components that make up leukocyte and Namalwa interferons, both from the direct analysis and sequencing of the actual peptides and from the nucleotide sequences of cDNA clones. ZOON et al. (1980) published the sequence of the first 20 NH_2 amino acids of one of the components of Namalwa interferon (NH_2 terminal amino acid serine, probably incorrect: see GOEDDEL et al. 1981). ALLEN and FANTES (1980) determined partial sequences in a mixture containing at least five Namalwa interferon components (NH_2 terminal amino acid cysteine), and FANTES and ALLEN (1981) later found that this interferon consists of at least eight active components. NAGATA et al. (1980) showed that there were at least eight different genes coding for leukocyte interferon, and GOEDDEL et al. (1981) published the actual structures of eight such cDNAs. RUBINSTEIN et al. (1979), LEVY et al. (1980) and PESTKA und RUBINSTEIN (1980) described eight different peptides isolated by high pressure liquid chromatography from leukocyte interferon.

2. Antigenic Characteristics

Namalwa cells induced with Sendai virus produce both IFN-α and -β, the latter in amounts estimated as 10%–20% of the total (HAVELL et al. 1978; DALTON and PAUCKER 1979). HAYES et al. (1979) showed that the proportion of IFN-β and -α produced by human diploid fibroblasts in response to NDV depended on the multiplicity of infection and on how much the virus had been inactivated with ultraviolet light. There have as yet been no comparable studies with Namalwa cells. KLEIN and VILCEK (1980) reported that in the small amounts of interferon formed spontaneously by Namalwa cells and the much larger amounts found after superinfection with a transforming strain of EBV, there was no IFN-β, whereas both IFN-α and -β were formed by cells treated with IdUrd.

As already mentioned, STRANDER et al. (1975) noticed that leukocyte and Namalwa interferons were antigenically similar. This was confirmed by later results: ZOON et al. (1979b) used immobilised antileukocyte globulins for affinity chromatographic purification of Namalwa interferon and STEWART et al. (1980) similarly purified leukocyte interferon on an anti-Namalwa interferon column. PYHÄLÄ (1978) found that antibodies raised in rabbits or sheep against leukocyte interferon had higher neutralising titres against leukocyte than against Namalwa interferon, suggesting some difference in the two interferons. However, it seems possible that the higher IFN-β content of Namalwa interferon (HAVELL et al. 1978) was responsible for this difference, especially as an injection of fibroblast interferon boosted neutralising titres against both these interferons as well as against fibroblast interferon.

3. Monoclonal Antibodies to Components of Namalwa and Leukocyte Interferons

SECHER and BURKE (1980), isolated a clone of hybrid myeloma cells that secreted mouse monoclonal antibody to Namalwa interferon. An affinity column was prepared from the IgG fraction of this antibody, and it purified crude Namalwa interferon 5,000-fold in one step. Further work has shown that not all the interferons induced in Namalwa cells by Sendai virus are retained by this antibody (ALLEN et al. 1982), i.e. there are at least some antigenic differences between some of the many components in Namalwa interferon.

4. Specific Activity of Pure Namalwa Interferon

ZOON et al. (1980) calculated a specific activity of 2.5×10^8 IU per milligram protein for the 18,500 daltons component of Namalwa interferon, and FANTES and ALLEN (1981) found a similar value (approximately 2×10^8 IU per milligram protein) for the mixture of all components. These figures are very similar to those published for leukocyte interferon (e.g. RUBINSTEIN et al. 1979).

5. Other Properties

Because, until recently, leukocyte interferon has been the more readily available to investigators, HuIFN-α from this source has been more extensively studied than Namalwa cell interferon. The rather limited data with the latter are considered in the next sections.

a) Antiviral Action in Heterologous Cells

Like HuIFN-α from primary leukocytes, Namalwa interferons have pronounced antiviral activity in a number of heterologous cells, which is sometimes even higher than in human cells (GRESSER et al. 1974; DESMYTER and STEWART 1976), and this property is often used to distinguish these interferons from fibroblast interferon. This heterospecific activity seems to reside in the "lower molecular weight" components (BRIDGEN et al. 1980).

b) Anticellular Effects

Leukocyte interferon has been shown to inhibit the growth of many cell lines (e.g. STRANDER and EINHORN 1977; CREASEY et al. 1980) and there is no reason to believe that lymphoblastoid interferons will behave differently. CHRISTOFINIS and FINTER (1977) showed that the growth of Daudi cells was equally reduced by the two interferons. BALKWILL et al. (1978) found that Namalwa interferon inhibited the in vitro growth of normal human mammary epithelicial cells and breast cancer cells. Xenografts of the latter in hairless mice were also inhibited (BALKWILL et al. 1980).

c) Migration-Inhibitory Factor and RNase Activity

Partly purified leukocyte interferon did not inhibit the migration of guinea-pig macrophages (L. H. BLOCK, K. CANTELL, S. BAMBERGER, R. RUHENSTROH-BANEY, and H. STRANDER 1977, personal communication) and crude and partly purified Namalwa interferon failed to inhibit the migration of human leukocytes (K. H. FANTES, C. OWEN-DAVIES, and C. J. BURMAN 1977, unpublished work). One can conclude that these interferons and migration-inhibitory factor are different substances. WINCHURCH et al. (1977) reported that partially and "highly" (specific activity 3.4×10^6 IU per milligram protein) purified human leukocyte interferon had marked RNase activity and it was suggested that this might play a role in the antiviral and other activites of the interferon. In contrast, KARPETSKY et al. (1979) showed that partly (3.7×10^5 IU per milligram protein) and more highly (6.7×10^7 IU per milligram protein) purified Namalwa interferon was devoid of such activity. It is, however, unlikely that the two pure interferons will be found to differ in this respect: the RNase concentration in the crude leukocyte interferon preparation was approximately 20 times higher than in the crude Namalwa interferon, and it is probable that further purification of the leukocyte interferon would eliminate all RNase activity.

d) Stimulation of Natural Killer Cells

Like primary leukocyte interferon, Namalwa interferon was found to enhance the activity of natural killer cells (MOORE and POTTER 1980; MOORE et al. 1980).

References

Adams A, Lidin B, Strander H, Cantell K (1975) Spontaneous interferon production and Epstein-Barr virus antigen expression in human lymphoid cell lines. J Gen Virol 28:219–225

Adolf GR, Swetly P (1979a) Interferon production by human lymphoblastoid cells is stimulated by inducers of Friend cell differentiation. Virology 99:158–166

Adolf GR, Swetly P (1979b) Glucocorticoid hormones inhibit DNA synthesis and enhance interferon production in a human lymphoid cell line. Nature 282:736–738

Adolf GR, Swetly P (1980) Tumour-promoting phorbol esters inhibit DNA synthesis and enhance virus-induced interferon production in a human lymphoma cell line. J Gen Virol 51:61–67

Allen G, Fantes KH (1980) A family of structural genes for human lymphoblastoid (leukocyte-type) interferon. Nature 287:408–411

Allen G, Fantes KH, Burke DC, Morser J (1982) Analysis and purification of human lymphoblastoid (Namalwa) interferon using a monoclonal antibody. J Gen Virol 63:207–212

Baker PN, Bradshaw TK, Morser J, Burke DC (1979) The effect of 5-bromodeoxyuridine on interferon production in human cells. J Gen Virol 45:177–184

Baker PN, Morser J, Burke DC (1980) Effects of sodium butyrate on a human lymphoblastoid cell line (Namalwa) and its interferon production. J Interferon Res 1:71–77

Balkwill F, Watling D, Taylor-Papadimitriou J (1978) Inhibition by lymphoblastoid interferon of growth of cells derived from the human breast. Int J Cancer 22:258–265

Balkwill F, Taylor-Papadimitriou J, Fantes KH, Sebesteny A (1980) Human lymphoblastoid interferon can inhibit the growth of human breast cancer xenografts in athymic (nude) mice. Eur J Cancer 16:569–573

Besançon F, Bourgeade MF (1974) Affinity of murine and human interferons for concanavalin A, J Immunol 113:1061–1063

Bose S, Hickman J (1977) Role of carbohydrate moiety in determining the survival of interferon in the circulation. J Biol Chem 252:8336–8337

Bose S, Gurari-Rotman D, Ruegg VT, Corley L, Anfinsen CB (1976) Apparent dispensability of the carbohydrate moiety of human interferon for antiviral activity. J Biol Chem 251:1659–1662

Bridgen PJ, Anfinsen CB, Corley L, Bose S, Zoon KC, Ruegg UT, Buckler CE (1977) Human lymphoblastoid interferon: large scale production and partial purification. J Biol Chem 252:6585–6587

Bridgen PJ, Zoon KC, Smith ME (1980) Characterization of the two components of human lymphoblastoid interferon. Fed Proc 39:A2054

Cantell K, Hirvonen S (1977) Preparation of human leukocyte interferon for clinical use. Tex Rep Biol Med 35:138–144

Christofinis GJ, Finter NB (1977) The preparation of interferon from lymphoblastoid cell lines. Proc Symp Interferon, Yugoslav Acad Sci Arts, Zagreb, pp 39–47

Christofinis GJ, Steel CM, Finter NB (1981) Interferon production by human lymphoblastoid cell lines of different origin. J Gen Virol 52:169–171

Creasey AA, Bartholomew JC, Merigan TC (1980) Role of G_0-G_1 arrest in the inhibition of tumor cell growth by interferon. Proc Natl Acad Sci USA 77:1471–1475

Cundliffe B, Morser J (1979) The effect of inhibitors of glycosylation on interferon production in human lymphoblastoid cells. J Gen Virol 43:457–461

Dalton BJ, Paucker K (1979) Antigenic properties of human lymphoblastoid interferons. Infect Immun 23:244–248

De Ley M, Billiau A, De Somer P (1978) A semi-continuous system for the production of human interferon in lymphoblastoid cell cultures. J Gen Virol 40:455–458

Desmyter J, Stewart WE (1976) Molecular modification of interferon: Attainment of human interferon in a configuration active on cat cells but inactive on human cells. Virology 70:451–458

Fantes KH (1970) Purification and properties of human interferon. Ann NY Acad Sci 173:118–121

Fantes KH, Allen G (1981) The specific activity of pure human interferons and a non-biological method for estimating the purity of highly purified interferon preparations. J Interferon Res 1:465–421

Finter NB (1966) Interferons in animals and man. In: Finter NB (ed) Interferons. North-Holland, Amsterdam, p 232

Finter NB (1973) Interferons and inducers in vivo: I Antiviral effects in experimental animals. In: Finter NB (ed) Interferons and interferons inducers. North-Holland, Amsterdam, p 295

Finter NB (1982) Large scale production of human interferon from lymphoblastoid cells. Tex Rep Biol Med 41:175–178

Finter NB, Fantes KH (1980) The purity and safety of interferons prepared for clinical use: the case for lymphoblastoid interferon. Gresser I (ed) Interferon 1980. Academic, London, p 65

Goeddel DV, Leung DW, Dull TJ, Gross M, Lawn RM, McCandliss R, Seeburg PH, Ullrich A, Yelverton E, Gray PW (1981) The structure of eight distinct cloned human leukocyte interferon cDNAs. Nature 290:20–26

Gresser I, Bandu MT, Brouty-Boye D, Tovey M (1974) Pronounced antiviral activity of human interferon on bovine and porcine cells. Nature 251:543–545

Grob PM, Chadha KC (1979) Separation of human leukocyte interferon components by concanavalin A – agarose affinity chromatography and their characterization. Biochemistry 18:5782–5786

Haase AT, Johnson JS, Kasel JA, Margolis S, Levy HB (1970) Induction of interferon in lymphoblastoid cell lines. Proc Soc Exp Biol Med 133:1076–1083

Havell EA, Yip YK, Vilcek J (1978) Characteristics of human lymphoblastoid (Namalwa) interferon. J Gen Virol 38:51–60

Hayes TG, Yip YK, Vilcek J (1979) Leukocyte interferon production by human fibroblasts. Virology 98:351–363

Henle G, Henle W (1965) Evidence for a persistent viral infection in a cell line derived from Burkitt's lymphoma. J Bacteriol 89:252–258

Henle G, Henle W (1967) Immunofluorescence interference and complement fixation technics in the detection of the herpes-type virus in Burkitt tumor cell lines. Cancer Res 27:2442–2447

Heremans H, De Ley M, Volckaert-Vervliet G, Billia A (1980) Interferon production and virus replication in lymphoblastoid cells infected with different viruses. Arch Virol 63:317–320

Jankowski WJ, Davey MW, O'Malley JA, Sulkowski E, Carter WA (1975) Molecular structure of human fibroblast and leukocyte interferons: probe by lectin and hydrophobic chromatography. J Virol 16:1124–1130

Johnston MD (1979) European Patent 520

Johnston MD (1980) Enhanced production of interferon from human lymphoblastoid (Namalwa) cells pre-treated with sodium butyrate. J Gen Virol 50:191–194

Johnston MD (1981) The characteristics required for a Sendai virus preparation to induce high levels of interferon in human lymphoblastoid cells. J Gen Virol 56:175–184

Johnston MD, Fantes KH, Finter NB (1978) Factors influencing production of interferon by human lymphoblastoid cells. Adv Exp Med Biol 110:61–74

Karpetsky TP, Winchurch RA, Burman CJ, Fantes KH (1979) Ribonuclease activity of preparations of human lymphoblastoid interferon. J Gen Virol 44:241–244

Klein F, Ricketts RT, Jones WI, Dearmon IA, Temple MJ, Zoon KC, Bridgen PJ (1979) Large-scale production and concentration of human lymphoid interferon. Antimicrob Agents Chemother 15:420–427

Klein G, Vilcek J (1980) Attempts to induce interferon production by IdUrd induction and EBV superinfection in human lymphoma lines and their hybrids. J Gen Virol 46:111–117

Knight E (1976) Interferon: Purification and initial characterization from human diploid cells. Proc Natl Acad Sci USA 73:520–523

Levy WP, Shively J, Rubinstein M, Del Valle U, Pestka S (1980) Amino-terminal amino acid sequence of human leukocyte interferon. Proc Natl Acad Sci USA 17:5102–5104

Mizrahi A, Reuveny S, Traub A, Minai M (1980) Large scale production of human lymphoblastoid (Namalwa) interferon. Biotech Lett 2:267–271

Mogensen KE, Pyhala L, Torma ET, Cantell K (1974) No evidence for a carbohydrate moiety affecting the clearance of circulating human leukocyte interferon in rabbits. Acta Pathol Microbiol Scand [B] 82:305–310

Moore GE, Gerner RE, Franklin HA (1967) Culture of normal human leukocytes. JAMA 199:519–524

Moore M, Potter MR (1980) Enhancement of human natural cell – mediated cytotoxicity by interferon. Br J Cancer 41:378–387

Moore M, White WJ, Potter MR (1980) Modulation of target cell susceptibility to human natural killer cells by interferon. Int J Cancer 25:565–572

Morser J, Meager A, Colman A (1980) Enhancement of interferon mRNA levels in butyric acid-treated Namalwa cells. FEBS Lett 112:203–206

Nagata S, Mantei N, Weissmann C (1980) The structure of one of the eight or more distinct chromosomal genes for human interferon-α. Nature 287:401–408

Nilsson K, Pontén J (1975) Classification and biological nature of established human hematopoietic cell lines. Int J Cancer 15:321–341

Nilsson K, Giovanella BC, Stehlin JS, Klein G (1977) Tumorigenicity of human hematopoietic cell lines in athymic nude mice. Int J Cancer 19:337–344

Oxman MN (1973) Interferon, tumors and tumor viruses. In: Finter NB (ed) Interferons and interferon inducers. North-Holland, Amsterdam, p 391

Pestka S, Rubinstein M (1980) German Patent 2947134

Petricciani JC, Salk PL, Salk J, Noguchi PD (1982) Theoretical considerations and practical concerns regarding the use of continuous cell lines in the production of biologics. Dev Biol Standard 50:15–25

Pickering LA, Kronenberg LH, Stewart WE II (1980) Spontaneous production of human interferon. Proc Natl Acad Sci USA 77:5938–5942

Priestman TJ (1980) Initial evaluation of human lymphoblastoid interferon in patients with advanced malignant disease. Lancet 1:113–118

Pritchett R, Pedersen M, Kieff E (1976) Complexity of EBV homologous DNA in continuous lymphoblastoid cell lines. Virology 74:227–231

Pyhälä L (1978) Neutralising antibodies against human leukocyte, lymphoblastoid and fibroblast interferons elicited by immunisation with human leukocyte interferon. Acta Path Microbiol Scand Sect C 80:291–298

Rohatiner AZS, Balkwill FR, Griffin DB, Malpas JS, Lister TA (1982) A phase 1 study of human lymphoblastoid interferon administered by continuous intravenous infusion. Cancer Chemother Pharmacol 9:97–102

Rubinstein M, Rubinstein S, Familletti PC, Miller RS, Waldman AA, Pestka S (1979) Human leukocyte interferon: production, purification to homogeneity and initial characterization. Proc Natl Acad Sci USA 76:640–644
Secher DS, Burke DC (1980) A monoclonal antibody for large scale purification of human leukocyte interferon. Nature 285:446–450
Sklarz B (1967) Organic Chemistry of Periodates. Q Rev 21:3–28
Stewart WE, Desmyter J (1975) Molecular heterogeneity of human leukocyte interferon: Two populations differing in molecular weights requirements for renaturation and cross-species antiviral activity. Virology 67:68–73
Stewart WE, Lin LS, Wiranowska-Stewart M, Cantell K (1977) Elimination of size and charge heterogeneities of human leukocyte interferons by chemical cleavage. Proc Natl Acad Sci USA 74:4200–4204
Stewart WE, Wiranowska-Stewart M, Koistinen V, Cantell K (1979) Effect of glycosylation inhibitors on the production and properties of human leukocyte interferon. Virology 97:473–476
Stewart WE, Sarkar FH, Taira H, Hall A, Nagata S, Weissmann C (1980) Comparison of some biological and physicochemical properties of human leukocyte interferons produced by human leukocytes and by *E. coli*. Gene 11:181–186
Strander H, Cantell K (1966) Production of interferon by human leukocytes in vitro. Ann Med Exp Biol Fenn 44:265–273
Strander H, Cantell K (1967) Further studies on the production of interferon by human leukocytes in vitro. Ann Med Exp Biol Fenn 45:20–29
Strander H, Einhorn (1977) Effect of human leukocyte interferon on the growth of human osteosarcoma cells in tissue culture. Int J Cancer 19:468–472
Strander H, Mogensen KE, Cantell K (1975) Production of human lymphoblastoid interferon. J Clin Microbiol 1:116–117
Tovey MG, Begon-Lours J, Gresser I (1974) A method for the large scale production of potent interferon preparations. Proc Soc Exp Biol Med 146:809–815
Tovey MG, Begon-Lours J, Gresser I, Morris AG (1977) Marked enhancement of interferon production in 5-bromodeoxyuridine treated human lymphoblastoid cells. Nature 267:455–457
Volckaert-Vervliet G, Billiau A (1977) Induction of interferon in human lymphoblastoid cells by Sendai and measles virus. J Gen Virol 37:199–203
Volckaert-Vervliet G, DeClercq E, Billiau A (1980) Interaction of polyriboinosinic acid · polyribocytidylic acid with human lymphoblastoid cells. Biochem Biophys Res Comm 92:883–888
White RJ, Klein F (1980) Large-scale production of human lymphoblastoid interferon. Cancer Treatment Rev 7:245–252
Winchurch RA, Karpetsky TP, Levy CC, Cantell K (1977) Ribonuclease activity in human interferon preparations. J Virol 21:1247–1248
Yamane I, Sato T, Minamoto Y, Kudo T, Tachibana T (1982) Spontaneous and potential interferon producing cell line transformed from human cord blood and grown in a serum-free medium. In: Conference on clinical potential of interferons in viral diseases and malignant tumors, 2–4 Dec 1980. University of Tokyo Press, Tokyo
Zajac BA, Henle W, Henle G (1969) Autogenous and virus-induced interferons from lines of lymphoblastoid cells. Cancer Res 29:1467–1475
Zoon KC, Buckler CE (1977) Large-scale production of human interferon in lymphoblastoid cells. Tex Rep Biol Med 35:145–153
Zoon KC, Buckler CE, Bridgen PJ, Gurari-Rotman D (1978) Production of human lymphoblastoid interferon by Namalwa cells. J Clin Microbiol 7:44–51
Zoon KC, Smith ME, Bridgen PJ, Zur Nedden D, Anfinsen CB (1979) Purification and partial characterization of human lymphoblastoid interferon. Proc Natl Acad USA 76:5601–5605
Zoon KC, Smith ME, Bridgen PJ, Anfinsen CB, Hunkapiller MW, Hood LE (1980) Amino terminal sequence of the major component of human lymphoblastoid interferon. Science 207:527–528

CHAPTER 14

Fibroblast Interferons: Production and Characterization

V. G. EDY

A. Introduction

It is rather trite to point out that, as experiments are performed and results published, our understanding of a scientific problem usually becomes more sophisticated, and on occasion also more correct. This truism is especially applicable to the subject matter to this chapter, for much work on the production and characterisation of fibroblast interferon (IFN) was performed before it was understood that the interferon produced by fibroblast cells differed in any way other than source from the interferon produced by leukocytes, that the interferon produced by a single, apparently homogeneous, cell type could contain more than one component, that these components could differ slightly or significantly, let alone that fibroblast inferferon per se was not a homogeneous substance. This has made the interpretation of most of the early work on interferons quite difficult, as it is not evident what type, or types, of interferons were being worked with.

As the vast bulk of work on production and characterisation of interferons has been performed using material from two species, human and mouse, this review will concentrate on these types. Throughout the review, I will attempt, as far as seems sensible, to use the $\alpha, \beta, \gamma \dots$ nomenclature system for interferons (in essence, α = leukocyte, β = fibroblast, γ = immune) set up by the Ad Hoc Committee on Interferon Nomenclature, which has been very widely published (for example, STEWART et al. 1980).

In attempting a review of even a small facet of a subject that has received as much attention as interferon, the reviewer risks being overwhelmed by the sheer volume of published results. I confess to having been overwhelmed, and to have survived only by making an almost arbitrary selection of the papers to be discussed. Much of the earlier work on interferon is covered in the books of FINTER (1973) and STEWART (1979).

B. Production

I have limited this section to systems devised to produce relatively large quantities of interferon, or systems presented as having that potential.

I. Human

The large scale production of interferon from human amnion was described by FOURNIER et al. (1967), and this interferon differed from that produced by leukocytes. MERIGAN et al. (1966) discussed the use of diploid foreskin fibroblasts for interferon production.

1. Superinduction

A major advance in the production of interferons was the discovery and optimisation of the superinduction process by several groups of workers, based on an initial observation of VILCEK et al. (1969). This is a process whereby the addition of inhibitors of protein and RNA synthesis at the correct times after induction, followed by the removal of the block on translation, leads to a dramatic enhancement of interferon production. The most commonly used antimetabolites are cycloheximide, a reversible inhibitor of translation; and actinomycin D, an irreversible inhibitor of transcription. Superinduction is reviewed in more detail in Chap. 6. The application of this superinduction process to human cells (HO et al. 1972; BILLIAU et al. 1972; HAVELL and VILCEK 1972; BILLIAU et al. 1973) was a great advance in the feasibility of fibroblast-derived interferon production. This process has been used by numerous groups in the production of interferon, essentially without modification. (See Sect. B.I.2.)

Alternative Superinduction Methods

An alternative superinduction method, using the RNA synthesis inhibitor 5,6-dichloro-l-β-D-ribofuranosylbenzimidazole (DRB) was described by SEHGAL et al. (1975a, 1976a, b), and it has been reported that fibroblast cells can be repeatedly superinduced by using DRB (WIRANOWSKA-STEWART et al. 1977). (Cells treated with actinomycin D cannot be reinduced, as the block on transcription is irreversible.). A superinduction system using either neutral red or chloroquine to enhance human fibroblast interferon production 4–64-fold was also reported by SEHGAL et al. (1975b). Another group of published superinduction methods depend on the fact that ultraviolet irradiation of induced cells greatly enhances interferon production, provided that the correct dose of radiation is given at the correct time (MOZES and VILCEK 1974; LINDNER-FRIMMEL 1974; MOZES et al. 1974; MAEHARA et al. (1980).

Finally, it was shown that simply increasing the calcium concentration of the medium (from the 2 mM $CaCl_2$ present in normal medium to 12 mM) enhances the production of human fibroblast interferon as much as can be achieved with cycloheximide and actinomycin D superinduction. The calcium content had to be elevated from 12 h preinduction with poly(I)·poly(C) to harvest (20 h postinduction) (MEAGER et al. 1978). Despite the apparent simplicity of all the alternative methods discussed, none of the techniques yet appears to have found favour in large scale production work.

2. Large Scale Production Using Diploid Cells

"Large scale" and "mass" production are relatively flexibly defined terms, since the scale of interferon production has tended to expand over the past few years, and will probably continue to do so. Therefore, the selection of "large scale" methods for inclusion in this section has, of necessity, had to be rather arbitrary. Another problem in writing this section is that much of the work on large scale production is done under commercial auspices, and is therefore often kept rather secret. Although novel production methods may be hinted at in conferences, and described, usually in glowing terms, in press releases, etc., they are often not described in the scientific literature or in patents, making appraisal of the claims often difficult.

Initial production work on any sensible scale of human IFN-β was performed using cells grown either in stationary bottles or roller flasks, with a surface area available for cell growth of only a few hundreds of square centimetres in each vessel (DE SOMER et al. 1974; HAVELL and VILCEK 1974; KNIGHT 1976; EDY et al. 1978, EDY 1978; HOROSCEWICZ et al. 1978; BILLIAU et al. 1979; CARTER and HOROSCEWICZ 1980). Although such production systems are clearly successful, the costs associated with manipulating many bottles were a major factor in attempts to apply other large scale tissue culture systems to the production of IFN-β. Because diploid fibroblast cells are anchorage dependent, i.e., will not grow in suspension, work has concentrated on getting as much surface area (suitable for cell growth) as possible into a single vessel, and in keeping the ratio of surface area to volume as high as possible. LEVINE et al. (1978) give a table showing relative surface area:volume ratios for various cell culture systems, although the results are somewhat idealised.

A small vessel, containing spirally wound plastic film treated so as to be suitable for tissue culture use was described by HOUSE et al. (1972) and is commercially available. It was found suitable for the growth of cells required for interferon production (BILLIAU et al. 1979). However, because of its relatively low surface area:volume ratio, it was not economical to use in the final production stages (VAN DAMME and BILLIAU, 1981).

A second plastic devise, also commercially available, is the "Multitray" (R. SKODA 1977, unpublished work; R. SKODA, V. PAKOS, R. HORMANN and A. JOHANSSON 1977, unpublished work). Basically, this consists of a number of rectangular plastic trays, each of approximately 600 cm^2 surface area, fastened one on top of another, with communicating passages for gas and liquid. The commercially available units have ten such trays fastened together, and are about as large as can be conveniently handled by laboratory personnel. These "Multitrays" are used by Rentschler Arzneimittel GmbH, Laupheim, West Germany in its successful interferon production programme, although the cost of the device per unit growth area is quite high, and the device cannot readily be reused.

A conceptually rather similar device, where a series of glass plates is housed in a vessel containing medium, has been developed at Abbott Laboratories, North Chicago, Illinois and is apparently useful for interferon production (SCHLEICHER 1973). Other varieties of stacked plate device are being used for interferon production by other companies, although this information is largely gleaned from the popular press. Some of these devices achieve a quite considerable degreee of sophistication, for example, the stacked plate vessel developed by the Searle Company, High Wycombe, England. This would appear to consist of a series of stainless steel plates contained within a sealed vessel of some hundreds of litres capacity. The claimed advantages of the system as compared with roller bottles are that risks of bacterial contamination are much less, as vastly fewer vessels need to be handled to make a given volume of interferon, and an increased surface area per unit volume of medium makes for greater efficiency of fibroblast production.

Another group of methods of large scale tissue culture, that have been used in IFN-β production, depend on the breaking up of the required surface area into myriad small particles, placed in a vessel through which flows the necessary growth medium. The original concept appears to be that of MCCOY et al. (1962), whilst a system using glass beads was developed for the growth of normal diploid cells by WOHLER et al. (1972).

A system for the large scale growth of human fibroblasts on glass beads has been described by a group of workers from the Beecham Company, Epsom, England, and some results on IFN-β production have been given (BURBIDGE 1979, 1980; ROBINSON et al. 1980). The interferon induction scheme used (BURBIDGE 1979) did not include superinduction, and therefore it is not easy to compare the interferon yields found with those claimed by others.

An alternative version of this basic idea has been developed by MERK 1982, who uses a large stainless steel tank packed with 6 × 6 mm stainless steel helices. A 100-l-tank packed in this way apparently suffices to provide a growth area of approximately 80 m^2, which in turn when fully confluent with cells, yields 1,250 IU/cm^2, for a mean total yield of 10^9 IU IFN-β per run.

To get even more surface area into a given volume of medium, one must switch to so-called microcarrier systems, in which the growth substrate is divided into even smaller particles, which are maintained in suspension in the tissue culture medium. The original work on microcarriers was performed by VAN WEZEL (1967), using positively charged dextran beads prepared by coating Pharmacia diethylaminoethyl (DEAE)-Sephadex A-50 with a small amount of nitrocellulose. Although the system was relatively succesful, problems were experienced with long lag times, loss of inoculum, and undefined "toxicity". (VAN HEMERT et al. 1969; VAN WEZEL 1973; HORNG and MCLIMANS 1975; SPIER and WHITESIDE 1976; LEVINE et al. 1977 a, b). Using beads prepared according to VAN WEZEL (1967, 1973), A. L. VAN WEZEL and V. G. EDY (unpublished work) were unable to obtain reproducibly good growth of human diploid fibroblasts, and were unable to get the cells to make significant amounts of IFN-β.

A major advance in making the microcarrier system more generally usable was the discovery that the key to the apparent toxicity of the dextran beads lay in their excessive charge density. By controlling reaction conditions, LEVINE et al. (1977a, b) were able to produce beads with a positive charge of about 2 mequiv./g, about one-half the charge on commercially available DEAE-dextran beads. Using these microcarrier beads, HEL-299 human diploid fibroblasts could be grown to relatively high densities (3–4 × 10^6 cells/ml) without apparent toxicity problems. More extensive studies on the parameters of successful microcarrier culture have been published (LEVINE et al. 1979; THILLY and LEVINE 1979; HIRTENSTEIN et al. 1980; CLARK et al. 1980; NIELSEN and JOHANSSON 1980).

The application of the microcarrier system to human IFN-β production was first published by GIARD et al. (1979), where the poly(I)·poly(C)–cycloheximide–actinomycin D superinduction schedule described by HAVELL and VILCEK (1972) was applied to a variety of diploid fibroblast lines. Using the FS-4 line, yields of around 10^4 U/ml, or 5 U per 1,000 cells, were attained, about the same yield per cell as the authors were able to obtain with roller bottle cultures. Refinements of the technique, adjusting time of exposure and dose of inducer and of the antimetabolites increased the yields to more than 2 × 10^4 U/ml, and to about 20 U per 1,000 cells (GIARD and FLEISCHAKER 1980). The large scale application of this technique to the production of human IFN-β, on a scale of up to 48 l per run, and with peak yields of IFN-β in excess of 20,000 IU/ml, has been recently reported (EDY et al. 1982).

3. Cell Substrates for Human Interferon Production

For regulatory reasons amongst others, the bulk of the work on human IFN-β production has been performed using a variety of diploid lines, usually screened for interferon-producing capacity. For examples, see VILCEK et al. (1978), HOROSCEWICZ et al. (1979), and MEAGER et al. (1979). Such diploid lines are somewhat difficult to grow, grow relatively slowly, will only tolerate low split ratios, and, of course, are of finite life span. Therefore, there has been some impetus to find a transformed, immortal cell line capable of producing large amounts of human IFN-β. Two groups of workers have published results on nondiploid lines producing relatively large quantities of interferon. The MG-63 line, derived from an osteosarcoma, was found to produce somewhat more IFN-β than normal diploid fibroblasts, was very easy to cultivate and grew rapidly to high densities (BILLIAU et al. 1977). When superinduced, highly acceptable yields of interferon were produced, of the order of 10^5 IU/ml. TAN and his co-workers have derived a clone from an SV40-transformed ethylmethane sulphonate-treated human fibroblast, called C-10 (BERTHOLD et al. 1978), although details of the cell line do not seem to have been published. Yields of interferon were up to 3×10^5 IU/ml.

4. Production of Fibroblast Interferons in Microbial Cells

The "genetic engineering" approach to the production of interferons has generated considerable interest: scientific, commercial and public. This subject is reviewed in Chap. 7. Suffice it to say, at this juncture, that published yields of human IFN-β have not been as great as those achieved for IFN-α.

II. Mouse

The production of mouse fibroblast interferon has been somewhat less well studied than that of human IFN-β, perhaps because the commercial, as opposed to scientific, motivation was lacking. Also, relatively simple systems, such as will be described in the following discussion, give relatively large amounts of IFN, sufficient for characterisation studies or to treat some experimental condition in mice.

To write just about the production of mouse IFN-β is complicated by the fact that, in contrast to the human situation where human fibroblasts produce mostly IFN-β with only a trace of IFN-α under normal conditions of induction with polynucleotides (HAVELL et al. 1978), many mouse cell systems produce mixtures of interferons. This subject is dealt with in Sect. C.I.2. Therefore, in writing about production, and characterisation, of mouse IFN-β, some problems of interpretation of results can be expected, as it is often not clear what proportion of crude interferon is IFN-α and what IFN-β.

1. Virus-Induced Systems

A relatively simple system for the production of relatively large amounts of mouse interferon was described by STEWART et al. (1971). L929 cells grown in roller bottles were primed (pretreated with a small amount of mouse interferon) and then induced with the MM strain of encephalomyocarditis virus. This resulted in crude interferon preparations with a tritre of around 10^4 IU/ml. Because of the ease of growth of L-cells and the large amount of interferon produced in response to such a simple induction methodology, this method and variations of it, most notably using Newcastle disease virus (NDV), have been reported by numerous groups of authors. The most dramatic mouse interferon yields, however, were reported by Taira et al. (1980 b) using Ehrlich ascites tumour cells grown in roller bottles. Using NDV as the inducer and refeeding the cultures with medium containing a fraction of foetal bovine serum and theophylline, the authors were able to achieve interferon yields of $1–2 \times 10^6$ IU/ml, with a specific activity between 1 and 1.5×10^6 IU per milligram protein.

2. Large Scale Production Systems

A multisurface cell culture device was described by Knight (1977) for L-cell interferon production, consisting of five concentric glass cylinders inside a roller bottle. This resulted in a surface area available for growth approximately 9-fold greater than that of a normal roller bottle. Interferon yields were approximately 20-fold greater than had been found with normal roller bottles; no explanation of this 2-fold increase in efficiency of production was given.

Perhaps because it is relatively easy to produce L-cell derivatives that will grow in suspension culture, little other work has been published on large surface area systems for mouse interferon production. Reuveny et al. (1980) describe the production of interferon from L929 cells grown on DEAE-dextran and DEAE-cellulose microcarriers, with yields of around 4×10^4 IU/ml following induction with Sendai virus.

Pirt and his co-workers (Mogensen et al. 1972; Tovey et al. 1973) studied the production of L-cell interferon in serum-free suspension culture, using poly(I)·–poly(C) and soluble DEAE-dextran as the induction system. Perhaps because of the induction method chosen, or because of the use of serum-free medium for cell culture, yields were around 1,000 IU/ml, only about 10% of the yield achievable in roller bottles. However, by selecting a high yielding strain of L-cells capable of growing in suspension, and by using NDV as the inducer, Sano et al. (1974) were able to obtain very good yields of interferon in excess of 30,000 U/ml, on a scale of up to 20 l, and with a specific activity of $\geqq 10^5$ U per milligram protein. The key to obtaining high yields in this system was found to be removal of the inducer virus after induction of interferon synthesis had occurred.

3. Superinduction

The superinduction of mouse interferon production seems to have been reported by only two groups. Production of 50,000–100,000 IU/ml from a cell line MO57/2 following priming, induction with poly(I)·poly(C) and superinduction with cycloheximide and actinomycin D has been described (Edy et al. 1973). A cell line, C243-3, was introduced by Oie et al. (1972) which yielded, in monolayer culture, up to ten times more interferon per ml culture supernatant than L-cells are generally reported to produce. Using NDV as the inducer, and superinducing with cycloheximide and actinomycin D, yields greater than 4×10^5 IU/ml with a specific activity greater than 10^6 IU per milligram protein have been reported (TOVEY et al. 1974). The C243-3 cells were grown in suspension in relatively large volumes.

4. Cloning of Mouse Interferon

At the date of writing, no report of the successful cloning of a mouse interferon gene, nor of its expression in a prokaryote, has appeared.

C. Characterization of Fibroblast Interferons

Work on the characterisation of interferons was long impeded by the lack of purified interferons. Therefore, much work was performed on crude or partially purified interferon preparations, which, as will be described in Sect. C.III may have contained a heterogeneous mixture of various IFN-α and IFN-β species. Even initial work on highly purified interferons is somewhat suspect, for the yield on purification with early preparations was low, which may have meant that a nonrepresentative fraction of the original interferon was studied. Work on the more recent purification methods has given much better recoveries, several tens of percent rather than a few percent, so one may be more certain as to the applicability of the results. The characterisation of interferons has been succinctly reviewed by KNIGHT (1980).

Fibroblast interferons do not seem to have been clearly distinguished from other types of interferons until 1975, when it was shown that interferon preparations from human fibroblasts and leukocytes were largely not neutralised by antisera raised against interferon from the other source. (HAVELL et al. 1975a). This distinction had been shown earlier, by the different stability patterns of fibroblast- and leukocyte-derived interferons, although the implications of the results were not fully recognised (EDY et al. 1974). Detergent denaturation conditions were also shown to differ for fibroblast- and leukocyte-derived interferons (STEWART et al. 1975). The differences between human IFN-α and IFN-β has been recently reviewed by HAYES (1981). The demonstration that mouse interferon types could likewise by divided into leukocyte-derived/related and fibroblast-derived/related (the present-day α and β) seems to have been first fully described by YAMAMOTO and KAWADE (1980) although the assumption that mouse IFN-α and IFN-β existed was made earlier.

I. Molecular Weight Studies

1. Human Fibroblast Interferon

The molecular weight of IFN-β has been measured by several groups of workers, who have generally claimed that their preparations contain a single peak of activity with a molecular weight in the range of 20–25,000 (see, for example, REYNOLDS and PITHA 1975; KNIGHT 1976; TAN et al. 1979), although earlier workers had claimed molecular weights ranging from 20,000 to more than 100,000 (reviewed by FANTES

1973). In the light of this apparent heterogeneity, the finding of CARTER (1971) that human fibroblast interferon behaved as if 96,000 and 24,000 daltons components were aggregates of a 12,000 daltons monomer is interesting. Although many workers were unable to reproduce these results, and the subunit hypothesis involved to explain them was dubbed "imaginative" (STEWART 1979), FRIESEN etal. (1981) were able to detect a low molecular weight component in some of their preparations of human IFN-β. Although the great bulk of their interferon behaved as if it had a molecular weight of 20–21,000, small amounts of interferons were found with molecular weights of 10,000, 17–18,000, 35,000, and 40,000. FRIESEN et al. (1981) claim that the 17,000–18,000 daltons component is probably related to the 20–21,000 daltons component, differing in degree of glycosylation, and that the 35,000 and 40,000 daltons components are dimers. Occasionally they even saw tetramers, with an apparent molecular weight of 80,000. However, amino acid analysis of the 10,000 daltons component suffices to exclude the possibility that it is a fragment of one of the longer species. The homogeneity/heterogeneity controversy about human fibroblast interferon is reviewed in Sect. C.III. Molecular weight studies are also complicated further by the fact that human IFN-β (and mouse interferons also) are most probably glycoproteins, with perhaps varying degrees of glycosylation. Interferons as gylcoproteins are discussed in Sect. C.IV.

2. Mouse Interferons

Polyacrylamide gel electrophoresis (PAGE) of L-cell interferon showed at least two components, with molecular weights variously estimated as 20,000 and 32,000 (KNIGHT 1975) or 25,000 and 40,000 (YAMAMOTO and KAWADE 1976). The different components were shown to differ in stability and in cross-species activity (STEWART et al. 1977), and although they appear to share some common structure (IWAKURA et al. 1978), they are antigenically different (YAMAMOTO and KAWADE 1980), with the lower molecular weight species being identified as mouse IFN-α, and the higher molecular weight species as IFN-β (YAMAMOTO 1981). Finally, LENGYEL's group have shown mouse interferon from Ehrlich ascites tumour cells to consist of three components – molecular weights 20,000 (A), 26,000–33,000 (B), and 35,000–40,000 (C), two of which (A and B) have NH_2 terminal amino acid sequences which show some homology with that of human IFN-β, whilst the third (C) shows a high degree of homology with the NH_2 terminal amino acid sequence of a human IFN-α (TAIRA et al. 1980 a).

II. Stability

The physical lability of human fibroblast interferon preparations attracted early interest, as it seemed clear that if fibroblast-derived interferons were to be purified and tested in the clinic, their lack of stability had to be overcome. DE SOMER's group reported that crude fibroblast interferon, which was inactivated by shaking, could be protected by nonionic detergents (DE SOMER et al. 1974) or by low pH (EDY et al. 1974). The cause of inactivation on shaking was shown to be shear forces (CARTWRIGHT et al. 1977 a) and certain thiol reagents, most notably DL-thioctic acid, were found to stabilise IFN-β against this shear inactivation, although they increased the lability of IFN-β on heating (CARTWRIGHT et al. 1977 b). JARIWALLA et al. (1975, 1977) studied the thermal inactivation of mouse L-cell interferon, and used the data to generate a model of different molecular states of interferon, which of course, is subject to the caveat that their work was based on the assumption of the homogeneity of the material under study. The stabilisation of various mouse and human interferon preparations against thermal inactivation by the detergent sodium dodecylsulphate (SDS) was reported in a series of papers by STEWART (for example, STEWART 1974; STEWART et al. 1974, 1975). Both human fibroblast and mouse L-cell interferon had to be treated with SDS in the presence of urea and mercaptoethanol if activity was to be retained. This discovery has proved useful not in improving the stability of interferon preparations, but in allowing accurate molecular weight determinations by SDS PAGE. The mechanism of action of SDS stabilisation has been discussed by BRAUDE and DE CLERCQ (1979). The most impressive stabilisation system reported to date, however, is that of SEDMAK and GROSSBERG (1981), who showed that rare earth salts of the lanthanide series were highly effective in stabilising both human and mouse IFN-α and IFN-β against both shear and thermal inactivation. Under some conditions, they also observed significant enhancement of the activity of interferons when treated with lanthanides. The exact mechanism of these effects remains unknown.

III. Heterogeneity of Interferons

1. Human Fibroblast Interferon

Isoelectric focussing experiments on crude preparations of human fibroblast (and mouse L929 cell) interferons seemed to show that the materials were quite heterogeneous (STANCEK et al. 1970). However, because many experiments involving SDS PAGE of human IFN-β showed only a single band of activity (see STEWART 1979, for references), it was claimed that IFN-β was a single substance. Only a single NH_2 terminal amino acid sequence was detected (KNIGHT et al. 1980, STEIN et al. 1980), and studies on the cloning of IFN-β gene sequences also suggested that IFN-β was a homogeneous product (HOUGHTON et al. 1981; TAVERNIER et al. 1981) in contradistinction to human IFN-α, where numerous (eight or more) different, but closely related genes have been found (NAGATA et al. 1980). Thus, although only one species of IFN-β has been fully purified and sequenced, there is some evidence that a second or further species might exist.

When crude preparations of human IFN-β were inactivated by shaking or treatment with guanidine hydrochloride, a stable fraction of activity remained. This stable fraction was neutralised by antiserum to fibroblast interferon, but not to leucocyte interferon, and was claimed to be a second IFN-β component (EDY et al. 1977b). By thiol exchange chromatography, SENUSSI et al. (1979) were able to resolve IFN-β preparations into a stable and a labile component, stability being measured as shear sensitivity. More elegant experiments by SEHGAL and his co-workers have demonstrated the existence of two different size classes of messenger RNA coding for human IFN-β. They refer to the translation products of these two mRNAs as IFN-β_1 and IFN-β_2 (SEHGAL and SAGAR 1980; SOREQ et al. 1981). WEISSENBACH et al. (1980) demonstrated that the IFN-β_1 messenger was present in the greater amount, and was smaller than the IFN-β_2 mRNA. When these messengers were translated in vitro, the β_1 product had a molecular weight of 20,000, the β_2 23,000–

26,000. An antiserum raised against a single completely purified human IFN-β_1 was found to be effective at neutralising IFN-β_1, less effective with IFN-β_2. The β_2 product does not contain the NH_2 terminal amino acid sequence described by KNIGHT et al. (1980), although a region of homology was detected between the β_1 and β_2 sequences, lying in an area of the polypeptide that is highly conserved when comparing IFN-β_1 with the IFN-α species. Two IFN-β mRNAs, differing in size, have also been isolated from Sendai virus-induced human lymphoblastoid cells (SAGAR et al. 1981). So far, no mRNA coding for the 10,000 daltons species of human IFN-β described by FRIESEN et al. (1981) has been reported. Most recently, work with monoclonal antibodies is also compatible with the suggestion that two forms of IFN-β exist (HOCHKEPPEL et al. 1981).

2. Mouse Interferons

The heterogeneity of mouse interferons is discussed largely in Sect. C.I.2. Additional evidence for the heterogeneity of mouse IFN-β comes from the work of TAIRA et al. (1980 a) who were able to demonstrate two sizes of interferon sharing a common NH_2 terminal amino acid sequence, and from that a SAGAR et al. (1981), who showed that NDV-induced L929 made two size classes of interferon mRNA, and that an α and β message were present in each size class. In this regard it is interesting that whilst most workers have demonstrated 2–3 separate mouse interferons, α and β, made in a single system, KNIGHT (1975) found 10–11. KNIGHT (1980) suggests that this may be due to his studies being performed on interferon induced with MM virus; most other workers studying interferon induced by NDV infection.

IV. Glycosylation of Interferons

1. Human Fibroblast Interferon

A variable degree of glycosylation was often invoked to explain the heterogeneity of various interferon preparations when examined by a variety of means (for references see STEWART 1979). The evidence that interferons were glycoprotein in nature was reviewed by WEIL and DORNER (1973). D-Glucosamine and 2-deoxyglucose, which are both inhibitors of the normal glycosylation of glycoproteins, were shown to reduce the production of interferon by diploid human fibroblasts dramatically when induced with poly(I)·poly(C) (HAVELL et al. 1975 b). These authors point out, however, that although the reduced production of interferon could result from the interference with the proper glycosylation of the interferon polypeptide, it is also possible that some secondary side effect caused the reduction in yield. HAVELL et al. (1977) demonstrated that partially inhibitory concentrations of 2-deoxyglucose or glucosamine cause the IFN-β produced to be resolvable into two size classes, one with a molecular weight of about 20,000 (normal, glycosylated interferon) and the other around 16,000 (possibly the nonglycosylated polypeptide).

The carbohydrate component of human IFN-β was directly demonstrated by KNIGHT (1976), who showed that purified IFN-β in polyacrylamide gels could be stained with periodic acid–Schiff reagents. The role of the carbohydrate is a matter of some debate, and currently remains unknown. That nonglycosylated interferon, such as is made by genetically engineered strains of *Escherichia* coli, is active in vitro is self-evident, as its detection depends on such activity. How such nonglycosylated interferon will behave in vivo is a matter of considerable interest.

2. Mouse Interferons

Like human IFN-β, interferons made in mouse fibroblasts are perceived to be glycoproteins. As for human interferon, KNIGHT (1975) demonstrated by periodic acid–Schiff staining the carbohydrate content of at least 6 of the 10–11 components he was able to resolve in his MM virus-induced L9–29 cell interferon preparation. Studies with the antibiotic, tunicamycin (an inhibitor of glycosylation) have shown that inhibition of glycosylation results in the production of two components, both with a molecular weight ~17,000 (FUJISAWA et al. 1978; HAVELL and CARTER 1981).

V. Purification Studies

Much of the work on interferon characterisation came as a spin-off of work on purification. The most striking example of this is in hydrophobic affinity chromatography, which has shown that IFN-β will bind hydrophobically to, and can be eluted from, albumin–agarose (HUANG et al. 1974), concanavalin A–agarose (DAVEY et al. 1974), ω-carboxypentyl–agarose (DAVEY et al. 1975), hydrophobic amino acids and dipeptides immobilised on agarose (SULKOWSKI et al. 1976) octyl–agarose (DAVEY et al. 1976) and Cibacron Blue F3GA (JANKOWSKI et al. 1976; CESARIO et al. 1976; KNIGHT et al. 1980). This is not an exhaustive list of all the ligands that have been tested, almost all with good results.

Other purification methods are controlled pore glass adsorption chromatography (EDY et al. 1976) and metal chelate affinity chromatography (EDY et al. 1977a; CHADHA et al. 1979). Recently, it has been claimed that a combination of these two methods gives highly purified interferon with good recovery (HEINE et al. 1980, 1981). Similarly, good purification and recovery was obtained by KNIGHT et al. (1980) using Blue Sepharose (Cibacron Blue F3GA linked to agarose). Many of the methods developed for the purification of human fibroblast interferon have also been used, with slight modification, for mouse interferons. Mouse interferons have also been shown to have a high affinity for, and to be well purified by, adsorption chromatography on, certain homopolynucleotides (DE MAEYER-GUIGNARD et al. 1977). This is by no means a complete listing of the purification methods used for fibroblast interferons; indeed it occasionally seems as if each group of workers has its own method. The purification of fibroblast interferons has recently been reviewed by KNIGHT (1980).

VI. Amino Acid Composition and Sequence

1. Human Fibroblast Interferon

With the advent of apparently completely purified interferons, amino acid composition data were rapidly generated and published (TAN et al. 1979; KNIGHT et al. 1980; FRIESEN et al. 1981). The last two sets of data are compatible, but there appear to be differences with the data of TAN and his colleagues. This may, of course, reflect the different sources that these groups had for their IFN-β. The NH_2 terminal amino acid sequence of IFN-β was published by KNIGHT et al. (1980) and KNIGHT and HUNKAPILLER (1981), for the first 13 and 21 amino acids respectively. It is rather sad that this extremely difficult and laborious work has been overshadowed by the sudden blossoming of genetic engineering techniques. The cloning of DNA coding for human IFN-β has been reported by several groups, and the sequence of parts (HOUGHTON et al. 1980; TANAGUCHI et al. 1980 a), and the whole (TANAGUCHI et al. 1980 b), of this nucleic acid have been published. The predicted amino acid sequences agree perfectly with the actual sequence data so far published.

2. Mouse Interferons

The first amino acid compositions for mouse interferons were published on the three interferons made by Ehrlich ascites tumour cells (CABRER et al. 1979). Not suprisingly, the composition data differ from those published for human IFN-β. The NH_2 terminal amino acid sequences for these three interferons have now been determined (TAIRA et al. 1980) and, as mentioned in Sect. C.I.2, two show slight homology with human IFN-β whilst the third shows a quite high degree of similarity to human IFN-α. In this regard, it is interesting that mouse L929 cell interferon has been shown to possess a component antigenically related to human IFN-α (HAVELL 1979), and it has been suggested that human IFN-α, which has a reasonable degree of activity on mouse cells, resembles mouse interferon in its fit with its receptor (BRAUDE et al. 1980).

VII. Conclusions

As interferon preparations progressed from crude "soups" lightly contaminated with traces of interferon, to completely purified, electrophoretically homogeneous material, we have come to know more and more about less and less. "Pure" interferon has been sincerely, but mistakenly claimed in the past on many occasions, a phenomenon which is partially understandable in the light of the very high activity of the interferon molecule. However, the polypeptides now being produced by conventional techniques as well as via recombinant DNA methodology are almost certainly the "real thing", so that we will not have to learn yet more about even less.

References

Berthold W, Tan C, Tan YH (1978) Purification and in vitro labelling of interferon from a human fibroblastoid cell line. J Biol Chem 253:5206–5212

Billiau A, Joniau M, De Somer P (1972) Production of crude human interferon with high specific activity. Proc Soc Exp Biol Med 140:485–491

Billiau A, Joniau M, De Somer P (1973) Mass production of human interferon in diploid cells stimulated by poly I.C. J Gen Virol 19:1–8

Billiau A, Edy VG, Heremans H, Van Damme J, Desmyter J, Georgiades JA, De Somer P (1977) Human interferon: mass production in a newly established cell line, MG-63. Antimicrob Agents Chemother 12:11–15

Billiau A, Van Damme J, Van Leuven F, Edy VG, De Ley M, Cassiman JJ, Vanden Berghe M, De Somer P (1979) Human fibroblast interferon for clinical trials: Production, partial purification and characterisation. Antimicrob Agents Chemother 16:49–55

Braude IA, De Clercq E (1979) Mechanism of interaction of sodium dodecyl sulfate with mouse interferon. J Biol Chem 254:7758–7764

Braude IA, De Clercq E, Zhang ZX, Edy VG, De Somer P (1980) Neutralisation of interferon activity in homologous and heterologous cells with homologous and heterologous antibody. Proc Soc Exp Biol Med 165:161–166

Burbidge C (1979) Cell culture method. U.S. Patent No. 4, 144, 126

Burbidge C (1980) The mass culture of human diploid fibroblasts in packed beds of glass beads. Dev Biol Stand 46:169–172

Cabrer B, Taira H, Broeze RJ, Kempe TD, Williams K, Slattery E, Konigsberg WM, Lengyel P (1979) Structural characteristics of interferons from mouse Ehrlich ascites tumor cells. J Biol Chem 254:3681–3684

Carter WA (1971) Purification of mouse and human interferons: Detection of subunit structure. Prep Biochem 1:55–75

Carter WA, Horoscewicz JS (1980) Production, purification and clinical application of human fibroblast interferon. Pharmacol Ther 8:359–377

Cartwright T, Senussi O, Grady MD (1977a) The mechanism of the inactivation of human fibroblast interferon by mechanical stress. J Gen Virol 36:317–321

Cartwright T, Senussi O, Grady MD (1977b) Reagents which inhibit disulphide bond formation stabilise human fibroblast interferon. J Gen Virol 36:323–327

Cesario TC, Schryer P, Mandel A, Tilles JG (1976) Affinity of human fibroblast interferon for blue dextran. Proc Soc Exp Biol Med 153:486–489

Chadha KC, Grob PM, Mikulski AJ, Davis LR, Sulkowski E (1979) Copper chelate affinity chromatography of human fibroblast and leukocyte interferons. J Gen Virol 43:701–706

Clark J, Hirtenstein M, Gebb C (1980) Critical parameters in the microcarrier culture of animal cells. Dev Biol Stand 46:117–124

Davey MW, Huang JW, Sulkowski E, Carter WA (1974) Hydrophobic interaction of human interferon with concanavalin A-agarose. J Biol Chem 249:6354–6355

Davey MW, Huang JW, Sulkowski E, Carter WA (1975) Hydrophobic binding sites on human interferon. J Biol Chem 250:348–349

Davey MW, Sulkowski E, Carter WA (1976) Hydrophobic interaction of human, mouse, and rabbit interferons with immobilized hydrocarbons. J Biol Chem 251:7620–7625

De Maeyer-Guignard J, Thang MN, De Maeyer E (1977) Binding of mouse interferon to polynucleotides. Proc Natl Acad Sci USA 74:378–379

De Somer P, Joniau M, Edy VG, Billiau A (1974) Mass production of human interferon in diploid cells. In: Waymouth C (ed) The production and use of interferon for the treatment and prevention of human virus infections. Tissue Culture Association, Rockville, p 39

Edy VG (1978) Large-scale production of human interferon in monolayer cell cultures. Tex Rep Biol Med 37:132–137

Edy VG, Billiau A, De Somer P (1973) Enhancement of interferon production in a mouse cell line, a high-yielding source of mouse interferon. Appl Microbiol 26:434–436

Edy VG, Billiau A, Joniau M, De Somer P (1974) Stabilisation of mouse and human interferons by acid pH against inactivation due to shaking and guanidine hydrochloride. Proc Soc Exp Biol Med 146:249–253

Edy VG, Braude IA, De Clercq E, Billiau A, De Somer P (1976) Purification of interferon by adsorption chromatography on controlled pore glass. J Gen Virol 33:517–521

Edy VG, Billiau A, De Somer P (1977a) Purification of human fibroblast interferon by zinc chelate affinity chromatography. J Biol Chem 252:5934–5935

Edy VG, Desmyter J, Billiau A, De Somer P (1977b) Stable and unstable forms of human fibroblast interferon. Infect Immun 16:445–448

Edy VG, Van Damme J, Billiau A, De Somer P (1978) Human interferon: Large-scale production in embryo fibroblast cultures. Adv Exp Med Biol 110:55–60

Edy VG, Augenstein DC, Edwards CR, Cruttenden VF, Lubiniecki AS (1982) Large-scale tissue culture for human IFN-β production. Tex Rep Biol Med 41:169–174

Fantes KH (1973) Purification and physico-chemical properties of interferons. In: Finter NB (ed) Interferons and interferons inducers, 2nd edn. North-Holland, Amsterdam, p 171

Finter NB (ed) (1973) Interferons and interferon inducers, 2nd edn. North-Holland, Amsterdam
Fournier F, Falcoff E, Chany C (1967) Demonstration, mass production and characterisation of a heavy molecular weight human interferon. J Immunol 99:1036–1041
Friesen HJ, Stein S, Evinger M, Familletti PC, Moschera J, Meienhofer J, Shively J, Pestka S (1981) Purification and molecular characterisation of human fibroblast interferon. Arch Biochem Biophys 206:432–450
Fujisawa J, Iwakura Y, Kawade Y (1978) Nonglycosylated mouse L-cell interferon produced by the action of tunicamycin. J Biol Chem 253:8677–8679
Giard DJ, Fleischaker RJ (1980) Examination of parameters affecting human interferon production with microcarrier-grown fibroblast cells, Antimicrob Agents Chemother 18:130–136
Giard DJ, Loeb DH, Thilly WG, Wang DIC, Levine DW (1979) Human interferon production with diploid fibroblast cells grown on microcarriers. Biotechnol Bioeng 21:433–442
Havell EA (1979) Isolation of a subspecies of murine interferon antigenically related to human leukocyte interferon. Virology 92:324–330
Havell EA, Carter WA (1981) Effects of tunicamycin on the physical properties and antiviral activities of murine L cell interferon. Virology 108:80–86
Havell EA, Vilcek J (1972) Production of high-titered interferon in cultures of human diploid cells. Antimicrob Agents Chemother 2:476–484
Havell EA, Vilcek J (1974) Mass production and some characteristics of human interferon from diploid cells. In: Weymouth C (ed) The production and use of interferon for the treatment and prevention of human virus infections. Tissue Culture Association, Rockville, p 47
Havell EA, Bergman B, Ogburn CA, Berg K, Paucker K, Vilcek J (1975a) Two antigenically distinct species of human interferon. Proc Natl Acad Sci USA 72:2185–2190
Havell EA, Vilcek J, Falcoff E, Berman B (1975b) Suppression of human interferon production by inhibitors of glycosylation. Virology 63:475–483
Havell EA, Yamazaki S, Vilcek J (1977) Altered molecular species of human interferon produced in the presence of inhibitors of glycosylation. J Biol Chem 252:4425–4427
Havell EA, Hayes TG, Vilcek J (1978) Synthesis of two distinct interferons by human fibroblasts. Virology 89:330–334
Hayes TG (1981) Differences between human α (leukocyte) and β (fibroblast) interferons. Arch Virol 67:267–281
Heine JW, De Ley M, Van Damme J, Billiau A, De Somer P (1980) Human fibroblast interferon purified to homogeneity by a two step procedure. Ann NY Acad Sci 350:364–373
Heine JW, Van Damme J, De Ley M, Billiau A, De Somer P (1981) Purification of human fibroblast interferon by zinc chelate chromatography. J Gen Virol 54:47–56
Hirtenstein M, Clark J, Lindgren G, Vretblad P (1980) Microcarriers for animal cell culture: A brief review of theory and practice. Dev Biol Stand 46:109–116
Ho M, Tan YH, Armstrong JA (1972) Accentuation of production of human interferon by metabolic inhibitors. Proc Soc Exp Biol Med 139:259–262
Hochkeppel HK, Menge U, Collins J (1981) Monoclonal antibodies against human fibroblast interferon. Nature 291:500–501
Horng C, McLimans W (1975) Primary suspension culture of calf anterior pituitary cells on a microcarrier surface. Biotechnol Bioeng 17:713–732
Horoscewicz JS, Leong SS, Itio M, Di Berardino L, Carter WA (1978) Aging in vitro and large-scale interferon production by 15 new strains of human diploid fibroblasts. Infect Immun 19:720–726
Houghton M, Stewart AG, Doel SM, Emtage JS, Eaton MAW, Smith JC, Patel TP, Lewis HM, Porter AG, Birch JR, Cartwright T, Carey NH (1980) The amino terminal sequence of human fibroblast interferon as deduced from reverse transcripts obtained using synthetic oligonucleotide primers. Nucleic Acids Res 8:1913–1931
Houghton M, Jackson IJ, Porter AG, Doel SM, Catlin GH, Barber C, Carey NH (1981) The absence of introns within a human fibroblast interferon gene. Nucleic Acids Res 9:247–277

House W, Shearer M, Maroudas NG (1972) Method for bulk culture of animal cells on plastic films. Exp Cell Res 71:293–298

Huang JW, Davey MW, Hejna CJ, von Muenchhausen W, Sulkowski E, Carter WA (1974) Selective binding of human interferon to albumin immobilised on agarose. J Biol Chem 249:4665–4667

Iwakura T, Yonehara S, Kawade T (1978) Presence of a common structure in the two molecular species of mouse L cell interferon. Biochem Biophys Res Commun 84:557–563

Jankowski WJ, von Muenchhausen W, Sulkowski E, Carter WA (1976) Binding of human interferons to immobilised Cibacron blue F3GA: The nature of molecular interaction. Biochemistry 15:5182–5187

Jariwalla R, Grossberg SE, Sedmak JJ (1975) The influence of physicochemical factors on the thermal inactivation of murine interferon. Arch Virol 49:261–272

Jariwalla R, Grossberg SE, Sedmak JJ (1977) Effect of chaotropic salts and protein denaturants on the thermal stability of mouse fibroblast interferon. J Gen Virol 35:45–52

Knight E (1975) Heterogeneity of purified mouse interferons. J Biol Chem 250:4139–4141

Knight E (1976) Interferon: Purification and initial characterization from human diploid cells. Proc Natl Acad Sci USA 73:520–523

Knight E (1977) A multisurface glass roller bottle for growth of animal cells in culture. Appl Environ Microbiol 33:666–670

Knight E (1980) Purification and characterization of interferons. In: Gresser I (ed) Interferon 1980. Academic, London, p 1

Knight E, Hunkapiller MW (1981) Characterization of radioactive human fibroblast-derived beta interferon synthesized in vivo: J Interferon Res 1:297–303

Knight E, Hunkapiller MW, Korant BD, Handy RWF, Hood LE (1980) Human fibroblast interferon: Amino acid analysis and amino terminal amino acid sequence. Science 207:525–526

Levine DW, Wang DIC, Thilly WG (1977a) Optimising parameters for growth of anchorage dependent mammalian cells in microcarrier culture. In: Acton RT, Lynn JD (eds) Cell culture and its application. Academic, New York, p 191

Levine DW, Wong JS, Wang DIC, Thilly WG (1977b) Microcarrier cell culture: New methods for research-scale application. Somatic Cell Genet 3:149–155

Levine DW, Thilly WG, Wang DIC (1978) New microcarriers for the large scale production of anchorage-dependent mammalian cells. Adv Exp Med Biol 110:15–23

Levine DW, Wang DIC, Thilly WG (1979) Optimisation of growth surface parameters in microcarrier cell culture. Biotechnol Bioeng 2:821–825

Lindner-Frimmel SJ (1974) Enhanced production of human interferon by U.V. irradiated cells. J Gen Virol 25:147–150

Maehara N, Komatsu H, Shimoda K, Makino S, Nagano T, Matumoto M (1980) Enhanced production of virus-inhibiting factor (interferon) in human diploid cells by ultraviolet irradiation and temperature shift-down after stimulation with Newcastle disease virus. Microbiol Immunol 24:907–914

McCoy TA, Whittle W, Conway E (1962) A glass helix perfusion chamber for massive growth of cells in vitro. Proc Soc Exp Biol Med 109:235–237

Meager A, Graves ME, Bradshaw TK (1978) Stimulation of interferon yields from cultured human cells by calcium salts. FEBS Lett 87:303–307

Meager A, Graves ME, Shuttleworth J, Zucker N (1979) Interferon production: Variations in yields from human cell lines. Infect Immun 25:658–663

Merigan TC, Gregory DF, Petralli JO (1966) Physical properties of human interferon prepared in vitro and in vivo. Virology 29:515–522

Merk W (1982) Large-scale production of human fibroblast interferon in cellfermenters. Dev Biol Stand 50:137–140

Mogensen KE, Tovey MG, Pirt SJ, Mathison GE (1972) Induction of mouse interferon in a chemically defined system. J Gen Virol 16:111–114

Mozes LW, Vilcek J (1974) Interferon induction in rabbit cells irradiated with UV light. J Virol 13:646–651

Mozes LW, Havell EA, Gradoville ML, Vilcek J (1974) Increased interferon production in human cells irradiated with ultraviolet light. Infect Immun 10:1189–1191

Nagata S, Mantei N, Weissmann C (1980) The structure of one of the eight or more distinct chromosomal genes for human interferon-α. Nature 287:401–408
Nielsen V, Johansson A (1980) Biosilon, optimal culture conditions and various research scale culture techniques. Dev Biol Stand 46:131–136
Oie HK, Gazdar AF, Buckler CE, Baron S (1972) High interferon producing line of transformed murine cells. J Gen Virol 17:107–109
Reuveny S, Bino T, Rosenberg M, Mizrahi A (1980) A new cellulose-based microcarrier culturing system. Dev Biol Stand 46:137–145
Reynolds FH, Pitha PM (1975) Molecular weight study of human fibroblast interferon. Biochem Biophys Res Commun 65:107–112
Robinson JH, Butlin PM, Imrie RC (1980) Growth characteristics of human diploid fibroblasts in packed beds of glass beads. Dev Biol Stand 46:173–181
Sagar AD, Pickering LA, Sussman-Berger P, Stewart WE, Sehgal PB (1981) Heterogeneity of interferon mRNA species from Sendai virus-induced human lymphoblastoid (Namalva) cells and Newcastle disease virus-induced murine fibroblast (L) cells. Nucleic Acids Res 9:149–160
Sano E, Matsui Y, Kobayashi S (1974) Production of mouse interferon with high titers in a large-scale suspension culture system. Jpn J Microbiol 18:165–172
Schleicher JB (1973) Multisurface stacked plate propagators. In: Kruse PF, Patterson MK (eds) Tissue culture, methods and applications. Academic, New York, p 333
Sedmak JJ, Grossberg SE (1981) Interferon stabilisation and enhancement by rare earth salts. J Gen Virol 53:195–198
Sehgal PB, Sagar AD (1980) Heterogeneity of poly(I)·poly(C)-induced human fibroblast interferon mRNA species. Nature 288:95–97
Sehgal PB, Tamm I, Vilcek J (1975a) Human interferon production: Superinduction by 5,6-dichloro-l-β-D-ribofuranosylbenzimidazole. Science 190:282–284
Sehgal PB, Tamm I, Vilcek J (1975b) Enhancement of human interferon production by neutral red and chloroquine: Analysis of inhibition of protein degradation and macromolecular synthesis. J Exp Med 142:1283–1300
Sehgal PB, Tamm I, Vilcek J (1976a) Regulation of human interferon production I. Superinduction by 5,6-dichloro-l-β-D-ribofuranosylbenzimidazole. Virology 70:532–541
Sehgal PB, Tamm I, Vilcek J (1976b) Regulation of human interferon production II. Inhibition of messenger RNA synthesis by 5,6-dichloro-l-β-D-ribofuranosylbenzimidazole. Virology 70:542–544
Senussi OA, Cartwright T, Thompson P (1979) Resolution of human fibroblast interferon into two distinct classes by thiol exchange chromatography. Arch Virol 62:323–331
Soreq H, Sagar AD, Sehgal PB (1981) Translational activity and functional stability of human fibroblast β_1 and β_2 interferon mRNAs lacking 3′-terminal RNA sequences. Proc Natl Acad Sci USA 78:1741–1745
Spier RE, Whiteside JP (1976) The production of foot-and-mouth disease virus from BHK 21 C13 cells grown on the surface of glass spheres. Biotechnol Bioeng 18:649–657
Stancek D, Gressnerova M, Paucker K (1970) Isoelectric components of mouse, human, and rabbit interferons. Virology 41:740–750
Stein S, Kenny C, Frieden HJ, Shively J, Del Valle U, Pestka S (1980) NH_2-terminal amino acid sequence of human fibroblast interferon. Proc Natl Acad Sci USA 77:5716–5719
Stewart WE (1974) Distinct molecular species of interfons. Virology 61:80–86
Stewart WE (1979) The interferon system. Springer, Berlin Heidelberg New York
Stewart WE, Grosser LB, Lockart RZ (1971) Priming: a non-antiviral function of interferon. J Virol 7:792–801
Stewart WE, De Clercq E, De Somer P (1974) Stabilisation of interferons by defensive reversible denaturation. Nature 249:460–461
Stewart WE, De Somer P, Edy VG, Paucker K, Berg K, Ogburn CA (1975) Distinct molecular species of human interferons: Requirements for stabilisation and reactivation of human leukocyte and fibroblast interferons. J Gen Virol 26:327–331

Stewart WE, Le Goff S, Wiranowska-Stewart M (1977) Characterisation of two distinct molecular populations of type I mouse interferons. J Gen Virol 37:277–284

Stewart WE, Blalock JE, Burke DC, Chany C, Dunnick JK, Falcoff E, Friedman, RM, Galasso GJ, Joklik WK, Vilcek JT, Youngner JS, Zoon KC (1980) Interferon nomenclature: Report from the committee on interferon nomenclature. In: Gresser I (ed) Interferon 2. Academic, London, p 97

Sulkowski E, Davey MW, Carter WA (1976) Interaction of human interferons with immobilised hydrophobic amino acids and dipeptides. J Biol Chem 251:5381–5385

Taira H, Broeze RJ, Jayaram BM, Lengyel P, Hunkapiller MW, Hood LE (1980a) Mouse interferons: Amino terminal amino acid sequences of various species. Science 207:528–530

Taira M, Broeze RJ, Slattery E, Lengyel P (1980b) Large-scale production of mouse interferons from monolayers of Ehrlich ascites tumour cells. J Gen Virol 49:231–234

Tan YH, Barakat F, Berthold W, Smith-Johannsen H, Tan C (1979) The isolation and amino acid/sugar composition of human fibroblastoid interferon. J Biol Chem 254:8067–8073

Taniguchi T, Fujii-Kurayama T, Muramatsu M (1980a) Molecular cloning of human interferon cDNA. Proc Natl Acad Sci USA 77:4002–4006

Taniguchi T, Ohno S, Fujii-Kurayama T, Muramatsu M (1980b) The nucleotide sequence of human fibroblast interferon cDNA. Gene 10:11–15

Tavernier J, Derynck R, Fiers W (1981) Evidence for a unique human fibroblast interferon (IFN-β)chromosomal gene, devoid of intervening sequences. Nucleic Acids Res 9:461–471

Thilly WG, Levine DW (1979) Microcarrier culture: A homogeneous environment for studies of cellular biochemistry. Methods Enzymol 58:184–194

Tovey MG, Mathison GE, Pirt SJ (1973) The production of interferon by chemostat cultures of mouse LS-cells grown in chemically defined, protein-free medium. J Gen Virol 20:29–35

Tovey MG, Begon-Lours J, Gresser I (1974) A method for the large-scale production of potent interferon preparations. Proc Soc Exp Biol Med 146:809–815

Van Damme J, Billiau A (1981) Large-scale production of human fibroblast interferon. In: Pestka S (ed) Methods in enzymology, vol 78, interferons, part A. Academic, New York, p 101

Van Hemert D, Kilburn DG, Van Wezel AL (1969) Homogenous cultivation of animal cells for the production of virus and virus products. Biotechnol Bioeng 11:875–885

Van Wezel AL (1967) Growth of cell-strains and primary cells on microcarriers in homogenous culture. Nature 216:64–65

Van Wezel AL (1973) Microcarrier culture of animal cells In: Kruse PF, Patterson MK (eds) Tissue culture, methods and applications. Academic, New York, p 372

Vilcek J, Rossman TG, Varacalli F (1969) Differential effects of actinomycin D and puromycin on the release of interferon induced by double-stranded RNA. Nature 223:682–683

Vilcek J, Havell EA, Gradoville ML, Mika-Johnson M, Douglas WHJ (1978) Selection of new human foreskin fibroblast cell strains for interferon production. Adv Exp Med Biol 110:101–118

Weil R, Dorner F (1973) Interferon structure: Facts and speculations: In: Carter WA (ed) Selective inhibitors of viral functions. CRC, Cleveland, p 107

Weissenbach J, Chernajovsky T, Zeevi M, Shulman L, Soreq H, Nir U, Wallach D, Perricaudet M, Tiollais P, Revel M (1980) Two interferon mRNAs in human fibroblasts: In vitro translation and *Escherichia coli* cloning studies. Proc Natl Acad Sci USA 77:7152–7156

Wiranowska-Stewart M, Chudzio T, Stewart WE (1977) Repeated superinduction of interferon in human diploid fibroblast cultures. J Gen Virol 37:221–223

Wohler W, Rudiger HW, Passarge E (1972) Large-scale culturing of normal diploid cells on glass beads using a novel type of culture vessel. Exp Cell Res 74:571–573

Yamamoto T (1981) Antigenicity of mouse interferons: two distinct molecular species common to interferons of various sources. Virology 111:312–319
Yamamoto T, Kawade T (1976) Purification of two components of mouse L cell interferon: Electrophoretic demonstration of interferon protein. J Gen Virol 33:225–236
Yamamoto T, Kawade T (1980) Antigenicity of mouse interferons: Distinct antigenicity of the two L cell interferon species. Virology 103:80–88

CHAPTER 15

Immune Interferon

J. A. GEORGIADES, S. BARON, W. R. FLEISCHMANN, JR.,
M. LANGFORD, D. A. WEIGENT, and G. J. STANTON

A. Position of Human Immune Interferon in the Lymphokine System

ISAACS and LINDENMANN discovered interferon in 1957. During the last 26 years, a number of cellular products have been identified (COHEN et al. 1977, 1980; WAKSMAN and NAMBA 1976). Table 1 presents the growing list of recognized lymphokines, monokines, and cytokines, including interferon, which are biologically active mediators produced by cells (GEORGIADES et al. 1980a). At present, it is not clear whether these lymphokine functions listed in Table 1 represent different molecules or whether a few molecules have multifunctional properties. The lymphokine, human immune interferon (HuIFN-γ) illustrates this problem. IFN-γ may mediate many functions including suppressor T-cell effects (JOHNSON 1981; JOHNSON and BLALOCK 1980), antiviral effects (WHEELOCK 1965), anticellular effects (BLALOCK et al. 1980; FLEISCHMANN et al. 1980), natural killer (NK) cell activation (KUMAR et al. 1979; SENIK et al., to be published), and changes in normal cells which render them resistant to lysis by NK cells (PERUSSIA et al. 1980). Most of these functions can be induced by the same molecular population. IFN-γ can also suppress antibody production (SONNENFELD et al. 1977).

In this paper, we will consider selected aspects of the induction, production, purification, molecular properties, and functions of IFN-γ. The suppressor T-cell effects, antiproliferative effects, NK cell activations, and immunoregulatory functions of the IFN-γ will only be superficially covered since several excellent review articles covering the subjects have recently appeared (BARON et al. 1980; EPSTEIN 1975, 1979; JOHNSON and BARON 1976; SONNENFELD 1980).

Historically, interferon produced after T-cell stimulation (FALCOFF et al. 1972; GREEN et al. 1969; STABO et al. 1974; WHEELOCK 1965) was differentiated from other interferons in 1973 by SALVIN and YOUNGNER during studies of mice with delayed hypersensitivity. In contrast to previously described mouse and human interferons (HuIFN-α or HuIFN-β), IFN-γ was pH sensitive and was not neutralized by antibody to HuIFN-α or HuIFN-β (PAUCKER 1977; VOLLE et al. 1975). Soon afterwards, it was found that MuIFN was present in lymphokine preparations obtained from lymphocyte cultures stimulated by means of specific antigens and mitogens, and that this was also MuIFN-γ (YOUNGNER and SALVIN 1973).

B. Production of HuIFN-γ

I. Inducers

Among different IFN-γ inducers, the most popular are phytohemagglutinin (PHA), concanavalin A (con A), staphylococcal enterotoxin A (SEA) (LANGFORD

Table 1. Mediators produced by various cells during the immune response (GEORGIADES et al. 1980a)

AEF	Allogeneic effect factor
AgDMIF	Antigen-dependent macrophage-inhibiting factor
AIM	Antibody-inhibiting material
ANP	Antineoplaston A
ASE	Antigen-specific enhancer (of the T-cell-dependent antibody response)
ASF	Allotypic suppression factor
ASS	Antigen-specific suppressor (of the T-cell-dependent antibody response)
ASTCF	Antigen-specific T-cell factor
BAF	B-cell-activating factor
BCF	Basophil chemotactic factor
BF	Blastogenic factor
CHA	Chemotactic factor
CRP	C reactive protein
DBMCF	Differentiating B memory cell factor
DDHF	Desensitization of delayed hypersensitivity factor
DLF	Differentiating lymphocyte factor
DMMF	Depressor of monocyte migration
ECHF	Eosinophil chemotactic factor
FIF	Feedback inhibition factor
GAF	Glucocorticord-antagonizing factor
GRF	Genetically restricted factor
HFIgE	Helper factor for IgE
HRF	Histamine-releasing factor
IA1	Inflammatory activity factor
IDS	Inhibitor of DNA synthesis
IFC	Interferon complex
IFEF	Interferon-enhancing factor
IgESF	IgE suppressor factor
IIFIF	Immune interferon-inhibitory factor
IRA	Immunoregulatory globulin
ISF	Immunosuppressive factor from mastocytoma
IVPF	Increasing vascular permeability factor
LAF	Lymphocyte-activating factor
LAFTC	T-lymphocyte-activating factor
LAP	Soluble nondialyzable factor acting on PHA-stimulated thymocytes
LCHA	Lymphocyte chemotactic factor
LEM	Leukocyte endogenous factor
LF	Leukotactic factor
LIF_1	Leukocyte-inhibitory factor
LIF_2	Lymphocyte-inhibitory factor
LMF	Lymphocyte mitogenic factor
LT	Lymphotoxin
LTF	Lymphocyte-trapping factor
MAF	Macrophage-activating factor
MAGF	Macrophage aggregation factor
MCF	Monocyte chemotactic factor
MDF	Macrophage disappearance factor
MIF	Migration-inhibitory factor
MILF	Macrophage-inhibitory-like factor
MLRS	Mixed lymphocyte reaction suppressor
NAF	Normal cell-activating factor
NALE	Nonadherent lymphocyte suppressor acting early in leukocyte response
NALL	Nonadherent lymphocyte suppressor acting late in leukocyte response
NIP	Normal immunosuppressive protein
NSM	Nonspecific mediator (T-cell derived)
OAF	Osteoclast-activating factor
PAIF	Peritoneal adherence inhibitor
PEF	Phagocytosis-enhancing factor
PSF	Polymorphonuclear-stimulating factor
SCDF	Stem cell-differentiating factor
SIIR	Suppressor of the initiation of primary immune response
SIREF	Specific immune response-enhancing factor
SIRS	Soluble immune response suppressor
SMAF	Specific macrophage-arming factor
SRF	Skin-reactive factor
SSF	Soluble suppressor factor
TCSDPT	T-cell suppressor depressing passive transfer (of contact sensitivity)
TEF	Thymus extract factor
TF	Transfer factor
TI	Tumor inhibitor (from fibroblast cultures)
TNF	Tumor necrosis factor
TRF	T-cell-replacing factor
XRF	Xenogenic reconstruction factor

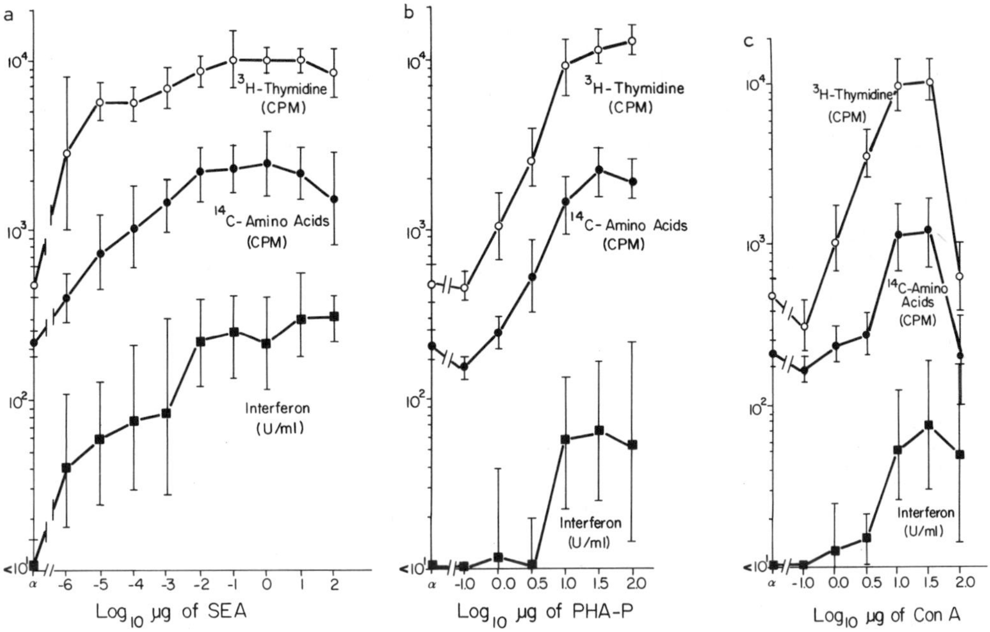

Fig. 1 a–c. Mean dose–response and 95% confidence limits of thymidine ^3H incorporation, amino acid ^{14}C incorporation, and immune interferon production in lymphocyte cultures stimulated with (**a**) SEA, (**b**) PHA-P, and (**c**) con A, for 20 individuals. LANGFORD et al. (1978)

et al. 1978), and antilymphocyte serum (FALCOFF et al. 1972). As may be seen in Fig. 1, PHA and con A are mitogens which are used to induce IFN-γ in mouse spleen cells over a relatively narrow concentration range because higher levels of these compounds are toxic for cells (LANGFORD et al. 1978). In contrast, SEA could induce IFN-γ synthesis over a relatively broad concentration range since this peptide inducer is relatively nontoxic for cells while exhibiting high mitogenic activity. In addition to PHA, con A, and SEA, pokeweed mitogen (PWM), tuberculin purified protein derivative (PPD), diphtheria toxoid, tetanus toxoid, herpes simplex antigen, galactose oxidase, and calcium ionophore induce lymphoid cells to produce IFN-γ (DIANZANI et al. 1979, 1980a; EPSTEIN 1977; FRIEDMAN and COOPER 1969; GREEN et al. 1969; JOHNSON and BARON 1976; JOHNSON et al. 1977). FALCOFF et al. (1972, 1981) demonstrated that antilymphocyte serum is also a good inducer of HuIFN-γ. These inducers varied widely in the concentration needed for maximal production of IFN-γ. In addition, donor "sensitization" was required for antigen induction of IFN-γ (EPSTEIN 1977).

The ability of SEA to produce high levels of IFN-γ over a broad concentration range in murine splenocytes and human peripheral blood leukocytes (PBL) (JOHNSON et al. 1977; LANGFORD et al. 1978) suggested its potential for IFN-γ production. We also compared the IFN-γ inducibility of SEA with PHA and con A in cultures of human PBL. Among the tested inducers, SEA was found to be the most potent (LANGFORD et al. 1979). It exhibited maximal mitogenic and interferon inducibility over a broad concentration range (10^{-5}–10^{-2} μg/ml); and induced 3–5 times more IFN-γ than the other inducers tested. Maximal production of IFN-γ by SEA was not significantly affected by age, sex, or race of donors. SEA was not cytotoxic at any concentration tested; and could be removed from the IFN-γ preparations (LANGFORD et al. 1979). In addition, we have found that other staphylococcal enterotoxins (i.e., SEB, SED, and SEE) are potent IFN-γ inducers. Because SEB has been shown to be as effective as SEA and to have less emetic effects than SEA (BERGDOLL 1970), it may prove to be the inducer of choice for large scale IFN-γ production for clinical trials. Unfortunately, all these mitogens are highly toxic for humans, and IFN-γ produced for clinical use must be exhaustively purified. To solve this problem, DIANZANI et al. (1979) undertook a search for other less toxic inducers. This attempt led to the discovery that peripheral human lymphocytes exposed to an enzyme, galactose oxidase, produced large quantitites of HuIFN-γ. Cleavage of galactose from the cell surface with α-galactosidase prevented induction of the HuIFN-γ by galactose oxidase. Extending these studies, they found that HuIFN-γ synthesis also might be induced by treating lymphocytes with a calcium ionophore (DIANZANI et al. 1980). Furthermore, use of antilymphocyte serum (FALCOFF et al. 1972) as an inducer offered several advantages, especially during the purification process. A mixed lymphocyte reaction could also be used for IFN-γ induction (VIRELIZIER et al. 1977a).

FALCOFF et al. (1980) suggested that IFN-γ should be separated into two subclasses, one subgroup represented by IFN-γ molecules produced by immunocompetent cells stimulated by specific antigens and the other subgroup, represented by interferon produced by T-cells stimulated with nonspecific stimulants like mitogens and lectins. The first subgroup of HuIFN-γ was produced by B-lymphocytes and for that reason resembled those of virus interferon to pH 2.0 sensitivity and antigenic cross-reactivity. The second subgroup, produced mainly by T-cells was pH sensitive and showed no cross-reactivity with virus interferons (IFN-α and IFN-β).

II. IFN-γ System

Studies on the mechanism of induction of IFN-γ revealed that production of IFN-γ by T-cells requires the collaboration of Macrophages. It was found that thymocytes, in the absence of macrophages, were inhibited in the synthesis of IFN-γ following mitogen stimulation (SONNENFELD 1980). The evidence showed that macrophages stimulated by antigen or mitogen released a mediator essential for IFN-γ synthesis. Subsequently, GERY and WAKSMAN (1972) defined the macrophage-derived factor as leukocyte activation factor (LAF), also called interleukin-1 (IL-1). Induced both proliferation of thymocytes and substituted for macrophage function in the production of IFN-γ from stimulated T-lymphocytes. As part of the process of IFN-γ production, IL-1 initiated a cascade of cell–cell interactions resulting in the synthesis of many additional lymphokines. Among the lymphokines released was T-cell growth factor (TCGF) or interleukin-2 (IL-2), a physiologic mitogen for activitated T-cells, which induces their clonal expansion (WAGNER et al. 1980). Interactions between IL-1 and IL-2 and specific antigen or mitogen were essential elements for interferon synthesis.

Relatively little is known about the lymphokine system, its chemistry and the biologic role of different molecules. Even less is known about disorders in the lymphokine system. Among better-known molecules is IFN-γ which is, by definition, a lymphokine (COHEN et al. 1980). Evidence suggesting the existence of malfunctions of the lymphokine systems come from indirect and direct observations of the synthesis of lymphokines during the course of a disease (DECLERCQ 1979).

One of the sources of information about malfunctions of the lymphokine system included studies of NK cell activity in patients with different diseases. An accumulated body of evidence suggests that interferons might be selective activators of the NK cells. If that is true, the interferon system may be impaired in several human genetic disorders such as Chédiak–Higashi syndrome, Wiskott–Aldrich syndrome, ataxia–teleangiectesia (RADER and HALIOTIS 1980), IgA deficiency (EPSTEIN and AMMAN 1974), hypogammaglobulinemia (STRANNEGARD et al. 1980), and Crohn's disease (VANTRAPPEN 1980) because in all these diseases a profound defect in NK cell activity has been observed (EPSTEIN and AMMAN 1974; RADER and HALIOTIS 1980). It is important to point out that among all these categories of diseases there is a high incidence of malignancy (RADER and HALIOTIS 1980). Also, depression of NK activity was observed in patients with neoplasia (HOKLAND and ELLEGAARD 1981; PROSS and BAINS 1976). There are also indirect indications that production of another member of the lymphokine family, IL-2, is impaired in certain genetic disorders and neoplasias, namely: disglobulinemia, acute and chronic lymphocytic leukemia, lymphosarcoma, and Hodgkin's disease (DAO et al. 1978). Since IL-2 is one of the essential factors involved in IFN-γ synthesis (as described earlier in this section, impairment in IL-2 production automatically effects HuIFN-γ synthesis. Furthermore, pretreatment of embryonic cells with proven carcinogens resulted in reduced production of interferon (BARNESS et al. 1980). Indirect evidence such as examples we have mentioned, strengthen observations that in certain types of leukemias (ALL, AML, CLL) and non-Hodgkin's lymphomas, the production of HuIFN-α is maintained at the normal level, but HuIFN-γ synthesis is impaired (G. JACKSON, A. MIZRAHI, J. FREEMAN, J. O'MALLEY 1980, personal communication).

HOOKS et al. (1979, 1980) reported that HuIFN-γ was present in the blood of patients with autoimmune diseases such as lupus erythematosus, rheumatoid arthritis, scleroderma, and Sjögren's syndrome. Normal individuals and patients with aphthous stomatitis show no detectable level of interferon. SCHNITZER and YITTERBERG (1981) confirmed HOOK's original observations. Therapeutic administration of anti-IFN globulin to patients with allergic disorders considerably improved their clinical status (SKURKOVICH and EREMKINA 1975).

In animals, similar findings were observed. For example, New Zeal and Black (NZB) mice and F_1 hybrids (NZB/NZW) as they age, spontaneously develop a syndrome similar to human systemic lupus erythematosus. Such mice trated with MuIFN-α showed an increased incidence of glomerulonephritis, proteinuria, and anemia (HEREMANS et al. 1978; SERGIESCU et al. 1979). A similar acceleration of the initial disease was observed following administration of the MuIFN-γ (SERGIESCU et al. 1979).

Mice infected neonatally with lymphocytic choriomeningitis (LCM) virus developed autoimmune diseases similar to that which naturally occurred in NZB mice (GRESSER et al. 1980). Treatment of LCM-infected mice with MuIFN-α augments the severity of the clinical manifestations (GRESSER et al. 1980). Administration of a potent anti-IFN globulin to LCM-infected mice inhibited development of both the early and late syndromes. This indicated that an excess of IFN-γ in the blood circulation might induce lesions in different organs by formation of immunocomplexes (BOROS and CARRICK 1980; WIGZELL 1981).

Similarly excessive production of other lymphokines might cause diseases. This subject will not be further elaborated as several excellent reviews are available (ADELMAN et al. 1973; SYNDERMAN et al. 1979). However, from this short review and articles already mentioned, it is possible that dysfunction in lymphokine systems might cause a variety of severe diseases. Some dysfunctions may lead to the progressive degeneration of cells and organs while others may lead to uncontrolled cell growth.

III. Large Scale Production of HuIFN-γ

Studies of lymphokines and their interactions require their production in sufficient quantities for purification and biologic characterization. This will help ascertain their primary and secondary functions. In order to achieve this goal, large scale methods for the production of mouse and human IFN-γ were devised (DE LEY et al. 1980; FALCOFF et al. 1980; LANGFORD et al. 1979; OSBORNE 1979). The methods were based on the induction of lymphocytes with the T-cell mitogens, SEA (LANGFORD et al. 1979) and con A (DE LEY et al. 1980), or antilymphocyte serum (FALCOFF et al. 1972). In our hands, HuIFN-γ was produced optimally (10^3 U/ml) when cultures at concentrations of $1–2 \times 10^6$ cells/ml were incubated at pH 7.2 for 3 days at a concentration of SEA of 0.02 μg/ml. Substitution of human albumin or plasma to the medium (1%–5%), instead of fetal calf serum (FCS) simplified HuIFN-γ purification for possible clinical trials. Removal of HuIFN-γ-containing culture medium and resuspension of the viable cells to 1×10^6/ml in fresh medium for an additional 2 days (4–5 days) with SEA resulted in further IFN-γ production at reduced yield (10^2 U/ml). An additional repeat stimulation at 6–8 days resulted in even less IFN-γ synthesis ($10^{1.5}$ U/ml). However, this negative trend could be reversed by application of a different mitogen, resulting in full production. By criteria such as pH 2.0 sensitivity, kinetics of antiviral action, and antibody neutralization, the bulk of the detectable interferon produced under these conditions was HuIFN-γ.

Our experience indicates that approximately 1 U IFN-γ was obtained from 1,000 lymphocytes. In comparison, 3 U HuIFN-β (BILLIAU et al. 1977) and 1–10 U HuIFN-α (CANTELL et al. 1974) were reported to be produced by 1,000 cells. Since we do not know which subpopulation of cells produces the different interferons, this production by mixed populations has limited meaning.

C. Properties of IFN-γ

IFN-γ produced by leukocytes stimulated with SEA and other mitogens was acid labile (90%–95% inactivation by pH 2.0 at room temperature for 5 h). The remaining acid-stable interferon was not neutralized by antisera to human leukocyte interferon (LANGFORD et al. 1981), but was neutralized by antibodies to HuIFN-γ (M. P. LANGFORD et al. 1980, unpublished work). SEA-induced HuIFN-γ was inactivated by heating (56 °C for 1 h) and could be stabilized by lyophilization. Lyophilized crude preparations retained full activity for more than 1 year. Crude or partially purified HuIFN-γ was not active on rabbit kidney cells, rat (WIRA) cells, mouse L929 cells, baby hamster kidney cells, or bovine cells (LANGFORD et al. 1979). It was active on human WISH, HeLa, and foreskin fibroblast cells and on monkey Vero cells. The molecular weight range was from 35,000 to 70,000 (GEORGIADES et al. 1979; LANGFORD et al. 1979). In addition, SEA-induced IFN-γ induced the antiviral state in human cells at a much slower rate than other interferons which suggested that it may have a different mode of activation (LANGFORD et al. 1979). It was also a potent anticellular agent and enhanced NK cell activity (BLALOCK et al. 1980; FALCOFF et al. 1980; LANGFORD et al. 1981; PERUSSIA et al. 1980; SENIK et al. to be published). Partially purified SEA-induced IFN-γ was antigenically distinct in that antisera made to it did not cross-neutralize human or mouse leukocyte (IFN-α) or fibroblast (IFN-β) interferons (LANGFORD et al. 1981). The antisera to SEA-induced IFN-γ neutralized the IFN activity induced by several mitogens, such as PHA, con A, PWM, by galactose oxidase and calcium ionophore (LANGFORD et al. 1981).

Treatment of human fibroblast cells with HuIFN-γ, crude and purified preparations, induced in cells the synthesis of proteins similar to those induced by HuIFN-α and HuIFN-β (EPSTEIN et al. 1981; HOVANESSIAN et al. 1980; RUBIN and GUPTA 1980). More specifically, IFN-γ induces the same two enzymes: 2′5′-oligo (A) polymerase (also reterred to as synthetase) (BAGLIONI and MARDNEY 1980; EPSTEIN et al. 1981; FALCOFF et al. 1980), and protein kinase (EPSTEIN et al. 1981), which have been postulated to play a role in the expression of IFN-α and IFN-β activity. Since the amount of induced proteins by HuIFN-γ differed significantly from that induced by HuIFN-α and HuIFN-β, we believe that the observed quantitative changes were responsible for the higher antiproliferative activity of IFN-γ (RUBIN and GUPTA 1980). These observations are in agreement with our earlier observations that HuIFN-γ has stronger antitumor activity than HuIFN-α and HuIFN-β (BLALOCK et al. 1979).

In addition, it has been found that in contrast to IFN-α and β, IFN-γ showed no affinity to gangliosides (ANKEL et al. 1980). That aspect might be of medical significance, since tumors are frequently surrounded by an elevated level of gangliosides, which in effect might bind HuIFN-α and HuIFN-β (KLAPPEL et al. 1977). Treatment of patients with elevated ganglioside levels in the blood or in the vicinity of the tumor might not be very effective. In such cases, HuIFN-γ may be the interferon of choice.

The observations of GRESSER et al. (1974) that mouse L1210 cells exposed for long periods of time to virus-induced interferon became resistant to interferon, might also be relevant to interferon therapy (GRESSER 1980). Those resistant cells still remained sensitive to MuIFN-γ treatment. This suggests that alternate administration of viral interferon and HuIFN-γ might be a useful approach in preventing the selection of interferon-resistant neoplastic cells.

There are several additional areas where IFN-γ may play an important role and are therefore worth mentioning. MISRAHI et al. (1978) found that the level of the

IFN-γ activity induced in PBL by by PHA in the presence of tunicamycin was similar to control preparations. However, tumicamycin treatment established all HuIFN-γ heterogenicity, when measured by affinity to different chromatographic matrices. IFN-γ preparations also depressed the cytochrome P-450 drug metabolism system of the liver (Sonnenfeld et al. 1980). Depression of the cytochrome P-450 system correlated with the level of IFN-γ. The activity of the cytochrome P-450 system also decreased significantly when IFN-γ was induced in vivo (Harned et al. 1982). Unfortunately, nothing is known yet about the mechanism of the depression of the cytochrome P-450 system. Studies of the underlying mechanisms would be extremely important.

Also, IFN-γ preparations (mouse and human) increased or decreased macrophage phagocytosis, depending on the interferon concentration (Degre et al. 1981). The importance of these observations is not yet known; however, this subject was recently reviewed by Schultz (1980). Modulation of the immune system by IFN-γ was also recently reviewed (Epstein 1979; Sonnenfeld 1980; Wigzell 1981) and for that reason, only the most crucial and significant properties of the IFN-γ will be mentioned. IFN-γ exhibited immunomodulatory properties similar to IFN-α and IFN-β. IFN-γ also exhibited prodound effects on the suppression of antibody formation (Epstein et al. 1981; Falcoff et al. 1980; Green et al. 1969; Sonnenfeld 1977, 1980; Virelizier et al. 1977a), enhancement of antibody formation (Sonnenfeld 1980), and enhancement of lymphocyte surface antigen expression. This last phenomenon was observed independently in mouse and human systems (Heron et al. 1978; Sonnenfeld 1980). Also, specific T-cell cytotoxicity was increased following IFN-γ treatment (Simon et al. 1979).

D. Purification of IFN-γ

A purification scheme was developed as a result of the extensive evaluation of various purification steps. We found (Georgiades et al. 1979) that SEA-induced HuIFN-γ did not bind to hydrophobic matrices under ordinary conditions. However, adsorption of crude HuIFN-γ to a Matrex Blue (Amicon, Danvers, Massachusetts) hydrophobic column at the initiation of purification resulted in an increase of antiviral activity, perhaps due to removal of an inhibitor of interferon. Such inhibitors were found in the mouse system (Fleischmann et al. 1980a). Controlled pore glass (CPG) beads appeared to be a superior substrate for concentration of HuIFN-γ. HuIFN-γ could be eluted from CPG with buffer consisting of 1 *M* NaCl and 50% ethylene glycol dissolved in phosphate buffered saline (PBS) (elution buffer). In addition to concentration, a modest 20–30-fold purification was achieved. IFN-γ displaced from CPG could be further purified on an Ultrogel AcA54 gel filtration column (LKB, Rockville, Maryland) equilibrated with a PBS elution buffer consisting of 1 *M* NaCl plus 18% ethylene glycol. The bulk of HuIFN-γ activity was present in the fractions of molecular weight range 35,000–70,000. Results of a typical purification are presented in Table 2 and Figs. 2 and 3. The specific activity of the starting material was 10^2 U HuIFN-γ per milligram protein, while that of the AcA54 pools was about $10^{5.6}$ U per milligram protein, with the peak fraction containing $10^{6.88}$ U per milligram protein.

Table 2. Purification of human immune interferon (J. A. GEORGIADES 1980, unpublished work)

Treatment	Volume (ml)	Total protein (mg)	IFN titer (U/ml)	Total IFN (U)	Specific activity (log_{10} U per milligram protein)
Starting material	9,935	2,722	1,000	9,935,000	$10^{2.56}$
Eluted from MB[a]	660	2,831	8,250	5,445,000	$10^{3.28}$
Not bound to MB	1,200	2,039	300	360,000	$10^{2.25}$
Eluted from CPG[b]	168	470.0	132,371	22,238,328	$10^{4.67}$
Not bound to CPG	1,400	1,817	>10		
AcA54 pool (MB)	420	617.4	9,548	40,010,160	$10^{4.81}$
AcA54 pool (CPG)	220	112.5	319,789	70,353,580	$10^{5.79}$
Peak fraction AcA54 (CPG)	10	1.3	1,000,000	10,000,000	$10^{6.88}$

[a] Matrex Blue
[b] Controlled pore glass beads

Several additional purification methods have been recently designed using CPG, silicic acid, chromatography on immobilized con A, and partition chromatography (DE LEY et al. 1980; OSBORNE et al. 1979; WITZERBIN et al. 1978; YIP et al. 1981). YIP et al. (1981) obtained relatively high purification of his PHA–forbol ester-induced HuIFN-γ. WIRANOWSKA-STEWART and associates (1980) utilized a purification scheme involving adsorption on CPG followed by further purification of a poly(U)–sepharose column.

Both J. VILCEK and W. E. STEWART (1980, personal communication) reported that preparations of HuIFN-γ exceeding a specific activity of 10^6 U/ml became unstable and the addition of inert proteins was essential for their stability. Several other modifications of the purification procedures have also been published (DELEY et al. 1980; FALCOFF et al. 1980).

E. Characterization of IFN-γ Induced by Staphylococcal Enterotoxin A

Interferon purified by the method described by us (GEORGIADES et al. 1979) was used in the studies listed in this section.

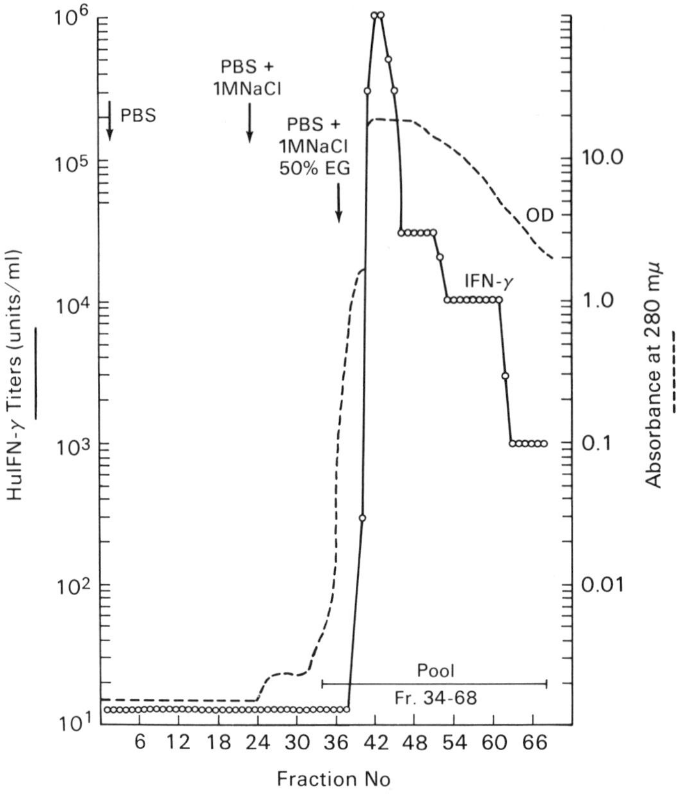

Fig. 2. Elution profile of HuIFN-γ from CPG beads. HuIFN-γ not adsorbed to Matrex Blue beads was mixed with CPG (5 mg/ml) and stirred at +4 °C for 3 h. The CPG beads were allowed to sediment. The supernatant was discarded by decanation. The sedimented beads were washed twice with cold PBS and packed into the column. In the column, the beads were further washed with PBS and PBS + 1 *M* NaCl. IFN-γ was eluted with PBS + 1 *M* NaCl + 50% ethylene glycol (EG). J. A. GEORGIADES (1979, unpublished work)

I. Transfer of the Antiviral Activity Between Leukocytes and Epithelial Cells

Cell culture studies indicated that interferon-induced transfer of antiviral activity between cells in tissues might be responsible for significant amplification of the interferon system. It was initially shown that interferon treated mouse L-cells could transfer virus resistance to cocultivated cells of another species (BLALOCK et al. 1977). Subsequently, the cell species shown to transfer interferon-induced antiviral activity were expanded to two additional species, human and rabbit; and the resipient cells to four species, human, hamster, chicken, and monkey (HUGHES et al. 1978). The magnitude of the antiviral response in cocultivated mixtures of cloned mouse L-cells was shown to be controlled by as few as 10% of the most sensitive cells. The rate of development of the antiviral response in the cocultures was controlled by the fast reacting human amnion WISH cells (BLALOCK and STANTON

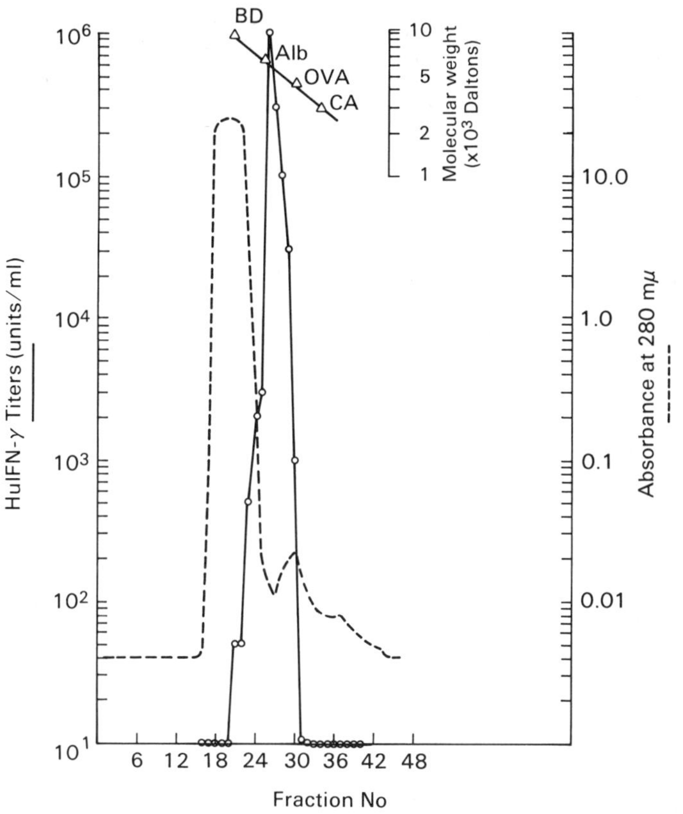

Fig. 3. Filtration of HuIFN-γ by AcA54 chromatography. The column (2.5×90 cm) was loaded with IFN-γ from pooled fractions obtained from CPG column. Fractions 34–68 from CPG column were concentrated on Amicon stirred cells with YM-10 membrane to 20 ml. AcA54 column was equilibrated with buffer consisting of 18% ethylene glycol and 1 *M* NaCl in PBS: 10-ml fractions were collected. Molecular weight standards: Blue dextran (BD), bovine serum albumin (Alb), ovalbumin (OVA), carbonic anhydrase CA. J. A. GEORGIADES (1981, unpublished work)

1980). Taken together, these studies suggested that interferon induced transfer of antiviral activity could occur between cells of different species and between cells of the same species. The transfer system which might result from transfer of signal molecules between cells (BLALOCK and BARON 1979) was efficient, rapid, and could occur in the absence of interferon. Thus, it probably accounts for a significant part of the overall antiviral activity that develops in membranes as a result of exposure to endogenous or exogenous interferons. Interferon itself appears to diffuse poorly through certain body membranes (WEISSENBACHER et al. 1970). More recently, mobile cells of the immune system have been shown to transfer antiviral activity to exogenous and allogeneic recipient epithelial and fibroblastic cells (BLALOCK et al. 1980). Since these cells were capable of migrating, it was plausible that they could be exposed to early, locally produced interferon at sites of infection or in lymphoid tissues and subsequently migrate from these tissues to transfer protection to adjacent or distal tissues. In this regard, MuIFN-γ has been shown be more efficient

Table 3. Comparison of the antiviral and anticellular activity of human interferons (BLALOCK et al. 1980 a)

Human interferon	WISH cells	Hep-2 cells	Titer (U/ml)		Antiviral/anticellular titer
			Antiviral	Anticellular	
Fibroblast	+	–	20	1	20
	–	+	30	< 2	> 15
Leukocyte	+	–	100	1	100
	–	+	100	< 2	> 50
Immune	+	–	30	20	1.5
	–	+	30	10	3.5

in inducing transfer of antiviral activity in cocultures of WISH and L-cells than IFN-α (BLALOCK et al. 1979). Similar studies with IFN-γ-induced leukocytes are in progress.

II. Anticellular Properties of IFN-γ

A comparison of the anticellular activites of highly purified HuIFN-α, HuIFN-β, and HuIFN-γ carried out by BLALOCK et al. (1980) showed that HuIFN-γ preparations were about 20–100 times more active than HuIFN-α and HuIFN-β (Table 3). The more potent anticellular activity of the HuIFN-γ was not likely to be due to the presence of contaminating lymphokines since the slope of the anticellular dose–response curves for crude and 13,800-fold purified HuIFN-γ were similar. These data strongly support the suggestion (GEORGIADES et al. 1980) that HuIFN-γ itself has unusually potent anticellular activity.

III. Potentiation of IFN-γ Action

Combinations of MuIFN-γ and mouse L-cell interferon have been shown to potentiate the antiviral and antitumor properties of interferon by factors of ten or more (FLEISCHMANN et al. 1979, 1980). For example, as shown in Table 4, 3 U MuIFN-γ caused a 2.6-fold reduction of virus yield and 26 U L-cell interferon caused a 43-fold reduction of virus yield. The combination of these interferons might have been expected to cause a 50-fold reduction of virus yield, consistent with a total of 29 U interferon activity. However, the observed level of virus reduction was 714-fold, a level consistent with 320 U. Thus, the two interferons, employed in combination, demonstrated an 11-fold greater than expected activity. Similar results were obtained in a human system. Mixed preparations of HuIFN-γ and HuIFN-β showed a potentiation of interferon antiviral activity [J. A. GEORGIADES, W. R. FLEISCHMANN, JR. 1979, independent unpublished work; E. FALCOFF, J. VILCEK 1980, independent personal communications). However, mixed preparations of HuIFN-α and HuIFN-β gave only an additive effect. Thus, IFN-γ appeared to be a critically important interferon for the demonstration of potentiation by mixed preparations. Potentiation properties of the HuIFN-γ were recently utilized by us for classification of interferon isospecies (see Sect. E.VII; GOLDSTEIN et al. 1981).

Table 4. Potentiation of interferon activity by mixed preparation of IFN-γ[a] (FLEISCHMANN et al. 1979)

IFN sample	Virus yield (PFU/ml)[b]	Fold inhibition	IFN titer (U/ml)		Fold potentiation[e]
			Actual[c]	Expected[d]	
No IFN	$1.0 \times 10^9 \pm 0.1 \times 10^9$				
Immune IFN	$3.8 \times 10^8 \pm 0.4 \times 10^8$	2.6	3		
Fibroblast IFN	$2.3 \times 10^7 \pm 0.1 \times 10^7$	43	26		
Immune IFN + fibroblast IFN	$1.4 \times 10^6 \pm 0.03 \times 10^6$	714	320	29	11

[a] Mouse L-cell monolayers were treated for 12 h with growth medium – no interferon (IFN) – immune interferon, fibroblast interferon, and immune interferon and fibroblast interferon in combination. The monolayers were challenged with Mengo virus at a multiplicity of infection of 10 PFU/cell, and virus yields were harvested 24 h later

[b] PFU plaque-forming units; values are mean ± standard deviation

[c] Actual interferon titers were determined by comparison of virus yield with a standard yield reduction curve of interferon activity determined concurrently

[d] Expected interferon titer was determined by adding the actual titers of the interferons present in the mixed interferon preparation

[e] The potentiation factor was determined by dividing the actual interferon titer by the expected interferon titer

Potentiation of the antitumor activity of interferon has also been demonstrated (FLEISCHMANN et al. 1980). P388 tumors developed more slowly in mice treated with a combination of MuIFN-γ and virus interferons than in untreated mice or in mice treated with either interferon alone. In vitro studies of mouse B16 melanoma cell cloning demonstrated: (a) that potentiation of the direct anticellular effect was a property of MuIFN-γ and virus interferons themselves; (b) that clones resistant to combined interferon treatment did not develop; and (c) that the potentiation level was dependent on the concentration of the two interferons and continued to increase as the concentrations increased (FLEISCHMANN 1982).

IV. Antigenic Classification of IFN-γ

Antibodies to HuIFN-γ were produced in rabbits after multiple intramuscular or subcutaneous injections of $\geq 10^5$ U MuIFN-γ and HuIFN-γ at different sites, once or twice a month for 4–6 months (LANGFORD et al. 1981). Approximately 75% of the rabbits produced neutralizing antibodies. Studies with antibodies to HuIFN-γ conducted by LANGFORD et al. (1981) revealed that antibody to HuIFN-γ did not neutralize HuIFN-α or HuIFN-β. Furthermore, HuIFN-γ induced by various T-lymphocyte mitogens and by specific antigens shared several sommon molecular species, but also showed species which might be distinct (GOLDSTEIN et al 1981; LANGFORD et al. 1981).

Antibodies to MuIFN-γ were also induced in rabbits after intramuscular injections of the SEA-induced and partially purified IFN. Immunized rabbits received seven injections of MuIFN-γ averaging 14,000 U per dose. All MuIFN-γ was suspended in complete Freund adjuvant and given at monthly intervals at multiple

Table 5. Distribution of crude HuIFN-γ activity resolved by analytic isoelectrofocusing (IFPAG)[a] (GOLDSTEIN et al. 1981)

	Gel slice number	Induction (% of total activity)[b]		
		SEA	PHA	Con A
Cathode (−)	1	0.2	4.8	0.2
	2	2.2	4.8	0.2
	3	2.2	0.0	5.4
	4	0.2	12.7	5.4
	5	2.2	15.9	4.3
	6	21.6	0.0	1.6
	7	2.2	15.9	16.3
	8	21.6	15.9	5.4
	9	4.3	0.0	5.4
	10	6.5	0.0	5.4
	11	6.5	0.0	1.6
	12	21.6	0.0	5.4
	13	2.2	1.6	5.4
	14	2.2	12.7	5.4
	15	0.7	1.6	5.4
	16	0.0	0.0	5.4
	17	0.7	0.0	5.4
	18	0.7	4.8	5.4
	19	0.7	4.8	5.4
Anode (+)	20	1.7	4.8	5.4

[a] Samples applied at anodic (+) end (equivalent to gel slice numbers 16, 17, and 18) of a preestablished pH gradient directly on the gel surface

[b] Data are expressed as % of total activity eluted from gel slices relative to the total IFN activity recovered from all slices (total IFN activity recovered was always ≧100%, perhaps owing to separation from inhibitors)

sites; 10 days after the seventh inoculation, the antibodies were found. Prior to evaluation in neutralization tests, serum was absorbed with mouse spleen and L-cells to remove anticellular antibodies. The resulting serum neutralized all MuIFN-γ preparations tested, including MuIFN-γ induced in vitro by SEA, con A, PHA, PMN, and in mixed lymphocyte cultures. MuIFN-γ produced in vivo with specific antigen was also neutralized. The antiserum was equally potent against all of these preparations. The serum did not neutralize any virus interferon preparations tested. Described data suggest that MuIFN-γ produced under diverse conditions were antigenically the same or closely related (OSBORNE et al. 1980a, b).

V. Electrodynamic Characterization of IFN-γ

When crude SEA-induced HuIFN-γ was subjected to analytic isoelectrofocusing on ultrathin polyacrylamide gel (IFPAG) with a broad range pH gradient (3.5–10.0) GEORGIADES et al. 1980; GOLDSTEIN et al. 1979, 1981), several apparently different species of HuIFN-γ were discovered. The proportion of each isospecies did tend to vary from preparation to preparation; however, the pattern was consistent. Similar patterns of isospecies were observed when crude and highly purified SEA-

Table 6. Affinity of different mitogen-induced HuIFNs to MB and CPG[a] (GOLDSTEIN et al. 1981)

Interferon	Starting material	Antiviral activity bound[b]	
Source	Total (U)	MB (%)	CPG (%)
SEA (fresh)	71,004,236	1.87	98.13
PHA (fresh)	23,650,908	98,94	1.06
Con A (fresh)	14,310,750	43.70	56.30

[a] Crude interferon supernatants were treated with Matrex Blue (MB). Material not bound was then mixed with controlled pore glass beads (CPG)
[b] Essentially 100% of the IFN activity not binding to MB was bound to CPG

induced HuIFN-γ samples were fractionated on the same gel by IFPAG. In addition, changes were insignificant when focusing times were extended from 55 to 220 min. Furthermore, comparative studies with crude preparations of SEA-, con A, and PHA-induced HuIFN-γ using IFPAG suggested numerous isospecies having significant HuIFN-γ activity distributed throughout almost the entire pH gradient. This broad distribution was observed for HuIFN-γ induced by all three inducers (Table 5). It appeared that different mitogens might generate distinct isospecies, many common to each inducer, but occurring in different proportions (GOLDSTEIN et al. 1981). The broad distribution of the antiviral activity might be explained by different degrees of glycosylation of the HuIFN-γ molecule (MIZRAHI et al. 1978). Other possible explanations of the nature of the heterogenicity of the HuIFN-γ revealed by analytic isoelectrofocusing are as follows:

1. HuIFN-γ species may be distinct molecular forms having different biologic functions.
2. The isospecies may reflect differences in their association with different carrier protein molecules.
3. The isospecies may represent association with a lipid moiety at different levels of association.
4. Different forms may be due to other lymphokines that mimic the antiviral properties of the HuIFN-γ in the bioassay.

To study this problem further, we developed methods for preparative isoelectrofocusing separation of the IFN-γ (PIEF). This method allowed us to obtain larger quantities of the HuIFN-γ isospecies essential for more in-depth studies (GOLDSTEIN et al. 1981).

VI. Physicochemical Properties of IFN-γ

As mentioned earlier, HuIFN-γ induced by SEA did not significantly bind to hydrophobic column such as: Matrex Blue beads (Amicon, Danvers, Massachusetts), Phenyl Sepharose beads (Pharmacia, Newark, New Jersey), Albumin Bio-gel 10 beads (Bio-Rad, Richmond, California). However, the hydrophobic interaction

Table 7. Binding of HuIFN-γ to lipid-treated Matrex Blue columns (GEORGIADES et al. 1980)

Matrex Blue columns	Interferon applied (U)	Interferon not adsorbed (%)	Interferon adsorbed (%)	Total recovered (% of added)	Total protein applied (mg)	Protein recovered in region of eluted interferon (mg)
New beads	10,000	60,672 (95.7)[a]	2,752 (4.3)	63,424 (634.2)	343	35
Used beads[b]	20,000	38,400 (37.9)	62,784 (62.0)	101,184 (505.9)	406	33
Lipid-treated beads[c]	20,000	24,000 (16.6)	120,320 (83.4)	144,320 (721.6)	337	37

[a] These values were derived from % recovered interferon adjusted to 100%
[b] These beads were used in six consecutive purification experiments
[c] Lipid fraction obtained from methanol–chloroform extraction of used beads, was diluted in methanol–chloroform and mixed with new Matrex Blue beads. The methanol–chloroform solution was evaporated and dried beads were suspended in PBS, pH 7.2, for chromatography of interferon preparations

Table 8. Sensitivity of interferons to different detergents[b] (GEORGIADES et al. 1981)

Detergent	Interferons ($\log_{10}$ U/ml)							
	HuIFN-α Experiment		HuIFN-β Experiment		HuIFN-γ Experiment			
	I	II	I	II	I	II	III	IV
Ionic								
SDS	4.0	4.0	3.5	3.5	1.3	0.56	< 1.0	< 1.0
Sarcosil	> 4.0	4.0	3.5	3.3	0.72	0.56	< 1.0	< 1.0
Nonionic								
Triton X-100	4.0	4.0	3.5	3.5	2.9	1.7	N.D.[b]	2.5
Np 40	4.0	4.0	3.5	3.0	2.9	1.7	1.95	3.0
Tween 80	4.0	4.0	4.0	3.5	3.0	2.47	1.9	3.0
Control	4.0	4.0	3.5	3.5	3.0	2.3	2.3	3.0

[a] Detergents dissolved in distilled water were mixed with IFN in proportions of 1:10. Mixture was vortexed for 10–15 s and after incubation for 1 h at room temperature, samples were assayed for interferon activity. A 0.5 $\log_{10}$ step dilution and four replicates of each sample were used

[b] N.D. not done

Table 9. Sensitivity of different human interferons to lipid solvents (GEORGIADES et al. 1981)

Solvent	Polarity[b]	IFN titer		
		HuIFN-α	HuIFN-β	HuIFN-γ
Control		3.7	3.0	2.8
Hexane	0.1	3.5	3.0	2.1
Benzene	2.7	3.5	3.0	1.9
Ethyl ether	2.8	3.5	3.0	1.0
Isobutanol	4.0	2.5	N.D.[c]	0.5
Ethyl acetate	4.4	2.8	2.7	0.8
Chloroform–methanol 2:1	5.2	3.7	3.0	0.7

[a] Solvents were cooled to 0 °C in an ice bath and then mixed in proportions of 1:1 with human interferons. After incubation for 1 h at room temperature, interferons were separated from lipid solvents and assayed for antiviral activities. A 0.5 $\log_{10}$ step dilution and four replicates of each sample were used. Experiments were repeated at least twice. Units were expressed as $\log_{10}$ U/ml

[b] High purity solvent guide, by Burdick and Jackson Laboratories, Muskegon, Michigan

[c] N.D. not done

properties of HuIFN-γ induced by other inducers were considerably different. Table 6 illustrates this point. Matrex Blue beads bound only about 2% of SEA-induced HuIFN-γ, while they bound 99% and 49% of the total IFN-γ activity induced by PHA and con A, respectively (GEORGIADES et al. 1979; GOLDSTEIN et al. 1981).

Repeated use of the Matrex Blue beads (GEORGIADES et al. 1980) for purification of HuIFN-γ resulted in a significant change in their properties; the bound

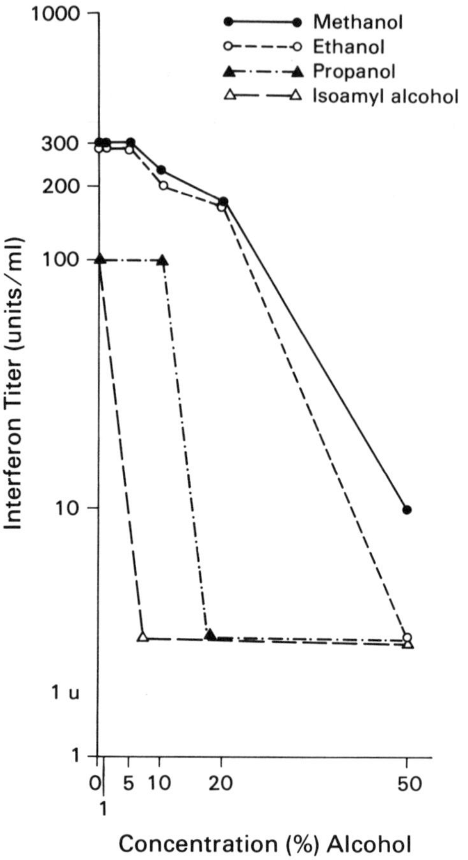

Fig. 4. The influence of alcohol on HuIFN-γ. Crude HuIFN-γ was mixed in equal proportion with 0.1 ml of each of the individual alcohols. The solutions were mixed at room temperature on a vortex mixer for 10–20 and then allowed to incubate for 15 min at 37 °C. Aliquots of each mixture were assayed for antiviral activity on WISH cells. J. A. GEORGIADES (1980, unpublished work)

more SEA-induced HuIFN-γ. Chloroform–methanol (2:1) extraction of the beads with increased binding capacity resulted in the removal of lipids with chromatographic properties similar to those of sterol esters, waxes, and apolar lipids and simultaneously reversed the binding properties of the Matrex Blue beads to their initial properties. Addition of lipids extracted from used Matrex Blue to fresh Matrex Blue beads resulted in binding of HuIFN-γ (Table 7). This suggested that lipids might modulate the biologic activity of SEA-induced HuIFN-γ by complex formation and dissociation.

To better define the variables governing this interaction, we continued to investigate the relationship of lipid and HuIFN-γ (GEORGIADES et al. 1980). To this end, we tested the sensitivity of HuIFN-γ to various detergents, urea, lipid solvents, alcohols, and hydrolytic enzymes. In addition, the binding properties of HuIFN-γ

Table 10. Influence of different hydrolases on HuIFN-γ[a] (GEORGIADES et al. 1981)

Enzymes SEA-induced HuIFN-γ	Phospholipases						
	None	Lipase	A2	C	D	Lysozyme	Neuraminidase
1 h	200	100	100	1,000	100	100	100
6 h	10	200	100	10	80	100	100
Enzyme control	0	0	0	0	0	0	0

[a] HuIFN-γ was mixed with enzyme in proportions of 10:1; the mixture was vortexed for 10–15 s and incubated in a water bath for 60 min at 37 °C. Immediately thereafter, mixtures were assayed for antiviral activity

to lipophilic matrices were examined (GEORGIADES et al. 1981). Of the several detergents tested, only ionic detergents inactivated HuIFN-γ. Nonionic detergents showed only a slight inhibitory effect (Table 8). The inactivation of interferon by ionic detergents might have been due to the solubilization of a putative lipid portion of the HuIFN-γ molecule. Thus, HuIFN-γ is lipoprotein in nature.

Further support for this idea was provided by experiments in the lipid solvents as shown in Table 9. In contrast to HuIFN-α and HuIFN-β, the HuIFN-γ appeared to be sensitive to all polar solvents tested. Nonpolar or very weakly polar solvents such as *n*-hexane or benzene showed a less marked effect on the reduction of the antiviral titer of HuIFN-γ. Alcohols in concentrations greater than 20% drastically reduced IFN-γ activity (Fig. 4). This reduction was irreversible. The degree of inhibition of HuIFN-γ activity by the alcohols increased with increasing carbon chain length of the alcohol. To confirm the involvement of the lipids in the HuIFN-γ molecule, we also tested the effect of different hydrolases on its antiviral activity. Table 10 summarizes the results obtained following treatment of HuIFN-γ with different enzymes. Phospholipase C gave in initial increase in HuIFN-γ activity followed by a decreasing activity with further incubation. Other lipid hydrolases, such as phospholipases A and D and lipase had no effect on HuIFN-γ (Table 10). Since phospholipase C had a profound effect on HuIFN-γ activity, one possibility was that the enzyme acted on a phospholipid localized on the surface of the HuIFN-γ molecule (a hydrophobic region). To determine if one or more large hydrophobic regions were accessible, we tested the behavior of the SEA-induced HuIFN-γ on lipid-binding matrices (Fig. 5). HuIFN-γ does not show affinity to any of the matrices studied. These results suggested that the essential lipid component, if it exists, might be small, or localized within the molecular structure. The surface of the HuIFN-γ was apparently free of large hydrophobic elements.

During purification procedures, we observed considerable losses in HuIFN-γ. One of the reasons might have been delipidation of HuIFN-γ occurring upon chromatography on Matrex Blue and CPG. Removal of the protective lipid layer may cause in alteration in the quarternary structure of the HuIFN-γ molecule and lead ultimately to its inactivation. Experiments directed toward this problem revealed that HuIFN-γ was sensitive to different glycols and glycerol (Fig. 6). J. J. SEDMAK

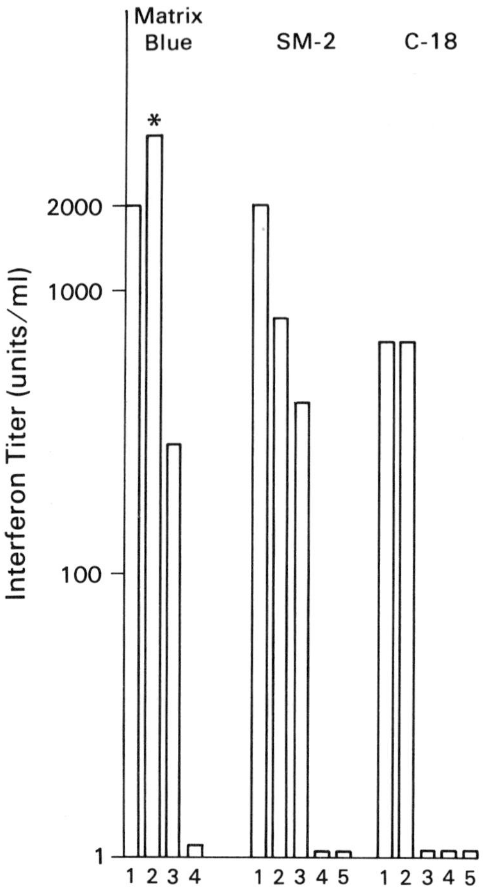

Fig. 5. Elution profile of crude HuIFN-γ on Matrex Blue, SM-2, and C-18 hydrophobic columns. Before use, columns were equilibrated with PBS, pH 7.2. 10 ml crude HuIFN-γ was loaded on each column. The bars represent: (1) the total amount of HuIFN-γ loaded; (2) unbound to the column; (3) HuIFN-γ eluted with PBS; (4) and (5) HuIFN-γ eluted with 1 *M* NaCl. Samples were stored at +4 °C until assayed. Interferon titers were determined in WISH cells. Asterisk represents the protentiation of HuIFN-γ titer described in the text. J. A. GEORGIADES (1980, unpublished work)

et al. (1980, personal communication) observed that ethylene glycol inactivates HuIFN-γ. Our studies with ethylene glycol and its analogs suggested that sensitivity seemed to depend on the position of the hydroxyl group in the carbon chain of the glycol. Removal of ethylene glycol from the IFN-γ preparation considerably improved the stability of HuIFN-γ.

However, upon prolonged incubation at 37 °C, the decay of HuIFN-γ activity was still observed. Proteases or hydrolases might have been responsible for this decay. Since addition of protease inhibitors such as L-1-tosylamide-2-phenylethylchloromethyl ketone (TPCK) and phenylmethylsulfonylfluoride (PMSF) did

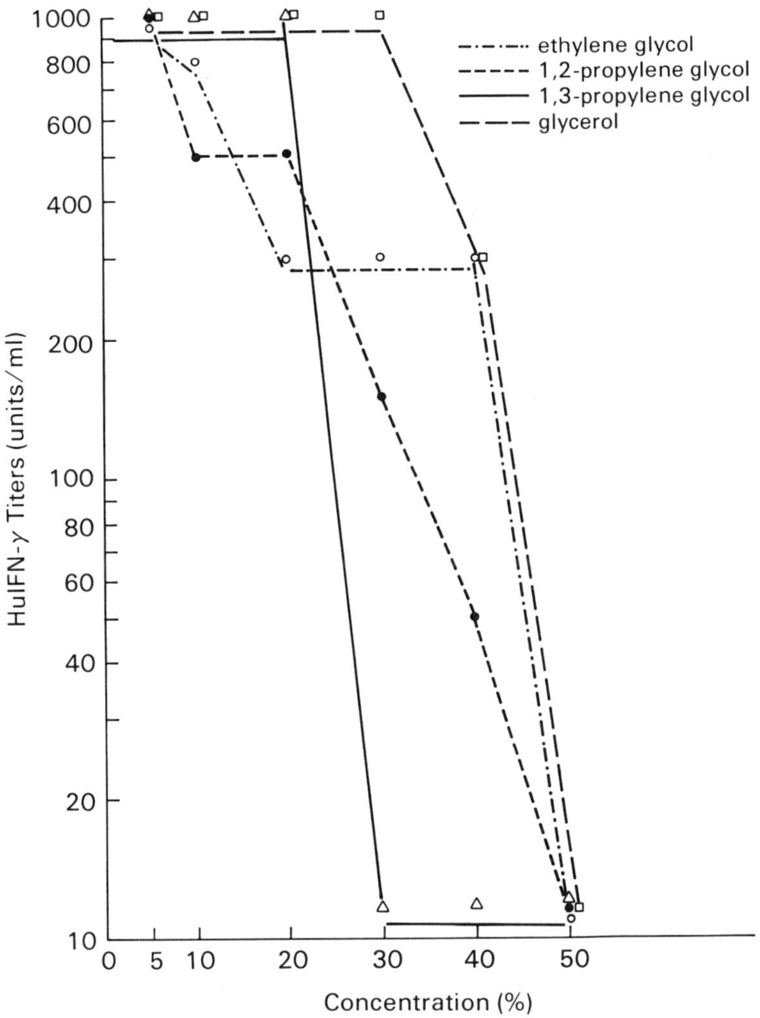

Fig. 6. Inactivation of crude HuIFN-γ by ethylene glycol, 1,2-propylene glycol, 1,3-propylene glycol, and glycerol. Crude HuIFN-γ was mixed in equal proportions with 0.5 ml of each of the individual reagents. Each compound was previously properly diluted in PBS to reach the desired concentrations. The solutions with crude HuIFN-γ were mixed at room temperature on a vortex mixer for 10–20 s and than allowed to incubate for 1 h at 37 °C. Immediately after incubation, aliquots of each mixture were assayed for antiviral activity on WISH cells. J. A. Georgiades (1980, unpublished work)

not inhibit interferon decay, we decided to test the possibility that hydrolases resistant to these inhibitors might be present in our HuIFN-γ preparations. This problem was attacked by analyzing changes in AcA54 elution profiles of HuIFN-γ after incubation at 37 °C. Figure 7a presents the elution profile of SEA-induced HuIFN-γ purified on CPG and stabilized by dialyzing against PBS and 1.0 *M* NaCl. Apparently different molecular weight species ranging in size from 20,000 to 100,000 were observed. Figure 7b shows elution profiles of the same HuIFN-γ incubated for about 8 h at 37 °C. A profound change in protein and HuIFN-γ activities was noted. These changes were connected with considerable losses in HuIFN-γ activity. If the same HuIFN-γ preparations were treated for 30 min with phospholipase C, similar changes occured, suggesting that addition of phospholipase C to interferon accelerated the decay process (Fig. 7c). Even more dramatic changes were seen when the incubation period was further prolonged (Fig. 7d). Results presented in Fig. 7 suggested the presence in IFN-γ preparations of endogenous enzymes which cleave the HuIFN-γ molecule. Further experiments confirmed our finding that endogenous phospholipase may be responsible for HuIFN-γ decay (J. A. GEORGIADES 1981, unpublished work). A colorilmetric assay (KURIOKA and MATSUDA 1975) with *p*-Nitrophenylphosphorylcholine as a substrate for phospholipase C demonstrated the presence of such activities in concentrated HuIFN-γ preparations (GEORGIADES et al. 1982). The enzyme was absent from media from noninduced cultures. Additional studies also revealed presence in interferon preparations of a group of proteases resistant of inhibition by trypsin inhibitor, 1,2-phenantroline, NaN_3, TPCK, and PMSF. This has been revealed by using the SCHUMACHER and SCHILL (1972) method. The presented data demonstrate multiple causes of HuIFN-γ decay.

VII. Classification of IFN-γ Subspecies

Data accumulated from an immunologic classification of HuIFN-γ suggested the existence of more than one species (FALCOFF et al. 1980; GOLDSTEIN et al. 1979, 1981; LANGFORD et al. 1981). Physicochemical properties of HuIFN-γ reported by us and others also support these observations (ANKEL et al. 1980; MIZRAHI et al. 1978; WIETZERBIN et al. 1978). Furthermore, purification of the HuIFN-γ induced by different mitogens revealed that these HuIFN-γ interacted differently with Matrex Blue beads (see Table 6; GOLDSTEIN et al. 1981). These preliminary observations, together with analytic electrodynamic studies by us (GEORGIADES et al. 1980a; GOLDSTEIN et al. 1979, 1981), suggested the existence of multiple HuIFN-γ species which shared different physicochemical properties. To further investigate this possibility, larger quantities of highly purified HuIFN-γ were prepared by means of the PIEF technique (GOLDSTEIN et al. 1981).

SEA-induced HuIFN-γ, prior to separation on PIEF, was purified on Matrex Blue, CPG, and AcA54. Isospecies of HuIFN-γ isolated by means of PIEF were characterized further using the following criteria:

1. Adsorbtion to Matrex Blue beads
2. pI range in which HuIFN-γ activity was found
3. Sensitivity to pH 2.0 treatment
4. Sensitivity to lipid solvents
5. Potentiation of HuIFN-β antiviral activity
6. Neutralization by antibody to SEA-induced HuIFN-γ
7. Neutralization by antibody to con A-induced HuIFN-γ

Antiserum against the major species (56,000 daltons) of SEA-induced HuIFN-γ was prepared in rabbits (LANGFORD et al. 1981). Antiserum to con A-induced in-

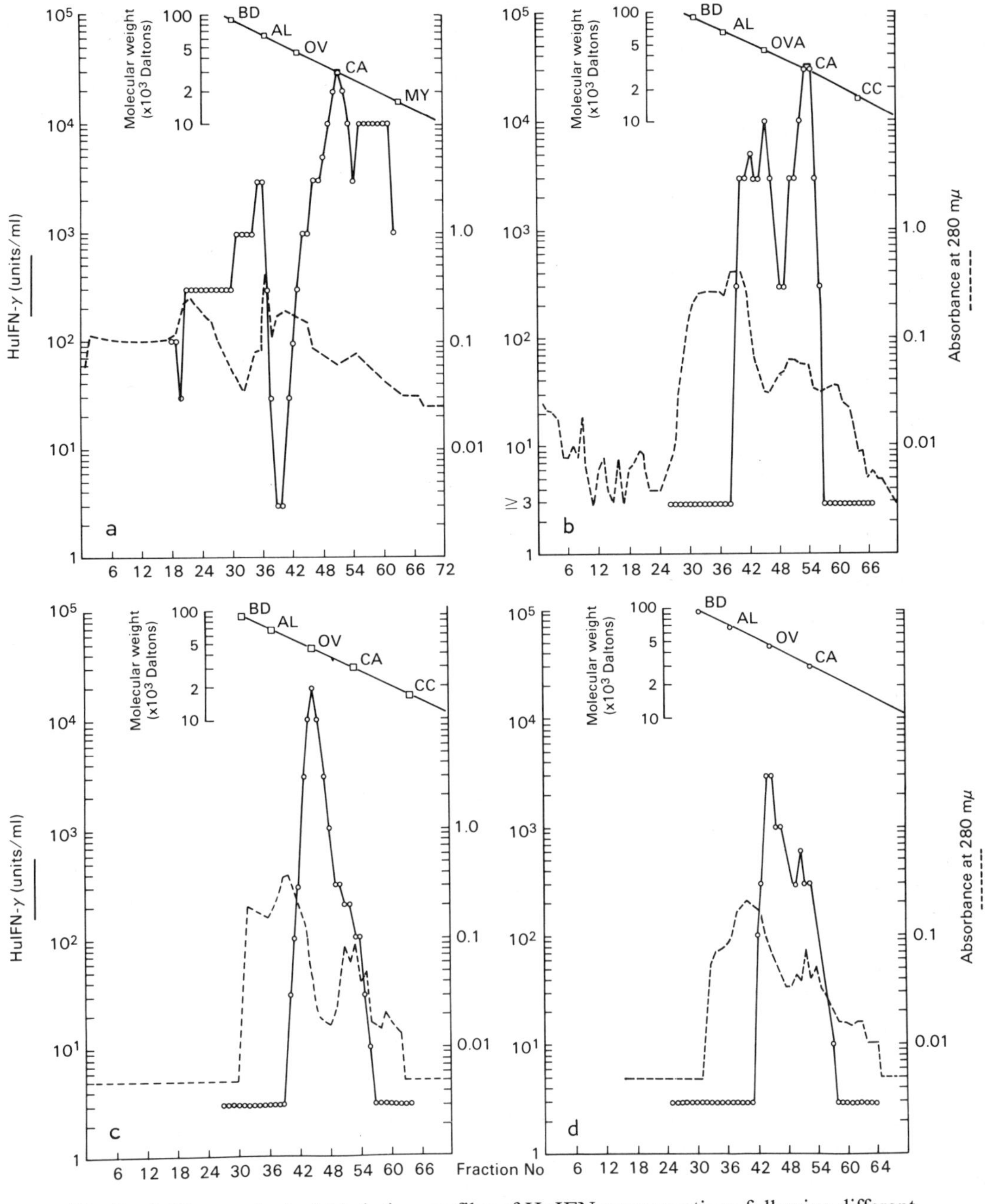

Fig. 7 a–d. Changes in AcA54 elution profiles of HuIFN-γ preparations following different treatments. HuIFN-γ purified on CPG was dialyzed overnight against PBS buffer with 1 *M* NaCl, and 5 ml interferon was loaded: **a** immediately onto AcA54 column (90 × 2.5 cm); **b** after incubations for 8 h to 37 °C; **c** after incubation for 30 min at 37 °C with phospholipase C; **d** after incubation for 1 h at 37 °C with phospholipase C. AcA54 column was equilibrated with buffer-connected PBS supplemented with 1 *M* NaCl and 5% ethylene glycol, 10-ml fractions were collected. Molecular weight standards: Blue dextran (*BD*), bovine serum albumin (*AL*), ovalbumin (*OV*), carbonic anhydrase (*CA*), and cytochrome *c* (*CC*). J. A. Georgiades (1980, unpublished work)

Table 11. Interferon species recognized following application of different criteria (GOLDSTEIN et al. 1981)

HuIFN-γ subclasses	2	11	3	12	6	14
Adsorption to Matrex Blue	Yes	No	Yes	No	Yes	NO
pI range	10.2–9.6	10.0–9.3	9.2–8.9	9.1–8.7	7.4–7.1	7.2–6.9
pH 2.0 sensitivity [a]	R	R	S	R	S	R
Lipid solvent sensitivity [a]	R	S	S	S	S	R
Sensitivity to SEA-induced IFN antibodies [a]	S	R	R	R	R	R
Sensitivity to con A-induced IFN antibodies [a]	R	S	S	S	S	S
Potentiation of HuIFN-β [b]	No	No	Yes	Partial	Yes	No

[a] R = resistant; S = sensitive (about 100% loss of interferon activity)
[b] Potentiation was measured by mixing equal concentration of HuIFN-β with HuIFN-γ in a plaque reduction assay system

terferon provided by Dr. M. DE LEY, Rega Institute, Catholic University of Leuven, Leuven, Belgium (DE LEY et al. 1980). This antiserum was obtained following immunization of rabbits against the major HuIFN-γ species present in 18-h-old leukocyte cultures induced by con A. Antiserum to SEA-induced IFN at a dilution of 1:1,000 neutralized 10 reference units HuIFN-γ. Dr. DE LEY's antiserum had 32,000 neutralization units per milliliter. Neutralization tests with isospecies of the HuIFN-γ isolated by means of the PIEF method were performed by mixing equal volumes of various dilutions of interferon with 150 neutralization units antibody. Results showing ≧10-fold reduction of the interferon titer were considered statistically significant. IFN separated by PIEF and characterized by the criteria already mentioned revealed the presence of a number of apparently different classes of the HuIFN-γ (GOLDSTEIN et al. 1981). Three isospecies, selected as examples from Matrex Blue and three isospecies from CPG-bound material, are shown in Table 11. It is apparent that differences exist not only among the species within each group (Matrex Blue or CPG), but also between groups when similar pI species are compared.

During these investigations, we found isospecies which were resistant to pH 2.0 treatment, and failed to potentiate HuIFN-β (Table 11, subclass 14). However, they were neutralized by antiserum to HuIFN-γ. The question a rises whether such species can be classified as HuIFN-γ or whether they represent another antigenic group. This observation is in good agreement with other reports (FALCOFF et al. 1980; GOLDSTEIN et al. 1979; LANGFORD et al. 1981).

Identification of many different HuIFN-γ isospecies immediately raises ts are in progress to answer this question. Also, it will be of interest to determine whether maximal HuIFN-γ activity is regulated by specific stoichiometric interactions among different HuIFN-γ species. Evaluation of the biologic role of these many possible forms is also necessary.

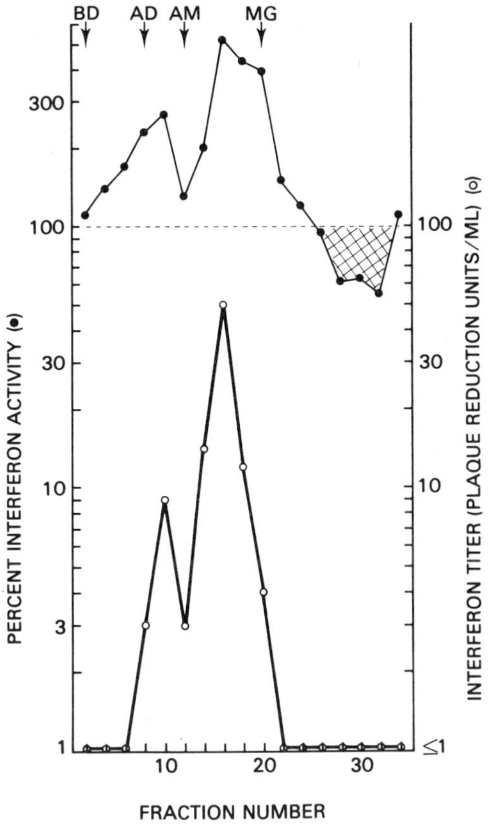

Fig. 8. Separation of interferon and inhibitor activities by AcA34 purification. Crude immune interferon was passed through an AcA34 gel filtration column (2.5×60 cm). Fractions (5 ml) were collected and assayed for interferon (IFN) and inhibitor activities. Interferon titers were determined by plaque reduction assay. For inhibitor titration, column fractions were combined with fibroblast interferon (final concentration, 25 U fibroblast interferon per milliliter), and the protective capacity of the mixture was determined by yield reduction assay. The data are expressed as the percentage of the added interferon activity which was detectable. Values less than 100% represent inhibitor-containing fractions. Values greater than 100% represent potentiator-containing fractions. *Arrows* indicate the elution position of the protein standards used for calibration of the column (BD blue dextran, >350,000 daltons; AD albumin dimer, 134,000 daltons, AM albumin monomer, 67,000 daltons; MG myoglobin, <20,000 daltons). FLEISCHMANN et al. (1979)

VIII. Detection of Other Biologically Active Molecules in IFN-γ Preparations

Migration-inhibitory factor (MIF) is probably the earliest discovered lymphokine. Early attempts at separating MIF from MuIFN-γ failed (YOUNGNER and SALVIN 1973). The question has arisen, then, as to whether MIF and MuIFN-γ might be different biologic expressions of the same molecule. We attempted to solve this problem starting with crude MuIFN-γ preparations. Following sequential precipitation with ammonium sulfate, we found that at least 95% of the MuIFN-γ activity was found in protein fraction precipitated by 55%–80% saturation of ammonium sulfate, whereas most of MIF activity was found in the reconstituted 55% ammonium sulfate precipitate. Furthermore, the remaining MIF activity present in MuIFN-γ fractions were separated by bovine serum albumin–Affi-gel 10 (Bio-Rad, Richmond, California) affinity chromatography (GEORGAIDES et al. 1979 a).

Among the lymphokines previously mentioned is present an inhibitor of MuIFN-γ action. This molecule (or molecules) is seen in preparations where the lymphocytes were in contact with SEA for 3 days or longer. The inhibitor of MuIFN-γ (FLEISCHMANN et al. 1979 a, 1980 a) was first detected because it lowered the protective capacity of MuIFN-γ preparations. The inhibitor was separable from MuIFN-γ by gel filtration chromatography and partially purified by hydrophobic and gel filtration chromatography (Fig. 8). It has also been seen in PHA- or con A-stimulated MuIFN-γ preparations. Its biologic significance is not yet clear, but apparently it plays a role in regulating the activity of IFN. As mentioned earlier, HuIFN-γ exhibit higher anticellular activities than HuIFN-α or HuIFN-β. This anticellular activity was found to copurify with HuIFN-γ (BLALOCK et al. 1980).

To determine the possible role of lymphotoxin in the mediation of the anticellular activity of partially purified HuIFN-γ, cytotoxic activity was monitored during the IFN-γ purification. Over 50% of the lymphotoxin activity of the starting material failed to bind to CPG beads (TRIVERS et al., to be published). The remaining lymphotoxin activity had an elution profile significantly different than HuIFN-γ by AcA54 chromatography. This was evidenced by the presence of lymphotoxin activity in fractions which lacked antiviral activity.

IX. Mechanism of Induction of the Antiviral State by IFN-γ

A striking difference between IFN-γ and other interferons is its slow induction of the antiviral state. As may be seen in Fig. 9, HuIFN-α and HuIFN-β rendered cells resistant to virus rapidly, as compared with HuIFN-γ (LANGFORD et al. 1979). This slow action of IFN-γ might suggest that it acts indirectly as an inducer of the antiviral state and that its true biologic function is other than antiviral. Working with DIANZANI et al. (1980 a), we studied the mechanisms of induction of the antiviral state using human and mouse models. it has been generally accepted that interferon itself is not the direct inhibitor of viral replication. Instead, interferon acts by inducing the cells to produce one or more secondary proteins, which are needed for ultimate antiviral activity by cells. It has been shown by using metabolic inhibitors that HuIFN-α and HuIFN-β directly induce the production of these "antiviral proteins". Specifically, mammalian cells treated with virus-induced interferons in the presence of cycloheximide (an inhibitor of protein synthesis) developed the antiviral state immediately after reversal of the drug action. This finding indicated that a mRNA leading to the production of the antiviral protein was transcribed in the presence of interferon and cycloheximide and was translated only after reversal of cycloheximide action. The addition of actinomycin D before removal of cycloheximide did not block the development of viral resistance. This sug-

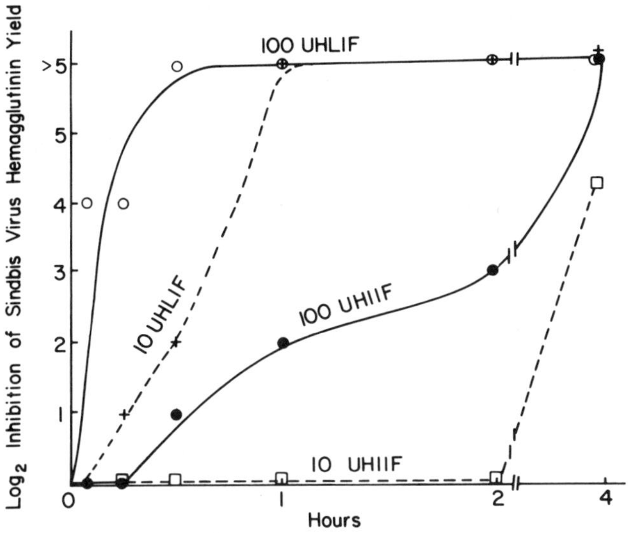

Fig. 9. Development of antiviral activity in human WISH cells treated for various periods of time with the indicated concentrations (U/ml) of HuIFN-γ and HuIFN-α. Interferon activity was measured by a decrease in the hemagglutinin yield of Sindbis virus as described in the text. LANGFORD et al. (1979)

gested that HuIFN-α and HuIFN-β directly induced the antiviral protein or proteins without the need of intermediary proteins. The same experimental plan was used to study the mechanism of activation of the antiviral state by IFN-γ. In contrast to cells treated with virus-induced interferons, cells treated with IFN-γ in the presence of cycloheximide and then actinomycin D failed to develop a significant level of antiviral activity, implying that there are two sequential derepressional events in the mechanism by which IFN-γ activates the antiviral state. Thus, IFN-γ may induce intermediary proteins before the antiviral proteins are made. Similar suggestions were formulated by BAGLIONI and MARONEY (1980).

F. The Prospect of Using IFN for Treatment of Viral and Neoplastic Diseases

The possible application of HuIFN to control certain human diseases was examined immediately after its discovery, and it was strongly supported by successful studies in laboratory animals and also in some localized human infections. It soon became evident, however, that a systemic interferon effect was achieved only with administration of very high doses of exogenous interferon with prolonged levels in the bloodstream. This goal was made more difficult, not only by the scarcity of potent interferon preparations, but also by the rapid clearance of the administered interferon. This problem will be apparently overcome by large scale production of interferon.

The potential for medical application of HuIFN-γ is particularly high since it appears to have a much stronger antitumor activity than HuIFN-α and HuIFN-β (BLALOCK et al. 1980). Furthermore, HuIFN-γ can potentiate the antiviral and antitumor effects of the other two interferons (FLEISCHMANN et al. 1979, 1980). It is possible that this effect may be related to the different mechanisms by which HuIFN-γ and other types of interferon activate cells. In addition, HuIFN-γ preparations, similar to HuIFN-α and HuIFN-β, render target cells resistant to lytic activity of the NK cells (PERUSSIA et al. 1980).

The potentiating capability of mixed preparations of HuIFN-γ and HuIFN-α or HuIFN-β may increase the potency of administered interferon, thus increasing its efficacy. In addition, the use of HuIFN-γ as an alternative treatment, in cases where a high level of gangliosides in blood (KLAPPEL et al. 1977) may make IFN-α or IFN-β ineffective might have obvious advantages (ANKEL et al. 1980). Finally, the observations of FALCOFF et al. (1980) that mouse tumor cells resistant to virus interferon remain sensitive to IFN-γ, might be relevant to interferon therapy. HuIFN-α therapy might select resistant cells that would escape from treatment. Application of HuIFN-γ in such situations might be of great value. Also, alternate therapy with HuIFN-αand HuIFN-γ might be a useful approach in preventing relapse due to selection of resistant cell populations.

Interferons, including HuIFN-γ, promise eventually to be medically relevant. Studies at the molecular, cellular, and whole animal level may lead to such application and will lead to a mechanistic understanding of an essential body system. It is our deep conviction that this goal can be achieved best by studies of highly purified, physicochemically undamaged individual isospecies of HuIFN-γ.

Acknowledgments. The work was supported from the W. Lanier Foundation and the National Cancer Institute. We thank Mrs. DIANE WEIGENT for her skillful secretarial help in typing this manuscript.

References

Adelman EW, Hammond ME, Cohen S, Dvorak FD (1973) Lymphokines as inflammatory mediators. In: Cohen S, Pick E, Oppenheim JJ (eds) Biology of the lymphokines. Academic, New York, pp 13–58

Ankel H, Krishuamurti C, Besancon F, Steafnos S, Falcoff F (1980) Mouse fibroblast (type 1) and immune (type II) interferons: Pronounced differences in affinity to gangliosides and in antiviral and anti-growth effects on mouse leukemia L1210 R cells. Proc Natl Acad Sci USA 77:2528–2532

Baglioni C, Maroney AP (1980) Mechanism of action of human interferon. Induction of 2′5′-oligo A polymerase. J Biol Chem 255:8390–8393

Barness CM, Streips NU, Sonnenfeld G (1980) Effect of carcinogen and analogs on interferon induction. SAG Oncology MS 198. Carcinogen and Interferon, p 1–4

Baron S, Blalock JE, Dianzani F, Fleischmann WR Jr, Georgiades JA, Johnson HM, Stanton GJ (1980) Immune interferon. Some properties and functions. Ann NY Acad Sci 350:130–144

Bergdoll MS (1970) Enterotoxins. In: Martin TC, Kodis S (eds) Toxins. Academic, New York, pp 265–321

Billiau A, Edy VG, Heremans H, van Damme J, Desmyter J, Georgiades JA, de Somer P (1977) Human interferon: Mass production in a newly established cell line. MG63. Antimicrob Agents Chemother 12:11

Blalock JE, Baron S (1977) Interferon-induced transfer of viral resistance between animal cells. Nature 269:422–425

Blalock JE, Baron S (1979) Mechanisms of interferon induced transfer of viral resistance between animal cells. J Gen Virol 42:363–372
Blalock JE, Stanton GJ (1980) Efficient transfer of interferon-induced virus resistance between human cells. J Gen Virol 41:325–331
Blalock JE, Georgiades J, Johnson HM (1979) Immune-type interferon-induced transfer of viral resistance. J Immunol 122:1018–1021
Blalock JE, Georgiades JA, Langford MP, Johnson HM (1980) Purified human immune interferon is a more potent anticellular agent than leukocyte or fibroblast interferons. Cell Immunol 49:390–394
Blalock JE, Weigent DA, Langford MP, Stanton GJ (1980) Transfer of interferon-induced viral resistance from human leukocytes to other cell types. Infect Immun 39:356–360
Boros LD, Carrick LJ (1980) The artificial granuloma II induction of pulmonary granuloma formation by exogenous, circulating and localized granumloma-derived lymphokines. In: De Weck LA, Kristensen F, Landy M (eds) Biochemical characterization of lymphokines. Academic, New York, pp 599–604
Cantell K, Hirvonen S, Mogensen KE, Pyhala L (1974) Human leukocyte interferon: production, purification, stability and animal experiments. The production and use of interferon for the treatment of human virus infections. In Vitro 3:35–38
Cohen S, Bigassi P (1980) Lymphokines, cytokines and interferon(s). In: Gresser J (ed) Interferon 2. Academic, London, pp 81–95
Cohen S, David J, Feldmann U, Glade PR, Oppenheim JJ, Papermaster WB, Pick E, Pierce CW, Rosenstreick DL, Waksman BH (1977) Current state of studies of mediators of cellular immunity: a progress report. Cell Immunol 33:233–244
Dao CD, Bernadau JPM, Bilski-Pasquir (1978) T lymphocyte colonies in the lympho proliferative disorders. Immunology 34:741–750
DeClercq E (1979) New trends in antiviral chemotherapy. Soc Belge Biochem 87:353–359
De Ley M, Van Damme J, Clacys H, Deering H, Heine JW, Billiau A, Vermylen C, De Somer P (1980) Interferon induced in human leukozytes by mitogens: production, partial purification and characterization. Eur J Immunol 10:877–883
Degre M, Pollag H, Mopland B, Sonnenfeld G, De Ley M (1981) Interferon effects on phagocytic cells. Antiviral Res (Abstr 1) 1:14
Dianzani F, Monahan TM, Scupham A, Zucca M (1979) Enzymatic induction of interferon production by galactose oxidase treatment of human lymphoid cells. Infect Immun 26:879–882
Dianzani F, Monahan TM, Georgiades JA, Alperin JB (1980) Human immune interferon: induction in lymphoid cells by a calcium ionophore. Infect Immun 29:561–563
Dianzani F, Zucca M, Scupham A, Georgiades JA (1980a) Immune and virus-induced interferons may activate cells by different derepressional mechanism. Nature 283:400–402
Epstein LB (1975) Mitogen stimulated interferon: the role of human T and B lymphocytes and macrophages. In: Geraldes A (ed) Effects of interferon on cells, viruses and immune system. Academic, New York, pp 393–408
Epstein LB (1977) Mitogen and antigen induction in vitro and in vivo. Tex Rep Biol Med 35:42–56
Epstein LB (1979) The comparative biology of immune and classical interferons. In: Cohen S, Pick E, Oppenheim JJ (eds) Biology of the lymphokines. Academic, New York, pp 443–514
Epstein LB, Ammann AJ (1974) Evaluation of T lymphocyte effector function in immunodeficiency diseases: abnormality in mitogenstimulated interferon in patients with selective IgA deficiency. J Immunol 112:1617–1626
Epstein LB, Cox DR, Lucas DO, Weil J, Epstein CJ (1981) The biology and properties of interferon-gamma: an overview. Antiviral Res (Abstr 1) 1:21
Falcoff E, Falcoff R, Catinot L, Vomecourt A, Sanceau J (1972) Synthesis of interferon in human lymphocytes stimulated in vitro by antilymphocyte serum. Rev Eur Etud Clin Biol 17:20–26
Falcoff E, Wietzerbin J, Stefanos S, Lucero M, Billardin C, Catinot L, Besonson F, Ankel H (1980) Properties of mouse immune T interferon (type II). Ann NY Acad Sci 350:145–156

Falcoff R, Vequero C, Rabourdin C, Sanceau J, Catinot L, Senik A, Andrew G, Fridman W, Falcoff E (1981) Induction of human interferon and lymphokine activites. Antiviral Res (Abstr 1) 1:21

Fleischmann WR Jr (1982) Potentiation of the direct anticellular activity of mouse interferon: Mutual sinergism and interferon concentration dependence. Cancer Res 42:869–875

Fleischmann WR Jr, Georgiades JA, Osborne LC, Johnson HM (1979) Potentiation of interferon activity by mixed preparations of fibroblast and immune interferon. Infect Immun 26:248–253

Fleischmann WR Jr, Georgiades JA, Osborne LC, Dianzani F, Johnson HM (1979a) Induction of an inhibitor of interferon action in a mouse lymphokine preparation. Infect Immun 26:949–955

Fleischmann WR Jr, Kleyn KM, Baron S (1980) Potentiation of antitumor effect of virus-induced interferon by mouse immune interferon preparations. J Natl Cancer Inst 65:936–966

Fleischmann WR Jr, Lefkowitz EJ, Georgiades JA, Johnson HM (1980a) Production and function of an inhibition of interferon action found in mouse lymphokine preparations. In: Khan H, Hill NO, Gordon G (eds) Interferon: properties and clinical uses. L Fikes Foundation, Dallas, pp 195–209

Friedman RM, Cooper JI (1969) Stimulation of interferon production in human lymphocytes by mitogen. Proc Soc Exp Biol Med 125:901–905

Georgiades JA, Langford MP, Stanton GJ, Johnson HM (1979) Purification and potentiation of human immune interferon. IRCS Med Sci 7:559

Georgiades JA, Osborne LC, Moulton RG, Johnson HM (1979a) Separation of immune interferon and MIF. Proc Soc Exp Biol Med 161:167–170

Georgiades JA, Teng JI, Przyjemski J, Smith LL, Johnson HM (1980) Immune interferon and lipid interactions in the purification of interferon. J Appl Biochem 2:81–84

Georgiades JA, Langford MP, Goldstein LD, Blalock JE, Johnson HM (1980a) Human immune interferon: purification and activity against a transformed cell line. In: Khan A, Hill NO, Dorn GL (eds) Interferon: properties and clinical uses. L Fikes Foundation, Dallas, pp 97–108

Georgiades JA, Goldstein LD, Teng J (1981) Human gamma interferon exhibits properties of lipoprotein. Antiviral Res (Abstr 1) 1:85

Georgiades JA, Teng JL, Smith LL (1982) Phospholipase C activity in human interferons in human lymphokines. In: Khan A, Hill NO (eds) The biological immune response modifiers. Academic, New York, pp 519–525

Gery I, Waksman BH (1972) Potentiation of T-lymphocyte response to mitogens. II. The cellular source of potentiating mediator(s). J Exp Med 136:143–155

Goldstein LD, Georgiades JA, Langford MP, Stanton GJ, Johnson HM (1979) Human immune interferon: isoelectrofocusing analysis. IRCS Med Sci 5:560

Goldstein LD, Langford MP, Stanton GJ, De Ley M, Georgiades J (1981) Human gamma interferon: different molecular species. Antiviral Res (Abstr 1), p 43

Green JA, Cooperband SR, Kibrick S (1969) Immune specific induction of interferon production in culture of human blood leukocytes. Science 164:1415–1418

Gresser I, Bandu MT, Brouty-Boye D (1974) Interferon and cell division. IX. Interferon resistant L1210 cells: characteristic and origin. J Natl Cancer Inst 52:558–559

Gresser I. Morel-Manager L, Riviere Y, Guillan J, Towey GU, Woodrow D, Sloper JC, Moss J (1982) Interferon-induced diseases in mice and rats. Ann NY Acad Sci 350:12–20

Harned CJ, Nerland ED, Sonnenfeld G (1982) Effects of positive transfer and induction of gamma type II immune interferon preparations on the interaction of diphenylhydantoin by murine cytochrome P450. Interferon Res 2:5–10

Heremans H, Billiau A, Columbatti A, Hilgers J, De Somer P (1978) Interferon treatment of NZB mice: accelerated progression of autoimmune disease. Infect Immunol 21:925–930

Heron T, Hokland M, Berg K (1978) Enhanced expression of B_2-microglobulin and HLA antigens on human lymphoid cells by IFN. Proc Natl Acad Sci USA 75:6215–6219

Hokland P, Ellegaard J (1981) The effect of α interferon on the natural killer and antibody-dependent cellular cytotoxicity of malignant and nonmalignant lymphocyte subsets in chronic lymphocytic leukemia. Antiviral Res (Abstr 1), 1:84
Hooks JJ, Montsopoulos MH, Gers SA, Stahl IN, Decker HL, Notkins LA (1979) Immune interferon in the circulation of patients with autoimmune disease. New Eng J Med 301:5–8
Hooks JJ, Montsopoulos MH, Notkins LA (1980) The role of interferon in immediate hypersensitivity and autoimmune diseases. Regulatory functions of interferons. Ann NY Acad Sci 350:21–32
Hovanessian AG, Meurs E, Aujean O, Vaquero C, Stefanos S, Falcoff E (1980) Antiviral response and induction of specific proteins in cells treated with immune-T (type III) interferon analogous to that from viral interferon (type I) treated cells. Virology 104:195–204
Hughes TK, Blalock JE, Baron S (1978) Various heterologous cells exhibit interferon induced transfer of viral resistance. Arch Virol 58:77–80
Isaacs A, Lindenmann J (1957) Virus interference. I. The interferon. Proc R Soc London [Biol] 147:258–267
Johnson HM (1981) Cellular regulation of immune interferon production. Antiviral Res 1:37–46
Johnson HM, Baron S (1976) Interferon: effects on the immune response and the mechanism of activation of the cellular responses. CRC Critical Rev Biochem 4:203–227
Johnson HM, Blalock JE (1980) Interferon immuno suppression: mediation by a suppressor factor. Infect Immun 39:301–305
Johnson HM; Stanton GJ, Baron S (1977) Relative ability of mitogen to stimulate production of interferon by lymphoid cells and to induce suppression of the in vitro immune response. Proc Soc Exp Biol Med 154:138–141
Klappel TM, Keenan TD, Freeman MJ, Morre DJ (1977) Glycolipid-bound sialic acid in serum: Increased levels in mice and human bearing mammary carcinomas. proc Natl Acad Sci USA 74:3011–3013
Kumar V, Benz-Ezra J, Bennet M, Sonnenfeld G (1979) NK cell in mice treated with strontium 89. Normal target binding cell numbers but inability to kill even after interferon administration. J Immunol 123:1832–1838
Kurioka S, Matsuda M (1975) Phospholipase C assay using p-nitrophenyl-phosphoryl choline together with sorbitol and its application to studying the metal and detergent requirement of the enzyme. Ann Biochem 75:281–289
Langford MP, Stanton GJ, Johnson HM (1978) Biological effects of staphylococcal enterotoxin A on human peripheral lymphocytes. Infect Immun 22:62–68
Langford MP, Georgiades JA, Stanton GJ, Dianzani F, Johnson HM (1979) Large scale production and physicochemical characterization of human immune interferon. Infect Immun 26:36–41
Langford MP, Weigent DA, Georgiades JA, Johnson HM, Stanton GJ (1981) Antibody to staphylococcal enterotoxin A-induced human immune interferon. J Immunol 126:1620–1623
Mizrahi A, O'Malley J, Caster WA, Takatsuka A, Tamura G, Sulkowski E (1978) Glycosylation of interferons. Effects of tunicamycin on human immune interferon. J Biol Chem 253:7612–7615
Osborne LC, Georgiades JA, Johnson HM (1979) Large scale production and partial purification of mouse immune interferon. Infect Immun 23:80–86
Osborne LC, Georgiades JA, Johnson HM (1980a) Antibody to mouse immune interferon. IRCS Med Sci Biochem 8:212
Osborne LC, Georgiades JA, Johnson HM (1980b) Classification of interferons with antibody to immune interferon. Cell Immunol 53:65–70
Paucker K (1977) Antigenic properties. Tex Rep Biol Med 35:23–28
Perussia B, Santoli D, Trinchieri G (1980) Interferon modulation of natural killer cell activity. Ann NY Acad Sci 350:55
Pross HF, Baines MG (1976) Spontaneous human lymphocyte mediated cytotoxicity against tumor cells. I. The effect of malignant disease. Int J Cancer 18:593–604

Rader CJ, Haliotis T (1980) Do NK cells play a role in anti-tumor surveillance. Immunol Today 2:96–100

Rubin YB, Gupta LS (1980) Differential efficiencies of human type I and type II interferons as antiviral and antiproliferative agents. Proc Natl Acad Sci USA 77:5928–5932

Salvin SB, Youngner JS, Lederer WH (1973) Migration inhibitory factor and interferon in the circulation of mice with hypersensitivity. Infect Immun 7:68

Schmitzer JT, Yitterberg RS (1981) Serum interferon levels in patients with systemic lupus erythematosus. Antiviral Res (Abstr 1) 1:64

Senik A, Lucero M, Castagna M, Steafanos S, Falcoff R (to be published) T interferon (type II) enhances NK cell activity.

Schumacher GFB, Schill WB (1972) Radial diffusion in gel for micro determination of enzymes. II. Plasminogen activator, elastase, and nonspecific proteases. Anal Biochem 48:9–26

Schultz RM (1980) Macrophage activation by interferons. In: Pick E (ed) Lymphokine reports, vol 1. Academic, New York, pp 63–97

Sergiescu D, Cerutti I, Efthymiou E, Kahn A, Chany C (1979) Adverse effects of IFN treatment on the life span of NZB mice. Biomed Express 31:48–51

Simon CL, Farrar JJ, Kind PD (1979) Enhancement by IFN lymphocyte cytotoxicity in normal individuals to cells of human lymphoblastoid lines. J Immunol 121:1173–1176

Skurkovich SV, Eremkina EI (1975) The probable role of IFN in allergy. Ann Allergy 35:356–360

Stabo J, Green F, Jackson L, Baron S (1974) Identification of mouse lymphoid cells required for interferon production following stimulation with mitogens. J Immunol 112:1589–1593

Strannegard O, Bjonkander J, Hermodsson S, Lundgren E, Strannegard IL, Westberg G (1980) Production of interferon in lymphocyte cultures from patients with abnormal immune function. Ann Acad Sci 350:589–590

Sonnenfeld I (1980) Modulation of immunity by interferon. In: Pick E (ed) Lymphokine reports, vol 1. Academic, New York, pp 63–97

Sonnenfeld G, Mandel DA, Merigan CT (1977) The immunosuppressive effect of type II mouse interferon preparations on antibody production. Cell Immunol 34:193–206

Sonnenfeld G, Harned LC, Thaniyavern S, Huff T, Markel DA, Nerland ED (1980) Type II interferon induction and passive transfer depress the murine cytochrome P-450 drug metabolism system. Antimicrob Agents Chemother 17:969–972

Synderman R, Meadows L, Pike CM (1979) Quantification of lymphokine production in human disease. In: Cohen S, Pick E, Oppenheim JJ (eds) Biology of the lymphokines. Academic, New York, pp 181–208

Vantrappen G, Coremans G, Billiau A, De Somer P (1980) Treatment of Crohn's disease with interferon. A preliminary clinical trial. Acta Clin Biol 35:238–242

Virelizier J, Allison AC, De Maeyer E (1977a) Production by mixed lymphocyte cultures of a type II interferon able to protect macrophages against virus infections. Infect Immun 17:282–285

Virelizier LJ, Chan LE, Allison C (1977b) Immunosuppressive effects of lymphocyte (type II) and leukocyte (type I) interferon on primary antibody responses in vivo and in vitro. Clin Exp Immunol 30:299–304

Volle MJ, Jordan GW, Hoahr S, Merigan TC (1975) Characteristics of immune interferon produced by human lymphocyte cultures compared to other human interferons. J Immunol 115:230–233

Waksman BH, Namba Y (1976) Commentary on soluble mediators of immunologic interaction. Cell Immunol 21:161–1761

Wagner H, Hardt C, Hely K, Pfizenmeier K, Solbad W, Bartell R, Stockinger H, Rollinghoff M (1980) T-T cell interactions during cytotoxic T lymphocyte (CTL) responses: T cell derived helper factor (interleukin 2) as a probe to analyze CTL responsiveness and thymic maturation of CTL progenitors. Immunol Rev 51:215

Weissenbach M, Schachter N, Galin M, Baron S (1970) Intraocular production of interferon. Arch Ophthal 84:495–498

Wietzerbin J, Stefanos S, Lucero M, Falcoff E (1978) Presence of polynucleotide binding site on murine immune interferon (T-type). Biochem Biophys Res Comm 85:480–489
Wietzerbin J, Stefanos S, Lucero M, Falcoff E, O'Malley J, Sulkowski E (1979) Physico-chemical characterization and partial purification of mouse immune interferon. J Gen Virology 44:773–781
Wigzell H (1981) Interferon and natural killer cells. Antiviral Res (Abstr 1) 1:16
Wiranowska-Stewart M, Lin LS, Broude JA, Stewart WE II (1980) Production, partial purification, and characterization of human and murine interferons-type II. Mol Immunol 17:625–633
Wheelock EF (1965) Interferon-like virus inhibitor induced in human lymphocytes by phytohemagglutinin. Science 169:310–311
Yip YK, Roy HL, Urban C, Vilcek J (1981) Partial purification and characterization of human (immune) interferon. Proc Natl Acad Sci USA 78:1601–1605
Youngner JS, Salvin SB (1973) Production and properties of migration inhibitory factor and interferon in the circulation of mice with delayed hypersensitivity. J Immunol 111:1914

CHAPTER 16

Comparative Biologic Activities of Human Interferons

P. K. WECK and P. E. CAME

A. Introduction

Interferons have been shown to have a number of biologic activities other than the antiviral properties which first led to their discovery. Since the identification of interferon by ISSACS and LINDENMANN in 1957, numerous studies have been directed toward understanding the multiple effects these proteins have on cellular functions and immune responses (STEWART 1981). Although virus-induced interferons, the classical interferons, have been studied more extensively, primarily because of their availability, it is now well recognized that interferon induced as a result of immune reactions is also a potent antiviral agent (GREEN et al. 1969). This immune interferon first described by WHEELOCK (1965) also has antiproliferative and immunoregulatory activities. However, it differs in its stability at low pH and the conditions required to induce it.

The major classes of interferons can be distinguished by their antigenic properties, stabilities, molecular weights, and cross-species activities. These differences have resulted in the identification of at least three major interferon types with unique biologic properties (VILCEK et al. 1981) and have recently led to the use of a new nomenclature to refer to them as IFN-α (leukocyte), IFN-β (fibroblast), or IFN-γ (immune) interferon (WIRANOWSKA-STEWART and STEWART 1981). The application of recombinant DNA technology has confirmed these differences by showing that there are multiple unique gene sequences for human IFN-α (GOEDDEL et al. 1981) and that these are distinct from the genes coding for human IFN-β or IFN-γ (GOEDDEL et al. 1980a; GRAY et al. 1982). Chapters 4 and 5 of this volume, by SEHGAL and SAGAR and by ZOON and WETZEL, respectively, address a comparative analysis of interferon structural genes and molecular structures of interferons. Whether one type of interferon will prove more effective than another is yet to be determined; however, the availability of sufficient quantities of highly purified materials should permit that analysis. The varied biologic properties ascribed to the three major types of human interferon are indeed numerous and this chapter will compare some of them.

B. Native Interferons: Cell Source

Interferons were originally classified according to the cell type from which a particular interferon was obtained. Hence, interferons induced by viruses in leukocyte cultures or fibroblast cell cultures were referred to as leukocyte or fibroblast interferons, respectively; subsequently they were shown to be antigenically distinct

(HAVELL et al. 1975). For ease of reference in this chapter, any interferons obtained from leukocytes, fibroblasts, or other mammalian tissues are referred to as native interferons and are to be distinguished from interferons derived from bacteria via recombinant DNA technology. The latter interferons are referred to as recombinant DNA-derived interferons. Protocols relying on virus induction have been used to produce large quantities of human leukocyte interferon (CANTELL and HIRVONEN 1977); however, it is difficult to ascertain which of the cell subsets found in the mixed population of leukocytes are responsible for the production of the interferon. Studies by YAMAGUCHI et al. (1977) have shown that a non-T-cell lymphocyte is the source of Sendai virus-induced interferon, but whether this is the case for all viral inducers is not known. Cultured fibroblasts liberate interferon following induction not only with viruses, but with the synthetic polynucleotide poly(rI)·–poly(rC) which induces high titers of human IFN-β (HAVELL and VILCEK 1972). Determining the precise nature of the cell producing this interferon has proven elusive since only 30%–50% of the cells treated with poly(rI)·poly(rC) make interferon (KRONENBERG 1977). Because there are many different viral and nonviral substances which induce the production of IFN-α or IFN-β, it is difficult to reach any general conclusions about which particular cell type might be responding under the influence of each inducing agent (BARON et al. 1979).

Human IFN-γ can be induced by a variety of immune response stimulators. For example, lymphocytes produce IFN-γ in response to such agents as antilymphocyte serum (FALCOFF et al. 1972), purified protein derivative (PPD) (EPSTEIN et al. 1971 a), *Corynebacterium parvum* (SUGIYAMA and EPSTEIN 1978), vaccinia antigen (EPSTEIN et al. 1972), herpes simplex antigens (RASMUSSEN et al. 1974; VALLE et al. 1975), or *Listeria monocytogenes* (NAKANE and MINAGAWA 1981). Inducers such as influenza virus can also cause the induction of high titers of HuIFN-γ in lymphocytes (ENNIS and MEAGER 1981). Recently, inducers such as diterpene esters (YIP et al. 1981 a) or staphylococcal enterotoxins (LANGFORD et al. 1979) have been used in the large scale production and partial purification of human IFN-γ (WIRANOWSKA-STEWART et al. 1980; YIP et al. 1981 b). The synthesis and secretion of this interferon from lymphocytes apparently requires more than a single population of cells and may require direct cell interaction. IFN-γ has been shown to be produced in mixed lymphocyte reactions and protects macrophages against virus infection (VIRELIZIER et al. 1977). EPSTEIN et al. (1971 b) have shown that macrophage and lymphocyte interaction are needed for the production of phytohemagglutinin-stimulated interferon, and more recent studies indicate that a T-lymphocyte subset is responsible for IFN-γ production (EPSTEIN and GUPTA 1981). The use of monoclonal antibodies to cell surface markers has proven that a helper T-cell secretes HuIFN-γ, but that monocytes are required as accessory cells (CHANG et al. 1982). This interferon is unstable at low pH and is not neutralized by antisera directed against human IFN-α or -β.

C. Biologic Activity

I. Antiviral Properties

Native interferons, irrespective of their cellular origin, were discovered as a result of their ability to inhibit virus replication. Human IFN-α and IFN-β have been shown to have activity against a wide spectrum of animal (HILFENHAUS et al. 1975) and human viral agents including such common pathogens as herpes simplex viruses (HSV)-1 and -2 (OVERALL et al. 1980) and rhinoviruses (CAME et al. 1976). The full breadth of antiviral spectrum has recently been reviewed by SEHGAL et al. (1982). Human IFN-γ, which inhibits vesicular stomatitis virus (VSV), has also been shown to inhibit herpesvirus replication (OVERALL et al. 1980).

Human IFN-α and IFN-β have different dose–response curves when titrated in certain assays, which provides further evidence of nonidentity of these interferons (EDY et al. 1976). A separate comparative study using partially purified IFN-α and IFN-γ demonstrated that VSV and encephalomyocarditis virus (EMCV) are inhibited to a greater degree by IFN-α, whereas reovirus and vaccinia virus were more sensitive to IFN-γ (RUBIN and GUPTA 1980). A possible explanation of why the human body would make three different interferons in response to virus infections can be obtained by analysis of in vitro experiments which suggest that the antiviral activities of IFN-β and IFN-γ can be enhanced by mixing these two interferons (FLEISCHMANN et al. 1979).

One of the technical barriers that remains in the way of directly comparing the in vitro activities of interferons from different cell sources is that interferon preparations often contain a mixture of interferon subtypes. For example, certain inducers of IFN-γ also cause the concomitant production of IFN-α (NAKANE and MINAGAWA 1981). Similarly, preparations of human IFN-γ can contain interferon with α-like properties (WIRANOWSKA-STEWART 1981). Furthermore, even highly purified human IFN-α preparations consist of a mixture of heterogeneous molecules that differ in their biophysical and biochemical properties as well as their activities on different cell types (PAUCKER et al. 1977, 1978; LIN et al. 1978; STEWART and DESMYTER 1975; DESMYTER and STEWART 1976). Studies conducted with recombinant DNA-derived IFN-α reveal that each of these subtypes apparently has different potency when tested in cell cultures of different species (WECK et al. 1981 a). It now seems likely that the presence of subtypes in unpurified preparations of native interferons led to earlier observations that interferons can cross species barriers (DESMYTER et al. 1968) and show activity on bovine or procine cells (GRESSER et al. 1974). In contrast to IFN-α, human IFN-β and IFN-γ have exhibited considerably less cross-species activity (DESMYTER and STEWART 1976; GRESSER et al. 1974; STEWART 1981). In addition to a difference in breadth of species specificity, the antiviral acitivity of IFN-γ also differs from the other two types in that it must be in contact with cells for a greater period of time for it to exert its activity. IFN-γ apparently activates cells more slowly than virus-induced interferon (DIANZANI et al. 1978).

In vivo studies designed to compare the antiviral properties of native human IFN-α and IFN-β have demonstrated that both are active in nonhuman primate systems. Work by LVOVSKY et al. (1981) has shown that primate viruses such as herpesvirus saimiri are sensitive to IFN-α. Human IFN-α and IFN-β were equally effective in preventing HSV-1-induced keratitis in African green monkeys treated with preparations containing 1.9×10^6 U/ml, and slight differences in efficacy of the two interferons at lower doses did not prove to be significantly different (NEUMANN-HAEFLIN 1977). These two interferons have also been used effectively to treat rabies virus-infected monkeys (HILFENHAUS et al. 1977 b). In in vitro studies conducted earlier it was demonstrated that oncogenic herpesviruses are affected by human IFN-α preparations and this activity is reflected in vivo in nonhuman primates (LAUFS et al. 1974). Quantitative comparative studies with human IFN-α, IFN-β, and IFN-γ should be possible using these animal models.

II. Growth Inhibition

Interferons induce an antiviral state in cells, and these polypeptides also inhibit or slow cell replication. Such effects on cellular function are apparent on both normal and transformed cell types (WILLIAMS et al. 1981) and many reports exist concerning the inhibition of cell division by human interferons. Thus, the biologic characteristic of interferon as a growth inhibitor has been examined in many systems and tested for inhibition of normal and neoplastic cells including hemopoietic cell colony growth (BALKWILL and OLIVER 1977; MCNEILL and GRESSER 1973), human tumor colony formation (BRADLEY and RUSCETTI 1981), and Daudi cell growth (GEWERT et al. 1981). Also, human bone marrow cell and fibroblast cell proliferation is reduced when these cells are cultured in the presence of either human IFN-α or -β (NISSEN et al. 1977; VAN'T HULL et al. 1978). Studies by BLALOCK et al. (1980) with partially purified IFN-α, -β or -γ demonstrated that the IFN-γ preparation they used was 20 or 100 times more potent than the IFN-β or IFN-α preparations, respectively, in inhibiting WISH or Hep-2 cell colony formation. It is noteworthy that these interferon preparations were of similar specific activities in antiviral units on WISH cells ($1-2 \times 10^6$ U/per milligram protein), therefore essentially equal amounts of proteins were added to the cell cultures.

Testing of native human IFN-α and IFN-β for anticellular activity has also been conducted against a series of transformed human fibroblast cell lines and has shown these cells to be more sensitive to IFN-β than to IFN-α (KUWATA et al. 1979). However, they reported equivalence of the antiviral potency of the two interferons, indicating that there is not a direct relationship between antiviral and antiproliferative activities, even though these diverse properties reside in the same polypeptide molecule (KNIGHT 1976; STEWART et al. 1976). Other experiments have demonstrated that human IFN-β is more suppressive than IFN-α on the growth of osteosarcoma cells while IFN-α showed greater activity against a lymphoblastoid cell line (EINHORN and STRANDER 1977). In contrast, the Daudi lymphoblastoid line showed little difference in its sensitivity to these two interferons (HILFENHAUS et al. 1976, 1977a). Comparison of the effects of IFN-α and -β on growth of normal and chronic myelogenous leukemic cells has shown that IFN-β is more inhibitory against granulocytic progenitor cells from hematologically normal individuals (WILLIAMS et al. 1981).

Results from experiments performed even with partially purified materials must be interpreted with some caution owing to the possible presence of other biologically active components. Lymphocytes readily synthesize other cellular proteins such as lymphotoxin (KLIMPEL et al. 1975, 1977) or migration-inhibitory factor (BLOCK et al. 1977) when induced to make interferon, and lymphotoxin and other lymphokines also possess cell growth-inhibitory activities (WARE and GRANGER 1979). The recent availability of purified native IFN-β preparations which possess significant anticellular properties (ITO and BUFFETT 1981), demonstrate that the antiproliferative property resides in the interferon molecule. However, not until purified preparations of the subtypes of IFN-α, -β or -γ are available will it be possible to quantify with precision the growth-inhibitory properties of interferons.

The biochemical mechanism for the regulation of cell growth by interferons is not well understood. Most of the data available at present indicate that interferon delays the traverse of a cell through the various phases of the cell cycle. This delay is dose dependent in cells that are sensitive to interferon and correlates with expected reductions in cellular macromolecular synthesis. For example, GEWERT et al. (1981) have shown that lymphoblastoid interferon profoundly decreases membrane transport and subsequent phosphorylation of thymidine in Daudi cells. Studies on glioma cells have shown that interferon treatment blocks the cell in S phase (LUNDBLAD and LUNDGREN 1981) and that both IFN-α and IFN-β also alter the duration of other phases of the cell cycle (LUNDGREN et al. 1979). Work with several melanoma cell lines has revealed considerable heterogeneity as to where they were blocked in the cell cycle following interferon treatment (CREASEY et al. 1980). That is, certain lines were stopped at G_0/G_1 whereas others were blocked in G_1, S_1, or G_2+M. Evidence also exists to indicate that treated cells progress slowly through one cell cycle and then fail to enter a new cycle. This is supported by the observation that, in the presence of interferon, Daudi cells which are dividing exponentially are less sensitive to inhibition than cells which have been resting and then stimulated to proliferate (HOROSZEWICZ et al. 1979). This effect of interferon on cell cycling is apparently a reversible event that is cytostatic and not cytocidal in nature; since after a lag period cells removed from interferon will resume dividing at a rate similar to control cultures (KNIGHT 1976). Whether all three types of human interferons alter cell proliferation via similar mechanisms is unknown, as is the relationship between such mechanisms and antiviral activities.

III. Immunoregulatory Properties

One of the most interesting and potentially important properties of interferons is their activities as immunomodulatory agents (EPSTEIN 1977; VILCEK et al. 1980a; DEMAEYER and DEMAEYER-GUIGNARD 1981). While numerous studies have been undertaken to measure the effects of human interferon on the immune response in vitro, very few experiments have been specifically designed to compare the activities of human IFN-α, -β, and -γ directly. Even with the recent availability of purified native IFN-α and -β, insufficient quantities of purified human IFN-γ have limited comparative immunoregulatory studies. However, separate studies have clearly demonstrated that all three types of interferon markedly enhance human natural killer (NK) cell activity in vitro. IFN-γ preparations can increase both antibody-dependent cell-mediated cytotoxicity (ADCC) against human liver cells and NK cell activity against K562 human leukemia target cells (CATALONA et al. 1981). Similar results have been obtained using purified fibroblast interferon in systems measuring cytotoxic T-cell responses or NK cell activity (ZARLING 1981). NK cell activity and ADCC are also augmented by the presence of purified native IFN-α in cell cultures (HERBERMAN et al. 1981) as is T-lymphocyte killer cell efficiency (HERON et al. 1976). Whether these increased cellular functions require the synthesis of new polypeptides is not clear. Furthermore, the role and relative potencies of subtypes within the native interferon preparations is still difficult to define.

Treatment of human lymphocytes with interferon generates enhanced synthesis of at least eight proteins in T-cell populations (Cooper et al. 1982) and lymphokine production in mitogen-stimulated cells is also enhanced by interferon (Blomgren and Einhern 1981). The biosynthesis of these new cell products may be responsible for the enhanced cell activity. For example, the cytocidal activity of macrophages from cancer patients is augmented by the addition of interferon or other lymphokines to cell cultures (Peri et al. 1981).

Just as interferons enhance the activity of lymphoid cell functions, they can also cause marked immunosuppression (Kadish et al. 1980). Human IFN-α significantly supresses the response of human lymphocytes to various mitogens, specific antigens, or allogeneic lymphocytes (Blomgren et al. 1974). Both IFN-α and IFN-β are capable of causing reduced DNA synthesis in mitogen-treated cultures, but dose responses to the interferons are quite different (Miorner et al. 1978). Lymphoblastogenesis in cells from patients with Down's syndrome can also be inhibited by human interferons (Guarari-Rotman et al. 1978) and IFN-α and IFN-β are equally effective in inhibiting ^{3}H thymidine incorporation by cultured cells (Cupples and Tan 1977).

The direction of the cellular responses may be related to the dose or to the time at which the addition of interferon is made to the responder cells. One index of the ability of human IFN-α to modulate human immune response in vitro has been determined by measuring the number of antibody-synthesizing cells to red cell antigen (Parker et al. 1981). Addition of interferon 24 h prior to the antigen caused a significant enhancement in the number of plaque-forming cells, whereas simulatenous addition resulted in a marked suppression. These opposite responses could be elicited with as little as 10 U interferon. Similarly, the effect of human IFN-α on pokeweed mitogen-induced B-cell differentiation varies with interferon concentration (Choi et al. 1981). That is, 100 U/ml cause an enhancement, in contrast to 10,000 U/ml which suppress the response. Such differences are also related to the cell type responding to interferon treatment. These experiments indicated that enhancement was mediated by activation of monocytes, but suppression was the result of an increased T-cell population (Choi et al. 1981). Immunoglobulin synthesis by pokeweed mitogen-stimulated human lymphocytes also varies according to the time of addition of interferon (Harfast et al. 1981). Pretreatment of cells with partially purified IFN-α resulted in greater than 100% increase in total IgG production, but when interferon was present throughout the incubation period of 7 days, immunoglobulin synthesis was significantly reduced. Separation of lymphocyte subpopulations followed by independent treatment of each cell type revealed that pretreatment of B-cells was needed for enhanced antibody synthesis and mixtures containing IFN-treated T-cells or monocytes and untreated B-cells did not produce increased amounts of IgG (Harfast et al. 1981).

Thus, interferon can have multiple and diverse effects on human lymphocyte functions and apparently can alter both humoral and cellular immune responses. However, a variety of experimental models now exist that enable qualitative and quantitative comparisons of the major types and α subtypes of interferons. It will be especially interesting to see if highly purified IFN-γ, a product of a particular lymphocyte population, is a more potent mediator of lymphocyte function than the α and β counterparts. The previous identification of numerous lymphokine activities in culture fluids from mitogen- or antigen-stimulated human lymphocytes will make an accurate assessment of interferons' immunoregulatory properties an extraordinarily difficult, but exciting challenge. It may be that interferons act in concert or synergy with other lymphocyte products to exert their effects on immune cell functions.

IV. Other Biologic Properties

In addition to the antiviral (STEWART 1981) and growth-inhibitory (GRESSER and TOVEY 1978) properties of native interferons, many other biologic activities associated with interferons have been described and reviewed more extensively elsewhere (EPSTEIN 1979; STEWART 1981). Some of the activities described include effects on the membrane and cytoskeletal components of cells following treatment with interferon (MUNIZ and CARRASCO 1981; CHANY 1981). "Priming" of interferon action on cells was one of the first activities described that is not directly related to virus replication (STEWART et al. 1971; FLEISCHMANN 1977). Interferon can inhibit cell fusion induced by Sendai virus (TOMITA and KUWATA 1981), cause increases in the number of lupus inclusions in certain cell lines (RICH 1981), and alter the fatty acids in uninfected cells (APOSTOLOV and BARKER 1981). Unfortunately, there is little information available on the effects of the major types of interferons in such systems and further study is required to predict whether these properties are common to all interferons or primarily the function of one or more subtypes.

V. Absorption and Distribution

An interesting property of the interferons is the relatively short circulating half-life observed when they are administered exogenously. Intravenous injections of human interferons to either experimental animals or human patients have shown that native human IFN-α or IFN-β is removed from the circulation with an initial half-life of approximately 15–20 min and a second phase clearance rate of about 1–2 h (CANTELL and PHYALA 1973; SKREKO et al. 1973; HABIF et al. 1975; EMODI et al. 1975; BOCCI 1977). Human IFN-α administered intramuscularly results in a slower appearance of interferon in the bloodstream, but a prolonged serum interferon half-life is observed (CANTELL et al. 1974). Similar results have been obtained using a number of different species including guinea pigs, rabbits, and sheep injected intramuscularly with human IFN-α (CANTELL et al. 1974; VILCEK et al. 1980) as well as nonhuman primates injected both intravenously and intramuscularly (SKREKO et al. 1973; HABIF et al. 1975). In contrast, intramuscular administration of native human IFN-β results in nearly undetectable serum levels of interferon activity (BILLIAU et al. 1979; VILCEK et al. 1980b). Investigators have suggested that a low blood level seen following intramuscular administration of IFN-β is due to binding or breakdown of interferon at the site of injection; however, no experiments have been reported to demonstrate such events clearly. Alternatively, it is possible that tissues have a greater abundance of receptor sites for IFN-β than for IFN-α which could explain the apparently more rapid clearance of IFN-β.

It has been suggested that the impurities in interferon preparations used in pharmacokinetic studies may affect clearance rates, but recent work with purified materials has not supported that view. It has been reported that IFN-α enters body fluids more readily and is stable whereas IFN-β diffuses more slowly and appears somewhat unstable in serum (HANLEY et al. 1979; CESARIO et al. 1979), but several other interpretations are available. The pharmacokinetic behavior of human IFN-γ is unknown at present. However, with the recent production of this material for use in human clinical trials new information should be generated soon. It will be of interest to learn if the circulating half-life for this lower molecular weight interferon will be similar to that reported for IFN-α and -β and whether renal clearance approximates that indicated for the other types (BOCCI 1981; BOCCI et al. 1981). Additional studies will also be needed to determine what effect, if any, inactivation, tissue binding, or catabolism at the site of injection has on the bioavailability of all types of interferon since these molecules are of varied chemical composition and stability (EDY et al. 1979; STEWART et al. 1975). Experiments using radioisotopically labeled purified major interferon types and subtypes may aid in distinguishing between binding and breakdown of interferons.

D. Recombinant DNA-Derived Interferons

The development of recombinant DNA technology in recent years has added a new dimension to interferon research and has resulted in the production of two human IFN-α subtypes (IFN-α_1 and IFN-α_2) which are presently in human clinical trials. The cloning of human genetic information into bacterial plasmids has resulted in the identification of at least 13 unique coding sequences for human IFN-α (GOEDDEL et al. 1980b; LAWN et al. 1981a, 1981c; STREULI et al. 1980; YELVERTON et al. 1981). Subsequent expression of these genes in *Escherichia coli* has revealed the existence of a family of human IFN-α consisting of 165 or 166 amino acid residues and the subtypes appear to have slightly different potencies when assayed in a series of mammalian cell cultures (WECK et al. 1981a). Because interferon derived from human leukocyte cultures is known to be composed of a heterogeneous population of molecules, it is most likely that this naturally derived material is a mixture of these many subtypes. Thus, it was questioned whether the bacteria-derived interferon would display biologic activity similar to the leukocyte-derived material. A limited study in squirrel monkeys challenged with EMCV clearly demonstrated that recombinant DNA-derived human IFN-α_2 was as active as native leukocyte interferon in reducing viremia and mortality (GOEDDEL et al. 1980b). In vitro studies have shown that some subtypes of bacteria-derived human IFN-α species show greater cross-species activity than natural material (STEWART et al. 1980; WECK et al. 1981a) and that native human IFN-α is heterogeneous in size (19–24,000 daltons) while *E. coli*-derived material is homogeneous (STEWART et al. 1980). Differences in size and cross-species antiviral activities of natural material are most probably related to the presence of multiple subtypes in such preparations, but it is not presently possible to determine which of the subtypes is more prevalent. Experiments designed to compare the subtypes in natural material, which can be separated by high pressure liquid chromatography, with those derived from cloning will add greatly to our understanding of the roles of the many subtypes of IFN-α.

Unlike the α subtypes, there is at present strong evidence for only a single species of human IFN-β and IFN-γ as determined by cDNA cloning techniques (DERYNCK et al. 1980; GOEDDEL et al. 1980a; TANIGUCHI et al. 1980b; GRAY et al. 1982). The IFN-β gene resembles the IFN-α genes in that it contains no intron regions (HOUGHTON et al. 1981; LAWN et al. 1981b) and is located on human chromosome 9 (OWERBACH et al. 1981). However, both these genes differ from the human IFN-γ gene which has extensive intervening sequences (GRAY et al. 1982).

Two different systems of nomenclature for the human IFN-α gene sequences have been employed by interferon workers, one by the Genentech group, South San Francisco, California and the other by WEISSMANN's laboratory, Zürich, Switzerland and this has led to some confusion in the description of these molecules. Although all cloned human IFN-α species have not yet been assigned a number, it is now apparent that human IFN-α_1, -α_2, -α_5, and -α_8 according to the nomenclature employed by WEISSMANN and colleagues correspond to LeIF D, A, G, and B respectively as described by the Genentech group (GOEDDEL et al. 1981; WEISSMANN 1981).

As a result of cloning of human IFN-α, -β, and -γ interferon genes in *E. coli*, it is evident that the IFN-α genes have 80%–95% DNA sequence homology and 40%–50% nucleic acid sequence homology with the IFN-β gene (TANIGUCHI et al. 1980a). In addition, the size of these proteins as predicted from their DNA sequences are 20,000, 20,500, and 17,110 daltons for IFN-α, -β, and -γ, respectively (GOEDDEL et al. 1980, 1981; GRAY et al. 1982). These molecular masses differ from those determined for native interferons and it is possible that these and other differences are responsible for some variations of biologic properties observed with the natural proteins. Experiments performed to date indicate that there may be no striking differences between the biologic characteristics of these molecules and the polypeptides derived from mammalian cells, but considerable analysis remains to be accomplished. Human IFN-α, -β, and -γ from *E. coli* are antigenically distinct and in the published reports display in vitro and in vivo antiviral properties very similar to those ascribed to naturally derived interferons (WECK et al. 1981b; STEBBING et al. 1981; GRAY et al. 1982). In addition, bacteria-derived IFN-α_1 has been shown to enhance NK cell activity, enhance ADCC, suppress mitogen-induced leukocyte migration inhibition, and inhibit in vitro tumor cell growth (MASUCCI et al. 1980; STEBBING et al. 1981; LEE et al. 1982).

A comparative study with recombinant DNA-derived IFN-α_1 and -α_2 demonstrated that both interferons caused inhibition of Daudi cell growth in vitro, but had no antiproliferative activity on a human amnion cell line (LEE et al. 1982). Recombinant DNA-derived human IFN-α_2 and buffy coat interferon are both effective in reducing herpetic keratitis in rabbits when applied topically, and intramuscular injection of either had no effect on the course of infection (SMOLIN et al. 1982). In these studies, topical administration of cloned human IFN-α_2 was as effective as native leukocyte-derived interferon in suppressing epithelial damage by day 7, regardless of whether treatment commenced 1 day prior to infection or 2 days postinfection. In vivo studies also showed that cloned IFN-α_1 has limited antiviral activity in a mouse model with EMCV challenge (WECK et al. 1982) and that bacteria-derived IFN-α_1 is more effective than recombinant DNA-derived IFN-α_2 when administered intravenously to EMCV-infected squirrel monkeys

Table 1. Relative antiviral activities[a] of bacteria-derived human interferons in mammalian cell cultures

Cell type		Interferon titers (U/ml)[b]			
		HuIFN-α_1	HuIFN-α_2	HuIFN-β_1	HuIFN-γ_1
Human	HeLa	1,000,000	1,600,000	1,000,000	1,200,000
Bovine	MDBK	13,000,000	3,600,000	N.A.	N.A.
Murine	L929	450,000	N.A.	300	N.A.
Rabbit	RK-13	240,000	18,000	1,600	N.A.
Monkey	Vero	430,000	590,000	100,000	370,000

[a] Interferon activities were determined with materials of greater than 95% homogeneity as measured by polyacrylamide gel electrophoresis

[b] Interferon titers are expressed as determined in microtiter CPE inhibition assays using VSV and standardized against the NIH human leukocyte (G023-901-527), for HuIFN-α and -γ, or human fibroblast (G023-902-527) standards. N.A. indicates no detectable activity

(STEBBING et al., to be published). In similar studies with recombinant DNA-derived human IFN-β_1, no antiviral activity was detected in the mouse EMCV model although it proved as effective as native IFN-β_1 in squirrel monkeys infected with lethal doses of EMCV (HARKINS et al., to be published). The use of nonhuman primate systems may permit direct comparison of the antiviral properties of recombinant DNA-derived human interferons with their native counterparts in vivo.

E. Conclusions

There are a number of very important potential advantages to producing the entire spectrum of human interferons by recombinant DNA methodology. One is the production of large amounts of highly purified material which has enabled the determination of the chemical and biologic properties of cloned human IFN-β_1 (HARKINS et al., to be published) or the assignment of the disulfide bridges of human IFN-α_2 (WETZEL 1981). Second, the presence of common restriction enzyme sites in the IFN-α genes has faciliated the construction and expression of unique genetic hybrids of IFN-α (WECK et al. 1981 b). One of these hybrids, IFN-α_2(B)α_1, is extremely potent as an antiviral and antitumor agent in mice and thus has allowed a number of expriments to examine the activity of this unique interferon in vivo (WECK et al. 1982; LEE et al., to be published). Third, the availability of highly purified preparations of nonglycosylated forms of human IFN-α, -β, and -γ should allow a direct comparison of these three interferons with their native counterparts which may elucidate the role of the carbohydrate embellishment. The data presented in Table 1 are a comparison of the antiviral activity and spectrum of some types and subtypes of interferons in five different mammalian cell cultures. As described earlier for natural material, bacteria-derived human IFN-β_1 and IFN-γ_1 exhibit a greater degree of species specificity than either recombinant DNA-derived IFN-α_1 or -α_2 and suggest that future experimental work examining the biologic activities of these interferons will require nonhuman primate or human systems.

The rapid generation of new information concerning the biologic characteristics of human interferons during the past several years has added greatly to our understanding of the interferon system. However, many questions remain unanswered. One of the most benificial outcomes of the production of human interferons by cloning techniques will be the availability of highly purified single subtypes and combinations of them which will allow a critical assessment of the many and varied properties of interferons. Additionally, for the first time it should make it possible to evaluate the pharmacology of these three major types of human interferon systematically. The direct comparison of highly purified IFN-α, -β, and -γ in different biologic systems will clarify their contributions to host defense mechanisms against viral and neoplastic diseases as well as their roles in regulation of cell division and immunoregulation.

Acknowledgment. The authors wish to thank JEANNE ARCH for her skills in the preparation and critical reading of this chapter.

References

Apostolov K, Barker W (1981) The effects of interferon on the fatty acids in uninfected cells. FEBS Lett 126:261–264

Balkwill FR, Oliver RTD (1977) Inhibitory effects of interferon on normal and malignant human haemopoietic cells. Int J Cancer 20:500–505

Baron S, Brunell PA, Grossberg SE (1979) Mechanisms of action and pharmacology: the immune and interferon systems. In: Galasso GJ, Merigan TC, Buchanan RA (eds) Antiviral agents and viral diseases of man. Raven, New York, pp 151–209

Billiau A, De Somer P, Edy VG, De Clercq E, Heremens H (1979) Human fibroblast interferon for clinical trials: pharmacokinetics and tolerability in experimental animals and humans. Antimicrob Agents Chemother 16:56

Blalock JE, Georgiades JA, Langford MP, Johnson HM (1980) Purified human immune interferon has more potent anticellular activity than fibroblast or leukocyte interferon. Cell Immunol 49:390–394

Block LH, Cantell K, Jamberger S, Ruhevstroth-Bauer G, Strander H (1977) Lack of correspondence between human leukocyte type I interferon and human migration inhibitory factor. Arch Virol 56:341–344

Blomgren H, Einhorn S (1981) Lymphokine production by PHA-stimulated human lymphocytes is enhanced by interferon. Int Arch Allergy Appl Immunol 66:173–178

Blomgren H, Strander H, Cantell K (1974) Effect of human leukocyte interferon on the response of lymphocytes to mitogenic stimuli in vitro. Scand J Immunol 3:697–705

Bocci V (1977) Distribution of interferon in body fluids and tissues. Tex Rep Biol Med 35:436–442

Bocci V (1981) Pharmacokinetic studies of interferons. Pharmacol Ther 13:421–440

Bocci V, Pacini A, Muscettola M, Paulesu L, Pessina GP (1981) Renal metabolism of rabbit serum interferon. J Gen Virol 55:297–304

Bradley EC, Ruscetti FW (1981) Effect of fibroblast, lymphoid and myeloid interferons on human tumor colony formation in vitro. Cancer Res 41:244–249

Came PE, Schafer TW, Silver GH (1976) Sensitivity of rhinoviruses to human leukocyte and fibroblast interferons. J Infect Dis 133:Suppl A136–139

Cantell K, Hirvonen S (1977) Preparation of human leukocyte interferon for clinical use. Tex Rep Biol Med 35:138–144

Cantell K, Phyala L (1973) Circulating interferon in rabbits after administration of human interferon by different routes. J Gen Virol 20:97–104

Cantell K, Phyala L, Strander H (1974) Circulating human interferon after intramuscular injection into animals and man. J Gen Virol 25:453–458

Catalona WJ, Ratliff TL, McCool RE (1981) Gamma interferon induced by Staphylococcus aureus protein A augments natural killing and antibody-dependent cell-mediated cytotoxicity. Nature 291:77–79

Cesario T, Vaziri N, Slater L, Tilles J (1979) Inactivators of fibroblast interferon found in human serum. Infect Immun 24:851

Chang TW, Testa D, Kung PC, Perry L, Dreskin HJ, Goldstein G (1982) Cellular origin and interactions involved in gamma-interferon production induced by OKt3 monoclonal antibody. J Immunol 128:585–589

Chany C (1981) Reorganization of the cytoskeleton by interferon in MSV-transformed cells. J Interferon Res 1:323–332

Choi YS, Lim KH, Sanders FK (1981) Effect of interferon alpha on pokeweed mitogen-induced differentiation of human peripheral blood lymphocytes. Cell Immunol 64:20–28

Cooper HL, Fagnani R, London J, Trepel J, Lester EP (1982) Effect of interferons on protein synthesis in human lymphocytes: enhanced synthesis of eight specific peptides in T cells and activation-dependent inhibition of overall protein synthesis. J Immunol 128:828–833

Creasey AA, Bartholomew JC, Merigan TC (1980) Role of G_0–G_1 arrest in the inhibition of tumor cell growth by interferon. Proc Natl Acad Sci USA 77:1471–1475

Cupples CG, Tan YH (1977) Effect of human interferon preparations on lymphoblastogenesis in Down's syndrome. Nature 267:165–167

De Maeyer E, De Maeyer-Guignard J (1981) Interferons as regulatory agents of the immune system. CRC Crit Rev Immunol 2:167–188

Derynck R, Remaut E, Saman E, Stanssens P, DeClercq E, Content J, Fiers W (1980) Expression of human fibroblast interferon gene in *Eschericha coli*. Nature 287:193–197

Desmyter J, Stewart WE II (1976) Molecular modification of interferon: attainment of human interferon in a conformation active on cat cells but inactive on human cells. Virology 70:451–458

Desmyter J, Rawls WE, Melnick JL (1968) A human interferon that crosses the species line. Proc Natl Acad Sci USA 59:69–76

Dianzani F, Salter L, Fleischmann JR WR, Zucca M (1978) Immune interferon activates cells more slowly than does virus-induced interferon. Proc Soc Exp Biol Med 159:94–99

Edy VG, Billiau A, De Somer P (1976) Human fibroblast and leukocyte interferons show different dose-response curves in assay of cell protection. J Gen Virol 31:251–255

Edy VG, Billiau V, Joniau M, De Somer P (1979) Stabilization of mouse and human interferons by acid pH against inactivation due to shaking and guanidine hydrochloride. Proc Soc Exp Biol Med 146:249–253

Einhorn S, Strander H (1977) Is interferon tissue specific. Effect of human leukocyte and fibroblast interferons on the growth of lymphoblastoid and osteosarcoma cell lines. J Gen Virol 35:573–577

Emodi G, Just M, Hernandez R, Hirt HR (1975) Circulating interferon in man after administration of exogenous human leukocyte interferon. J Natl Cancer Inst 54:1045–1048

Ennis FA, Meager A (1981) Immune interferon produced to high levels by antigenic stimulation of human lymphocytes with influenza virus. J Exp Med 154:1279–1289

Epstein LB (1977) The effects of interferons on the immune response in vitro and in vivo. In: Stewart WE II (ed) Interferons and their actions. CRC, Cleveland, p 91

Epstein LB (1979) The comparative biology of immune and classical interferons. In: Cohen S, Pick E, Oppenheim JJ (eds) Biology of the lymphokines. Academic New York, p 443

Epstein LB, Gupta S (1981) Human T-lymphocyte subset production of immune (gamma) interferon. Clin Immunol 1:186–194

Epstein LB, Cline MJ, Merigan TC (1971 a) PPD-stimulated interferon: in vitro macrophage-lymphocyte interaction in the production of a mediator of cellular immunity. Cell Immunol 2:602–613

Epstein LB, Cline MJ, Merigan RC (1971 b) The interaction of human macrophages and lymphocytes in the phytohemagglutinin stimulated production of interferon. J Clin Invest 50:744–753

Epstein LB, Stevens DA, Merigan TC (1972) Selective increase in lymphocyte interferon response to vaccinia antigen after revaccination. Proc Natl Acad Sci USA 69:2632–2636

Falcoff E, Falcoff R, Catinot L, Vomecourt A, Sanceau J (1972) Synthesis of interferon in human lymphocytes stimulated in vitro by antilymphocytic serum. Rev Eur Etud Clin Biol 17:20–26

Fleischmann Jr WR (1977) Priming of interferon action. Tex Rep Biol Med 35:316–325

Fleischmann WR, Georgiades JA, Osborne LC, Johnson HM (1979) Potentiation of interferon activity by mixed preparations of fibroblast and immune interferon. Infect Immun 26:248–253

Gewert DR, Shah S, Clemens MJ (1981) Inhibition of cell division by interferons. Changes in the transport and intracellular metabolism of thymidine in human lymphoblastoid (Daudi) cells. Eur J Biochem 116:487–492

Goeddel DV, Shepard HM, Yelverton E, Leung D, Crea R, Sloma A, Pestka S (1980 a) Synthesis of human fibroblast interferon by *E. coli*. Nucleic Acids Res 8:4057–4074

Goeddel DV, Yelverton E, Ullrich A, Heyneker HL, Miozzari G, Holmes W, Seeburg P, Dull T, May L, Stebbing N, Crea R, Maeda S, McCandliss R, Sloma A, Tabor JM, Gross M, Familletti PC, Pestka S (1980 b) Human leukocyte interferon produced in *E. coli* is biologically active. Nature 287:411–416

Goeddel DV, Leung DW, Dull TJ, Gross M, McCandliss R, Lawn RM, Seeburg PH, Ullrich A, Yelverton E, Gray PW (1981) The structure of eight distinct cloned human leukocyte interferon cDNAs. Nature 290:20–26

Gray PW, Leung DW, Pennica D, Yelverton E, Najarian R, Simonsen CC, Derynck R, Sherwood PJ, Wallace DM, Berger SL, Levinson AD, Goeddel DV (1982) Expression of human immune interferon cDNA in *E. coli* and monkey cells. Nature 295:503–508

Green JA, Cooperband SR, Kibrick S (1969) Immune specific induction of interferon production in cultures of human blood lymphocytes. Science 164:1415–1417

Gresser I, Tovey MG (1978) Antitumor effects of interferon. Biochim Biophys Acta 516:231–247

Gresser I, Bandu MT, Brouty-Boye D, Tovey M (1974) Pronounced antiviral activity of human interferon on bovine and porcine cells. Nature 251:543–545

Guarari-Rotman D, Revel M, Tartakovsky B, Segal S, Hahn T, Handzel Z, Levin S (1978) Lymphoblastogenesis in Down's syndrome and its inhibition by human interferon. FEBS Lett 94:187–190

Habif DV, Lipton R, Cantell K (1975) Interferon crosses blood-brain barrier in monkeys. Proc Soc Exp Biol Med 149:287–293

Hanley DF, Wiranowska-Stewart M, Stewart II WE (1979) Pharmacology of interferons I. Pharmacologic distinctions between human leukocyte and fibroblast interferons. Int J Immunopharmacol 1:219–226

Harfast B, Huddlestone JR, Casali P, Merigan TC, Oldstone MB (1981) Interferon acts directly on human B lymphocytes to modulate immunoglobulin synthesis. J Immunol 127:2146–2150

Harkins R, Hass PE, Aggarwal BB, Apperson S, Weck PK (to be published) Structural and biological properties of purified bacteria-derived human fibroblast interferon. Proc Natl Acad Sci USA

Havell EA, Vilcek J (1972) Production of high-titered interferon in cultures of human diploid cells. Antimicrob Agents Chemother 2:476–484

Havell EA, Berman B, Ogburn CA, Berg K, Pancker K, Vilcek J (1975) Two antigenically distinct species of human interferon. Proc Natl Acad Sci USA 72:2185–2190

Herberman RB, Ortaldo JR, Rubinstein M, Pestka S (1981) Augmentation of natural and antibody-dependent cell-mediated cytotoxicity by pure human leukocyte interferon. J Clin Immunol 1:149–153

Heron I, Berg K, Cantell K (1976) Regulatory effect of interferon on T cells in vitro. J Immunol 117:1370–1373

Hilfenhaus J, Thierfelder H, Barth R (1975) Sensitivity of various primate cells and animal viruses to the antiviral activity of human leukocyte interferon. Arch Virol 48:203–211

Hilfenhaus J, Damm H, Karges HE, Manthey KF (1976) Growth inhibition of human lymphoblastoid Daudi cells in vitro by interferon preparations. Arch Virol 51:87–97

Hilfenhaus J, Damm H, Johannsen R (1977 a) Sensitivity of various human lymphoblastoid cells to the antiviral and anticellular activity of human leukocyte interferon. Arch Virol 54:271–277

Hilfenhaus J, Weinmann E, Major M, Barth R, Jaeger O (1977 b) Administration of human interferon to rabies virus-infected monkeys after exposure. J Infect Dis 135:846–849

Horoszewicz JS, Leong SS, Carter WA (1979) Noncycling tumor cells are sensitive targets for the antiproliferative activity of human interferon. Science 206:1091–1093

Houghton M, Jackson IJ, Porter AG, Doel SM, Catlin GH, Barber C, Carey NH (1981) The absence of introns within a human fibroblast gene. Nucleic Acids Res 9:247–266

Isaacs A, Lindenmann J (1957) Virus interference I. The interferon. Proc R Soc Lond [Biol] 147:268–273

Ito M, Buffett RF (1981) Cytocidal effect of purified human fibroblast interferon on tumor cells in vitro. J Natl Cancer Inst 66:819–826

Kadish AS, Tansey FA, Yu GS, Doyle AT, Bloom BR (1980) Interferon as a mediator of human lymphocyte suppression. J Exp Med 151:637–650

Klimpel GR, Day KD, Lucas DO (1975) Differential production of interferon and lymphotoxin by human tonsil lymphocytes. Cell Immun 20:187–189

Klimpel GR, Dean JH, Day KD, Chen PB, Lucas DO (1977) Lymphotoxin and interferon production by rosette-separated human peripheral lymphocytes. Cell Immun 32:293–297

Knight E (1976) Antiviral and cell growth inhibitory activities reside in the same glycoprotein of human fibroblast interferon. Nature 262:302–303

Kronenberg LH (1977) Interferon production by individual cells in culture. Virology 76:634–642

Kuwata T, Fuse A, Suzuki N, Morinaga N (1979) Comparison of the suppression of cell and virus growth in transformed human cells of leukocyte and fibroblast interferon. J Gen Virol 43:435–439

Langford MP, Georgiades JA, Stanton GJ, Dianzani F, Johnson HM (1979) Large scale production and physicochemical characterization of human immune interferon. Infect Immun 26:36–41

Laufs R, Steinke H, Jacobs C, Hilfenhaus J, Karges H (1974) Influence of interferon on the replication of oncogenic herpes viruses in tissue cultures and in nonhuman primates. Med Microbiol Immunol 160:285–294

Lawn RM, Adelman J, Dull TJ, Gross M, Goeddel DV, Ullrich A (1981 a) DNA sequence of two closely linked human interferons. Science 212:1159–1162

Lawn RM, Adelman J, Franke AE, Houck CM, Gross M, Najarian R, Goeddel DV (1981 b) Human fibroblast interferon gene lacks interons. Nucleic Acids Res 9:1045–1052

Lawn RM, Gross M, Houck CM, Franke AE, Gray PW, Goeddel DV (1981 c) DNA sequence of a major human leukocyte interferon gene. Proc Natl Acad Sci USA 78:5435–5439

Lee SH, Kelley S, Chiu H, Stebbing N (1982) Stimulation of natural killer cell activity and inhibition of proliferation of various leukemic cells by purified human leukocyte interferon sub-types. Cancer Res 42:1312–1316

Lee SH, Weck PK, Moore J, Chen S, Stebbing N (to be published) Pharmacological comparison of two hybrid recombinant DNA-derived human leukocyte interferons. In: Merigan TC, Friedman R, Fox CF (eds) Chemistry and biology of interferons: relationship to therapeutics, UCLA symp mol cell biol 25. Academic, New York

Lin LS, Wiranowska-Stewart M, Chudzio T, Stewart WE II (1978) Characterization of the heterogeneous molecules of human interferons: differences in cross-species antiviral acitivities of various molecular populations in human leukocyte interferons. J Gen Virol 39:125–130

Lundblad D, Lundgren E (1981) Block of glioma cell line in S by interferon. Int J Cancer 27:749–754

Lundgren E, Larsson I, Miorner H, Strannegard O (1979) Effects of leukocyte and fibroblast interferon on events in the fibroblast cell cycle. J Gen Virol 42:589–595

Lvovsky E, Levine DH, Fucillo D, Ablashi DV, Bengal ZH, Armstrong GR, Levy HB (1981) Epstein-Barr virus and herpes virus saimiri: sensitivity to interferons and interferon inducers. J Natl Cancer Inst 66:1013–1019

Masucci MG, Szigeti R, Klein E, Gruest J, Montagnier L, Taira H, Hall A, Nagata S, Weissmann C (1980) Effect of interferon-α1 from *E. coli* on some cell functions. Science 209:1431–1435

McNeill TA, Gresser I (1973) Inhibition of haemopoietic colony growth by interferon preparations from different sources. Nature 244:173–174

Miorner H, Landstrom LE, Larner E, Larson I, Lundgren E, Strannegard O (1978) Regulation of mitogen-induced lymphocyte DNA synthesis by human interferon of different origins. Cell Immunol 35:15–24

Muniz A, Carrasco L (1981) Protein synthesis and membrane integrity in interferon-treated HeLa cells infected with encephalomyocarditis virus. J Gen Virol 56:153–162

Nakane A, Minagawa T (1981) Alternative induction of interferon alpha and interferon gamma by *Listeria monocytogenes* in human peripheral blood mononuclear leukocyte cultures. J Immunol 126:2139–2142

Neumann-Haeflin D, Sundmacher R, Skoda R, Cantell K (1977) Comparative evaluation of human leukocyte and fibroblast interferon in the prevention of herpes simplex virus keratitis in a monkey model. Infect Immun 17:468–470

Nissen C, Speck B, Emodi G, Iscove NM (1977) Toxicity of human leukocyte interferon preparations in human bone-marrow cultures. Lancet i:203–204

Overall JC, Tze-Jou Y, Kern ER (1980) Sensitivity of herpes simplex virus types 1 and 2 to three preparations of human interferon. J Infect Dis 142:943

Owerbach D, Rutter WJ, Shows TB, Gray P, Goeddel DV, Lawn RM (1981) Leukocyte and fibroblast interferon genes are located on human chromosome 9. Proc Natl Acad Sci USA 78:3123–3127

Parker MA, Mandel AD, Wallace JH, Sonnenfeld G (1981) Modulation of the human in vitro antibody response by human leukocyte interferon preparations. Cell Immunol 58:464–469

Paucker K, Dalton BJ, Torma ET, Osburn CA (1977) Biological properties of human leukocyte interferon components. J Gen Virol 35:341–351

Paucker K, Dalton BJ, Torma ET (1978) Antigenic properties and heterospecific antiviral activities of human leukocyte interferon species. Adv Exp Med Biol 110:75–84

Peri G, Polentarutti N, Sessa C, Mangioni C, Mantovani A (1981) Tumoricidal activity of macrophages isolated from human ascitic and solid ovarian carcinomas: augmentation by interferon, lymphokines and endotoxin. Int J Cancer 28:143–152

Rasmussen LE, Jordan GW, Stevens DA, Merigan TC (1974) Lymphocyte interferon production and transformation after herpes simplex infections in humans. J Immunol 112:728–736

Rich SA (1981) Human lupus inclusions and interferon. Science 213:772–775

Rubin BY, Gupta SL (1980) Differential efficacies of human type I and type II interferons as antiviral and antiproliferative agents. Proc Natl Acad Sci USA 77:5928–5932

Sehgal PB, Pfeffer LM, Tamm I (1982) Interferon and its inducers. In: Came PE, Caliguiri LA (eds) Chemotherapy of viral infections. Springer, Berlin Heidelberg New York, pp 205–311 (Handbook of experimental pharmacology, vol 61)

Skreko F, Zajac T, Bahnsen HP, Haff RF, Cantell K (1973) The kinetics of human interferon clearance in gibbons. Proc Soc Exp Biol Med 142:946–947

Smolin G, Stebbing N, Friedlander M, Friedlander R, Okumoto M (1982) Natural and cloned human leukocyte interferon in herpes virus infections of rabbit eyes. Arch Opthalmol 100:481–483

Stebbing N, Weck PK, Fenno JT, Apperson S, Lee SH (1981) Comparison of the biological properties of natural and recombinant DNA derived human interferons. In: Shellekens H (ed) Biology of the interferon system. Elsevier-North Holland, New York, p 25

Stebbing N, Weck PK, Fenno JT, Rinderknecht E, Estell DA (to be published) Antiviral effects of bacteria derived human leukocyte interferons against encephalomyocarditis virus infection of squirrel monkeys. Arch Virol

Stewart WE II (1981) The interferon system. Springer, Wien New York

Stewart WE II, Desmyter J (1975) Molecular heterogeneity of human leukocyte interferon: two populations differing in molecular weights, requirements for renaturation and cross-species antiviral activity. Virology 67:68–78

Stewart WE II, Gresser LB, Lockart RZ (1971) Priming: a non-antiviral function of interferon. J Virol 1:792–801

Stewart WE II, De Somer P, Edy VG, Paucker K, Berg K, Osburne CA (1975) Distinct molecular species of human interferons: requirements for stabilization and reactivation of human leukocte and fibroblast interferons. J Gen Virol 26:327–331

Stewart WE II, Gresser I, Tovey MG, Bandu MT, Goff SL (1976) Identification of the cell multiplication inhibitory factors in interferons. Nature 252:300–302

Stewart WE II, Sarkar FH, Taira H, Hall A, Nagata S, Weissmann C (1980) Comparisons of several biological and physicochemical properties of human leukocyte interferons produced by human leukocytes and *E. coli*. Gene 11:181–186

Streuli M, Nagata S, Weissmann C (1980) At least three human type alpha interferons: structure of alpha-two. Science 209:1343–1347

Sugiyama M, Epstein LB (1978) Effect of *Corynebacterium parvum* on human T-lymphocyte interferon production and T-lymphocyte proliferation in vitro. Cancer Res. 38:4467–4473

Taniguchi T, Mantei N, Schwarzstein M, Nagata S, Muramatsu M, Weissmann C (1980a) Human leukocyte and fibroblast interferons are structurally related. Nature 285:547–549

Taniguchi T, Ohno S, Fuji-Kuriyama Y, Muramatsu M (1980b) The nucleotide sequence of human fibroblast interferon cDNA. Gene 10:11–15

Tomita Y, Kuwata T (1981) Suppressive effects of interferon on cell fusion by Sendai virus. J Gen Virol 55:289–295

Valle MJ, Jordan GW, Haahr S, Merigan TC (1975) Characteristics of immune interferon produced by human lymphocyte cultures compared to other human interferons. J Immunol 115:230–233

Van't Hull E, Schellekens H, Lowenberg B, De Vries MJ (1978) Influence of interferon preparations on the proliferative capacity of human and mouse bone marrow cells in vitro. Cancer Res 38:911–914

Vilcek J, Gresser I, Merigan TC (1980a) Regulatory functions of interferons. Ann NY Acad Sci 350:1–157

Vilcek J, Sulea IT, Zerebeckyj IL, Yip YK (1980b) Pharmacokinetic properties of human fibroblast and leukocyte interferon in rabbits. J Clin Microbiol 11:102–105

Vilcek J, Yip YK, Pang RHL, Kimberly T, Henriksen D, Zerebeckyj-Eckhardt I, Urban C, Taniguchi T (1981) How many interferons are there. Miami Winter Symp 18:331–345

Virelizier JL, Allison AC, De Maeyer E (1977) Production by mixed lymphocyte cultures of a type II interferon able to protect macrophages against virus infection. Infect Immun 17:282–285

Ware CF, Granger GA (1979) A physicochemical and immunological comparison of the cell growth inhibitory activity of human lymphotoxins and interferons in vitro. J Immunol 122:1763–1768

Weck PK, Apperson S, May L, Stebbing N (1981a) Comparison of the antiviral activities of various cloned human interferon-alpha subtypes in mammalian cell cultures. J Gen Virol 57:233–237

Weck PK, Apperson S, Stebbing N, Gray PW, Leung D, Shepard HM, Goeddel DV (1981b) Antiviral activities of hybrids of two major human leukocyte interferons. Nucleic Acids Res 9:6153–6166

Weck PK, Rinderknecht E, Estell DA, Stebbing N (1982) Antiviral activity of bacteria derived human leukocyte interferons against EMC virus infection of mice. Infect Immun 35:660–665

Weissmann C (1981) The cloning of interferon and other mistakes. In: Gresser I (ed) Interferon. Academic, London, p 101

Wetzel R (1981) Assignment of the disulfide bonds on leukocyte interferon. Nature 289:606–607

Wheelock EF (1965) Interferon-like virus inhibitor induced in human leukocytes by phytohemagglutinin. Science 149:310–311

Williams CK, Svet-Moldavskaya, Vilcek J, Ohnuma T, Holland JF (1981) Inhibitory effects of human leukocyte and fibroblast interferons on normal and chronic myelogenous leukemic granulocytic progenitor cells. Oncology 38:356–360

Wiranowska-Stewart M (1981) Heterogeneity of human gamma interferon preparations: evidence for presence of alpha interferon. J Interferon Res 1:315–322

Wiranowska-Stewart M, Stewart WE II (1981) Interferons: types alpha, beta and gamma. In: Hadden JW, Stewart WE II (eds) Lymphokines: Biochem Biol Act. Humana, Clifton, p 133

Wiranowska-Stewart M, Lin LS, Brande IA, Stewart WE II (1980) production, partial purification and characterization of human and murine interferons type II. Mol Immunol 17:625–633

Yamaguchi T, Handa K, Shimizu Y, Abo T, Kumagai K (1977) Target cell for interferon production in human leukocytes stimulated by Sendai virus. J Immunol 118:1931–1946

Yelverton E, Leung D, Weck P, Gray PW, Goeddel DV (1981) Bacterial synthesis of a novel human leukocyte interferon. Nucleic Acids Res 9:731–741

Yip YK, Pang RH, Oppenhein JD, Nachbar MS, Henricksen D, Zerebeckyj-Eckhardt I, Vilcek J (1981 a) Stimulation of human gamma interferon production by diterpene esters. Infect Immun 34:131–139

Yip YK, Pang RHL, Urban C, Vilcek J (1981 b) Partial purification and characterization of human gamma (immune) interferon. Proc Natl Acad Sci USA 78:1601–1605

Zarling JM (1981) Enhancement of human cytotoxic T cell responses and NK cell activity by purified fibroblast interferon and polynucleotide inducers of interferon. Prog Cancer Res Ther 19:167–180

CHAPTER 17

Manufacture and Safety of Interferons in Clinical Research

J. C. PETRICCIANI, E. C. ESBER, H. E. HOPPS, and A. ATTALLAH

A. Introduction

Leukocyte interferon for clinical trials became available in the early 1970s, the bulk of which was provided from Finland by CANTELL et al. (1974) and STRANDER and CANTELL (1966). Fresh buffy coat cells from human blood were stimulated to produce interferon by induction with Newcastle disease or Sendai viruses. Since the production process involved fresh, primary human cells suspended in serum-containing tissue culture medium and infected with an inducing virus, many of the tests used in examining live and inactivated tissue culture-derived vaccines were considered appropriate for application to leukocyte interferon. At first, these included only sterility, general safety, pyrogenicity, and potency. Also, the manufacturer was asked to provide data which identified the product as interferon, e.g., low pH stability, sedimentation characteristics, and biologic activity. As procedures became available for hepatitis B surface antigen (HB_sAg) testing, it was reasonable to require that buffy coats used in production should be derived only from blood shown to be negative for the presence of HB_sAg. It is quite likely that as tests for hepatitis virus A and for the agents of non-A and non-B hepatitis are developed, these would also be required for source leukocytes used in interferon production. With the refinement of interferon production procedures, experimental materials were also tested for protein and moisture content.

A second type of cell culture system useful for interferon production was introduced by HAVELL and VILCEK (1972) i.e., human neonate foreskin fibroblasts grown first as stationary cultures and later in roller bottles. Since cell lines of this type were analogous in many respects to the well-characterized WI-38 and MRC-5 lines, similar methodologies were recommended for their characterization and certification, including tumorigenicity tests and extensive karyologic monitoring. In 1979, the International Association for Biological Standardization/World Health Organization (IABS/WHO) Ad Hoc Committee on Karyology outlined an efficient, practical procedure for characterizing new diploid cell lines, and recommended the establishment of a manufacturs working cell bank (MWCB) from an approved seed stock MOORHEAD (1979). The Committee also recognized that interferon is different from replicating microbial agents and that karyologic monitoring production is unnecessary.

BEALE (1979) AND CHRISTOFINIS and FINTER (1977) described the production of interferon in Epstein–Barr virus (EBV)-transformed lymphoblastoid cells (Namalwa) growing in suspension. Prior to the acceptance of lymphoblastoid-derived interferon for use in clinical trials in Great Britain, a variety of biochemical and biologic tests were performed on the cell line and the purification process was also examined rigorously in an effort to assure safety of the product insofar as possible with "state of the art" testing. A very different kind of substrate for interferon production involves the use of bacteria and recombinant DNA technology (GOEDDEL et al. 1980). Recombinant DNA-derived interferon is now being tested clinically and informal guidelines are being formulated for this unique material. It is clear that not all of the old procedures will necessarily apply, and that several new ones will be required.

The development of guidelines for interferon testing has been an evolutionary process. As more sophisticated changes have occurred in methods of production, so too have changes and improvements occurred in testing. In the ensuing sections a description will be given of the current recommended test procedures as well as an explanation of why such tests are considered to be extremely important in establishing overall safety and efficacy of interferon products in the treatment of human diseases.

B. Manufacture

I. Introduction

The production and characterization of interferons derived from leukocytes, lymphoblastoid cells, fibroblasts, and immunocompetent cells have already been discussed in Chaps 12, 14, 15, and 17 from the point of view of scientific and technical requirements. In addition to those considerations, there are other factors with which a manufacturer must be concerned when the interferon is intended for use in clinical research in humans. These additional manufacturing considerations relate primarily to the purity, potency, and stability of the interferon. There are two basic reasons for these special concerns: (a) using experimental material which meets at least minimal standards; and (b) reducing risks and protecting the welfare of human subjects who participate in the research. By establishing minimal standards of purity, potency, and stability there is a much greater likelihood that the data generated in the study will be meaningful and reliable than if no standards were used. Directly related to the concern for using material which is likely to give reliable data is the need to reduce risks to those who will receive the interferon. By paying particular attention to the quality of the interferon in terms of its purity, potency, safety, and stability, the risks to human subjects are reduced and subjects are protected from receiving experimental material which has lost activity or which contains impurities which are known to be harmful. These are basic principles which apply to all investigational biologic agents, and represent both common sense and good medical practice in an experimental setting. It is important to recognize, however, that in the investigational stages of a biologic agent such as interferon, rigid criteria or standards are inappropriate both because the amount of product available for testing may be very limited and because of the constant development of new technology and new information. There will inevitably be improvements in the production of an experimental product which will make it possible to use more highly purified and potent material than at some previous time. As a result, there usually emerges a new consensus on what is acceptable. For example, in 1979 there was general agreement at an international workshop that interferon to be used in clinical trials should have a potency of at least 10^6 U per milligram protein (ATTALLAH et al. 1980). On the other hand, there may be rather abrupt and dramatic technologic-breakthroughs which offer the potential for levels of purity and potency which are orders of magnitude higher than what was previously possible. This may be the case with interferon produced by recombinant DNA technology. In those instances, it would be precipitous to require that all interferon preparations meet those new levels of purity and potency without first examining comparative clinical data and the consequences of such a requirement for ongoing clinical studies. In other words, changes in minimal standards usually take an evolutionary course based on consensus, even when rather large changes suddenly become possible.

In contrast to biologic products which are still in the investigational stage and limited in their use, licensed products which are available for general commercial distribution and use by the medical profession must meet a variety of regulatory requirements including, in the United States, those for Good Manufacturing Practice (GMP) and the General Provisions for Licensed Biologicals (GPLB) CODE OF FEDERAL REGULATIONS (1980a, b). These requirements include tests for potency, general safety, sterility, purity, residual moisture, pyrogenicity, identity, and constituent materials such as diluents, preservatives, extraneous proteins, and antibiotics. The strict application of those regulatory requirements to investigational biologic agents would unnecessarily restrict both research itself and the settings in which the research for new products could be undertaken. At the same time, the public must have assurance that the investigational products in use have met at least some minimal standards and that the potential benefits of the products outweigh the known risks. Because by its very nature an investigational biologic agent may carry unknown and unforeseen risk, that benefit:risk ratio may change during the course of product evaluation. However, by applying as many of the GMP and GPLB provisions as are practical, many, if not most, of the known potential risks associated with the manufacture of a biologic agent can be eliminated. For that reason, manufacturers of interferon have been encouraged to review the applicability of both the GMP and GPLB regulations to their procedures. Some of the specific suggestions for final container testing, for example, are discussed in Sect. C.

II. Purity

The concept of purity in the context of an investigational biologic agent such as interferon takes on quite a different meaning from what we usually think of as purity in the case of a chemically synthesized drug. As we have noted, the level of purity which may be acceptable usually increases as technologic improvements are incorporated into the production process. There are three fundamental points to be considered in any discussion of the purity of interferon: (1) characterization of the material as interferon; (2) removal of unwanted materials which were necessary during production; and (3) demonstration that the purification procedure is capable of removing (or not introducing) potential contaminants of particular concern.

Basic to any manufacturing process is the demonstration that the process results in the desired product. In the case of IFN-α (type I), for example, it would be necessary for a new manufacturer to show that the material described as interferon actually has antiviral activity which is: (a) nonsedimentable at 100,000 × *g* for 2 h; (b) inactivated by treatment with protease; and (c) stable at pH 2 for 24 h at 4 °C. Other types of interferon such as IFN-γ (type II or immune interferon) would be characterized by other or additional properties as described in Chaps. 15 and 17. The antigenic characterization of interferon is rapidly becoming possible with the development and increasing availability of specific antisera. It should therefore soon be feasible routinely to determine the antigenic specificities and their relative proportions in a given lot of interferon. Under those circumstances, the new nomenclature for interferon (STEWART 1980) could be used as part of the identification of the material intendend for human use, in addition to identifying the cell substrate used to produce the interferon.

There are several materials which are unwanted in the final product, but which are necessary during interferon production; however, because each of them is unique, the method for dealing with them must be individualized. One example is Sendai virus which, as discussed in Chaps. 13 and 14, is used to induce interferon in leukocytes and lymphoblastoid cells. While the need for Sendai virus in the production of interferon from those cells is well established, one would like to be sure that active or infectious Sendai virus is absent from the final interferon product intended for human use. A Notice of Claimed Investigational Exemption for a New Drug (IND) for clinical studies with such interferon would therefore reasonably include data demonstrating that the purification procedure consistently eliminates infectious Sendai virus. A second example of a reagent intentionally added during manufacture of interferon, but which should be markedly reduced, if not eliminated, from the final product is the bovine serum used to grow the cell cultures from which interferon is harvested. Here again the need for bovine serum in the cell culture system is well recognized. On the other hand, it has been a long-standing policy and practice to reduce the amount of bovine serum in final products to very low levels. For example, current United States Federal regulations for licensed cell culture-produced viral vaccines (CODE OF FEDERAL REGULATIONS 1980), require that:

> Extraneous protein known to be capable of producing allergenic effects in human subjects shall not be added to a final virus medium of cell culture produced vaccines intended for injection. If serum is used at any state, its calculated concentration in the final medium shall not exceed 1:1,000,000.

It would therefore be reasonable to make a similar effort to reduce the potential of producing an allergic response to bovine serum or other foreign proteins when interferon is produced from cell culture systems.

The use of antibiotics is an additional example of something which may be necessary during the production of interferon, but which should be reduced in concentration in the final product intended for humans. This is another area where the current Federal regulations for licensed cell culture-produced viral vaccines give both specific and general guidance. Penicillin may not be used in the medium for viral vaccine cell substrates because of the potential for sensitizing recipients of the vaccines to penicillin, and because some recipients may already be sensitized and would develop an allergic reaction. Other antibiotics may be used in the cell culture medium, but only at their minimum effective concentrations. This same general approach to the use of antibiotics should be employed in the production of interferon.

The final category of potential impurities includes those which could be introduced into the interferon product by any of the elements of the production process itself. Some purification procedures, for example, use concanavalin A (con A) columns. It is possible for con A to leach from the columns into the interferon, and therefore, it would be important to test the final product to determine the amount, if any, of con A that is present. Here again, it may not be necessary to repeat this test on every batch; but a logical testing program should be established based on such factors as previous experience, the indroduction of a new lot of con A, or other changes in procedure which might affect the amount of con A in the final product.

III. Potency

The potency of a biologic product has been defined (CODE OF FEDERAL REGULATIONS 1980 d) for regulatory purposes as:

... the specific ability or capacity of the product, as indicated by appropriate laboratory tests or by adequately controlled clinical data obtained through the administration of the product in the manner intended, to effect a given result.

In practical terms, that means the product must be able to do something, and that "something" can be measured by in vitro or in vivo tests. It is obviously preferable for potency tests to be defined by measuring an in vitro parameter which correlates whith efficacy or a defined human response rather than to have to rely on human clinical tests each time potency is to be measured. The most widely accepted assays for defining activity are those in vitro bioassays which measure antiviral activity (See Chap. 2 for additional detail). With the availability of standard preparations and international reference standards, the antiviral test systems can more uniformly define interferon unitage with comparability among laboratories. There are also several assays which reflect other biologic properties of the interferon, such as inhibition of cell proliferation, measurement of cell cytotoxicity, or the alteration of the expression of cell surface antigens. None of the latter assays, however, lends itself easily to quantitation nor have they been correlated with a well-defined human response following the administration of exogenous interferon in vivo.

With the increasing availability of highly purified interferons and of highly specific antisera to interferons, it is probable that the potency of interferon will soon be determined by using a radioimmunoassay. Before such assays would be acceptable, however, data from them will need to be related to biologic activities. If the results are found to correlate with the antiviral assays and/or clinical activity, those tests would be a major advance and would lend themselves to standardization among laboratories because of the ability to calibrate the assays with reference standards and reagents, as is done in many other radioimmunoassays.

The importance of having available a reference standard bioassay which is reproducible, standardized, and calibrated, and with well-defined international reference reagents includes: (a) assuring that patients have received the amount of interferon described in the clinical investigation protocol by measuring the potency of each lot of interferon; (b) assuring consistency between lots of material made by the manufacturer; and (c) ensuring the stability of the product during short- or long-term storage. These points have been given added importance as a result of increasing availability of supplies of human interferon for clinical trials and because of the increasing variety of disease conditions (viral, neoplastic, neurologic, etc.) in which the products are being tested.

The concern regarding the tests of interferon potency in standardized systems have been expressed at the international workshops held at Woodstock, Illinois, in September, 1978 and at the Bureau of Biologics, Bethesda, Maryland, in October, 1979 (ATTALLAH et al. 1980; WOODSTOCK INTERNATIONAL WORKSHOP 1979). Because of the many biologic variables which have been found to affect interferon bioassays, a number of recommendations were made at each conference. Attention should be given to the following variables in establishing interferon potency assay: (a) the source and sensitivity of the cell substrate selected to produce a dose–response curve; (b) the definition of the endpoint determination to be used for assigning the unitage; (c) the source and characteristics of the virus which determine that the system selected is of adequate sensitivity; (d) the dose of virus, dilution steps, and number of replicates which will provide 95% confidence limits; (e) the selection of the external (international) and internal (laboratory) reference standards; (f) the basis on which potency values in titers and international units will be assigned; and (g) the critical importance of establishing parallelism between the dose–response curves of the test sample and the selected internal laboratory and international standards.

C. Safety

The issue of safety of interferon represents a very broad area in which some aspects remain in the realm of theoretical considerations while others are of immediate and practical concern. For purposes of discussion, safety can be divided into the two broad categories of cell substrate and the final product since the issues in each area are relatively well defined and separable. However, it is important to remember there is nothing absolute about safety, and that, particularly in the clinical research setting, one must evaluate safety, in the context of a benefit:risk assessment, case by case.

I. Cell Substrates

1. Primary Human Leukocytes

Primary human leukocytes are the cell substrate with which there has been the longest and most widespread experience of the production of interferon. In addition, it should be recalled that there is enormous experience of the use of human blood and blood products, and that experience forms a large part of the background against which the safety of this cell substrate must be considered. There are basically two safety issues associated with the use of primary human leukocytes, i.e., the potential presence of microbial agents, and the possibility that some of the cells from some of the donors may be in a preleukemic state, or at the extreme, may be overtly neoplastic.

Humans may act as the host for a very large number of microbial agents, many of which cause disease and can be isolated from blood. For example, hepatitis and syphilis are agents which can be transferred from one individual to another through blood transfusion (SPARKLING 1979). The potential for the transmission of disease through the use of blood and blood fractions in clinical medicine was recognized long ago, and a procedure gradually evolved which balanced the amount of donor and blood testing which should be performed against the clinical needs for blood and the risks based on past experience. As a result, there are current Federal regulations (CODE OF FEDERAL REGULATIONS 1980), which require that blood donors be in good health based on information obtained by taking a medical history, performing a limited physicial examination, and doing certain laboratory tests. The regulations further specify that there must be the following evidence for good donor health: (a) normal temperature; (b) a blood hemoglobin level no less than 12.5 g/100 ml; (c) freedom from acute respiratory diseases; (d) freedom from any infectious skin disease at the site of phlebotomy and from any such disease generalized to such an extent as to create a risk of contamination of the blood; (e) freedom from any disease transmissible by blood transfusion, insofar as can be determined by history and examination; and (f) freedom of the arms and forearms from skin punctures or scars indicative of addiction to self-injected narcotics. Moreover, no individual may be used as a blood donor if he or she has: (a) a history of viral hepatitis; (b) a history of close contact within 6 months of donation with an individual having viral hepatitis; and (c) a history of having received within 6 months human blood, or any derivative of human blood, which the U.S. Food and Drug Administration has advised the licensed establishment is a possible source of viral hepatitis. The blood obtained from donors which meet these criteria must then be tested for syphilis and for HB_sAg.

With this screening procedure which is based on a combination of medical history, physical examination, and laboratory testing, the incidence of transmission of infectious diseases by transfusion has been reduced to extremely low levels. Since the leukocytes used to produce interferon are obtained from blood and plasma donors, it follows that the probability of microbial agents being present in those leukocytes is extremely low. In the case of some types of interferon, as opposed to blood transfusions, the production procedure itself further reduces the risk of microbial contaminants because the crude material is taken to a low pH early in the process, and that step is likely to inactivate most agents of any significance. A possible exception would be hepatitis virus B which is known to be very resistant to inactivation, although specific data are not available on its possible inactivation by low pH.

The safety of primary human leukocytes, per se, presents a rather different problem from that of microbial contaminants, but here again the general clinical experience with blood transfusions can be used to give some assessment of the levels of risk. The theoretical risk of using leukocytes from preleukemic or undiagnosed leukemic individuals to produce interferon is that DNA of cellular or viral origin which might posses oncogenic potential would be released from the leukocytes, carried through the interferon production process, and finally inoculated into humans along with the interferon, with the possibility of inducing neoplastic disease in the recipients. A long-term follow-up of donors and recipients helps to put this theoretical risk into perspective (GREENWALD et al. 1976). The study identified 105 recipients of blood from donors who subsequently developed neoplasms of the lymphatic or hematopoietic tissues, and followed those blood recipients for an average of 7 years. The results showed that no recipient of the precancerous cells had developed leukemia or lymphoma. Because of the relatively small size of the recipient group, those negative results must be considered preliminary, but they do suggest that even in the extreme case where intact preleukemic or prelymphomatous cells are transfused into humans there is no marked increase in the incidence of neoplastic disease in the transfused individuals. These data, taken together with the fact that the incidence of leukemia and lymphoma is only about 1 per 10,000 in the general population, argues strongly that while there may be a theoretical risk in using primary human leukocytes to produce interferon, the available information points to the level of that risk being extremely small.

2. Lymphoblastoid Cells

The safety issue here deals with a practical assessment of the risks of transmitting the tumor-producing potential of the EBV-transformed lymphoblastoid cells to the recipient of the interferon. Our basic understanding of tumor cell biology and the factors which are causally related to tumorigenesis is so incomplete that any attempt to assess risk must necessarily be based on a relatively simplistic, but at the same time pragmatic approach. The first question which needs to be addressed is whether or not there are data to suggest that the tumor-producing potential of overtly neoplastic cells can be transferred to normal cells by the genetic material of the cancer cells. Recent experiments (SHIH et al. 1979, 1981) with mouse 3T3 cells incubated with DNA that was extracted from normal and malignant mouse cell lines showed that DNA from malignant cells gave rise to a higher proportion of transformation than normal DNA. Additional experiments with DNA extracted from human tumor cells (SHIH et al. 1981) are of special interest because DNAs from only two cell lines were able to transform mouse 3T3 cells, even though the DNAs of many different tumors were tested. While these results will need confirmation and extension in other laboratories, it is intriguing to speculate that the transfer of malignancy by DNA may have at least some species barriers and that human cells may be particularly resistant to this very special type of carcinogenesis in the same way that human cells in vitro appear to be resistant to classical chemical carcinogens.

There are a number of factors operating in vivo which are protective against foreign cells as well as against the incorporation of biologically active foreign genetic material. In the case of direct cell transfer by transfusion, the normal immunologic defense mechanism probably accounts for the destruction and clearance of the tumor cells from the circulation. This is consistent with unpublished results of a small exploratory study done about 10 years ago in which no tumors developed in two infant rhesus monkeys which had been inoculated directly into the left ventricle with 10^8 human leukemic cells. This route of inoculation was chosen so that there would be a general distribution of the malignant cells throughout the body with a large fraction going to the central nervous system. Even under such extreme conditions favorable to the development of leukemia, there was no evidence of leukemia or lymphoma after several years of obserevation. In addition to this specific experiment, the scientific literature is replete with data showing that unless the animal host is immunosuppressed and/or "privileged sites" are used for the tumor cell inoculation, it is extraordinarily difficult to generate tumors in animals when they are inoculated with human tumor cells.

The transfer of genetic material to cells in vitro is a very inefficient process unless special conditions are imposed such as complexing the DNA with DEAE-dextran. Even then, the efficiency of getting the exogenous DNA into the cells with subsequent gene expression may be only about 1 in 10^6. The situation is made even more difficult for effective gene transfer in vivo. Any tumor cell nucleic acid inoculated in vivo would immediately encounter nuclease activity in the serum at the site of inoculation and thoroughout the circulatory system as the nucleic acid is dispersed and diluted. Primate sera have been shown to be especially high in nuclease activity (LEVY et al. 1977). The diluted and at least partially degraded DNA would then have to get into cells without the help of agents such as DEAE-dextran. Those few molecules which might enter cells would next be exposed to cytoplasmic nucleases such as DNase I and II. Lysosomes are known to contain nucleases and are thought to be the primary intracellular sites for the hydrolysis and digestion of many classes of macromolecules, including DNA, following the incorporation of the molecules into the cell by pinocytosis. Considering all of the biologic obstacles associated with the transfer of undegraded and functional DNA into cells in vivo, it is not surprising to find an absence of reports in the literature demonstrating success. The risk, then, of inducing a tumor in a recipient of interferon produced from lymphoblastoid cells must remain only a theoretical consideration because of the large body of evidence in the literature which suggests that, even if a small amount of lymphoblastoid DNA did escape through the interferon purification process, the likelihood of its being able to exert to tumorigenic effect in vivo is infinitesimally small.

The second major safety consideration for lymphoblastoid cells is the possible presence of microbial agents, and those fall into two types: (a) those which are known and for which tests have been devised; and (b) those which are theoretically possible, but which have yet to be identified in any human tissue. Because a cell seed system is used for lymphoblastoid cells as well as for fibroblasts, it is possible to characterize the cell bank up to and beyond the passage level at which they would be used for interferon production, and to assure that the cell stock is free of viral and other known microbial agents including EBV. The problem of theoretical agents is, of course, impossible to address experimentally in any complete manner, but as a minimum, "state of the art" techniques can be applied to the cells in an effort to identify agents such as a human leukemia virus.

3. Fibroblast Cells

The in vitro propagation of human fibroblast cells to produce interferon has been discussed in Chapt. 15. The cells themselves are usually derived from human foreskin, but other tissues have also been used to establish cell banks at early population doublings. By using a cell seed system for fibroblast cells it is possible to pretest the cell line at various stages of its in vitro life to assure that it is free of detectable microbial agents. The use of such cell systems in vaccine production has now been widely accepted in the United States and many other countries for over 10 years. The question of whether or not the chromosomal constitution of such cell populations should be a major safety consideration has been discussed on a number of occasions. The most recent position was expressed in the report of the Ad Hoc Committee on Karyological Controls of Human Cell Substrates (MOORHEAD 1979) as follows:

> The relevance to product safety of karyological monitoring of cell substrates in the production of non-replicating biological products such as interferon is open to question. The potential risks of using karyologically abnormal cells are related to the possible contamination of the product with cellular nucleic acid. Control authorities should therefore consider the purification procedures used in the manufacturing process and the confidence with which one can exclude the presence of cellular nucleic acid in the final product. Current technology may allow the elimination of cellular nucleic acids from non-replicating biological products produced in cell culture systems, in which case karyological monitoring of the cell substrate is considered unnecessary.

In other words, abnormal karyology per se need not be a deterrent to the consideration of cell lines for the production of interferon. Implicit in this approach is the need to document the extent to which the purification procedure eliminates nucleic acid from the final product.

4. Bacteria (Recombinant DNA)

At first glance, one might think that if there are any safety issues associated with the use of bacteria to synthesize interferon, they must be minor and certainly less than those associated with lymphoblastoid cells. While that first impression may ultimately prove to be correct, there are at least two theoretical risks which are unique to the use of this cell substrate in the production of interferon. One relates to the fidelity with which the bacteria transcribe and translate the interferon genes, while the other risk is associated with potential for non-interferon human proteins in the final product.

Recombinant DNA technology is still in its infancy, even though tremendous progress has been made in a very short time. Now that human interferon genes have been cloned and expression of those genes in bacteria has been demonstrated, it is important to establish how closely those interferon products correspond to naturally occurring interferons. To the extent the recombinant molecules differ from the natural molecules, there should be increased caution over the introduction of those experimental materials into human subjects because of the possibility of new and potentially harmful effects from those novel molecular species.

The second theoretical risk is more directly related to recombinant DNA technology and human genes than it is to the bacteria themselves. If the interferon genes which were introduced into plasmids were derived from lymphoblastoid cells, then it is possible that in addition to the interferon genes other human genetic material could be taken along as a passanger. If that passanger DNA contains oncogene sequences, there is a risk that those genes will also be expressed in the bacteria, and that transforming proteins will be synthesized along with the interferon. With the recent demonstration that normal mouse DNA sheared to 0.5–3 kilobases can transform 3T3 cells in vitro (SHIH et al. 1979), it is possible that the same theoretical risk which we have described for human lymphoblastoid cells also applies to human fibroblasts and primary leukocytes. If, as current theories suggest, all cells contain oncogenes, then any human cells from which genes are extracted carry with them the potential for contaminating the appropriate genes, such as interferon, with oncogene sequences. Since the specific risk fo those theoretical events is that transforming proteins may be introduced with the interferon, purification of the interferon and the identification of contaminating proteins become especially important aspects of the production process.

II. Final Product

The safety of investigational biologic products such as interferon is established at several different points in the manufacturing process and during the course of the development of the product itself. For example, in 1983 the safety of using leukocyte interferon is rather different from that of the leukocyte interferon used in the first clinical trial because technologic advances now make possible the exclusion of potential contaminants such as hepatitis virus B, and the cumulative human experience with interferon over the past decade gives further assurance of at least its short-term safety in humans. In other words, there is a large body of data on the safety of leukocyte interferon in the generic sense which is based on both preclinical animal studies and clinical work in humans. To the extent that there are no data on the safety of a specific type of interferon at a given dose, route, or frequency, appropriate animal studies should be conducted to support the safety of that use of the material in humans. The question regarding to what extent interferon should undergo general long-term toxiocology tests is a difficult one to address. As in the case of tests performed on cell substrates, those tests are generic issues which, once they are settled, need not be performed over and over again, in contrast to tests like the final container sterility tests, which must be done on each lot. At one extreme, it could be argued that human interferon, like insulin, is a natural biologic product which all of us produce during the normal course of our entire lifetime. It therefore makes little sense to subject either insulin or interferon to an artificial assessment of safety in animal systems when we already have the ultimate data base for making that judgment – experience in humans. An alternate view would be that, even though interferon is a natural substance, its current clinical use is at concentrations and for periods of time which are far beyond normal physiologic limits, and we therefore need to be concerned about toxiocologic studies. Complicating the picture even further is the problem of species specificity and the resulting question of whether or not injection of human interferon into rodents would give meaningful information. There is also the additional question of whether or not one could reasonably extrapolate back to humans from long-term studies in rodents with rodent interferon. One final area about which little is known is the effect of therapeutic levels of interferon on embryogenesis and postnatal growth and development. If the potential usefulness of interferon for clinical conditions during pregnancy (e.g., cytomegalovirus infection) and childhood (e.g., juvenile laryngeal papilloma) becomes convincing, safety data in this area will have to be developed.

In addition to those elements of safety, there is good reason to be concerned with the safety of specific production lots from the point of view of assuring that each lot is free of extraneous toxic contaminants which may have inadvertently been introduced during the manufacturing process. This part of the safety evaluation of all biologic products is referred to as the final container tests. These tests are conducted on representative samples of interferon final containers from each lot which are intended for distribution for clinical use, and are listed in Table 1 (Pe-

Table 1. Suggestions for final container sterility, pyrogenicity, and general safety tests for interferon preparations to be used in human clinical studies

Test system	Volume and route	Units to be tested or animals used	Observation period	Comment
1. Bacterial and fungal sterility [a]	Total contents of 1 vial/tube of each medium (up to a maximum of 1 ml/tube)	10% of vials in a lot or 20 vials maximum	14 days	21 CFR 610.12 [c]
2. Rabbit pyrogenicity	1.5×10^6 U/kg or 0.1 ml, whichever is greater; i.v. [b]	3 rabbits	3 h	21 CFR 610.13(b)
3. General safety	1.5×10^6 U/kg or 0.1 ml, whichever is greater; i.p. [b]	2 guinea pigs (<400 g each)	7 days	21 CFR 610.11
	0.1 ml; i.p.	2 mice (<22 g each)	7 days	

[a] A membrane filtration procedure can be substituted as an alternate method following appropriate validation

[b] The rabbit pyrogen and general safety test volumes indicated are based on three times the maximum single human dose ($3 \times 30 \times 10^6$ U $= 9 \times 10^7$ U), assuming a 60 kg human patient (9×10^7 U/60 kg $= 1.5 \times 10^6$ U/kg). To obtain the dose per rabbit or guinea pig, 1.5×10^6 U is multiplied by the weight of the individual animal in kg. Because this calculation for mice results in a dose of less than 0.1 ml and the minimum acceptable dosage volume is 0.1 ml, the test in mice should be done with 0.1 ml per mouse. Abbreviations: i.p. intraperitoneal; i.v. intravenous

[c] Refers to Title 21 of the Code of Federal Regulations. Further details for these test procedures can be found in the indicated sections of these regulations

TRICCIANI 1981). They include tests for bacteria, fungi, pyrogenicity, and general safety. The latter test is aimed at identifying any gross toxicity which may be associated with a specific lot of interferon owing to human or mechanical errors during production and filling.

Tests for pyrogenic substances present an especially difficult problem because there is suggestive evidence that pyrogenicity may be an inherent property of at least some types of interferon rather than being due to contaminating endotoxins. Studies are now in progress to attempt to establish the relationship, if any, among rabbit pyrogenicity test data, purity of the interferon, and clinical effect. However, until this issue is resolved, it is recommended that the rabbit pyrogen assay be performed even though a positive test need not necessarily be a basis for rejection of an interferon lot for clinical use. The degree of pyrogenicity, the patient population, and the route of administration should all be considered in the assessment of the acceptability of any given lot of interferon. For example, much more caution should be exercised in the intravenous, intraarterial, intrathecal, and intraspinal routes of administration than when interferon is given by the intramuscular or subcutaneous routes.

In summary, there are a variety of factors to be considered in assessing the safety of interferon preparations, and some of those are intimately interrelated with the purity of the product. Although the focus of this discussion has been on tests which should be done on interferon preparations before they are used in clinical studies, we should point out that even though perfectly reasonable guidelines for testing interferon might be developed, the ultimate assessment of the safety of this biologic product will not come from in vitro tests or even in vivo animal tests, but rather from its clinical use in humans. And while it is beyond the sçope of this chapter, it is nevertheless appropriate to conclude this section by reemphasizing the importance of the design of clinical trials of interferon not only with regard to determining efficacy, but also for assessing safety.

D. Summary

This chapter comprises a review of those test procedures currently recommended for use in the control testing of interferons derived from: (a) source leukocytes (human); (b) human diploid fibroblast cells; (c) human lymphoblastoid cells; and (d) recombinant DNA technology. Certain basic tests can be applied to all types of interferon, e.g., sterility, potency, pyrogenicity, and general safety. However, with interferon derived from lymphoblastoid cells and from recombinant DNA systems, additional tests specific to the production mode should be utilized. One of the important goals of this chapter has been to explain why each of the tests has been suggested. The U. S. Bureau of Biologics has attempted to avoid imposing procedures that are not useful and that may also be expensive and time consuming. In large measure, this has been accomplished by encouraging Bureau scientists to work with the various sponsors and clinical investigators to develop methodologies which can best assure the public of the maximum safety of experimental interferons while at the same time not acting as a hindrence to further product development.

In summary, we would like to emphasize that the test procedures which seem necessary and reasonable at the present are not immutably fixed. In view of the rapid technologic developments of the past several years, there needs to be flexibility in terms of appropriate testing, and that flexibility must carefully balance concern for safety with the need for clinical research.

References

Attallah AM, Petricciani JC, Galasso GJ, Rabson AS (1980) Report of a workshop on standards for human interferon in clinical trials. J Infect Dis 142:300–301

Beale AJ (1979) Choice of cell substrate for biological products. Adv Exp Med Biol 118:83–97

Cantell K, Hirvonen S, Mogensen KE (1974) Human leukocyte interferon: production, purification, stability and animal experiments. In: Waymouth C (ed) The production and use of interferon for the treatment and prevention of virus infections. In Vitro 35–38

Christofinis GJ, Finter NB (1977) The preparation of interferon from lymphoblastoid cell lines. In: Proceedings of symposium: preparation, standardization and clinical use of interferon, Zagreb, June 8—9

Code of Federal Regulations (1980a) Title 21, part 211, Current good manufacturing practice for finished pharmaceuticals. Government Printing Office, Washington DC
Code of Federal Regulations (1980b) Title 21, part 610.10 et seq., General provisions for licensed biologicals. Government Printing Office, Washington DC
Code of Federal Regulations (1980c). Title 21, part 610.15 (b), constituent materials: extraneous protein; cell culture produced vaccines. Government Printing Office, Washington DC
Code of Federal Regulations (1980d) Title 21, part 600.3(r), Biological products: general provisions: definition. Government Printing Office, Washington DC
Code of Federal Regulations (1980e) Title 21, part 606.160, Records and reports. Government Printing Office, Washington DC
Goeddel DV, Yelverton E, Ullrich A, Heyneker HL, Miozzari G, Holmes W, Seeburg PH, Dull T, May L, Stebbing N, Crea R, Maeda S, McCandliss R, Sloma A, Tabor JM, Gross M, Familletti PC, Pestka S (1980) Human leukocyte interferon produced by E. coli is biologically active. Nature 287:411–416
Greenwald P, Woodward E, Nasca PC, Hempelmann L, Dayton P, Maksymowicz G, Blando P, Hanrahan LR, Burnett WS (1976) Morbidity and mortality among recipients of blood from preleukemic and prelymphomatous donors. Cancer 38:324–328
Havell EA, Vilcek J (1972) Production of high-titered interferon in cultures of human diploid cells. Antimicrob Agents Chemother 2:476–484
Levy HB (1977) Induction of interferon in vivo by polynucleotides. Tex Rep Biol Med 35:91–95
Moorhead P (1979) Report of Ad Hoc Committee on Karyological Controls of Human Cell Substrates. J Biol Stand 7:397–404
Petricciani JC (1981) Interferon test procedures. Bureau of Biologics, Food and Drug Administration, Bethesda
Shih C, Shilo B, Goldfarb MP, Dannenberg A, Weinberg R (1979) Passage of phenotypes of chemically transformed cells via transfection of DNA and chromatin. Proc Natl Acad Sci USA 76:5714–5718
Shih C, Padhy LC, Murray M, Weinberg RA (1981) Transforming genes of carcinomas and neuroblastomas introduced into mouse fibroblasts. Nature 290:261–264
Sparkling PF (1979) Syphilis. In: Besson PB, McDermolt W, Wyngaarden JB (eds) Textbook of medicine. Saunders, Philadelphia, p 506
Stewart WE II (1980) Report of the interferon nomenclature committee. Nature 286:110
Strander H, Cantell K (1966) Production of interferon by human leukocytes in vitro. Ann Med Exp Biol Fenn 44:265–273
Woodstock International Workshop (1979) Interferon standards: a memorandum. J Biol Stand 7:383–395

CHAPTER 18

Nonpolynucleotide Inducers of Interferon

D. A. STRINGFELLOW

A. Introduction

Following the discovery of interferon, a great deal of interest centered around developing methods of clinically utilizing this interesting material. During the 1950s and early 1960s, attention was given to the problem of producing interferon in cultured cells in vitro which could be purified and concentrated for exogenous transfer to the exposed or infected host. In the early 1960s, a small number of workers became interested in the possibility that an animal's own cells could be stimulated to produce their own endogenous interferon in vivo. These studies were stimulated by the discovery of STEINEBRING and YOUNGNER (1964) that an extract of gram-negative organisms, a lipopolysacchride (endotoxin), would induce a detectable interferon response when injected into mice. Consequently, interest centered around the potential use of molecules such as lipopolysaccharide to induce detectable levels of interferon in vivo.

In 1967, a group of workers at Merck, West Point, Pennsylvania (FIELD et al. 1967) found that double-stranded polyribonucleotides could also induce high levels of circulating interferon in mice as well as other animal species. They subsequently discovered the double-stranded RNA, polyriboinosinic · polyribocytidylic acid [poly(I) · poly(C)], which is one of the most potent interferon inducers ever discovered. Although this focused attention on polynucleotides, it did not decrease interest in the search for other molecular species that could stimulate an in vivo interferon response. These studies reached a milestone with the report of MAEYER and KRUEGER (1970) that a low molecular weight fluoronone compound, tilorone hydrochloride, induced high levels of serum interferon in mice after oral administration. This was the first synthetic, orally active interferon inducer.

During the early 1970s, several clinical reports were published which suggested that poly(I) · poly(C) did not induce high levels of interferon in humans at doses that were well tolerated HILL et al. (1971). Likewise, tilorone hydrochloride, although capable of inducing interferon in rodents, did not induce interferon in other animal species, for example, dogs or cats, and was not an active interferon inducer in humans KAUFMAN et al. (1971). These results decreased interest in the search for low molecular weight inducers even though during the mid-1970s a group of workers at the Pfizer Corporation, Gratton, Connecticut, in conjunction with investigators at the University of Illinois College of Medicine, Urbana, Illinois, demonstrated that a propanediamine CP20961, when given intranasally to volunteers, induced high levels of local nasal interferon (HOFFMAN et al. 1973;

GATMAITAN et al. 1973; GATMAITAN et al. 1973; PANUSARN et al. 1974). These studies, however, were dampened by the clinical observation that, even though interferon was induced, the clinical signs and symptoms of rhinovirus-infected volunteers were not appreciably affected. In retrospect, some of the negative clinical results with the propanediamine may be attributable to the variability of the clinical course of rhinovirus infections. The propanediamines might have been more successful against a virus infection with more reproducible clinical features. The combined effect of these results was a decrease in interest in inducers as a potential way of utilizing the interferon system. Much of the research effort with inducers was routed back into exogenous interferon production because of the positive clinical studies achieved by MERIGAN (1973, 1977); EINHORN and STRANDER (1977); STRANDER and EINHORN (1977), and STRANDER et al. (1979) using interferon in the treatment of virus and neoplastic diseases. Research emphasis during the last 5–6 years has been predominantly on exogenous interferon, although a small number of laboratories have pursued the possible use of low molecular weight inducers as a means of utilizing the interferon system.

This chapter is intended to highlight the progress so far made, the problems being encountered, and the state of clinical trials and preclinical development of low molecular weight interferon inducers.

At this point, however, it should be emphasized that, even though these compounds are capable of inducing an interferon response and are therefore referred to as interferon inducers, they do have a pronounced effect upon other immune parameters. They stimulate macrophage, natural killer cell, T-lymphocyte, and antibody response in experimental animals. Taken in this context, they should be broadly classified as immune modulators and not just in the restrictive sense of interferon inducers.

B. Chemical Structures

During the past 20 years, a variety of chemicals has been found capable of inducing interferon. The structures of some of the most prominent molecular species reported to be interferon inducers are illustrated in Fig. 1. Propanediamines (HOFFMAN et al. 1973), tilorone hydrochloride (MAYER and KRUEGER 1970), acradines (GLAZ et al. 1973), basic dyes (STRINGFELLOW 1980), anthraquinones (STRINGFELLOW et al. 1979), and pyrimidinones (STRINGFELLOW et al. 1980) have been the principal molecules studied. There is a variety of other chemical structures which have been reported to be capable of inducing interferon, but little is known about structure–activity relationships. That is, what types of structural modifications of the basic molecule can be made either to increase or to decrease interferon-inducing, antiviral, or antitumor activity. The comparative ability of several molecules to induce interferon and establish antiviral activity is summarized in Table 1. In mice, each molecule that induced circulating interferon levels of greater than 50 U/ml protected animals against a lethal dose of an interferon-sensitive virus (Semliki Forest virus or encephalomyocarditis virus). Interestingly, the simple fact that a compound did not induce an interferon response was no guarantee that molecule would not mediate antiviral activity. For example, one of the anthraquinones and several of the pyrimidinones which did not

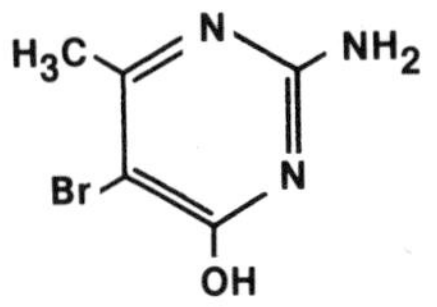

2-amino-5-bromo-6-methyl-4-pyrimidinol
(U-25, 166)

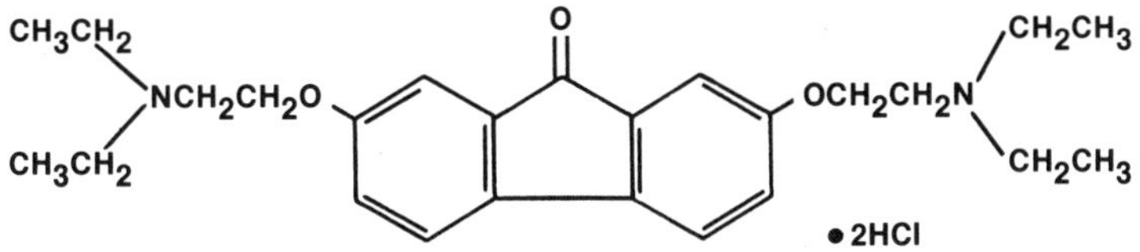

Bis-diethyl amino ethoxy-Fluorenone
(Tilorone Hydrochloride)

polyriboinosinic · polyribocytidylic acid
(poly (I) · poly (C)

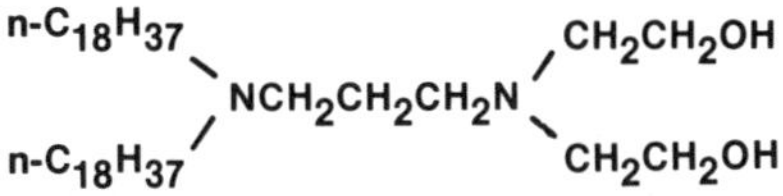

N, N-dioctadecyl-N', N'-bis (2-hydroxyethyl) propanediamine
(CP-20,961)

Fig. 1. Chemical structures of four classic interferon inducers

induce interferon were still capable of mediating antiviral activity; and, in some cases, were more potent antiviral agents than the best interferon inducers. These results again indicate that, even though referred to as interferon inducers, these molecules are active in a broader context and should be considered as biologic response or immune modulators.

I. Structure–Activity

What type of structural modification can be made and what effect will these modifications have on an ability of molecules to induce interferon or mediate antiviral activity? Data for the pyrimidinones as examples are summarized in Fig. 2. Any modification of the pyrimidinone molecule at the 1, 2, and 3, or 4 position

Table 1. Comparative interferon-inducing and antiviral properties of several „inducers" given intraperitoneally

Compound [a]	Dosage (mg/kg)	Maximum [b] interferon response (U/ml)	Antiviral protection [c] SFV	EMCV
Tilorone	200	6,500	+	+
	100	1,300	+	+
	50	500	+	+
	25	1,200	+	+
	12	25	−	−
ABPP	500	3,800	+	+
	250	2,300	+	+
	100	350	+	+
	50	35	±	−
	10	< 10	−	−
AIPP	500	< 10	+	+
	250	< 10	+	+
	100	< 10	+	+
	50	< 10	−	+
Poly(I)·poly(C)	5	5,500	+	+
	1	4,000	+	+
	0.5	510	+	+
	0.1	80	+	+
	0.05	< 10	−	−
BAA	200	7,500	+	+
	100	900	+	+
	50	150	+	+
	25	10	−	−
Placebo		< 10	−	−

[a] Tilorone, poly(I)·poly(C), 2-amino-5-bromo-6-phenyl-4(^{3}H)-pyrimidinone (ABPP), 2-amino-5-iodo-6-phenyl-4(^{3}H)-pyrimidinone (AIPP), and 1,5-bis[(3-morpholinopropyl) amino]anthraquinone (BAA) were given 18 h prior to EMCV or SFV infection (10 LD_{50})
[b] Maximum levels of circulating interferon detected after inducer injection
[c] Abbreviations: +, protection of 50% of infected mice; −, protection of less than 50% of infected mice

resulted in a loss of interferon-inducing or antiviral activity. This portion of the molecule had to remain intact to preserve the biologic activity of the molecule. However, modifications, could be made at the 5 and 6 position without losing antiviral activity, although making the alkyl side chain at the 6 position longer than ethyl or propyl severely reduced antiviral and interferon-inducing activity. The 5 position could be occupied by a halogen or short alkyl side chain and preserve biologic activity. WIERENGA et al. (1979) synthesized several molecules that had a phenyl group at the 6 position which were found to have markedly enhanced antiviral and a split in interferon-inducing activities. Again, however, only modest modification of the molecule could be made without losing the antiviral and

PYRIMIDINONES*

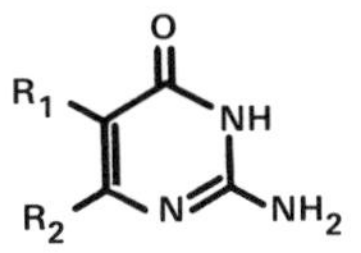

Abbreviation	R_1	R_2	IF**	AV***
ABMP	Br	CH_3	++++	+++
ABEP	Br	C_2H_5	++	++
ABPrP	Br	C_3H_7	+	+
ABPrP	Br	$CH(CH_3)_2$	–	–
ABPP	Br	C_6H_5	++++	++++
AIMP	I	CH_3	+++	+++
ACMP	Cl	CH_3	–	–
AIPP	I	C_6H_5	+	++++
ACPP	Cl	C_6H_5	++++	++++

(Substitutions: R_1, R_2)

*Compounds were injected i.p. at 1000 mg/kg i.p. Serum was collected at 8 hr for interferon assay. (Mice 20/group) were challenged with Semliki Forest virus 18 hr after compound.

**Serum interferon response: (–) = <10 units/ml, + = 10-50, ++ = 50-100, +++ = 100-1000, ++++ = 1000-10,000 units/ml.

***Antiviral activity: (–) = <50% of animals protected, + = 50%, ++ = 50-65%, +++ = 65-80%, and ++++ = 80-100% of animals protected.

Fig. 2. Structure–activity relationship of substituted pyrimidinones

interferon-inducing activity. This appears to be the rule rather than the exception with most classes of low molecular weight inducers. Only minor modification of the molecule will drastically affect antiviral and interferon-inducing activity.

It is not clearly understood how these molecules trigger interferon induction, whether the molecule needs to bind to a cellular receptor site or if it must be taken into the cell to trigger an interferon response by some intracellular mechanism. Whatever mechanism is involved appears to require very specific structural characteristics. In a broader sense it might be asked what type of molecules would be expected to induce an interferon response. Although this question has been asked by many laboratories, a clear answer has not been achieved in terms of predicting what type of molecular structures are more active inducers. The one thing that is clear from the data in Fig. 1 is that many of these molecules (i.e., tilorone, anthraquinones, and acradines) can bind to DNA and proteins and this might be involved in triggering the interferon response. However, the pyrimidinone molecules and the propanediamines do not bind to DNA or proteins.

Table 2. Antiviral, antitumor, and interferon-inducing activity of inducers

Compound [a]	Minimum interferon-inducing dose [b] (mg/kg)	Maximum serum interferon response [c] (U/ml)	Anti-SFV activity [d] (mg/kg)	Antitumor activity [e] (%)
Poly(I)·poly(C)	0.1	5,000	0.1	10
Tilorone	25	7,500	50	80
Pyran	20	200	20	50
ABPP	50	5,000	100	60
AIPP	800	100	50	50
ACPP	200	6,000	70	50
ABMP	200	5,000	200	30

[a] Compounds administered intraperitoneally (i.p.). Abbreviations defined in Table 1 and Fig. 1

[b] Minimum dose of compound needed to induce a detectable (> 50 U/ml) serum interferon response

[c] Maximum level of circulating interferon after administration of an optimal dose of compound

[d] Minimum i.p. dose of compound needed to protect 50% of mice against 10 LD_{50} Semliki Forest virus (SFV)

[e] Percentage survivors of mice injected i.p. with 2×10^5 B16 melanoma cells and treated i.p. daily for 9 days beginning 24 h, after cell injection with an optimal dose of drug (30 mice per group)

C. Comparative Interferon, Antiviral, and Antitumor Activity

The previous section dealt with the chemical structures which are active interferon inducers. It was mentioned that many of the molecules, even though they did not induce a detectable interferon response, still mediated antiviral and antitumor activity in experimental animals. The obvious question then is: what is the correlation between their ability to induce interferon and mediate antiviral and antitumor activity? This is a fairly difficult question to answer broadly for all of the low molecular weight interferon inducers, but an idea concerning comparative activities can be obtained using the pyrimidinones as examples. The data presented in Table 2 summarizes the antiviral/antitumor interferon-inducing capabilities of several of the pyrimidinones. Simply because a molecule could induce an interferon response was no guarantee that that molecule would have greater antiviral or antitumor activity than molecules which were poor interferon inducers. In fact, the quantity of interferon induced, that is, the maximum amount of interferon induced by a particular molecule, did not correspond to the antiviral and antitumor activity of that molecule. A molecule that would induce 100–500 U/ml interferon was just as capable of mediating an antiviral or antitumor state as a molecule which could induce 5,000–10,000 U/ml. The magnitude of the interferon response was not nearly as important as the minimum amount of compound needed to induce an interferon response. There was a consistent correlation between the ability to induce interferon at very low concentrations and ability to mediate an antiviral state under those same conditions, but there was not a correlation between magnitude of the interferon response and the degree of antiviral or antitumor activity. In the past, some investigators have used the magnitude of the interferon

Table 3. Summary of immune modulating activity of AIPP, ABPP, and ACPP

1. Increased:	murine natural killer cells in vivo
2. Increased:	murine macrophage mediated cytotoxicity increased after in vivo or in vitro addition
3. Increased:	in vivo antibody formation in unimmunized and immunized mice
4. Decreased:	in vitro spleen cell response to sheep red blood cells
5. Decreased:	killer T-cell cytotoxicity inhibited in vitro
6. Increased:	bone marrow colony-forming units
7. No effect:	in vitro compounds not mitogenic nor did they affect mitogen response

response as a predictor of antiviral or antitumor activity, suggesting that if a molecule could induce 500,000 or 1,000,00 U/ml interferon it would be the most effective in mediating antiviral or antitumor activity. This has not been the case. From the biological activity of interferon, it is not surprising that a small amount of circulating interferon could mediate as strong an antiviral state as large amounts of serum interferon.

If there was not a correlation between ability to induce interferon and the antiviral or antitumor activity of the pyrimidinones, then what mediated the antiviral activity? With the pyrimidinones we have evidence from studies of RENIS and EIDSON (1980) that the cellular immune response is critical in mediating the antiherpesvirus activities of these molecules. They demonstrated that administration of antithymocyte serum with the pyrimidinones decreased the antiherpesvirus activity of the molecules without affecting their interferon-inducing activity. These data suggested that T-lymphocytes were particularly important in mediating antiherpesvirus activity and led to an evaluation of the immune potentiating properties of these molecules. What was found was that the ability of the molecules to potentiate the immune response was not correlated with the ability of the molecules to induce an interferon response (FAST and STRINGFELLOW 1980). In fact, the three molecules in Table 3 had similar immune potentiating activity even though the iodophenyl compound AIPP was not capable of inducing a circulating interferon under these conditions. These results further enforce the hypothesis that, even though referred to as interferon inducers, low molecular weight inducers should be considered broadly as biologic response or immune response modifiers.

I. Antitumor Activity

In a variety of studies designed to explore the antineoplastic activity of inducers, the antitumor activity has been consistently tumor-load dependent. That is, after administration of the compound, animals were quite resistant to intraperitoneal injection of B16 melanoma cells at concentrations as high as 10^4 or 10^5 cells, but higher tumor loads completely overwhelmed the antitumor activity of these molecules (Table 4). To determine if various interferon inducers had comparable antitumor activity and were also comparable to interferon itself, each was injected into mice daily for 9 days beginning 24 h after intraperitonedal injection of B16 melanoma cells (2×10^4). Results summarized in Table 4 suggest that each of the molecules had similar antitumor activity and, in each case, the antitumor activity

Table 4. Comparative anti-B16 malignant melanoma activity of inducers and interferon

Agent[a]	Dose (i.p.)	MDD[b]	Survivors (%)[c]
ABPP	400 mg/kg	39	60
Poly(I)·poly(C)	100 mg/day	43	70
Tilorone	200 mg/kg	43	60
Pyran	15 mg/kg	40	80
Interferon[d]	5×10^5 U/day	42	30
Placebo	0.2 ml/day	38	20

[a] 2 × 10 B16 cells injected i.p.; mice were treated daily for 9 days beginning 24 h after B16 cell injection
[b] Mean day of death of mice that died due to melanoma
[c] Percent survivors (30 mice per group)
[d] Murine interferon-α (1×10^7 U per milligram protein); 5×10^5 U injected daily for 9 days

Table 5. Combination therapy with ABPP and surgery in mice injected in the footpad with B16 malignant melanoma cells

Days before surgery[a]	Survivors (%)[b]			
	ABPP alone	ABPP + surgery	Surgery + placebo	Placebo alone
7	30	100	50	0
14	20	70	10	0
21	0	60	0	0

[a] 2×10^3 B16 cells were injected into the left hind footpad; 7, 14, or 21 days later the left leg was amputated and therapy with placebos or ABPP (500 mg/kg, i.p.) was initiated 24 h later and continued once weekly for 9 weeks
[b] 30 mice per group

was tumor-load dependent. The data with the inducers were compared with exogenously transferred interferon (10^5 U murine L929 interferon daily). The inducers were more active than interferon in mediating antitumor activity. This may have been because the compounds mediated other cellular events independent of interferon. Macrophage activity and the antibody response were enhanced in inducer-treated animals, but not animals treated with interferon.

The tumor-load dependency found in the previous studies with B16 malignant melanoma was also observed in mice carrying leukemias or other solid tumors. These data suggest that inducers do have antitumor activity but, like interferon and other immune modulators, have a limited tumor-load capability and may be most effective if administered following surgery or in conjunction with cytotoxic agents. Results using pyrimidinones administered after surgical removal of a primary tumor are summarized in Table 5. Animals were injected with B16 malignant melanoma in the footpad and then 7, 14, or 21 days later the leg was amputated. Treatment was begun 1 day after surgery, using placebo or ABPP. Surgery consistently enhanced the antitumor activity of the pyrimidinone.

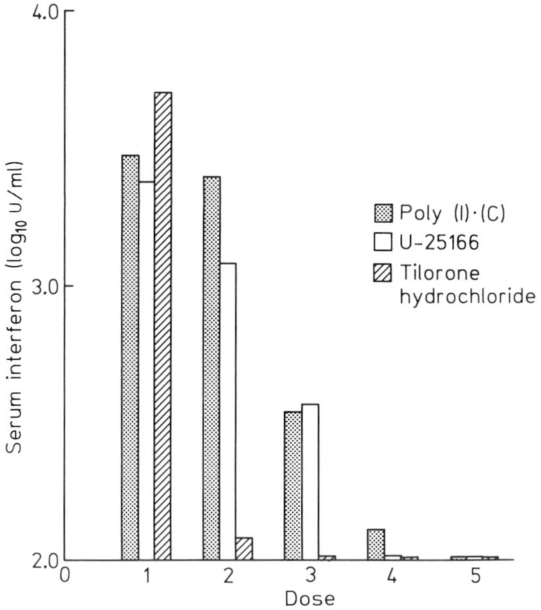

Fig. 3. Development of hyperactivity to interferon induction in mice to repeated daily doses of the same inducer

D. Hyporeactivity

The data presented so far suggest that interferon inducers are good immune potentiators and have antiviral and antitumor activity which may or may not be related to the interferon they induce. Yet, they do have a unique set of problems which is not observed with many other chemotherapeutic agents. That is, after animals are exposed to repeated daily injections of an interferon inducer, they lose their ability to respond to further interferon induction. In Fig. 3, mice received daily injections of a single interferon inducer and developed a severely impaired ability to respond to each of the inducers. This occurred with every interferon inducer and in every animal species that we have evaluated so far. Furthermore, mice infected with any of several viruses or carrying neoplastic diseases also develop a hyporeactive state. For example, as illustrated in Fig. 4, mice infected with encephalomyocarditis and then given a single injection of an interferon inducer 1, 2, 3, or 4 days later become less responsive to induction. The hyporeactive state was, however, inducer dependent. Mice were hyporeactive to tilorone hydrochloride as early as the second day of infection whereas poly(I)·poly(C) and the pyrimidinone could induce interferon through the fourth day of disease. These results suggest that virus infection and neoplastic disease may severely restrict use of such agents. Animals infected with encephalomyocarditis virus did not develop signs and symptoms of illness until the fourth or fifth day of disease. By the time they had developed signs of illness, they were hyporeactive to interferon induction.

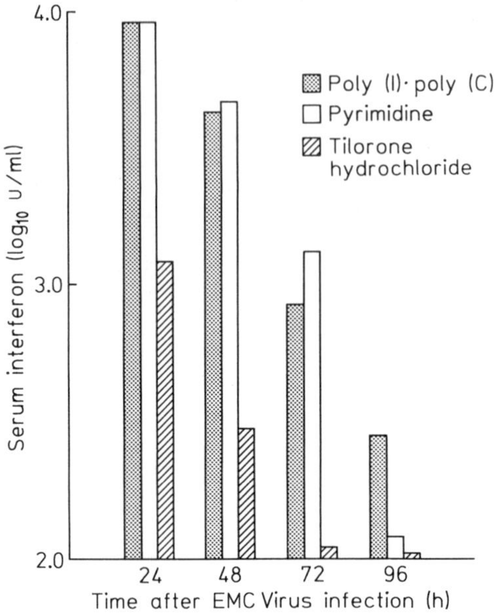

Fig. 4. Development of hyporeactivity to interferon induction in mice infected with encephalomyocarditis virus; mice received a single dose of inducer 1, 2, 3, or 4 days after infection

Results from efforts to overcome or avoid the hyporeactive state caused by multiple doses of an inducer suggest that treatment regimens can be developed which will decrease the severity of this phenomenon. Spacing injections of inducers over a long enough period will allow the animal to maintain a normal interferon response. For example, cats are able to respond to weekly administration of one of the pyrimidinone compounds (ABMP) over extended periods of time and remain responsive. If the compound is given daily, however, the animals become hyporeactive by the third day. By allowing an appropriate interval between injections of an inducer, the hyporeactive state was avoided. Many of the low molecular weight compounds discussed in this chapter can mediate an antiviral state that will persist for as long as 14 days. That is, after a single injection animals are resistant to virus infection for 14 days. This suggests that it may be possible to use such compounds in a once-weekly treatment regimen and maintain the desired biologic response indefinitely. Furthermore, administration of inducers in alternating sequences has overcome development of the hyporeactive state. As illustrated in Table 6, once animals were hyporeactive to tilorone hydrochloride, they were still responsive to injection of an unrelated inducer such as poly(I)·poly(C) or one of the pyrimidinone compounds. Likewise, once animals had become hyporeactive to pyrimidinones, they could be stimulated to produce interferon with an unrelated interferon inducer such as tilorone hydrochloride.

The problem of onset of hyporeactivity as a result of virus infection or neoplastic diseases has been a little more difficult to overcome, but studies reported in the past 2 years indicate that coadministration of inducers with prostaglandins

Table 6. Development of hyporeactivity to interferon induction in mice given daily doses of the same or another inducer[a]

Dose 1	Interferon (U/ml)	Dose 2	Interferon (U/ml)	Dose 3	Interferon (U/ml)	Dose 4	Interferon (U/ml)
ABMP	1,200						
ABMP		ABMP	500				
ABMP		Tilorone	4,600				
ABMP		BAA	4,500				
ABMP		PBS	< 50				
ABMP		ABMP		ABMP	300		
ABMP		ABMP		Tilorone	4,100		
ABMP		ABMP		BAA	3,100		
ABMP		ABMP		PBS	< 50		
ABMP		ABMP		ABMP		ABMP	< 50
ABMP		ABMP		ABMP		Tilorone	4,000
ABMP		ABMP		ABMP		BAA	2,500
ABMP		ABMP		ABMP		PBS	< 50
BAA	3,500						
BAA		BAA	400				
BAA		ABMP	5,000				
BAA		Tilorone	50				
BAA		BAA		BAA	550		
BAA		BAA		ABMP	730		
BAA		BAA		Tilorone	< 50		
BAA		BAA		BAA		BAA	< 50
BAA		BAA		BAA		ABMP	900
BAA		BAA		BAA		Tilorone	< 50

[a] ABMP = 2-amino-5-bromo-6-methyl-4-pyrimidinol; BAA = 1,5-bis[(3-morpholinopropyl)amino]anthraquinone

can restore the interferon response of hyporeactive cells and animals. Coadministration of an inducer with prostaglandin has correspondingly enhanced the antiviral activity of interferon inducers (STRINGFELLOW 1980).

E. Summary

Nonpolynucleotide interferon inducers represent a unique group of potential chemotherapeutic agents, possessing unique properties and problems. At present, predicting what molecules will be active interferon inducers is not possible. The only thing known is that once a molecule is found that is capable of inducing an interferon response, minor modification of that molecule can drastically alter biologic activity. Although referred to as interferon inducers, they are potent immune potentiators, increasing various immune parameters. Instead of being considered only as interferon inducers, they should be considered in a broader context of biologic response modifiers. This may explain why the ability of these molecules to mediate antiviral and antitumor activity is independent of their ability to induce interferon. The observation that a molecule cannot induce an interferon response is no guarantee it will not mediate antiviral or antitumor activity in vivo. The antitumor and antiviral activity of biologic response modifiers such as the low molecular weight inducers and interferon itself is very tumor-load or virus-load dependent. That is, the biologic activity can be overwhelmed by increasing the challenge inoculum. Interestingly, however, inducers uniformly have greater antitumor activity than exogenously transferred interferon. This may be because more circulating interferon was stimulated by the inducers than could be transferred exogenously or may be attributed to the additional immune potentiating properties of these molecules

The obvious question remaining is: where are we now and where do we go from here? Many of the molecules, particularly the pyrimidinones, are well tolerated by experimental animals and appear to have much less toxicity than inducers which have previously been evaluated clinically. The pyrimidinones are currently undergoing clinical studies, and answers on their tolerance and efficacy in the treatment of virus infections and neoplastic diseases should be available soon. The prospects are bright for the use of molecules like interferon inducers. They have, in many cases, properties that seem to be completely independent of the circulating interferon response, and availability of interferon produced through recombinant DNA technology should not affect their clinical development and utilization. In fact, there are situations where interferon and inducers have separate and distinct advantages, and use of one or the other, or both, may be indicated.

References

Einhorn S, Strander H (1977) Is interferon tissue specific? Effect of human leukocyte and fibroblast interferons on the growth of lymphoblastoid and osteosarcoma cell lines. J Gen Virol 35:573–580

Fast PE, Stringfellow DA (1980) Immune modulation by two antiviral isocytosines with different abilities to induce interferon. In: Nelson JD, Grassi C (eds) Current chemotherapy and infectious disease. Am Soc Microbiol Washington DC, pp 1396–1398

Field AK, Tytell AA, Lampson GP, Hilleman MR (1967) Inducers of interferon and host resistance, II. Multistranded synthetic polynucleotide complexes. Proc Natl Acad Sci USA 58:1004–1010

Gatmaitan BG, Stanley ED, Jackson GG (1973) The limited effect of nasal interferon induced by rhinovirus and a topical chemical inducer on the course of infection. J Infect Dis 127:401–407

Glaz ET, Szologay E, Stoger I, Talas M (1973) Antiviral activity and induction of interferon-like substance by Quinacrine and Acranil. Antimicrob Agents Chemother 3:537

Hill DA, Baran S, Levy HB, Bellanti J, Buckler CE (1971) Clinical studies of induction of interferon by polyinosinic-polycytidylic acid. Perspect Virol 7:197–222

Hoffman WW, Korst JJ, Niblack JF, Cronin TH (1973) N, N-dioctadecyl-N′, N′-bis(2-hydroxyethyl) propanediamine: antiviral activity and interferon stimulation in mice. Antimicrob Agents Chemother 3:498

Kaufman HE, Centifanto YM, Ellison ED, Brown DC (1971) Tilorone hydrochloride: human toxicity and interferon stimulation. Proc Soc Exp Biol Med 137:357–360

Mayer GD, Krueger RF (1970) Tilorone hydrochloride: mode of action. Science 169:1214

Merigan TC, Reed SE, Hall TS, Tyrell D (1973) Inhibition of respiratory virus infection by locally applied interferon. Lancet i:563–566

Merigan TC, Rand KH, Pollard RB, Abdallah PS, Jordan GW, Fried RP (1978) Human leukocyte interferon for the treatment of herpes zoster in patients with cancer. New Engl J Med 18:981–987
Panusarn C, Stanley ED, Dirda V, Rubenis M, Jackson GG (1974) Prevention of illness from rhinovirus infection by a topical interferon inducer. New Engl J Med 291:57–61
Renis HE, Eidson EE (1980) Protection of mice from herpes simplex virus infection by 5-halo, 6-arylisocytosines. In: Nelson JD, Grassi C (eds) Current chemotherapy and infectious disease. Am Soc Microbiol, Washington, DC
Strander H, Cantell K, Jakobsson PA, Nilsonne U, Soderber G (1974) Exogenous interferon therapy of osteogenic sarcoma. Acta Orthop Scand 45:958–961
Steinenbring WR, Youngner JS (1964) Patterns of interferon appearance in mice injected with bacteria or bacterial endotoxin. Nature 204:712
Strander H, Einhorn S (1977) Effect of human leukocyte interferon on the growth of human osteosarcoma cells in tissue culture. Int J Cancer 19:468–473
Strander H, Adamson U, Aparisi T, Broström A, Cantell K, Einhorn S, Hall K, Ingimarsson S, Nilsonne U, Söderberg G (1979) Adjuvant interferon treatment of human osteosarcoma. In: Bonadonna G, Mathe G, Salmon SE (eds) Adjuvant therapies and markers of post-surgical minimal residual disease II. Springer, Berlin Heidelberg New York, pp 40–44 (Recent results in cancer research, vol 68)
Stringfellow DA, Weed SD, Underwood GE (1979) Antiviral and interferon-inducing properties of 1,5-diamino anthraquinones. Antimicrob Agents Chemother 15:111
Stringfellow DA, Vanderberg HC, Weed SD (1980) Interferon induction by 5-halo-6-phenyl pyrimidinones. J Interferon Res 1:1–16
Stringfellow DA (1980) Interferon inducers: theory and experimental application. In: Stringellow DA (ed) Interferon and interferon inducers: clinical applications. Dekker, New York, pp 145–164
Wierenga W, Skulnick HI, Stringfellow DA, Weed SD, Renis HE, Eidson EE (1979) 5-Substituted 2-amino-6-phenyl-4(3H)-pyrimidinones. Antiviral- and interferon-inducing agents. J Med Chem 23:237–239

CHAPTER 19

Agents Which Modulate the Activity of Interferon

D. R. STRAYER and W. A. CARTER

A. Introduction

Interferons are obviously well-established physiologic substances which exert their biologic actions by a multiplicity of intracellular events, often carried out by intracellular substances whose synthesis is controlled by cell exposure to interferon. Such substances are, however, not well characterized and often are simply termed "interferon-associated intracellular mediators." Several are described in detail in various chapters of this volume. There are a variety of other physiologic substances, such as glucocorticoids and growth factors, whose biologic actions also seem to center, in a major way, on their ability to modulate the intracellular concentrations of various other effector substances (mediators). Cyclic nucleotides, as well as proteins which modulate levels of intracellular RNA, are just two examples of the biochemical spectrum of intracellular mediating substances whose concentrations can wax and wane, dependent on exposure of the cell to interferon, glucocorticoids, etc.

It should thus come as no surprise that there are a variety of established drugs, as well as potential new human medicinal substances, which alter the biologic properties of interferons. In some instances, these alterations afford enhanced biologic activity of the interferon polypeptide while, in others, the properties of interferon are simply altered or altogether eliminated. Clearly, it behooves the laboratory researcher, as well as the clinical pharmacologist, to be aware of the potential for interplay of the interferon effect with that of other chemotherapeutic agents. We are especially concerned herein with other drugs which may be used in situations of human neoplasia and viral disease. In other words, clinical situations in which interferon is also being evaluated.

Our chapter describes a group of examples demonstrating these modulation phenomena, ranging over those that occur with antineoplastic agents, antiviral drugs, and various physiologic substances. In many cases, the molecular basis for modulation of the properties of interferon still remains obscure. Nonetheless, we believe that it is timely to catalog these data even in their present rudimentary from, because this may help set the stage for a more systematic study of a potentially very important area of research. We have observed that such a compilation of experiments has apparently not been previously advanced, despite the significant number of treatises on interferon itself.

We believe that the ability to orchestrate a variety of intracellular effects simultaneously, such as by the coadministration of interferon with other medicinal substances, may prove eventually to be a potent way to control and direct the intrinsic power of the interferon system; indeed, there is already some evidence that one can improve the therapeutic outcome in certain animal tumor models by judicious use of interferon in combination with other well-established chemotherapeutic regimens. It is obviously our hope that this line of research, in its accelerated form, can also lead to improved therapeutic outcomes in humans treated with interferon.

B. Antineoplastic Agents

I. Antiviral Effects

Antineoplastic therapy in patients with certain malignant diseases, especially leukemia, may increase the severity of viral infections. For example, adrenocorticosteroid therapy has been implicated in favoring dissemination of herpes zoster (MERSELIS et al. 1964) and methotrexate, 6-mercaptopurine, and adrenocorticosteroid therapy may play a causal role in the severe and often fatal nature of chickenpox in patients with acute leukemia (PINKEL 1961).

CESARIO and SLATER (1980) studied the effects of seven antineoplastic agents (methotrexate, 5-fluorouracil, adriamycin, vincristine, 6-mercaptopurine, hydrocortisone, and estradiol) on the antiviral activity of human interferons-α and -β. Results of their in vitro studies are summarized in Table 1. Methotrexate and 5-fluorouracil had no effect on the titers of either interferon. Adriamycin and 6-mercaptopurine lowered the titers only when used during a pretreatment phase while vincristine decreased the titers of both interferons in both pretreatment and simultaneous treatment schedules. No consistent effect of hydrocortisone was detected. In contrast, ST. GEME et al. (1969), using a different system, failed to block the antiviral action of a chicken interferon with 6-mercaptopurine (3–30 μg/ml) in a 4-h preincubation plus 24-h simultaneous exposure with interferon. BOURGEADE et al. (1980) showed that cytochalasin-B, colchicine, and vinblastine, agents which disrupt the cytoskeletal network, reduced the antiviral effect of both type I and II mouse interferons.

II. Antitumor Effects

Clinical studies of human interferon-α in patients with malignancy have demonstrated antineoplastic activity against a number of tumor types including breast cancer, multiple myeloma, poorly differentiated nodular lymphoma, and acute lymphatic leukemia (MERIGAN et al. 1978; GUTTERMAN et al. 1980). Although several patients with poorly differentiated nodular lymphoma have had complete remissions (CR), the majority of responders have had partial (PR), or less than partial remissions. We believe that one approach for boosting the response rate will be to use interferon in combination with other antineoplastic agents. Clearly, the goal will be to develop combinations with additive or even synergistic activities while avoiding combinations which are antagonistic.

Antineoplastic drugs can often modulate the effectiveness of exogenous interferon preparations. Presumably, this phenomenon derives in part from the fact that interferon action entails the requirements for "effector" protein synthesis, such protein (or proteins) being implicated in actually carrying out, at an intracellular level, the biochemical actions initially triggered at the cell surface by exposure to, and binding of, the interferon molecule. Accordingly, drugs which interfere

Table 1. The effects[a] of various antineoplastic drugs on the antiviral activity of human interferons

Drug	Concentration (μg/ml)	Titer reduction (%)			
		Simultaneous		Pretreatment plus simultaneous	
		α	β	α	β
Methotrexate	16.0	0	0	0	0
	160.0	N.R.	0	N.R.	N.R.
5-Fluorouracil	40.0	0	0	0	0
	400.0	N.R.	0	N.R.	N.R.
Adriamycin	0.40	0	0	50–88	50–88
Vincristine	0.08	50–75	50	75–88	75–88
6-Mercaptopurine	3.2	0	0	50–75	50–75
	32.0	N.R.	0	N.R.	N.R.
Hydrocortisone	80.0	0	0–50	0	0
Estradiol	0.08	0	0	0	0
	0.80	N.R.	50	N.R.	N.R.

[a] The effects of each antineoplastic drug were observed either by adding the drug to cell culture simultaneously with the interferon (Simultaneous) or by overnight exposure of the cell monolayers to the drug followed by addition of interferon (Pretreatment plus simultaneous). The interferon assays were performed using human fibroblasts in a microassay using vesicular stomatitis virus as the challenge virus (CESARIO and SLATER 1980). N.R. refers to experimental blocks not reported

with transcription of mRNA or the mechanisms of protein biosynthesis may therefore modulate the ability of a target cell to propagate a biochemical signal it receives from administered interferon. Antitranscription and antiprotein synthesis activities are commonly associated with the action of anticancer drugs. Accordingly, the coadministration of anticancer drugs with interferon preparations must always be carefully thought through such that the desired effects are not readily cancelled out by incompatible intracellular events. L-cell interferon in combination with other antineoplastic agents was tested against L1210 leukemia (SLATER et al. 1981). Although L-cell interferon failed to increase the survival of BDF/1 mice with L1210 leukemia, which had been treated with 6-mercaptopurine, cyclophosphamide, cytosine arabinoside, or adriamycin, the survival time was significantly increased by the addition of L-cell interferon to methotrexate alone or in combination with 6-mercaptopurine ($P < 0.05$). These increased antitumor effects were additive rather than synergistic. BROSTRÖM (1980) studied the growth-inhibitory action of human interferon-α in combination with methotrexate on three human tumor cell lines which were sensitive to both agents. No definite synergistic or inhibitory effects were seen. The Daudi cell line appeared to be inhibited to a greater extent by the combination of 1.0 U/ml interferon-α plus 10 n*M* methotrexate than to either agent alone. Different results were obtained with the two osteosarcoma cell lines: a suggestion of increased growth inhibition by the combination was seen at one concentration level in only one of the two cell lines.

A synergistic antitumor effect was found by CHIRIGOS and PEARSON (1973) using BCNU in combination with interferon to treat mice injected with LSTRA leukemia cells. BCNU treatment was used as initial therapy to decrease the tumor burden (mass of tumor cells) followed by interferon in an attempt to eradicate the remaining leukemic cells. This effect was apparently achieved in that the overall cure rate of 71% ($P = 0.005$) was obtained in the combination treated group compared to only a 25% cure rate obtained with BCNU treatment alone. Importantly, interferon treatment alone did not prolong survival time. Similar results for simultaneous interferon and cyclophosphamide therapy have been obtained by GRESSER et al. (1978) in treating the spontaneous lymphoma of AKR mice. Their results suggest that therapy with interferon and cyclophosphamide, after diagnosis of lymphoma, contribute in an additive way to increased survival of AKR virus-infected mice.

C. Antiviral Agents

I. Acyclovir

Acyclovir, 9-(2-hydroxyethoxymethyl)guanine, a new antiviral drug, has antiherpes activity in several animal models as well as in human clinical trials. Human interferon-α administration following surgical manipulation of the trigeminal nerve roots has been shown to prevent reactivation of herpes simplex infection (PAZIN et al. 1979). These observations formed the basis for a study by STANWICK et al. (1981) who demonstrated that acyclovir and human interferon-β have an additive, possibly synergistic, effect against herpes simplex viruses 1 and 2 in Vero cells. Acyclovir alone was not active against vesicular stomatitis virus (VSV) and did not affect the activity of interferon-β against VSV.

II. Isoprinosine

Isoprinosine, an immunostimulant, has been reported to increase the antiviral activity of interferon against encephalomyocarditis virus (EMCV) infection in mice (CHANY and CERUTTI 1977). However, several specific conditions, including the route of administration of virus and interferon, as well as the time sequence of injections, are apparently critical for success. In general, the isoprinosine has to be given several hours prior to the interferon. More recently, FOMINA et al. (1980) observed an increased efficacy of a combination treatment using isoprinosine and mouse interferon against experimental viral encephalitis as compared with the effectiveness of either substance used alone. Again, the timing of drug administration was important with maximum effect being observed when the interval between administration of isoprinosine and interferon was prolonged up to 24 h.

Isoprinosine, in addition to augmenting the antiviral activity of interferon, has been shown to increase the antitumor action of interferon (CERUTTI et al. 1979). Mice were inoculated with 10^6 sarcoma 180/TG cells, whereupon therapy was initiated immediately with interferon, followed by isoprinosine 3 h later. This regimen was continued three times a week for 1 month. Mean survival time was 26 days in the control group, 23 days in the isoprinosine only group, 45 days in the interferon only group, and 64 days ($P < 0.005$ compared with the interferon only group) in the group treated with both interferon and isoprinosine. In addition, the final survival rate for those treated with isoprinosine and interferon (21/50) was greater than those treated with interferon alone (10/50; $P<0.05$) or the untreated controls (1/50; $P<0.001$).

III. Trifluorothymidine

Topical treatment of dentritic keratitis with either human interferon-α or trifluorothymidine has been reported to be of benefit. A randomized clinical trial using daily topical human interferon-α (30×10^6 U/ml) plus 1.0% trifluorothymidine found a significantly increased healing rate ($P<0.01$) of 2.9 days for the drug combination compared with 5.7 days for the trifluorothymidine alone group (SUNDMACHER et al. 1978). Relatively high local concentrations of interferon may be required since addition of a lower concentration of interferon-α (1×10^6 U/ml) to the trifluorothymidine treatment did not improve the rate of healing significantly over trifluorothymidine alone.

IV. Adenine Arabinoside

The combined antiviral effects of interferon plus adenine arabinoside (9-β-D-arabinofuranosyladenine) have been studied against herpes simplex viruses. LERNER and BAILEY (1974) found that human leukocyte interferon and adenine arabinoside were synergistic against HSV-1 (Ket strain) in an in vitro Vero tissue culture system. However, the combination of interferon plus adenine arabinoside appeared to be only additive against HSV-2 (LERNER and BAILEY 1976; BRYSON and KRONENBERG 1977) and vaccinia virus (BRYSON and KRONENBERG 1977).

Recently, SCULLARD et al. (1981) have used human leukocyte interferon plus adenine arabinoside to treat patients with chronic hepatitis associated with hepatitis virus B infection. Their results suggest that combination therapy was superior to either interferon or adenine arabinoside therapy alone in reducing or eliminating hepatitis B core antigen (HB_cAg)-staining as well as hepatitis B surface antigen (HB_sAg)-staining cells in immunofluorescent assays obtained from liver biopsy of patients before and after treatment.

D. Ganglioside-Binding Agents

The initial event required for interferon action is thought to involve its binding to ganglioside or ganglioside-like oligosaccharide receptors located on the surface of cells. This interaction at the cell membrane triggers a variety of intracellular processes and biochemical events which in turn are responsible for induction of the antiviral state. The B protein of cholera toxin and the B subunit of thyroid-stimulating hormone (TSH) also possess determinants which promote their interaction with ganglioside-containing receptors on the cell membrane. FRIEDMAN and KOHN have shown that cholera toxin or TSH added prior to, or at the same time as, interferon inhibit the establishment of antiviral activity in mouse L-cells (FRIEDMAN and KOHN 1976; KOHN et al. 1976). Neither cholera toxin nor TSH influences antiviral activity established prior to their addition. Whether interferon and cholera toxin share the same receptors on the cell surface, or alternatively whether mere binding of cholera toxin to the plasma membrane inhibits establishment of the interferon-induced antiviral state, is unknown. However, various lines of evidence suggest to us that these two proteins may share homologous regions of amino acid sequence which can lead to competition for available cell-binding sites.

DEGRÉ (1978) obtained evidence that cholera toxin inhibited both the antiviral and antiproliferative activities of human leukocyte interferon-α. His antiproliferative assays utilized cell counts of human amnion cells following 3 days of exposure to interferon and cholera toxin. In contrast, FUSE and KUWATA (1979), using the inhibition of DNA synthesis in RSa cells as an assay for antiproliferative activity, found that cholera toxin added with interferon inhibited the antiviral action, but not the antiproliferative activity of human leukocyte interferon-α.

Cholera toxin or its B subunit block the augmentation of erythroid differentiation of dimethylsulfoxide (DMSO)-treated Friend cells induced by low doses of interferon (BELARDELLI et al. 1980). Since the purified B subunit of cholera toxin is unable to activate adenylate cyclase, these results suggest that cholera toxin-induced alterations of membrane components, rather than increased intracellular cyclic AMP levels, may explain these effects on the differentiation-promoting action of interferon. In contrast, recent results of GOLDFARB and HERBERMAN (1981) as well as FUSE and KUWATA (1981) suggest that cholera toxin-mediated inhibition of human natural killer (NK) cell activity was at least partly modulated by intracellular cyclic nucleotides. Cholera toxin, but not its B subunit, inhibited both interferon-directed as well as "spontaneous" NK cell activity. In addition, GOLDFARB and HERBERMAN (1981) showed that cholera toxin A subunit had no depressive effect on NK cell activity. Thus, cell surface binding and cyclic AMP stimulation may be required for cholera toxin inhibition of NK cell activity, both the "spontaneous" activity as well as that promoted by exposure to the interferon molecule. It is of course possible that the mechanism of "spontaneous" activity of NK cells also derives from stimulation by endogenous interferon production.

E. Hormones

I. Glucocorticoids

Reports by workers studying the effects of glucocorticoids on the antiviral activity of interferon have suggested variable results, depending on the particular test system used. KILBOURNE et al. (1961) studying interferon produced by intraallantoic inoculation of chick embryos, obtained evidence that a prior 2-h exposure of chorioallantoic membranes to cortisone decreased the subsequent antiviral effects of preformed interferon against influenza virus. CESARIO and SLATER (1980) saw now consistent effect of hydrocortisone on the antiviral activity of human interferons-α and -β (see Sect. B. Antineoplastic Agents).

DE MAEYER and DE MAEYER (1963) studied the influence of the glucocorticoid, cortisol, and the androgenic steroid, Δ^1, 17α-methyltestosterone, on the antiviral action of interferon against Sindbis virus in rat tumor cell cultures. Both steroids increased the antiviral activity of interferon after a prior overnight incubation of cells with the steroid alone or with interferon. No increase in interferon activity was seen if: (1) the interferon exposure occurred first and the steroid was added subsequently; or (2) the cultures, exposed to steroid plus interferon overnight, were washed free of both drugs prior to virus challenge. No change in interferon activity was seen with the treatment schedule reported by KILBOURNE et al. (1961).

MENDELSON and GLASGOW (1966) found that cortisol at 2, 4, or 10 mg/ml had no effect on the activity of either mouse or chicken interferon. WU et al. (1976) showed that dexamethasone partially inhibited the antiviral activity of murine interferon on xenotropic type C virus production induced by iododeoxyuridine from K-BALB cells. The dexamethasone (10^{-6} *M*) was present during a 12-h interval (36–48 h after induction) following a 12-h interferon exposure. Maximal stimulation of virus production by dexamethasone was obtained 24 h after removal of the interferon. However, viral production at maximal stimulation was only 30%–50% of that produced by dexamethasone in the absence of interferon. Such studies are reminiscent of various clinical observations, suggesting that treatment of viral myocarditis with corticosteroids may result in apparent overproduction of virus (and resultant heart cell damage) possibly due to the antagonistic effect of corticosteroids on the endogenous interferon defense mechanism triggered by viral infection.

In summary, the modulatory effects of glucocorticoids upon the antiviral activity of interferon are apparently complex and results will vary, depending upon: (1) the host cell and virus system studied; (2) the steroid concentration and schedule employed; and (3) the particular glucocorticoid chosen. Given the multiplicity of actions of both drugs when studied separately, and the variety of intracellular mediators associated with this diverse cellular effect, it would be likely that even more diversity will be reported in future studies on the interplay of these two drugs.

II. Estrogens

SEAMAN et al. (1979) have shown that chronic adminstration of 17β-estradiol to BALB/c female mice led to reduced levels of NK cell activity. In addition, estrogen-treated mice had less augmentation of natural killing in response to 50 μg poly(I-C) compared with sham-treated control mice. Serum interferon levels following poly(I-C) treatment were slightly, but not significantly, higher in the estrogen-treated mice. Thus, the reduction in natural killing observed after sustained high levels of 17β-estradiol treatment in mice is not completely abrogated by induction of high circulating levels of interferon. Estrogens are apparently not directly toxic to mature NK cells since they do not alter NK cell activity in vitro, and at least 2 weeks of estrogen administration is required for a reduction in vivo (SEAMAN et al. 1978). Whether estrogen treatment blocks the maturation of NK cell precursors, or leads to inhibition of natural killing by mature NK cells, has not been resolved. We have also recently observed (D. R. STRAYER and W. A. CARTER 1982, unpublished work) that, in normal human subjects, a statistically significant reduction in NK cell activity is observed in the female as compared with age-matched males.

F. Growth Factors

Antagonism in action between interferons and several growth factors including platelet-derived growth factor (PDGF), fibroblast growth factor (FGF), and epidermal growth factor (EGF) has been reported recently (INGLOT et al. 1980; OLESZAK and INGLOT 1980; LIN et al. 1980; and SREEVALSAN et al. 1980). In contrast, interleukin-2 (IL-2) and interferon appear additive in augmenting NK cell activity (HENNEY et al. 1981; KURIBAYASHI et al. 1981). INGLOT et al. (1980), using asynchronous cell cultures, crude preparations of PDGF, and partially purified preparations of interferon, obtained evidence for an antagonism between the action of PDGF and mouse or human interferon. Human leukocyte interferon (100–10,000 U/ml) abolished the mitogenic effect of human PDGF on T98G, a human glioblastoma multiforme cell line. Similarly, the mitogenic effect of bovine PDGF on mouse L929 cells was eliminated by mouse fibroblast interferon (100–1,000 U/ml). In addition, the antiviral and anticellular action of both forms of interferon was inhibited by bovine PDGF. Under certain conditions, OLESZAK and INGLOT (1980) showed that EGF and FGF also acted as antagonists to the action of interferon. The mitogenic action of EGF (100 ng/ml) on T98G cells was reduced 80% by human leukocyte interferon (1,000 U/ml). Similarly, pretreatment of T98G cells with the same concentration of EGF resulted in inhibition of the anticellular action of interferon. In addition, FGF (5–50 ng/ml) reduced the antiviral activity of mouse interferon by 30%–90%.

LIN et al. (1980) also studied the effects of interferon on EGF action. Pretreatment of human fibroblasts with human fibroblast interferon (1,000 U/ml) inhibited EGF-stimulated TdR ^{3}H incorporation by more than 80%. In addition, when interferon was added subsequent to the EGF stimulus, the interferon growth-inhibiting action appeared rapidly within 1 h, suggesting that de novo gene expression may not be required. In these studies, interferon abolished the mitogenic effect of EGF without affecting receptor binding of EGF and without blocking amino acid transport (γ-aminoisobutyrate uptake). SREEVALSAN et al. (1980) investigated the differential effect of mouse L-cell interferon on DNA synthesis, 2-deoxyglucose uptake, and ornithine decarboxylase (ODC) activity in 3T3 cells which had been stimulated by growth factors including EGF and tumor promoters. The mouse interferon inhibited DNA synthesis and ODC activity, but had no effect on 2-deoxyglucose uptake.

The lymphokine IL-2, also termed T-cell growth factor, has recently been shown to augment the cytotoxic activity of NK cells (HENNEY et al. 1981; KURIBAYASHI et al. 1981). When preparations of IL-2 (devoid of interferon activity) were added to increasing doses of purified mouse fibroblast interferon, natural killing activity was stimulated to a greater extent than that seen with optimal concentrations of fibroblast interferon alone. In addition, monoclonal anti-IL-2 antibody preparations were able to block the NK cell-augmenting activity of the IL-2 preparations. However, since FARRAR et al. (1981) have shown that IL-2 has the ability to stimulate T-cells to produce immune interferon, the possibility exists that immune interferon working in a cooperative manner with fibroblast interferon can also explain the increased natural killing seen with IL-2 preparations.

G. Prostaglandins

The prostaglandins comprise a group of naturally occuring cyclic fatty acids which have been shown to promote a wide variety of biologic responses. Moreover, recent observations have established several important relationships between prostaglandins and the interferon system. YARON et al. (1977) demonstrated that poly(I-C) (10–100 µg/ml) and human interferon-β (10–100 U/ml) stimulated prostaglandin E (PGE) production by human synovial and foreskin fibroblasts in culture. Cortisol (2 μg/ml), aspirin (200 μg/ml), and indomethacin (2 μg/ml) inhibited this PGE induction by over 90% (YARON et al. 1978). FITZPATRICK and STRINGFELLOW (1980) showed that interferon induction following viral infection in seven different cell lines correlated 95% of the time with cellular prostaglandin (PGE_2 and PGFα) secretion. In addition, exogenously added human interferon (10 U/ml) stimulated both PGE_2 and $PGF_2\alpha$ production by human lung fibroblasts. Thus, the results of both YARON et al. (1977) as well as FITZPATRICK and STRINGFELLOW (1980) demonstrate that interferon, whether added exogenously or induced endogenously by viruses, can stimulate prostaglandin formation by cultured cells.

One clue to the possible role of interferon-stimulated prostaglandin production was obtained by STRINGFELLOW (1978), who showed that certain prostaglandins (PGE_1, $PGF_1\alpha$, PGA_1, PGE_2, $PGF_2\alpha$, and PGA_2) restore the cellular interferon response in mice rendered hyporeactive by viral infection. Hyporeactivity refers to the inability of an animal, or cells thereof, to respond to an interferon inducer. Furthermore, certain prostaglandins (PGE_1 and $PGF_1\alpha$) enhanced both the interferon response and therapeutic efficacy of interferon inducers in Friend leukemia virus-infected mice (STRINGFELLOW 1980). To obtain a significant effect on mortality, inducer and prostaglandin therapy had to be increased from 5 to 10 weeks. Also, initial studies in mice with rapidly progressive virus infections (Semliki Forest virus and EMCV) failed to show a beneficial effect of prostaglandins on the therapeutic efficacy of these particular interferon inducers. The results suggest that the therapeutic efficacy of interferon inducers in certain diseases may be enhanced by prostaglandins and that this approach might be most appropriate for diseases requiring prolonged therapy with increased likelihood of developing a hyporeactive state. Examples of diseases encompassed by this concept would be the so-called slow viruses associated with various demyelinating and certain connective tissue diseases such as rheumatoid arthritis. The specific cellular events which mediate hyporeactivity and are presumably influenced by prostaglandins remain unknown, although these processes appear not to involve cyclic nucleotides or manipulations of overall cellular macromolecular synthesis (STRINGFELLOW 1978).

Another clue to the possible role of interferon-stimulated prostaglandin synthesis has been obtained by POTTATHIL et al. (1980) who discovered that the enzyme, fatty acid cyclooxygenase, which is essential for the biosynthesis of prostaglandins, in necessary in L-cells for the establishment of the interferon-induced antiviral state. Pretreatment of L-cells with inhibitors of fatty acid cyclooxygenase (i.e., 10 μM oxyphenylbutazone, 10 μM phenylbutazone, 10 μM aspirin, or 10 μM indomethacin) suppressed the antiviral activity of mouse interferon against subsequent VSV replication. Loss of interferon antiviral activity correlated with the degree of cyclooxygenase inhibition achieved. However, cyclooxygenase inhibitors did not reverse the antiviral state already established in L-cells by prior treatment with interferon. Paradoxically, the addition of PGE_1, PGE_2, or 6-keto-$PGF_1\alpha$ during the interferon pretreatment resulted in a further reversal of interferon's antiviral activity in the presence of cyclooxygenase inhibitors. Even in the absence of cyclooxygenase inhibitors, prostaglandin pretreatment with interferon resulted in an inhibition of interferon's protective effect. Furthermore, prostaglandin exposure following pretreatment with interferon did not reverse the antiviral protective effect of interferon.

In summary, cyclooxygenase activity appears necessary for the establishment of the interferon-induced antiviral state in L-cells. Since exogenously supplied prostaglandins do not substitute for the presence of cyclooxygenase activity, it appears that an unidentified cyclooxygenase metabolite may be required for the establishment of the interferon-mediated antiviral state in L-cells. Competition between exogenously added prostaglandins and this putative intermediate for a common receptor might then explain the prostaglandin-induced inhibition of interferon's action.

POTTATHIL et al. (1980) believed it was unlikely that increased cAMP was the primary cause of the anti-interferon effect because 6-keto-$PGF_1\alpha$ did not induce an increase in cAMP. In contrast, TROFATTER and DANIELS (1980) attributed to an increase in intracellular cAMP levels the reversal of the interferon-induced antiviral effect against herpes simplex virus (HSV) which they observed with prostaglandin treatment of human skin fibroblasts. Although prostaglandins PGA_1, PGB_1, PGE_1, PGE_2, and $PGF_2\alpha$, as well as other cAMP-elevating agents (isoproterenol, imidozale, carbamylcholine, and dibutyryl cAMP), had no direct effect on HSV growth, these compounds inhibited the antiviral activity of human interferon (TROFATTER and DANIELS 1980). Recently, additional evidence has been reported, suggesting a role for fatty acid cyclooxygenase activity in mediating the effects of interferon (CHANDRABOSE et al. 1981). A clone of L1210 mouse leukemia cells which was selected for interferon resistance (antiviral and antiproliferative) was found to lack cyclooxygenase activity. Mixing experiments failed to demonstrate the presence of a diffusible inhibitor specific for fatty acid cyclooxygenase in these interferon-resistant L1210 cells. Thus, evidence is accumulating which supports the hypothesis that fatty acid cyclooxygenase activity is required to mediate both the antiproliferative and antiviral effects of interferon in mouse cells.

However, recent studies suggest that cyclooxygenase activity may play a somewhat different role in the actions of human interferons as compared with mouse interferons. The studies in human systems come largely from Vanderbilt University (W. MITCHELL, R. FORTI, J. FORBES, R. WORKMAN and W. HUBBARD 1983, unpublished work). These authors observed in human fibroblasts *no* effect of aspirin, indomethacin, or phenylbutazone on the antiviral activity of human interferons-α, -β, or -γ, as judged by cytopathic effects of VSV or VSV release. They did, however, observe that oxyphenylbutazone blocked protection of interferon against VSV effects in these same cells. Thus, a functional cyclooxygenase enzyme may not always be required for the mediation of certain interferon effects.

Important interplay between the prostaglandin and interferon systems has also been demonstrated in host defense mechanisms involving cellular cytotoxicity. For example, SCHULTZ et al. (1978) demonstrated that the prostaglandins PGE_1 and PGE_2, but not $PGF_2\alpha$, inhibit reversibly the tumoricidal activity of interferon-activated macrophages from mice. If PGE_1 or PGE_2 at 10^{-5} *M* was added to the macrophage cultures during a 16-h preincubation step simultaneously with interferon (1,000 U/ml), or added during a brief 2-h pulse immediately following interferon treatment, the interferon activation of tumoricidal macrophages was inhibited 70%–94%. Dibutryl cAMP (10^{-3} *M*), but not dibutryl GMP (10^{-3} *M*), inhibited the cytotoxic activity of interferon-induced macrophages by 55%. These results are consistent with previously reported studies in macrophages demonstrating stimulation of adenylate cyclase by prostaglandins of the E-series (O'DONNELL 1974).

TARGAN (1981) evaluated some of the seemingly intricate interactions of prostaglandin PGE_2 and interferon upon NK cell augmentation. Sequential treatment of peripheral blood lymphocytes from normal donors with human interferon-α (10 U/ml for 1 h) followed by PGE_2 ($10^{-8} M$ for 30 min) synergistically enhanced NK cellular cytotoxicity. If PGE_2 was added too early following the interferon exposure (20 min or less), pre-NK lytic potential was inhibited. Thus, important temporal relationships apparently must be fulfilled to induce synergistic enhancement of NK cell recycling potential by interferon and PGE_2. A single-cell cytotoxicity assay indicated that interferon and PGE_2 acted on the same pre-NK cell population. The mechanism of interferon and PGE_2 synergism seems to involve one or more events which result in an increased frequency of lytic interactions between effector cells and target cells.

H. Vitamins

I. Vitamin A

Vitamin A has been shown to suppress the production as well as inhibit the antiviral action of interferon (BLALOCK and GIFFORD 1974, 1976a). This suppressive effect was blocked by cycloheximide and therefore may be secondary to protein-induced transcriptional controls (BLALOCK and GIFFORD 1977; BLALOCK 1977). The inhibition of the antiviral action of interferon appears to be a result of an interaction between vitamin A and the interferon molecule (BLALOCK and GIFFORD 1975). This inhibitory effect was decreased by increasing concentrations of calf serum which apparently prevented the interaction of retinoic acid and interferon. The loss of interferon activity was greatest when retinoic acid and retinol were present while retinyl acetate and retinol only slightly inhibited interferon activity. Thus, inhibition of interferon action seemed most dependent on the side chain of the vitamin A molecule, while the ring portion appeared to be most important for the suppression of interferon production (BLALOCK and GIFFORD 1976 b).

Retinoic acid (10^{-5}–10^{-7} *M*) enhances human NK cell activity in vitro (GOLDFARB and HERBERMAN 1981). Augmentation in killing activity between 50% and 100% was seen in lymphocyte preparations from approximately 60% of the individuals tested. This boosting of NK cell activity was inhibited by the tumor promotor, PMA (phorbol-12-myristate-13-acetate) and by cholera toxin. Human fibroblast interferon (1,000 U/ml) combined with retinoic acid (10^{-4}–10^{-8} *M*) produced less enhancement in killing than either drug alone.

II. Vitamin C

Several investigators have reported an enhancement of interferon response by vitamin C. SIEGEL (1974) fed BALB/cJ mice L-ascorbate (250 mg%) in their drinking water. After 3 months of this ad libitum diet, mice were inoculated with Rauscher leukemia virus. Animals were bled 72 h later and sera were assayed for interferon by measuring antiviral activity against VSV. Ascorbate-treated mice showed a 62%–145% increase in circulating interferon activity. Although blood ascorbate levels were not measured in these studies, additional in vitro experiments (SIEGEL 1975) showed that media from cultures of mouse L-cells or mouse embryo fibroblasts treated with 10^{-4} M ascorbate and poly(I-C) contained enhanced interferon antiviral activity compared with poly(I-C) treatment alone. Neither of these experiments addressed the question of whether ascorbate promoted the production of interferon or whether ascorbate enhanced the antiviral activity of mouse interferon. However, DAHL and DEGRÉ (1976) studied the effect of ascorbic acid on human interferon production and antiviral activity. Ascorbic acid (10–20 μg/ml) enhanced production of interferon by human embryo skin or lung fibroblasts induced by poly(I-C) or Newcastle disease virus, but did not alter interferon production in two lymphoblastoid cell lines induced by Sendai virus. In addition, human leukocyte interferon (a preparation from K. CANTELL and co-workers) assayed 1.6–2.5 times higher in the presence of ascorbic acid (5 μg/ml). These investigators carefully noted that the small concentrations of ascorbic acid, present in the original induced interferon preparation, had no effect on the antiviral titer.

J. Histamine Antagonists

Certain histamine antagonists, such as cimetidine, a histamine H_2 receptor antagonist, have been shown to exert antitumor activity in vivo in animal models, possibly through inactivation of suppressor T-cells (GIFFORD et al. 1981). Recently, the therapeutic potential of cimetidine in combination with interferon-α has been tested with very encouraging results. BORGSTRÖM et al. (1982) first reported on six patients with malignant melanoma treated with 4×10^6–12×10^6 U/day of leukocyte interferon who began receiving oral cimetidine (1,000 mg/day) as a complement some 3–8 weeks after the start of interferon therapy. No objective tumor regressions had been observed on interferon therapy alone. However, the combined therapy resulted in two complete remissions, one partial remission, and a stationary disease status in another patient. No severe side effects were observed in this small series of patients. HILL et al. (1983) recently confirmed and extended these studies with 17 patients who were entered onto a protocol consisting of intralesional interferon and oral cimetidine (1,200 mg/day). In 15 evaluable patients, they observed 5 objective regressions, 4 patients with stable disease, and 6 had disease progression. Interferon-α dosages ranged from 4×10^6 to 16×10^6 U/week. Thus, results from both groups suggest that interferon and cimetidine together may exert pronounced beneficial effects in certain cases of malignant melanoma.

K. Differentiation-Promoting Agents: DMSO, TPA, Insulin

The interferon system has the ability to modulate the terminal differentiation of eukaryotic cells in a number of model systems. One of the best-studied differentiation models is the DMSO-stimulated Friend erythroleukemic cell system. Relatively high concentrations of mouse interferon (500–1,000 U/ml) inhibited the

DMSO-induced erythroid differentiation of Friend leukemia cells in a dose-dependent manner (ROSSI et al. 1977a). The inhibitory effect was most pronounced when interferon and DMSO were given simultaneously and was reduced if the interferon was given 24–48 h after DMSO. Comparison of the inhibitory effects of pure and partially purified interferon preparations indicated that the inhibitory factor was interferon itself, rather than contaminants (ROSSI et al. 1980). Although the mechanism for induction of differentiation by DMSO is unknown, the inhibition of DMSO-stimulated differentiation of Friend cells by interferon appears to operate at both the level of transcription of globin into RNA and its translation (ROSSI et al. 1977b). In addition, the marked inhibition of hemoglobin production was not paralleled by an overall inhibition of protein synthesis and removal of interferon reversed the differentiation block (ROSSI et al. 1977a). While high concentrations of interferon inhibited DMSO-induced differentiation of Friend leukemia cells, low doses of interferon (5–250 U/ml) without DMSO actually stimulated erythroid differentiation. Moreover, low doses of interferon (12–30 U/ml) were able to enhance globin gene expression induced by submaximal concentrations of DMSO (i.e., 0.8%–1.2% compared with 1.5%, ROSSI et al. 1980).

Another model system in which the possible role of interferon in regulating cellular differentiation has been studied is mouse 3T3 fibroblasts that differentiate into adipose cells. KEAY and GROSSBERG (1980) recently reported that mouse fibroblast interferon (10 U/ml) inhibited the insulin-promoted (10 μg/ml) conversion of 3T3-L1 mouse fibroblasts into adipocytes. The increased incorporation of acetate ^{14}C into lipids induced by insulin was a sensitive indicator of the antidifferentiation effect of interferon with concentrations as low as 1 U being inhibitory. This inhibition appeared not to be secondary to a general cellular toxicity since no inhibitory effects were detected on DNA content or protein synthesis. CIOE' et al. (1980) found that mouse interferon (50–200 U/ml) inhibited the conversion of BALB/c3T3 cells into adipocytes as effectively as 12-*O*-tetradecanoylphorbol-13-acetate (TPA) and that, in combination, the two compounds acted synergistically to block differentiation. Available evidence suggests that interferon and TPA differ in the mechanism by which they inhibit differentiation of the 3T3 cells. In addition, in contrast to the Friend leukemia cell system, inhibition of differentiation alone or in combination with TPA did not affect cell growth as measured by final cell densities or viability of confluent cultures.

A third well-studied model system of differentiation is the mouse myeloid leukemia cell (M1). Treatment of M1 cells in vitro with various inducers, including D-factor (a protein factor contained in certain conditioned media), glucocorticoids, or lipopolysaccharide induced differentiation of the M1 cells into macrophages and granulocytes (HOZUMI et al. 1979). Double-stranded (ds)RNA (i.e., complexes of polyinosinic and polycytidylic acids) enhanced the introduction of differentiation promoted by D-factor, but did not induce differentiation alone (YAMAMOTO et al. 1979). In addition, the dsRNA induced significant levels of interferon and the addition of rabbit antiserum prepared against purified L-cell interferon to the culture abolished the differentiation-enhancing action of the dsRNA. Interestingly, interferon which was purified from dsRNA-treated M1 cells did not itself induce differentiations of M1 cells, but it did enhance the induction of differentiation by D-factor, lipopolysaccharide, or polyinosinic acid (TOMIDA et al. 1980a). These results suggested that this differentiation-promoting effect of dsRNA was mediated by interferon induced in the culture (YAMAMOTO et al. 1979).

Treatment with dsRNA [200 μg poly(I–C) twice weekly] of mice inoculated with M1 cells induced significant serum levels of both interferon and differentiation-stimulating activity and the dsRNA treatment markedly increased the survival of the mice compared with untreated controls (TOMIDA et al. 1980b). STRAYER et al. (1982) have reported that clinical results with mismatched dsRNA in a patient with chronic myelogenous leukemia (Philadelphia chromosome positive) in blastic crisis suggested that the mismatched dsRNA promoted in vivo terminal differentiation of myeloblasts into mature granulocytes. Thus, these results suggest that the promotion of normal differentiation in leukemic cells by the interferon system may become an important new clinical rationale. Enlarged clinical trials coupled with in vitro studies should further define the therapeutic potential of dsRNA and the interferon system in stimulating differentiation. We have also observed (D. R. STRAYER and W. A. CARTER 1982, unpublished work) that mismatched dsRNA, in the presence of hemin, augments differentiation of the human erythroid leukemia cell line, K562. Interestingly, interferon blocks this differentiation step when added to the K562–dsRNA–hemin system. Various lines of evidence are now emerging which indicate that certain dsRNAs, especially the mismatched dsRNAs of the general structure $rI_n \cdot r(C_{12},U)_n$, have biologic activities outside the scope of the interferon molecule. Especially intriguing, for example, are the distinguishing effects observed in cellular differentiation systems as well as in human tumor cell antiproliferative systems (LIN et al. 1982).

L. Conclusion

We have indicated various generic families of established drugs, or potential new drugs, which modulate the activity of interferon and vice versa. While the field of drug interaction is by no means a new one to the clinical pharmacologist, clinical and preclinical interferon researchers are still just beginning to uncover the multiplicity of ways whereby the interferon-induced cascade (clinically, we call it simply the interferon-effect) can be modified by other medicinal substances already within the target cells or about to be administered to the human body.

One can argue that such knowledge is too meticulous or too narrow ever to be of much clinical utility. We believe otherwise. The commonality of molecular targets, for example, between certain glucocorticoids, prostaglandins, and interferons leads us to believe that the potential therapeutic activities of interferons will become more strongly harnessed and directed as the molecular events which underscore "drug modulation" are progressively uncovered.

References

Belardelli F, Ausiello C, Tomasi M, Rossi GB (1980) Cholera toxin and its b subunit inhibit interferon effects on virus production and erythroid differentiation of Friend leukemia cells. Virology 107:109–120

Blalock JE (1977) Inhibition of interferon production by retinoic acid (Vitamin A acid). Tex Rep Biol Med 35:69–77

Blalock JE, Gifford GE (1974) Effect of "Aquasol A," Vitamin A, and "Tween 80" on vesicular stomatitis virus plaque formation and on interferon action. Arch Ges Virusforsch 45:161–164

Blalock JE, Gifford GE (1975) Inhibition of interferon action by vitamin A. J Gen Virol 29:315–324

Blalock JE, Gifford GE (1976a) Suppression of interferon production by vitamin A. J Gen Virol 32:143–147

Blalock JE, Gifford GE (1976b) Comparison of the suppression of interferon production and inhibition of its action by vitamin A and related compounds (39532). Proc Soc Exp Biol Med 153:298–300

Blalock JE, Gifford GE (1977) Retinoic acid (vitamin A acid) induced transcriptional control of interferon production. Proc Natl Acad Sci USA 74:5382–5386

Borgström S, von Eyben FE, Flodgren P, Axelsson B, Sjörgren HO (1982) Human leukocyte interferon and cimetidine for metastatic melanoma. N Engl J Med 307:1080–1081

Bourgeade MF, Chany C, Merigan TC (1980) Type I and type II interferons: differential antiviral actions in transformed cells. J Gen Virol 46:449–454

Broström LÅ (1980) The combined effect of interferon and methotrexate on human osteosarcoma and lymphoma cell lines. Cancer Lett 10:83–90

Bryson YJ, Kronenberg LH (1977) Combined antiviral effects of interferon, adenine arabinoside, hypoxanthine arabinoside, and adenine arabinoside-5′-monophosphate in human fibroblast cultures. Antimicrob Agents Chemother 11:299–306

Cerutti I, Chany C, Schlumberger JF (1979) Isoprinosine increases the antitumor action of interferon. J Immunopharmac 1:59–63

Cesario TC, Slater LM (1980) Diminished antiviral effect of human interferon in the presence of therapeutic concentrations of antineoplastic agents. Infect Immun 27:842–845

Chandrabose KA, Cuatrecases P, Pottathil R, Lang DJ (1981) Interferon-resistant cell line lacks fatty acid cyclooxygenase activity. Science 212:329–331

Chany C, Cerutti I (1977) Enhancement of antiviral protection against encephalomyocarditis virus by a combination of isoprinosine and interferon. Arch Virol 55:225–231

Chirigos MA, Pearson JW (1973) Cure of murine leukemia with drug and interferon treatment. J Natl Cancer Inst 51:1367–1368

Cioe' L, O'Brien TG, Diamond L (1980) Inhibition of adipose conversion of Balb/c 3T3 cells by interferon and 12-O-tetradecanoylphorbol-13-acetate. Cell Biol Int Rep 4:255–264

Dahl H, Degré M (1976) The effect of ascorbic acid on production of human interferon and the antiviral activity in vitro. Acta Pathol Microbiol Scand 84:280–284

Degré M (1978) Cholera toxin inhibits antiviral and growth inhibitory activities of human interferon (40032). Proc Soc Exp Biol Med 157:253–255

De Maeyer E, De Maeyer J (1963) Two-sided effect of steroids on interferon in tissue culture. Nature 197:724–725

Farrar WL, Johnson HM, Farrar JJ (1981) Regulation of the production of immune interferon and cytotoxic T lymphocytes by interleukin 2. J Immunol 126:1120–1125

Fitzpatrick FA, Stringfellow DA (1980) Virus and interferon effects on cellular prostaglandin biosynthesis. J Immunol 125:431–437

Fomina AN, Grigoryan SS, Nikolaeva OV, Ershov FI (1980) Combined use of isoprinosine and interferon inducer in treatment of experimental viral infection. Antibiotiki 25:857

Friedman RM, Kohn LD (1976) Cholera toxin inhibits interferon action. Biochem Biophys Res Commun 70:1078–1084

Fuse A, Kuwata T (1979) Effect of cholera toxin on the antiviral and anticellular activities of human leukocyte interferon. Infect Immun 26:235–239

Fuse A, Sato T, Kuwata T (1981) Inhibitory effect of cholera toxin on human natural cell-mediated cytotoxicity and its augmentation by interferon. Int J Cancer 27:29–36

Gifford RRM, Ferguson RM, Voss BV (1981) Cimetidine reduction of tumour formation in mice. Lancet 1:638–639

Goldfarb RH, Herberman RB (1981) Natural killer cell reactivity: Regulatory interactions among phorbol ester, interferon, cholera toxin, and retinoic acid. J Immunol 126:2129–2135

Gresser I, Maury C, Tovey M (1978) Efficacy of combined interferon cyclophosphamide therapy after diagnosis of lymphoma in AKR mice. Eur J Cancer 14:97–99

Gutterman JJ, Blumenschein GR, Alexanian R, Yap H, Buzdar AU, Cabanillas F, Hortobagyi GN, Hersh EM, Rasmussen SL, Harmon M, Kramer M, Pestka S (1980) Leukocyte interferon-induced tumor regression in human metastatic breast cancer, multiple myeloma and malignant lymphoma. Ann Intern Med 93:399–406

Henney CS, Kuribayashi K, Kern DE, Gillis S (1981) Interleukin-2 augments natural killer cell activity. Nature 291:335–338

Hill NO, Pardue A, Khan A, Hill RW, Aleman C, Hilario R, Hill JM, Osther K (1983) Interferon and cimetidine for malignant melanoma. N Engl J Med 308:286

Hozumi M, Honma Y, Tomida M, Okabe J, Kasukabe T, Sugiyama K, Hayashi M, Takenaga K, Yamamoto Y (1979) Induction of differentiation of myeloid leukemia cells with various chemicals. Acta Haematol Jp 42:941–952

Inglot AD, Oleszak E, Kisielow B (1980) Antagonism in action between mouse or human interferon and platelet growth factor. Arch Virol 63:291–296

Keay S, Grossberg SE (1980) Interferon inhibits the conversion of 3T3-L1 mouse fibroblasts into adipocytes. Proc Natl Acad Sci USA 77:4099–4103

Kilbourne ED, Smart KM, Pokorny BA (1961) Inhibition by cortisone of the synthesis and action of interferon. Nature 190:650–651

Kohn LD; Friedman RM, Holmes JM, Lee G (1976) Use of thyrotropin and cholera toxin to probe the mechanism by which interferon initiates its antiviral activity. Proc Natl Acad Sci USA 73:3695–3699

Kuribayashi K, Gillis S, Kern DE, Henney CS (1981) Murine NK cell cultures: effects of interleukin-2 and interferon on cell growth and cytotoxic reactivity. J Immunol 126:2321–2327

Lerner MA, Bailey EJ (1974) Synergy of 9-β-D-arabinofuranosyladenine and human interferon against herpes simplex virus, type 1. J Infect Dis 130:549–552

Lerner MA, Bailey EJ (1976) Differential sensitivity of herpes simplex virus types 1 and II to human interferon: antiviral effects of interferon plus 9-β-D-arabinofuranosyladenine. J Infect Dis 134:400–404

Lin SL, Ts'o POP, Hollenberg MD (1980) The effects of interferon on epidermal growth factor action. Biochem Biophys Res Commun 96:168–174

Lin SL, Greene JJ, Ts'o POP, Carter WA (1982) Sensitivity and resistance of human tumor cells to interferon and $rI_n \cdot rC_n$. Nature 297:417–419

Mendelson J, Glasgow LA (1966) The in vitro effects of cortisol on interferon production and action. J Immunol 96:345–352

Merigan TC, Sikora K, Breeden JH, Levy R, Rosenberg SA (1978) Preliminary observations on the effect of human leukocyte interferon in non-Hodgkin's lymphoma. N Engl J Med 299:1449–1453

Merselis JG, Kaye D, Hook EW (1964) Disseminated herpes zoster. Arch Intern Med 113:679–686

Oleszak E, Inglot AD (1980) Platelet-derived growth factor (PDGF) inhibits antiviral and anticellular action of interferon in synchronized mouse or human cells. J Interferon Res 1:37–48

Pazin GJ, Armstrong JA, Lam MT, Tarr GC, Jannetta PJ, Ho M (1979) Prevention of reactivated herpes simplex infection by human leukocyte interferon after operation on the trigeminal root. N Engl J Med 301:225–230

Pinkel D (1961) Chickenpox and leukemia. Pediatrics 58:729–737

Pottathil R, Chandrabose KA, Cuatrecasas P, Lang DJ (1980) Establishment of the interferon-mediated antiviral state: Role of fatty acid cyclooxygenase. Proc Natl Acad Sci USA 77:5437–5440

O'Donnell ER (1974) Stimulation and desensitization of macrophage adenylate cyclase by prostaglandins and catecholamines. J Biol Chem 249:3615–3621

Rossi GB, Dolei A, Capobianchi MR; Peschle C, Affabris E (1980) Interactions of interferon with in vitro model systems involved in hematopoietic cell differentiation. Ann NY Acad Sci 350:279–293

Rossi GB; Matarese GP, Grappelli C, Belardelli F, Benedetto A (1977a) Interferon inhibits dimethyl sulphoxide-induced erythroid differentiation of Friend leukemia cells. Nature 267:50–52
Rossi GB, Dolei A, Cioe' L, Benedetto A, Matarese GP, Belardelli F (1977b) Inhibition of transcription and translation of globin messenger RNA in dimethyl sulfoxide-stimulated Friend erythroleukemic cells treated with interferon. Proc Natl Acad Sci USA 74:2036–2040
Schultz RM, Pavlidis NA, Stylos WA, Chirigos MA (1978) Cytotoxic activity of interferon-treated macrophages studied by various inhibitors. Cancer Treat Rep 62:1889–1892
Scullard GH, Pollard RB, Smith JL, Sacks SL, Gregory PB, Robinson WS, Merigan TC (1981) Antiviral treatment of chronic hepatitis B virus infection. I. Changes in viral markers with interferon combined with adenine arabinoside. J Infect Dis 143:772–783
Seaman WE, Blackman MA, Gindhart TD, Roubinian JR, Loeb J, Talal N (1978) β-estradiol reduces natural killer cells in mice. J Immunol 121:2193–2198
Seaman WE, Merigan TC, Talal N (1979) Natural killing in estrogen-treated mice responds poorly to poly I·C despite normal stimulation of circulating interferon. J Immunol 123:2903–2905
Siegel BV (1974) Enhanced interferon response to murine leukemia virus by ascorbic acid. Infect Immun 10:409–410
Siegel BV (1975) Enhancement of interferon production by poly(rI)·poly(rC) in mouse cell cultures by ascorbic acid. Nature 254:531–532
Slater LM, Wetzel MW, Cesario T (1981) Combined interferon-antimetabolite therapy of murine L1210 leukemia. Cancer 48:5–9
Sreevalsan T, Rozengurt E, Taylor-Papadimitriou J, Burchell J (1980) Differential effect of interferon on DNA synthesis, 2-deoxyglucose uptake and ornithine decarboxylase activity in 3T3 cells stimulated by polypeptide growth factors and tumor promotors. J Cell Physiol 104:1–9
St. Geme JW Jr, Horrigan DS, Toyama PS (1969) The effect of 6-mercaptopurine on the synthesis and action of interferon. Proc Soc Exp Biol Med 130:852–855
Stanwick TL, Schinazi RF, Campbell DE, Nahmias AJ (1981) Combined antiviral effect of interferon and acyclovir on herpes simplex virus types I and II. Antimicrob Agents Chemother 19:672–674
Strayer DR, Carter WA, Brodsky I, Gillespie DH, Greene JJ, Ts'o POP (1982) Clinical studies with mismatched double-stranded RNA. Tex Rep Biol Med 41:663–671
Stringfellow DA (1978) Prostaglandin restoration of the interferon response of hyporeactive animals. Science 201:376–378
Stringfellow DA (1980) Antiviral and interferon-inducing properties of interferon inducers administered with prostaglandins. Antimicrob Agents Chemother 17:455–460
Sundmacher R, Cantell K, Neumann-Haefelin D (1978) Combination therapy of dendritic keratitis with trifluorothymidine and interferon. Lancet 2:687
Targan SR (1981) The dual interaction of prostaglandin E_2 (PGE_2) and interferon (IFN) on NK lytic activation: enhanced capacity of effector-target lytic interactions (recycling) and blockage of pre-NK cell recruitment. J Immunol 127:1424–1428
Tomida M, Yamamoto Y, Hozumi M (1980a) Stimulation by interferon of induction of differentiation of mouse myeloid leukemic cells. Cancer Res 40:2919–2924
Tomida M, Yamamoto Y, Hozumi M (1980b) Inhibition of the leukemogenicity of myeloid leukemic cells in mice and in vivo induction of normal differentiation of the cells by poly(I)·poly(C). Gan 71:457–463
Trofatter KF Jr, Daniels CA (1980) Effect of prostaglandins and cyclic adenosine 3′, 5′-monophosphate modulators on herpes simplex virus growth and interferon response in human cells. Infect Immun 27:158–167
Wu AM, Schultz A, Gallo RC (1976) Synthesis type C virus particles from murine-cultured cells induced by iododeoxyuridine. V. effect of interferon and its interaction with dexamethasone. J Virol 19:108–117
Yamamoto Y, Tomida M, Hozumi M (1979) Stimulation of differentiation of mouse myeloid leukemic cells and induction of interferon in the cells by double-stranded polyribonucleotides. Cancer Res 39:4170–4174

Yaron M, Yaron I, Gurari-Rotman D, Revel M, Lindner HR, Zor U (1977) Stimulation of prostaglandin E production in cultured human fibroblasts by poly(I)·poly(C) and human interferon. Nature 267:457–459
Yaron M, Yaron I, Wiletzki C, Zor U (1978) Interrelationship between stimulation of prostaglandin E and hyaluronate production by poly(I)·poly(C) and interferon in synovial fibroblast culture. Arthritis Rheum 21:694–698

CHAPTER 20

Effects of Interferon and Its Inducers on Leucocytes and Their Immunologic Functions

J. M. ZARLING

A. Introduction

In addition to the antiviral and anticellular effects caused by interferon, immunomodulation mediated by interferon undoubtedly contributes to the interferon-induced resistance to overwhelming and sometimes fatal viral infections and also to regression or retardation of growth of certain tumors in animals and humans.

Reviewed in this chapter are several of the diverse effects caused by interferon and its inducers on mouse and human lymphocytic and monocytic functions. The specific areas that are discussed are interferon's actions on: (a) antibody production; (b) cell surface antigen expression on lymphoid cells; (c) proliferative and cytotoxic responses of lymphocytes to mitogens and alloantigens; (d) delayed-type hypersensitivity responses; (e) macrophage functions, including phagocytic and tumoricidal activities; and (f) natural killer cell activity. The effects of interferon on some of these functions, as well as on allograft rejection and graft versus host disease which are not discussed herein, have been reviewed by EPSTEIN (1977) and STEWART (1981). Since there has recently been much interest, on the part of many investigators, in the role and regulation of cells involved in naturally occurring resistance to tumor and virus-infected cells, a relatively extensive discussion of natural killer cells and their responses in vitro and in vivo to interferon and a number of interferon inducers is included.

B. Effects of Interferon and Its Inducers on Antibody Production

From the results of studies reviewed in this section, it is apparent that interferon or its inducers can either suppress or enhance antibody production in vivo and in vitro. The differential effects observed have generally been dependent upon the time of administration of interferon in relationship to antigenic stimulation. Further, the relative concentration of interferon governs, to a great extent, whether a reduction or enhancement of antibody production will ensue.

Several years ago, BRAUN and LEVY (1972) reported that in vivo intraperitoneal administration of virus-induced interferon to mice can result in either a decrease or an increase in the number of plaque-forming cells (PFC) responding to sheep red blood cells (SRBC) measured 2 days later. The effect observed was dependent upon the dose of interferon administered. Low doses (250–1,500 U) enhanced the number of PFC while doses above 5,000 U reduced the number of plaques. In vivo inoculation of mice with approximately 2×10^5 U Newcastle disease virus (NDV)-induced interferon 2 days prior to SRBC immunization markedly suppressed the PFC response to SRBC (CHESTER et al. 1973; MERIGAN et al. 1975). Doses less than 5×10^4 U did not suppress the PFC response. These investigators likewise found that interferon administered 4–48 h prior to immunization with SRBC decreased circulating hemolysin and agglutinin titers of anti-SRBC antibodies (BRODEUR and MERIGAN 1975). In contrast, no suppression was observed if interferon was administered 1–2 days after immunization with SRBC; further, if interferon was given 2–4 days after SRBC challenge, there was an enhancement in antibody production. SONNENFELD et al. (1978) reported that low doses of interferon can augment PFC responses to SRBC, but that high doses suppress this response. Secondary antibody production to SRBC was found to be markedly suppressed if mice were treated with interferon prior to SRBC challenge (BRODEUR and MERIGAN 1975). VIRELIZIER et al. (1976) reported that the effects of infection of mice with an interferon-inducing virus, mouse hepatitis virus, on subsequent antibody production to SRBC was dependent upon the time of antigenic challenge in relation to the time when circulating levels of interferon were high. Thus, challenge with SRBC after the acquisition of circulating interferon levels resulted in decreased antibody production whereas challenge with the antigen prior to the increase in interferon levels was associated with enhanced antibody production.

In vitro exposure of mouse spleen cells to interferon was found, by many investigators, either to suppress or enhance antibody production, consistent with observations already discussed concerning the effects of in vivo administration of interferon. MAZZUR and PAUCKER (1967) reported that incubation of SRBC-sensitized spleen cells with a fairly crude interferon preparation resulted in an enhanced number of PFC. GISLER et al. (1974) found that treatment of SRBC high responding spleen cultures with very high concentrations of interferon from 6 h before to 4 h after addition of SRBC led to a decrease in antibody production. On the other hand, treatment of low responding cultures with relatively low concentrations of interferon led to an enhancement in antibody production. These investigators found that the addition of interferon 92 h after antigen stimulation led to a marked increase in numbers of PFC measured 4 h later, consistent with the early work of MAZZUR and PAUCKER (1967). JOHNSON et al. (1975c) reported that maximal inhibition of the number of PFC to SRBC occurred when interferon was added with the SRBC or 1 day later. Addition of interferon for as few as 4 h resulted in suppressed antibody production measured 5 days later, suggesting that interferon suppresses an early event in antibody production. In contrast, a slight enhancement in the number of PFC occurred when interferon addition was postponed until 2–3 days after the addition of SRBC.

Since these studies dealt with the effects of interferon on antibody production to SRBC, a T-cell-dependent antigen, it was not known whether interferon's effects would be restricted to T-cell-dependent antigens. Thus, the effect of interferon on antibody production to a T-cell-independent B-cell antigen, *Escherichia coli* lipopolysaccharide (LPS) was studied. BRODEUR and MERIGAN (1975) found that interferon administered in vivo prior to administration of LPS suppresses the PFC response to LPS. In in vitro studies of primary antibody responses to LPS, JOHNSON et al. (1975a) reported that interferon decreases PFC responses to LPS. This effect was also observed in spleen cell cultures from which macrophages were removed, suggesting that interferon can directly affect B-cell function. SONNENFELD et al. (1978) found that treatment of spleen cells with interferon 1 day prior to stimulation with LPS led to a decrease in PFC to LPS, but that treatment with interferon after LPS stimulation failed to decrease this response. These results, together with observations that interferon decreases PFC responses to LPS in athymic hairless mice, also indicated that interferon can directly suppress B-cell function. JOHNSON and BARON (1976) compared the concentrations of interferon necessary to suppress PFC responses to SRBC and to the T-cell-independent antigen LPS and found that one-half as much interferon is necessary to suppress the response to SRBC. They concluded that the antibody response to a T-cell-dependent antigen may be much more sensitive to the suppressive effects of interferon. Since interferon was found either to suppress or enhance antibody production to a T-cell-dependent antigen (SRBC) and to suppress, but not enhance antibody production to a T-cell-independent B-cell antigen (LPS), SONNENFELD et al. (1978) have speculated that the enhancing effect of interferon on antibody production to T-cell-dependent antigens may be due to inhibition of suppressor T-cell activity; however, this hypothesis has not been proven experimentally.

In addition to the effects of interferon on IgG and IgM production, NGAN et al. (1976) provided evidence that interferon can suppress the production or release of IgE. Mouse IgE-producing spleen cells, which can cause heterologous adoptive cutaneous anaphylaxis in rat skin, were markedly inhibited in causing this response when the spleen cells were cultured with NDV-induced interferon in vitro.

Polyribonucleotide inducers of interferon have also been shown to suppress antibody production to SRBC. Polyinosinic · polycytidylic acid [poly(I) · poly(C)] and polyadenylic · polyuridylic acid [poly(A) · poly(U)] were found to suppress primary PFC responses to SRBC (JOHNSON et al. 1975b). Whereas interferon can suppress PFC responses to the T-cell-independent antigen LPS of spleen cells from hairless mice, polyribonucleotide inducers of interferon suppress the responses of spleen cells from intact mice, but not from hairless mice. These results suggest that polyribonucleotides may induce interferon in T-cells and that the interferon can then directly suppress B-cell function.

C. Effects of Interferon on Cell Surface Antigen Expression on Lymphoid Cells

I. Mouse Cells

The first studies on the effects of interferon on the expression of cell surface antigens were performed with the murine leukemia cell line L1210. LINDAHL-MAGNUSSON et al. (1973) incubated L1210 cells for various lengths of time with interferon, then the cells were compared with untreated and mock-interferon-treated cells for their ability to absorb out anti-H-2 antibodies. Treatment of the cells for 18 h, but not for 6 h, with interferon led to an increased ability of the cells to decrease the titer of anti-H-2 antisera. It was calculated that there was a 45% and 180% increase in expression of H-2 on the surface of cells treated with interferon for 24 and 48 h, respectively. Procedures which inactivate interferon, i.e., trypsin, sodium periodate, and heat, suppressed the antiviral activity as well as the factor that enhances the expression of H-2 antigens, supporting the contention that the effect on the antigen expression is mediated by interferon. Interferon treatment of an L1210 cell line which is interferon resistant did not result in an effect on the expression of H-2 cell surface antigens. These investigators (KILLANDER et al. 1976) considered the possibility that interferon could cause an accumulation of L1210 cells in one particular phase of the cell cycle which is perhaps normally accompanied by a relatively large amount of histocompatibility antigens expressed on the cell surface. An alternative explanation put forth was that interferon exerts a direct effect on the expression of cell surface antigens which is independent of the position of the cells in the cell cycle. Using cytophotometric and autoradiographic techniques, they found that: (a) the distribution of interferon-treated cells in the different phases of the cell cycle was the same as that for untreated cells; and (b) enhanced expression of histocompatibility antigens was observed on interferon-treated cells in all phases of the cell cycle. It was concluded, therefore, that interferon directly increases histocompatibility antigen expression on L1210 cells which is independent of interferon's effects on cell division (KILLANDER et al. 1976).

LINDAHL et al. (1974) also asked whether interferon would affect the expression of histocompatibility antigens on the surfaces of normal thymocytes or spleen cells from mice. Thymocytes of 3-month-old DBA/2 mice were incubated with 800 U/ml interferon for 12 h. The interferon-treated cells were compared with untreated cells for their ability to absorb out anti-H-2 activity from anti-H-2-containing serum. An increase of approximately 460% of H-2 expression was observed on the whole thymus population. In contrast to the dramatic increase in H-2 expression on the unfractionated thymocyte population, the small number of thymocytes which are cortisone resistant and which ordinarily express a very high concentration of H-2 antigens did not show a further increase in the expression of H-2 antigens following interferon treatment. Compared with the whole thymocyte population, the effects of interferon on H-2 expression on spleen cells were less pronounced with increases ranging from 50% to 250%. Interferon did not effect the expression of Thy-1 antigen on spleen cells or thymocytes.

Having shown that in vitro treatment of thymocytes or spleen cells with interferon resulted in increased expression of H-2 antigens, LINDAHL et al. (1976) then asked whether in vivo treatment of mice with interferon would modify the expression of histocompatibility antigens on these cells. Spleen cells and thymocytes, obtained from mice injected intraperitoneally four times at 12-h intervals with interferon, were compared with cells from control mice for their ability to absorb anti-H-2 antibody. Approximately four times as many cells from control mice, compared with cells from interferon-treated mice, were required to remove the same amount of antibody activity. Inoculation of mice with the interferon inducer, NDV likewise led to an increased expression of H-2 on spleen cells. In these studies, interferon treatment did not significantly affect the total number of cells obtained from thymocytes of spleen, and there was no decrease in cell viability.

The availability of restricted antisera against determinants controlled by subregions of the H-2 complex enabled VIGNAUX and GRESSER (1977) to ask which particular antigens are affected in expression following interferon treatment. C3H mouse spleen cells, incubated with 3,000 U interferon, were compared with control-treated cells for their ability to quantitatively absorb anti-H-2Kk, anti-H-2Dk, and antibodies to I region-encoded antigens. Results obtained indicated that there is enhanced expression of H-2D and H-2K antigens but not of I region-encoded antigens. Likewise, LONAI and STEINMAN (1977) reported that there is a 2- to 8-fold increase in H-2Kk or H-2Dk antigen expression on C3H thymocytes, based on findings of 2- to 4-fold greater reduction in antibody titer after absorption with the interferon-treated cells as compared with the untreated cells. No reduction was seen in the titer of alloantibodies against I region differences following incubation with the interferon-treated cells. Since the effects on H-2 expression were observed following treatment of cells for only 2 h, this argued against the possibility that interferon caused selective survival or multiplication of cells having increased expression of H-2 antigens. In addition, these investigators found that interferon increased the ability of T-cells, but not B-cells, to bind a radiolabeled synthetic polypeptide antigen and that anti-H-2Kk or anti-H-2Dk, but not anti-Iak prevented the increased binding of antibody to the T-cells. Finally, it was found that treatment with anti-Ly-2.1 (reactive with cytotoxic suppressor cells), but not anti-Ly-1.1 (reactive with helper cells) in the presence of complement, eliminated the ability of interferon-treated cells to bind the antigen. These results suggest that the interferon-responsive T-cells are of the Ly-2 phenotype.

II. Human Cells

More recently, studies have been undertaken to determine whether human histocompatibility antigens are likewise increased in expression on normal lymphoid cells or lymphoblastoid cell lines following interferon treatment. HERON et al. (1978) incubated human peripheral blood lymphocytes with 500 U virus-induced human leukocyte interferon for 16 h. Cell survival and thymidine ^{14}C incorporation into untreated and interferon-treated cells were the same. Interferon-treated cells which were stained with anti-β_2-microglobulin and fluoresceinated anti-IgG showed an increase in the fluorescence intensity compared with untreated cells, but there was no difference in expression of surface immunoglobulin. Both T- and non-T-cell populations isolated from peripheral blood mononuclear cells showed an increased expression of β_2-microglobulin. Treatment for only 2 h led to the same increase in expression of β_2-microglobulin as did treatment for 16 h. Also, an increase in expression of the relevant HL-A antigens was observed. The increased expression of the cell surface antigens was dependent upon active protein synthesis. These investigators have suggested that at least some of interferon's effects on the immune response may be related to altered expression of histocompatibility antigens on lymphocytes (HERON et al. 1978).

FELLOUS et al. (1979) observed that lymphoblastoid cell lines, after treatment with interferon for at least 36 h, had a 4- to 5-fold increased capacity to absorb out relevant anti-HL-A-B activity and anti-β_2-microglobulin activity, but not anti-HL-A-DR activity. After 48 h incubation with 1,000 U human leukocyte interferon, peripheral blood lymphocytes expressed a four fold increase in β_2-microglobulin and approximately a two fold increase in HL-A-A, -B antigens. In contrast, no increase in expression of HL-A-DR (Ia-like) antigens on cells of the two donors tested was observed. The findings in both mouse and human thus suggest that there is an increase in expression in H-2 or HL-A-A, -B antigens whereas interferon does not effect the expression of I region-encoded or DR antigens in mouse or human.

D. Effects of Interferon on Mitogen- or Antigen-Induced Lymphocyte Proliferative and Cytotoxic Responses

I. Mouse Lymphocytes

Several investigators have found that interferon suppresses T-cell proliferative responses to mitogens, soluble antigens, and allogeneic stimulating cells. LINDAHL-MAGNUSSON et al. (1972) reported that NDV-induced interferon (800 U/ml) suppressed thymidine ^{3}H incorporation into phytohemagglutinin (PHA)-stimulated mouse cells by at least 75% when the interferon was added simultaneously with or 1 day before PHA. A lesser suppressive effect was observed if the addition of interferon was postponed until 1 day after exposure to PHA. Proliferative responses to allogeneic stimulating cells, measured by thymidine ^{3}H incorporation in spleen cells stimulated in one-way mixed leukocyte culture (MLC) was markedly reduced when interferon (2,500 U/ml) was added at the onset of MLC. Similar results were obtained by ROZEE et al. (1973) who studied proliferative responses to another T-cell mitogen, concanavalin A (con A). Concentrations of 500–1,000 U NDV-induced interferon reduced subsequent thymidine ^{3}H incorporation into the con A-stimulated spleen cells. In this study and in the study of LINDAHL-MAGNUSSON et al. (1972) the factor responsible for suppressing proliferative responses shared biochemical and biophysical properties with the antiviral factor, providing evidence that interferon mediates the effect on lymphocytes. WALLEN et al. (1975) not only found that interferon suppresses mouse lymphocyte responses to PHA and con A, but also to the B-cell mitogens, pokeweed mitogen and *E. coli* lipopolysaccharide (LPS). In this study, the addition of viral interferon (100 U/ml) 1 day prior to mitogenic stimulation was more suppressive than was the addition of interferon simultaneously with mitogens. Inhibition of thymidine ^{3}H incorporation from 73% to 98% was observed in cells stimulated with PHA, con A or the B-cell mitogens, LPS or pokeweed mitogen.

CLINTON et al. (1976) induced interferon in mice by in vivo injection of poly(I) · poly(C) or Bacille Calmette Guérin (BCG). They tested the interferon-containing serum on proliferative responses to con A, PHA, and allogeneic stimulating cells in MLC. Both poly(I) · poly(C)- and BCG-induced interferon preparations suppressed MLC responses, but only the poly(I) · poly(C)-induced interferon preparation suppressed proliferative responses to con A and PHA. In vivo treatment of mice with interferon 4 and 24 h before removal of the spleen was found to result in an impaired ability of mouse spleen cells to respond proliferatively to con A, PHA, or LPS (BRODEUR and MERIGAN 1974). Inoculation with 3×10^4 U caused no suppression, 6×10^4 U moderately decreased proliferative responses to PHA and con A and 1.5×10^6 U markedly diminished proliferative responses to PHA and con A and moderately suppressed responses to the B-cell mitogen, LPS.

II. Human Lymphocytes

1. Proliferative Responses of T- and B-Cells

Similar to results obtained in the mouse studies, interferon has been found generally to suppress T-cell proliferative responses to antigens and mitogens and to suppress B-cell proliferative responses to a lesser degree. BLOMGREN et al. (1974) tested the effects of the Sendai virus-induced leukocyte interferon preparation used in clinical trails for its effects on human lymphocyte proliferative responses to the mitogens PHA, con A, and pokeweed mitogen, to the bacterial antigen purified protein derivative (PPD), and to alloantigens. Interferon concentrations as low as 10 U/ml were sufficient to suppress proliferative responses to con A and PHA whereas higher concentrations (100–1,000 U/ml) were necessary to suppress proliferative responses to PPD and very high concentrations (1,000–10,000 U/ml) were required to suppress proliferative responses to allogeneic stimulating cells in MLC. The observation that more interferon is required to suppress proliferative responses to alloantigens than to con A is consistant with findings in the mouse of LINDAHL-MAGNUSSON et al. (1972). Extremely high concentrations of interferon (as high as 20,000 U/ml) were required to decrease thymidine ^{3}H incorporation into pokeweed mitogen-stimulated B-lymphocytes.

SMITH et al. (1974) tested the effect of in vivo administration of the interferon inducer, poly(I) · poly(C) on subsequent proliferative responses of peripheral blood lymphocytes to PHA, con A, and alloantigens. Intravenous inoculation of 13 cancer patients with poly(I) · poly(C) (6–8 mg/kg) resulted in the detection of serum interferon at 8 h with peak levels at 12–24 h. When lymphocytes were isolated from peripheral blood 18 h after poly(I) · poly(C) administration, they responded poorly to PHA. In attempts to determine whether interferon induced by poly(I) · poly(C) could be responsible for the impaired proliferative responses, NDV-induced fibroblast interferon was added to lymphocytes in vitro and responses to con A, PHA, and alloantigens were measured. The degree of inhibition of thymidine ^{3}H incorporation ranged from 25% to 75% if interferon, as low as 36 U/10^6 cells, was added at the same time as the mitogen or allogeneic stimulating cells. If the cells had been stimulated for 24 h prior to the addition of interferon, no inhibition of thymidine ^{3}H incorporation was observed. These findings suggest that the early events in the activation of cells by mitogens or antigens are susceptible to the suppressive effects of interferon.

Consistent with the results of SMITH et al. (1974), MIÖRNER et al. (1978) found that virus-induced leukocyte or fibroblast interferon suppresses proliferative responses to PHA and con A if the interferon-containing preparations are added before or with the mitogens, but no suppression was observed if interferon was added 1 day after stimulation. They also found that, with low concentrations of interferon and/or low concentrations of mitogen, interferon can enhance proliferative responses.

2. Cytotoxic Responses of T-Cells

The cytotoxic responsiveness of human lymphocytes to allogeneic stimulating cells in MLC has also been studied. Consistent with findings already discussed, HERON et al. (1976) reported that the addition of 100–1,000 U/ml Sendai virus-induced interferon to cultures of responding lymphocytes and allogeneic stimulating cells suppressed thymidine ^{14}C incorporation by 20%–50%; however, the effector cells harvested at the end of MLC were more cytotoxic for target cells derived from the stimulating cell donors than were effector cells generated in the absence of interferon. The simultaneous addition of interferon and allogeneic stimulating cells resulted in augmentation of cytotoxic responses whereas the addition of interferon 1–5 days after the onset of MLC had little, if any, augmenting effect. The addition of interferon during the effector phase of the cell-mediated lympholytic assay did not augment the cytotoxic activity of the cytotoxic T-lymphocytes. This finding contrasts with the early finding of LINDAHL et al. (1972) that the addition of mouse interferon to allosensitized cytotoxic T-cells augments the cytotoxic activity at the effector level. The differences observed could be due to the fact that the mouse cells were sensitized in vivo while the human cells were sensitized in vitro or could be due to differences in interferon preparations used.

ZARLING et al. (1978) asked whether the addition of highly purified poly(I)·poly(C)-induced human fibroblast interferon would similarly decrease proliferative responses and augment cytotoxic responses of human T-cells to alloantigens. It was found that concentrations of 40–145 U/ml decreased thymidine ^{3}H incorporation into responding cells by 30%–50% and decreased recovery of the stimulated cells harvested on day 7 after the onset of MLC by approximately 50%. The addition of 100–800 U/ml augmented cytotoxic responsiveness by 4- to 5-fold when the results are compared in terms of lytic units per 10^6 effector cells. Thus, not only virus-induced leukocyte interferon (HERON et al. 1976), but also highly purified fibroblast interferon (ZARLING et al. 1978) which lacks other lymphokines suppresses proliferative responses and enhances cytotoxic responses to allogenic stimulating cells.

The mechanism whereby interferon augments cytotoxic responses to alloantigens is not clear. As discussed in a previous section, interferon treatment of lymphocytes can result in increased expression of histocompatibility antigens on cell surfaces and it could be possible that interferon may enhance cytotoxic responses by increasing the expression of those antigens which elicit cytotoxic responses. However, HERON and BERG (1979) found that treatment of stimulating cells alone prior to their addition to responding cells did not result in the elicitation of higher cytotoxic responses, even though the conditions used for interferon treatment were those which had been shown by these investigators to enhance the expression of HL-A antigens (HERON et al. 1978). Another possibility to explain the enhanced generation of cytotoxic T-cells could be that interferon decreases the generation of suppressor cells which are normally generated during the course of an MLC. HERON and BERG (1979) thus compared the ability of PHA- or con A-activated lymphoblasts generated in the presence or absence of interferon to prevent autologous lymphocytes from responding to allogeneic stimulating cells. The activated cells generated in the presence of interferon were more suppressive, suggesting that interferon enhances the generation or action of suppressor cells induced by these mitogens. The results of these experiments must be cautiously interpreted because it is possible that interferon may decrease the generation of alloantigen-induced suppressor cells, even though it apparently does not decrease the generation of suppressor cells by the mitogens, con A and PHA. A question which remains to be answered is whether interferon can also enhance cytotoxic T-cell responses to syngeneic or autologous tumor- or virus-infected cells.

E. Effects of Interferon on Delayed-Type Hypersensitivity Responses

Studies primarily of DEMAEYER and colleagues have dealt with the effects of interferon and interferon inducers on delayed-type hypersensitivity responses (DTHR) in mice. DEMAEYER et al. (1975) reported that if interferon was administered to mice 1 day before or on the day of sensitization with picryl chloride or SRBC, decreases in ear swelling to picryl chloride and in footpad swelling to SRBC were observed. When NDV, an interferon inducer, was given before antigenic challenge, there was likewise a decrease in DTHR which correlated with the level of serum interferon. These investigators concluded that the decrease in cell-mediated immune responses often seen in viral infections may be due to induction of interferon which can decrease DTHR. These investigators found that if NDV is given on the same day or the day after sensitization with SRBC, there was no decrease in DTHR, in contrast to their findings that NDV when given prior to antigenic challenge, decreases DTHR (DEMAEYER-GUIGNARD et al. 1975). In addition to studies of the effects of interferon on DTHR to picryl chloride and SRBC, DEMAEYER (1976) asked whether interferon would affect DTHR to viral antigens as measured by a decrease in footpad swelling. It was found that if interferon was given intraperitoneally before sensitization with NDV, there was a significant decrease in footpad swelling. Also, if interferon was administered after sensitization with the virus there was a decrease in DTHR, suggesting that interferon can affect both the afferent and efferent pathways of DTHR to NDV. In this study, only one concentration of interferon was administered at only one time so it is conceivable that altering the interferon dose or time of administration in relationship to antigenic challenge could effect the outcome, since, variations of these parameters have differential effects on humoral antibody responses.

SZIGETI et al. (1980) studied the effect of interferon on antigen and mitogen-induced migration inhibition of human leukocytes which is considered an in vitro counterpart of DTHR in humans. In studies with separated granulocytes, interferon was found to prevent supernatant from PHA-stimulated lymphocytes from inhibiting migration; thus, interferon appeared to block the leukocyte migration-inhibitory factor activity. Similarly, when cells from Epstein–Barr virus seropositive individuals were incubated with Epstein–Barr viral antigens, migration inhibition was abolished by human leukocyte interferon. In addition to their observations that interferon blocks the activity of leukocyte migration-inhibitory factor, these workers found that the addition of interferon to cultures of lymphocytes and PHA suppresses the production of leukocyte migration-inhibitory factor.

F. Effects of Interferon and Its Inducers on Macrophage Functions

I. Phagocytic Activity of Mouse Macrophages

HUANG et al. (1971) tested the hypothesis, based on accruing evidence that macrophages and also interferon can contribute to host resistance against certain infectious agents, that interferon may enhance the phagocytic activity of macrophages. Several different NDV-induced mouse interferon preparations tested at 50 U/ml, were found to increase, 2- to 3-fold, the number of mouse peritoneal exudate macrophages capable of phagocytizing colloidal carbon particles. The antiviral activity and phagocytic-enhancing activity were lost concomitantly upon treatment of the interferon-containing preparations with trypsin or heat. Further, DONAHOE and HUANG (1973) tested additional interferon-containing preparations, including those induced by statolon and found that these preparations likewise augmented macrophage activity which was ablated by treatment of the preparations with anti-interferon antibodies.

DONAHOE and HUANG (1976) subsequently asked whether induction of interferon in vivo by NDV or passive transfer of interferon would enhance macrophage phagocytic activity as assessed by enumerating the number of peritoneal macrophages which had ingested carbon particles inoculated intraperitoneally. They observed a slight depression in phagocytic activity 18 h after NDV injection followed by a marked enhancement which persisted for at least 66 h. To determine whether the effects observed could be attributed to the action of NDV-induced interferon (as opposed to the virus itself) mice were injected intraperitoneally with NDV-induced interferon preparations from which the NDV was removed by ultracentrifugation. A 2- to 4-fold increase in phagocytic activity was observed. It had been reported that protection against various infectious agents could be conferred on mice by treatment with interferon inducers (REMINGTON and MERIGAN 1970), but it was concluded that the enhanced reticuloendothelial activity was caused by the inducer itself and not be interferon. Although certain interferon inducers might directly affect the reticulendothelial system independent of interferon production, it is apparent from the study of DONAHOE and HUANG (1976) that an interferon-containing preparation devoid of the interferon-inducing virus was able to enhance macrophage phagocytic activity in vivo. GRESSER and BOURALI (1970) had previously reported that treatment of mice with interferon prior to injection with leukemic cells rendered the macrophages more phagocytic for the leukemic cells. As discussed in Sect. F.II, other investigators have more recently found that interferon inducers or interferon itself can enhance macrophage tumoricidal activities, but the macrophage-mediated effect has, in general, not been ascribed to phagocytic activity.

II. Tumoricidal Activity of Mouse Macrophages

Normal or activated macrophages have been shown to kill malignant cells by nonphagocytic mechanisms and have been implicated in playing a role in immune surveillance (EVANS and ALEXANDER 1976; KELLER 1976 A) as well as a role in regulating primary or metastatic tumor growth (ZARLING and TEVETHIA 1973; PROSS and KERBEL 1976; RUSSELL and MCINTOSH 1977; MANTOVANI 1978). Dependent upon the tumor cells tested, normal mouse macrophages or human monocytes can mediate cytotoxic or cytocidal effects (KELLER 1978; TAGLIABUE et al. 1979; RINEHART et al. 1978; HORWITZ et al. 1979; MANTOVANI et al. 1980b, c). Whereas at relatively high ratios of macrophage effector cells to tumor target cells antitumor effects can often be observed, at low ratios of macrophages to tumor cells an enhancement of tumor cell proliferation can occur (KELLER 1976B; HEWLETT et al. 1977; MANTOVANI et al. 1980b).

Studies have been undertaken to determine means of augmenting macrophage tumoricidal activity. SCHULTZ et al. (1977) found that mouse macrophages can be rendered cytotoxic for L1210 cells if the macrophages were exposed to poly(I)·poly(C) for at least 24 h. Whereas the double-stranded polyribonucleotides, poly(I)·(C) and poly(A)·(U) augmented the antileukemic effects of macrophages, single-stranded polyribonucleotides were ineffective in this regard. These results suggested that activation of this macrophage function may be mediated through interferon which is produced by double-stranded poly(I)·poly(C) or poly(A)·poly(U), but not by single-stranded polyribonucleotides. Further support for this contention derives from these investigators' findings that highly purified mouse fibroblast interferon rendered uninduced peritoneal exudate macrophages cytotoxic for MBL-2 leukemic cells. Macrophages, MBL-2 leukemic cells, and interferon were coincubated and the number of leukemic cells was enumerated at daily intervals. The presence of interferon caused accelerated spreading of macrophages, similar to findings of RABINOVITCH et al. (1977), and an increase in granulation in the macrophage cytoplasm. A marked inhibition of leukemic cell replication was observed which could not be attributed to a direct antiproliferative effect of interferon since in the absence of macrophages, the interferon was not cytostatic. It was further concluded that the antileukemic cell effects were not due to toxic metabolites or other factors produced by the interferon-treated macrophages, since supernatants from the interferon-treated cells did not effect MBL-2 cell growth. In these studies, interferon concentrations of 1,000 U/ml caused 93% inhibition of MBL-2 growth and significant effects were observed with 100 U/ml. In a previous study, it was found that macrophages from BCG-immune mice, following exposure in vitro to BCG, were rendered cytotoxic for tumor cells (EVANS and ALEXANDER 1972). Since immune interferon is produced under these conditions, SCHULTZ et al. (1977) suggested that the apparent immunologically specific induction of nonspecifically tumoricidal macrophages is probably due to interferon production. More recently, these investigators reported that LPS, poly(I)·poly(C), pyran copolymer, as well as L-cell interferon rendered macrophages cytocidal for MBL-2 leukemia cells and that an antibody to L-cell interferon prevented macrophage activation by interferon and the interferon inducers (CHIRIGOS et al. 1980).

Using the system described, SCHULTZ et al. (1978) and CHIRIGOS et al. (1980) found that prostaglandin E_1 or E_2, but not $F_2\alpha$ suppressed the ability of interferon to activate cytotoxic activity in mouse macrophages against MBL-2 leukemic cells. Further, following interferon activation of the macrophages for 16 h, prostaglandin E_1 or E_2 diminished the tumoricidal function. In vivo administration of 5 or 20 μg prostaglandin E_1 and E_2 with interferon or 24 h prior to interferon treatment led to a significant decrease in macrophage antitumor cytocidal activity (CHIRIGOS et al. 1980). Since activated macrophages release prostaglandin E_2 these investigators hypothesized that this agent may cause negative feedback inhibition of the activated state to the resting noncytotoxic state. They also speculated that the elevated level of prostaglandin E in the immediate locale of the tumor (SYKES and MADDOX 1972) may suppress the tumoricidal efficacy of activated macrophages. Since 3′,5′-cyclic nucleotides are widely involved in many cellular regulatory processes and since prostaglandin E_1 increases cyclic adenosine monophosphate (AMP) levels in macrophages, experiments were undertaken to determine the effects of dibutyl cyclic AMP on interferon-treated macrophages. Treatment of activated macrophages with 10^{-3}–10^{-5} *M* dibutyl cyclic AMP, but not with cyclic guanosine monophosphate suppressed the tumoricidal activity of the macrophages.

III. Cytotoxic Activity of Human Monocytes and Macrophages Against Tumor and Virus-Infected Cells

Studies have recently been undertaken to asess the effects of interferon on human monocyte-mediated tumoricidal activity. Preincubation of monocytes for 18 h with interferon modestly augmented monocyte-mediated lysis of TU5 tumor cells, but no affect was seen following 1 h treatment with interferon (JETT et al. 1980). In addition, human monocytes incubated with interferon (33–333 U/ml) significantly augmented thymidine ^{3}H release from TU5 mouse tumor cells in a 48-h assay (HERBERMAN et al. 1980). MANTOVANI et al. (1980b, c) found that highly purified fibroblast interferon augments tumoricidal effects of human peripheral blood monocytes and peritoneal macrophages, but does not render lung alveolar macrophages tumoricidal. Marked enhancement of cytocidal effects was observed when blood monocytes or peritoneal macrophages were preincubated for 20 h with interferon (300–1,000 U/ml). In addition to augmented cytotoxic effects against established tumor cell lines, MANTOVANI et al. (1980b, c) found that freshly isolated malignant ascites cells from some patients with ovarian carcinoma are susceptible to lysis by activated human monocytes. It remains to be determined whether other types of freshly isolated human tumor cells will likewise prove to be susceptible to the cytotoxic effects of interferon-activated macrophages.

In addition to studies suggesting that interferon activates macrophages to lyse tumor cells, recent evidence has been presented suggesting that interferon also activates macrophages to lyse cells infected with Herpes simplex virus (HSV) and cytomegalovirus. STANWICK et al. (1980) have recently studied the effect of human leukocyte interferon on human adherent monocytes from peripheral blood to lyse HSV-infected fibroblasts. At effector : target ratios of 50–100 : 1, significant lysis of the HSV-infected, but not the uninfected fibroblasts was observed. When the adherent cells were preincubated for 12–24 h with interferon (100 or 1,000 U/ml), a dramatic enhancement in cytotoxicity against the infected targets was observed. The authors concluded that the cytotoxic activity against the virus-infected cells is mediated by macrophages rather than by natural killer (NK) cells or by specifically immune T-cells since: (a) the effector cell population consisted of 95% cells staining with acid α-naphthylacetate esterase; (b) 90% of the effector cells were phagocytic; (c) incubation of the effector cells with latex particles completely inhibited the cytotoxic activity; and (d) cells from both HSV seropositive and seronegative donors were equivalently cytotoxic, ruling out a specific immune cell-mediated mechanism. Interferon also augmented macrophage-mediated lysis of cytomegalovirus-infected targets and the addition of a rabbit antibody to human leukocyte interferon prevented the interferon-containing preparation from activating the macrophages.

G. Effects of Interferon and Its Inducers on Natural Killer Cell Activity

I. Discovery and Possible Roles of NK Cells

Less than a decade ago, several investigators observed that lymphocytes from normal mice (ZARLING et al. 1975; HERBERMAN et al. 1975; KIESSLING et al. 1975; SENDO et al. 1975), rats (NUNN et al. 1976; SHELLAM 1977; OEHLER et al. 1978); and humans (TAKASUGI et al. 1973; McCOY et al. 1973; ROSENBERG et al. 1974; PROSS and JONDAL 1975) can spontaneously lyse or inhibit the proliferation of a variety of malignant cells in vitro. It has become apparent, based on the following lines of evidence, that the spontaneously occurring cytotoxic cells generally referred to as NK cells may play a role in resistance to early tumor growth and also resistance to certain virus infections. First, mice differing with regard to their level of NK cell activity measured in vitro, likewise differ with regard to resistance to in vivo challenges with NK-sensitive tumor cell lines (HALLER et al. 1977). Second, as will be discussed in detail, many agents which have been shown to mediate antitumor effects in vivo have been shown to augment NK cell activity against various tumor cells. Third, it has recently been reported that the mutant C57BL/6 beige mice have a selective defect in NK cell activity and that these beige mice are more susceptible to tumor growth and metastases than are their syngeneic normal counterparts (KÄRRE et al. 1980; TALMADGE et al. 1980). Patients with Chédiak–Higashi syndrome have normal DTHR and humoral immunity, but have very low NK cell activity (RODER et al. 1980). Survivors from this disease generally develop lymphoproliferative diseases which may be malignant (DENT et al. 1966). Most patients studied with chronic lymphocytic leukemia have virtually no detectable NK cell activity (ZIEGLER et al. 1981) and have a relatively high incidence of secondary malignancies. Finally, ZARLING et al. (1979) have found that fresh human leukemia cells that have not been adapted to tissue culture are susceptible to lysis by interferon-activated NK cells and MANTOVANI et al. (1980a) have made similar observations with human ovarian carcinoma cells. Partly because of the growing evidence which supports the contention that NK cells contribute to tumor cell growth inhibition, there has been much interest in the past few years to elucidate means to augment NK cell activity. Results obtained by several investigators, discussed in Sects. G.II and G.III, indicate that numerous interferon inducers as well as interferon itself augment both mouse and human NK cell activities.

II. Mouse NK Cell Activity

BCG had received much attention as a potentially useful immunotherapeutic agent based primarily on animal studies in which it caused regression of local tumor nodules. It was assumed that the mechanism whereby BCG exerted its antitumor effects was through activation of macrophages. However, WOLFE et al. (1976) reported that peritoneal excudate cells from mice inoculated with 10^7 viable BCG organisms 4–8 days previously were cytotoxic for certain tumor cells and that the lysis was mediated by cells lacking macrophage characteristics. In addition, they found that the effector cells also lacked markers characteristic of mature T-cells or B-cells and they thus concluded that BCG activates NK cells. Following this report, several other agents including bacterial immunoadjuvants, viruses, double-stranded polyribonucleotides, and tumor cells have been shown to augment NK cell activity in vivo and in vitro.

Infection of mice with lymphocytic choriomeningitis virus (LCMV) and certain other viruses has been shown to result, at least 5 days later, in cytotoxic T-lymphocytes that are lytic for syngeneic cells infected with this specific virus (ZINKERNAGEL and DOHERTY 1974; PFIZENMAIER et al. 1975). WELSH and ZINKERNAGEL (1977), however, found that as early as 1 day after infection with LCMV, effector cells lytic for a variety of virus-infected cells and other cell lines are present. These apparently nonspecific effector cells could also be induced in congenitally athymic hairless mice upon virus infection. The effector cells were found to be nonadherent, surface immunoglobulin negative, and sensitive to heat treatment. Exposure of mice to ^{89}Sr prior to virus infection prevented the generation of the early cytotoxicity, but not the generation of cytotoxic T-lymphocytes (WELSH and KIESSLING 1980). All of these findings are consistent with the hypothesis that LCMV infection leads to rapid augmentation of NK cell activity in vivo. Similarly, MACFARLAN et al. (1977) reported that injection of mice with the togavirus, Semliki Forest virus resulted, 2 days later, in the detection of effector cells cytotoxic for virus-infected cells and certain tumor cells.

HERBERMAN et al. (1977) reported that intraperitoneal inoculation of conventional or athymic hairless mice with a wide variety of viruses including Moloney sarcoma virus, LCMV, lactic dehydrogenase virus, polyoma virus, Sendai virus, and mouse adenovirus leads to dramatic increases in the ability of spleen cells to lyse NK-sensitive leukemic cells. BCG and *Corynebacterium parvum* likewise augmented the cytotoxic activity. Injection of mice with certain tumor cell lines, primarily leukemic lines, led to augmentation of NK cell activity and there was a correlation between the ability of tumor cells to boost NK activity and their susceptibility to lysis by NK cells. The peak in cytotoxic activity was generally 3 days after inoculation with the viruses or tumor cells.

It has become apparent that the observed enhancement of NK cell activity by these agents can be explained on the basis that they induce interferon which can then boost NK cell activity. WELSH (1978) asked whether the in vivo activation of NK cells occurring after injection of mice with LCMV could be due to interferon induced by this virus. High levels of interferon were detected in the serum within the first 3 days of infection during which time NK cell activity was high. As the interferon titer dropped, so did NK cell activity. Further evidence to support the contention that interferon could have been responsible for the observed increase in NK activity following injection with LCMV derived from the findings that supernatants from virus-infected L-cells could augment NK cell activity in vivo.

GIDLUND et al. (1978) also tested several inducers of interferon for their ability to augment NK cell activity in vivo and in vitro. They found that NDV, tilorone, statolon, poly(I) · poly(C), and *C. parvum* all enhanced mouse spleen NK cell activity in vitro. Since anti-interferon antibodies ablated the ability of these agents to boost NK cell activity, they concluded that the effects on NK cells of the interferon-inducing agents may be attributable to the induction of interferon. They recognized the possibility, however, that since the interferon used for producing antibodies was not purified and could also contain other lymphokines, the antisera could also include antibodies to other lymphokines which could be mediating the effects on NK cells.

DJEU et al. (1979) reported that poly(I) · poly(C) and other interferon inducers, including pyran and endotoxin, can augment NK cell activity in mice with profound effects on older mice whose NK cell activity had dropped to almost undetectable levels. The kinetics of augmentation by these various agents were the same as the kinetics of interferon production. These investigators also found that mouse interferon-containing preparations could augment NK cell activity in vivo and in vitro.

The mechanisms whereby interferon augments NK cell activity have been probed. RODER et al. (1978) used the interferon inducer NDV to augment NK cell activity and then asked whether there is an increase in the fraction of spleen cells which bind to NK-sensitive targets or whether the fraction of target binding cells remains constant. They isolated conjugates of lymphocytes bound to NK-sensitive targets by velocity sedimentation and found that the fraction of target binding cells was the same for the untreated and nonactivated effector cells. It was thus concluded that interferon augments cytotoxic activity of existing NK cells rather than increasing the number of cells which can bind to and subsequently lyse NK-sensitive targets. SENIK et al. (1980) found that short exposure of mouse lymphocytes to interferon (10–1,000 U/ml) resulted in enhanced NK cell activity. The addition of a potent anti-interferon antibody as early as 30 s after addition of interferon to the cells did not prevent interferon from augmenting NK cell activity, implying that the action of interferon cannot be inhibited once it binds to the lymphocyte membrane. Evidence that interferon itself, rather than a factor produced from interferon-treated cells, augments NK cell activity derives from their findings that supernatants harvested 3 h after treatment of the spleen cells with interferon can enhance NK cell activity of fresh cells and that anti-interferon totally ablates this effect. Results of experiments involving the use of metabolic inhibitors strongly suggest that RNA and protein synthesis are required for interferon-induced augmentation of NK cell activity. The addition of 2 μg/ml cycloheximide, a protein synthesis inhibitor, suppressed NK cell activation by 70% and the addition of 10 μg/ml actinomycin D, an RNA synthesis inhibitor, inhibited actication by interferon by nearly 70%. HERBERMAN et al. (1979) found that emetine, another protein synthesis inhibitor, prevented interferon-induced augmentation of NK cell activity. In contrast to the apparent requirement for RNA and protein synthesis in interferon-induced augmentation of NK cell activity, DNA synthesis appears not to be required since the kinetics of augmentation are extremely rapid and since the presence of cytosine arabinoside does not inhibit interferon's ability to activate NK cells.

In addition to results showing that interferon activates NK cells to lyse tumor cells, interferon-activated NK cells also lyse virus-infected cells and may play a role in resistance to viral infections. With certain viruses that are resistant to antiviral effects of interferon in vitro, interferon treatment in vivo can be efficacious with regard to contributing to recovery from the viral infection. For example, whereas interferon does not inhibit replication of vaccinia virus in vitro, when interferon was injected intramuscularly into rhesus monkeys who were given vaccinia virus intradermally, complete inhibition of the development of skin lesions was observed (SCHELLEKENS et al. 1979). REID et al. (1979) found that whereas as few as 10 uninfected HeLa or BHK-21 cells can produce tumors in hairless mice, if the cells were persistently infected with a variety of RNA viruses including vesicular stomatitis, measles, influenza, or mumps viruses, 10^4 cells failed to produce tumors. Up to 10^7 persistently infected cells still did not produce progressively growing tumors, but rather produced small nodules (MINATO et al. 1979). Irradiation (550 R) of recipients of the virus-infected tumor cells rendered them susceptible to tumor growth, implying that the host normally provides resistance against tumor growth by the virus-infected cells. These investigators suggested the possibility that NK cells may be more reactive against persistently infected tumor cells than against the uninfected tumor cells. Indeed, they observed that HeLa cells, infected with measles, mumps, or vesicular stomatitis virus were much more susceptible to lysis by NK cells than were uninfected HeLa cells. It was found that supernatants from cultures of spleens from hairless mice and virus-infected cells contain substantial levels of interferon (MINATO et al. 1980), suggesting that interferon may be responsible for the augmentation of NK cell activity against the virus-infected target cells. These investigators then tested the effects of mouse interferon purified to homogeneity (2×10^9 U per milligram protein) and found marked increases in NK activity against virus-infected HeLa cells, but not against uninfected HeLa cells. Results of preliminary experiments suggested that anti-interferon allows mumps-infected BHK-21 cells to grow in hairless mice (BLOOM et al. 1980).

III. Human NK Cell Activity

1. In Vitro Studies

Human NK cell activity has been shown to be augmented by interferon-inducing agents as well as by interferons themselves. TRINCHIERI and SANTOLI (1978) reported that supernatants harvested from human lymphocytes cultured with NDV or with a variety of tumor cell lines augment human NK cell activity of fresh lymphocytes against human tumor cell lines and fetal fibroblast lines. The antiviral activity of these supernatants and NK-enhancing activity shared the same characteristics and it was therefore concluded that the enhancement of NK activity was mediated by interferon produced by the stimulated lymphocytes. Pretreatment of the effector cells augmented NK activity 2- to 4-fold, but pretreatment of certain target cells, primarily the normal fibroblast lines, with interferon rendered them resistant to lysis by the activated NK cells. Interferon-induced acquisition of resistance to NK-mediated lysis in the target cells was dependent on RNA and protein synthesis. In these studies, although NK activity was augmented, no augmentation of antibody-dependent cell-mediated cytotoxicity (ADCC) activity was detected using normal lymphocytes as effector cells and human target cells in the presence of anti-HLA antibodies. Marked augmentation of NK activity was observed following 4 h of incubation with interferon inducers including NK-sensitive tumor cells and poly(I) · poly(C) (50 µg/ml) or with NDV-induced interferon (TRINCHIERI and SANTOLI 1978; TRINCHIERI et al. 1978).

EINHORN et al. (1978a) tested the Sendai virus-induced leukocyte interferon preparation, which is used in clinical trials, for its ability to augment NK cell activity against different target cells using three types of cytotoxicity assays. Lymphocytes cultured with interferon (10–1,000 U/ml) for 2 days with the Raji Burkitt's lymphoma cells caused 40%–50% inhibition of thymidine ^{3}H uptake in the Raji cells. In a microcytotoxicity assay, effector cells treated with interferon (10–100 U/ml) reduced the number of adherent tumor cells growing in microwells by at least fivefold and, using a ^{51}Cr release assay, these investigators found approximately a fourfold increase in lysis of Chang cells. HERBERMAN et al. (1979) reported that human leukocyte and fibroblast interferon preparations augmented human NK cell activity against the NK-sensitive myeloid leukemia cell line K562 and also that ADCC activity was enhanced following treatment of the effectors with the interferon preparations. Their findings that interferon augments ADCC as well as NK activity contrast with those of TRINCHIERI and co-workers (TRINCHIERI and SANTOLI 1978; TRINCHIERI et al. 1978) who observed augmentation of NK activity without an effect on ADCC. However, the results of HERBERMAN et al. (1979) agree with those of others (DROLLER et al. 1979; MOORE and KIMBER 1980) who showed enhancement of both activities by interferon. DROLLER et al. (1979) found that treatment of effectors for 1 or 16 h with interferon resulted in 100%–600% increases in NK activity and 25%–75% increases in ADCC activity.

MOORE and KIMBER (1980) found that treatment of human lymphocytes with lymphoblastoid interferon at 250 U/ml for as little as 1 h augmented cytotoxicity against NK-sensitive targets, including K562, MOLT-4, and CCRF/DEM cell lines. B-cell lines, which are relatively resistant to spontaneous NK-mediated lysis, were lysed by interferon-treated lymphocytes. These investigators also found that ADCC against human erythrocytes in the presence of antibodies to blood group antigens A is increased by approximately 50% following pretreatment of the lymphocytes with interferon (200–600 U/ml).

Most of the studies discussed involved the use of leukocyte interferon preparations which can contain other lymphokines and, in cases of virus-induced interferon, products of virus infection. ZARLING et al. (1979) therefore asked whether highly purified human fibroblast interferon (2×10^7 U per milligram protein) induced by poly(I) · poly(C), which lacks lymphokines and viral products, would augment human NK cell activity. Interferon pretreatment of lymphocytes with 100–300 U/ml for as few as 10 min significantly augmented NK activity against the K562 leukemia cell line. Removal of macrophages did not impair the ability of interferon to augment NK activity whereas the depletion of lymphocytes bearing receptors for the Fc portion of IgG eliminated both nonactivated NK and interferon-activated NK activities. In all individuals tested, interferon augmented NK cell activity by at least 150%. In addition to these results showing that highly purified fibroblast interferon augments NK cell activity, further evidence has recently been presented, indicating that indeed interferon itself augments NK and ADCC activities. MASUCCI et al. (1980) tested the ability of interferon produced by *E. coli* transformed with a hybrid plasmid containing a human leukocyte complementary DNA insert for its effects on NK and ADCC activities. Treatment of human lymphocytes with 1,000 U/ml partially purified *E. coli*-produced interferon augmented human NK activity to the same level as did human lymphoblastoid interferon. The *E. coli*-produced interferon also augmented ADCC activity against a human lymphoblastoid cell line exposed to rabbit anti-human IgG.

These results indicate that interferon can, without question, augment human NK cell activity. Results of many studies in the mouse reviewed in an earlier section have suggested, in addition, that augmentation of NK cell activity by numerous agents, including viruses, tumor cells, and double-stranded polyribonucleotides is mediated through interferon which is induced by these agents. The availability of analogs of poly(I)·poly(C) which differ in their ability to induce interferon enabled ZARLING and collaborators to ask whether augmentation of human NK cell activity by double-stranded polyribonucleotides is dependent upon the ability of the molecules to induce interferon (ZARLING 1980; ZARLING et al. 1980). Treatment of human lymphocytes with poly(I)·poly(C), or its mismatched analogs, $rI_n \cdot r(C_{12}, U)_n$ or $rI_n \cdot r(G_{29}, U)_n$ markedly augmented human NK cell activity. All three of these double-stranded molecules induce interferon production. In contrast, treatment with a methylated analog of poly(I)·poly(C), namely $rI_n \cdot mC_n$ which fails to induce interferon, likewise fails to augment NK cell activity (ZARLING et al. 1980). It was proposed, therefore, that augmentation of NK cell activity is an integral component of the double-stranded polyribonucleotide interferon system rather than on secondary biologic property of certain polyribonucleotides.

Concerning the mechanism whereby interferon enhances human NK cell activity, TARGAN and DOREY (1980) asked whether there is an increase in the number of effector cells binding to NK-sensitive targets following interferon treatment or whether the number of binding cells remains constant with an increase in the lytic capacity of the binding cells. Using a single-cell assay involving conjugate formation between effectors and target cells, these investigators found that 11%–13% of peripheral blood lymphocytes bind to K562 cells and of these bound cells, only 20%–30% lyse the targets. Treatment of the lymphocytes with interferon led to no increase in the number of target binding cells, but to an increase in the proportion of the target binding cells which actually lysed the target cells. Recently, these workers reported that the kinetics of lysis by NK cells is enhanced by interferon; maximum cytotoxicity was observed after 30 min whereas in the absence of interferon, cytotoxicity plateaued at 3 h (SILVA et al. 1980).

All of the studies discussed in this section concerning the effects of interferon and interferon inducers on NK activity in mouse and human involved the use of normal donors' lymphocytes as effector cells and, as target cells, tumor cell lines, or cell lines persistently infected with viruses. With regard to any potential clinical benefit from attempting to augment NK cell activity in cancer patients or patients with presumed persistent viral infections it is important to know: (a) whether NK cells from such patients are susceptible to augmentation by interferon or its inducers; (b) whether abnormal cells that have not been established as cell lines, such as fresh malignant cells, are susceptible to lysis by interferon-activated NK cells;

and (c) whether in vivo administration of interferon to humans augment NK cell activity.

Concerning the ability of interferon to augment NK cell activity of cancer patients' lymphocytes, LUCERO et al. (1981) reported that NK cell activity of 173 cancer patients bearing primarily lymphomas, melanomas, lung tumors, and breast tumors was not significantly different from that of normal individuals and that interferon augmented NK activity of the patients' lymphocytes to approximately the same level as in lymphocytes from normal subjects. MANTOVANI et al. (1980 a) found that patients with advanced ovarian carcinoma had, in general, reduced NK cell activity compared with normal subjects and that interferon could boost the NK activity of the patients' lymphocytes. VÁNKY et al. (1980) reported that interferon augmented NK activity of lymphocytes from a variety of sarcoma patients. ZIEGLER et al. (1981) found that lymphocytes from most patients with B-cell chronic lymphocytic leukemia had minimal, if any, detectable NK activity, even following removal of the leukemic B-cells. Interferon treatment could not render most patients' cells detectably cytotoxic for the NK-sensitive targets. It thus seems that depression of NK cell activity accompanies certain malignancies, but insufficient numbers of studies with patients having a variety of malignancies have been performed to conclude whether susceptibility to interferon's augmenting effect on NK activity is correlated with certain histologic types of tumors or stages of disease.

As discussed in the previous section, MINATO et al. (1980) found that murine NK cells are highly cytotoxic for cells infected with certain viruses and that interferon treatment augments NK activity against the virus-infected cells. These workers then asked whether individuals with suspected persistent viral infections, such as patients with multiple sclerosis or systemic lupus erythematosus have impaired NK activity. In preliminary studies, these patients were found to exhibit very low levels of NK activity (BLOOM et al. 1980). Exposure of these patients' lymphocytes to NDV resulted in a very low level of interferon production compared with that in the lymphocytes of normal subjects and there was rarely augmentation of NK activity observed in the patients' cells. It is not clear whether the impaired NK activity and resistance to boosting precedes the onset of multiple sclerosis or systemic lupus erythematosus and therefore may contribute to the development of these diseases or whether the impaired NK activity may be a consequence of the diseases.

Studies have recently been directed at determining whether malignant cells that have not been adapted to tissue culture or established as cell lines can be lysed by interferon-activated NK cells. This question has been raised because it was not clear whether susceptibility to NK-mediated lysis may be restricted to long-established tumor cell lines or whether spontaneously occurring fresh tumor cells may also express recognition structures for activated NK cells. ZARLING et al. (1979) reported that treatment of normal lymphocytes with highly purified fibroblast interferon (150 U/ml) augmented NK activity against NK-sensitive K562 cells in all individuals tested and that in one-half of the individuals tested, the interferon-treated lymphocytes were significantly cytotoxic for fresh leukemic cells derived from patients with a variety of leukemias. In no case were interferon-activated NK cells cytotoxic for autologous or allogeneic normal lymphocytes, mitogen-induced blasts, or bone marrow cells (ZARLING et al. 1979; ZARLING 1980). Thus, whereas spontaneously occurring human leukemia cells that have not been adapted to tissue culture are rarely lysed by fresh lymphocytes, interferon can render lymphocytes cytotoxic for these malignant cells. The antileukemic effector cells activated by interferon were found to be nonadherent and expressed receptors for the Fc portion of IgG, consistant with the characteristics of NK cells, Recently, Zarling and Kung (1980) have found that monoclonal antibodies directed against human mononuclear cell subpopulations can distinguish NK cells and interferon-activated NK cells from cytotoxic T-lymphocytes. Specifically, monoclonal antibodies OKT3 or OKT8 in the presence of complement deplete cytotoxic T-lymphocytes and not NK cells whereas OKM1 and complement markedly reduces NK cell activity. Since interferon can augment the generation of cytotoxic T-lymphocytes and also activate NK cells, these antibodies are useful for discerning the type of effector cell that is responsible for mediating lysis of tumor cells or virus-infected cells (Zarling and Kung 1980; Zarling et al. 1981).

Other investigators have also found that fresh malignant cells are generally resistant to lysis by fresh peripheral blood lymphocytes, but that following treatment with interferon, the lymphocytes can be significantly cytotoxic for tumor cells. Mantovani et al. (1980a) found that ovarian carcinoma cells are resistant to lysis by NK cells, but that interferon-activated NK cells can lyse a proportion of the patients' malignant cells. Vánky et al. (1980) found that interferon treatment of normal lymphocytes or lymphocytes from cancer patients could render the cells cytotoxic for allogeneic tumor biopsy cells. Vose (1980) reported that treatment of normal lymphocytes with 250 U interferon augmented cytotoxicity against cells of five of six patients' tumors, four of which were lung tumors and one of which was a colon tumor. It thus seems that at least some patients' leukemic cells and solid tumor cells do express cell surface structures recognized by NK cells and that these cells are susceptible to lysis by NK cells if they are activated by interferon. Although additional studies are needed to determine whether it can be predicted which types of tumors may be susceptible to lysis by interferon-activated NK cells, it can be concluded that sensitivity to lysis by activated NK cells is not restricted to malignant cells which have been adapted to tissue culture or established as cell lines.

2. In Vivo Studies

Studies have been undertaken to determine whether administration of exogenous interferon can augment NK cell activity in vivo in humans. Einhorn et al. (1978b) measured NK activity before and at different times after intramuscular injection of 3×10^6 U human leukocyte interferon. In five osteosarcoma patients, 6 h after injection, there was a decrease in NK activity followed by a marked augmentation in 24 h. At 48 h after interferon injection, NK activity was still higher than prior to interferon administration. This initial study has been extended to 40 patients primarily with myeloma, osteosarcoma, and malignant melanoma and it was found that in most cases, NK cell activity was markedly increased within 24 h after interferon administration (Einhorn 1980). Huddlestone et al. (1979) found that following injection of 10×10^6 U leukocyte interferon intramuscularly, NK activity against MOLT-4 cells rose within 12–24 h with a peak in cytotoxic activity observed at 18 h. The level of NK activity then began to drop, but generally remained higher than pretreatment levels when the patients were treated for 7–30 days. EINHORN et al. (1980) found that daily administration of 3×10^6 U leukocyte interferon for at least 6 months resulted in a continuous elevation of NK cell activity in four myeloma and one malignant melanoma patient. In a patient with metastatic breast cancer who received approximately 1×10^6 U highly purified fibroblast interferon every 2 days, NK activity remained threefold higher than pretreatment levels for at least 3 weeks (J. M. ZARLING 1980, unpublished observations).

It is thus apparent from these studies that interferon can augment NK cell activity in vivo and that many patients' tumor cells are susceptible to lysis by interferon-activated NK cells. It still remains to be determined, however, whether any of the antitumor effects observed in cancer patients following interferon treatment can be attributed to interferon-induced activation of NK cells directed against the patients' autochthonous tumor cells.

H. Summary and Concluding Comments

Several of the diverse immunologic effects mediated by interferon-containing preparations and interferon inducers, that have been observed primarily during the past 10 years and have been discussed in this chapter, are summarized in Table 1. In reviewing these studies, the question was not repeatedly raised as to whether or not the effects observed following in vitro or in vivo treatment with interferon-containing preparations or interferon inducers were conclusively mediated by interferon. In many of the studies, relatively crude interferon preparations were used, rendering it impossible to conclude, with certainty, that all the effects observed were indeed mediated by interferon. Even in studies in which agents which inactivated the antiviral activity in the preparations likewise inactivated the immunomodulatory activity, the possibility remains that other lymphokines present in leukocyte or immune interferon preparations could have contributed to the reported effects. In experiments where antibodies to interferon ablated the immunomodulatory effects mediated by the interferon-containing preparations or interferon inducers, a certain degree of caution is warranted in interpreting this finding since the antibodies used could also contain antibodies to other lymphokines; purified interferon was not used as the immunogen in raising the antibodies used in those studies. The use of monoclonal antibodies to different interferons should be useful for discerning whether effects mediated by interferon-containing preparations or interferon inducers are indeed caused by interferon. Despite the present inability to rule out the possibility that some agents which are interferon inducers may affect immunologic functions directly, it would seem to be more than coincidental that all of the agents which have been found to augment NK cell activity, for example, have been found capable of inducing interferon. It has become clear, during the very recent past, that interferon is definitely capable of mediating several different immunologic effects. This is because highly purified interferon preparations as well as the *E. coli*-produced human interferon have recently been found capable of affecting several different immunologic functions. Whether the diverse immunologic effects of interferon are mediated by a common molecular mechanism has not been determined.

Table 1. Effects of interferon and its inducers on leukocytes and their immunologic functions

	References
Effects on antibody production	
Decreases or increases antibody responses depending on time of interferon treatment in relation to antigenic stimulation and relative interferon concentration	MAZZUR and PAUCKER (1967) BRAUN and LEVY (1972) CHESTER et al. (1973) GISLER et al. (1974) BRODEUR and MERIGAN (1975) JOHNSON et al. (1975 a, b, c) MERIGAN et al. (1975) JOHNSON and BARON (1976) NGAN et al. (1976) VIRELIZIER et al. (1976) SONNENFELD et al. (1978)
Effects on cell surface antigen expression	
Mouse cells	
Increases cell surface expression of H-2K or H-2D antigens, but not of Ia or Thy-1 antigens	LINDAHL-MAGNUSSON et al. (1973) LINDAHL et al. (1974) VIGNAUX and GRESSER (1977) LONAI and STEINMAN (1977)
Human cells	
Increases cell surface expression of β_2-microglobulin and HLA-A, -B antigens, but not of HLA-DR antigens or cell surface IgG	HERON et al. (1978) FELLOUS et al. (1979)
Effects on mitogen- and antigen-induced lymphocyte proliferative and cytotoxic responses	
Mouse cells	
Suppresses proliferative responses to the mitogens PHA, con A, LPS, and PWM if added with or before the mitogen; less, or no, suppression if added after the mitogen; suppresses proliferative responses to alloantigens	LINDAHL-MAGNUSSON et al. (1972) ROZEE et al. (1973) BRODEUR and MERIGAN (1974) WALLEN et al. (1975) CLINTON et al. (1976)
Human cells	
Generally suppresses proliferative responses to PHA, con A, PWM, PPD, and alloantigens; less or no suppression if added after stimulation	BLOMGREN et al. (1974) SMITH et al. (1974) MIÖRNER et al. (1978)
Augments cytotoxic responses of T-cells to alloantigens when added at the onset of mixed leukocyte cultures	HERON et al. (1976) ZARLING et al. (1978) HERON and BERG (1979)
Effects on DTHR	
Mouse	
Decreases DTHR if given prior to or with sensitizing antigen	DEMAEYER et al. (1975) DEMAEYER-GUIGNARD et al. (1975) DEMAEYER (1976)
Human	
Suppresses mitogen- and antigen-induced leukocyte migration inhibition; blocks production and action of leukocyte migration-inhibitory factor	SZIGETI et al. (1980)

Table 1 (continued)

Effects on macrophage functions	*References*
Mouse	
Enhances macrophage phagocytic activity	HUANG et al. (1971)
	DONAHOE and HUANG (1973)
	DONAHOE and HUANG (1976)
	REMINGTON and MERIGAN (1970)
	GRESSER and BOURALI (1970)
Enhances macrophage spreading	RABINOVITCH et al. (1977)
	SCHULTZ et al. (1977)
Enhances macrophage tumoricidal activity	SCHULTZ et al. (1977)
	SCHULTZ et al. (1978)
	CHIRIGOS et al. (1980)
Human	
Enhances macrophage tumoricidal activity	JETT et al. (1980)
	HERBERMAN et al. (1980)
	MANTOVANI et al. (1980 b, c)
Enhances macrophage cytotoxic activity against virus-infected cells	STANWICK et al. (1980)
Effects on NK cell activity	
Mouse	
Increase in NK cell activity in vivo or in vitro by interferon or interferon inducers	WOLFE et al. (1976)
	WELSH and ZINKERNAGEL (1977)
	MACFARLAN et al. (1977)
	HERBERMAN et al. (1977)
	WELSH (1978)
	GIDLUND et al. (1978)
	RODER et al. (1978)
	DJEU et al. (1979)
	HERBERMAN et al. (1979)
	SENIK et al. (1980)
	MINATO et al. (1980)
	BLOOM et al. (1980)
Human	
Increase in NK cell activity in vitro by interferon and interferon inducers	TRINCHIERI and SANTOLI (1978)
	TRINCHIERI et al. (1978)
	EINHORN et al. (1978 a)
	HERBERMAN et al. (1979)
	DROLLER et al. (1979)
	ZARLING et al. (1979)
	ZARLING (1980)
	ZARLING et al. (1980)
	MOORE and KIMBER (1980)
	MASUCCI et al. (1980)
	MANTOVANI et al. (1980 a)
	SILVA et al. (1980)
	VÁNKY et al. (1980)
	VOSE (1980)
	LUCERO et al. (1981)
	ZIEGLER et al. (1981)
Increase in NK cell activity in vivo by interferon	EINHORN et al. (1978 b)
	HUDDLESTONE et al. (1979)
	EINHORN (1980)
	EINHORN et al. (1980)

As discussed in this chapter, several types of effector cells can by cytocidal for virus-infected cells or tumor cells, including specifically immune cytotoxic T-lymphocytes, macrophages, and NK cells. The activity of all three of these types of effector cells can be augmented by interferon. The effector mechanism which may be most important in overcoming viral diseases or cancers may well be dependent upon the type of virus infection or tumor in question. Hopefully, from further in vitro and in vivo immunologic studies, perhaps involving the use of monoclonal antibodies which distinguish among these effector cells, it should be possible to ascertain which type of effector is most important in eliminating cells infected with particular viruses or cells of tumors of various histologic types. Results of such studies, together with studies aimed at determining whether the relevant effector mechanism can be augmented by interferon in cells from the virus-infected or tumor-bearing host, will hopefully provide insight for predicting in which patients immunomodulation by interferon may be clinically efficacious.

Acknowledgments. Work performed in the author's laboratory was supported by National Institutes of Health grant CA 26738. J. M. ZARLING is a Scholar of the Leukemia Society of America. This is paper number 274 from the Immunobiology Research Center, University of Minnesota, Minneapolis. The author is grateful to E. A. SEVENICH, M. S. DIERCKINS, J. RITTER, and J. WATSON for exceptional assistance in the preparation of this manuscript.

References

Blomgren H, Strander H, Cantell K (1974) Effect of human leukocyte interferon on the response of lymphocytes to mitogenic stimuli in vitro. Scand J Immunol 3:697–705

Bloom B, Minato N, Neighbour A, Reid L, Marcus D (1980) Interferon and NK cells in resistance to persistently virus-infected cells and tumors. In: Herberman RB (ed) Natural cell-mediated immunity against tumors. Academic, New York, p 505

Braun W, Levy HB (1972) Interferon preparations as modifiers of immune responses. Proc Soc Exp Biol Med 141:769–773

Brodeur BR, Merigan TC (1974) Suppressive effect of interferon on the humoral immune response to sheep red blood cells in mice. I Immunol 113:1319–1325

Brodeur BR, Merigan tC (1975) Mechanism of the suppressive effect of interferon on antibody synthesis in vivo. J Immunol 114:1323–1328

Chester TJ, Paucker K, Merigan TC (1973) Suppression of mouse antibody producing spleen cells by various interferon preparations. Nature 246:92–94

Chirigos MA, Schultz RM, Stylos WA (1980) Interaction of interferon, macrophage and lymphocyte tumoricidal activity with prostaglandin effect. Ann NY Acad Sci 350:91–101

Clinton BA, Magoc TJ, Aspinall RL, Rapoza NP (1976) The influence upon mitogenic and cellular immunologic reactive systems in vitro by Poly (I:C) and BCG murine interferons induced in vivo. Cell Immunol 27:60–70

DeMaeyer E (1976) Interferon and delayed-typed hypersensitivity to a viral antigen. J Infect Dis 133:A63–A65

DeMaeyer E, DeMaeyer-Guignard J, Vandeputte M (1975) Inhibition by interferon of delayed-type hypersensitivity in the mouse. Proc Natl Acad Sci USA 72:1753–1757

DeMaeyer-Guignard J, Cachard A, DeMaeyer E (1975) Delayed-type hypersensitivity to sheep red blood cells: inhibition of sensitization by interferon. Science 190:574–576

Dent PB, Fish LA, White JF, Good RA (1966) Chediak-higashi syndrome observations on the nature of the associated malignancy. Lab Invest 15:1634–1642

Djeu JY, Heinbaugh JA, Holden HT, Herberman RB (1979) Augmentation of mouse natural killer cell activity by interferon and interferon inducers. J Immunol 122:175–181

Donahoe RM, Huang KY (1973) Neutralization of the phagocytosis-enhancing activity of interferon preparations by anti-interferon serum. Infect Immun 7:501–503

Donahoe RM, Huang KY (1976) Interferon preparations enhance phagocytosis in vivo. Infect Immun 13:1250–1257

Droller MJ, Borg H, Perlmann P (1979) In vitro enhancement of natural and antibody-dependent lymphocyte-mediated cytotoxicity against tumor target cells by interferon. Cell Immunol 47:248–260

Einhorn S (1980) Enhancement of human NK activity by interferon. In vivo and in vitro studies. In: Herberman RB (ed) Natural cell-mediated immunity against tumors. Academic, New York, p 529

Einhorn S, Blomgren H, Strander H (1978a) Interferon and spontaneous cytotoxicity in man. I. Enhancement of the spontaneous cytotoxicity of peripheral lymphocytes by human leukocyte interferon. Int J Cancer 22:405–412

Einhorn S, Blomgren H, Strander H (1978b) Interferon and spontaneous cytotoxicity in man. II. Studies in patients receiving exogenous leukocyte interferon. Acta Med Scand 204:477–484

Einhorn S, Blomgren H, Strander H (1980) Interferon and spontaneous cytotoxicity in man. V. Enhancement of spontaneous cytotoxicity in patients receiving human leukocyte interferon. Int J Cancer 26:419–428

Epstein LB (1977) The effects of interferon on the immune response in vitro and in vivo. In: Stewart WE II (ed) Interferons and their actions. CRC, Cleveland, p 91

Evans R, Alexander P (1972) Mechanism of immunologically specific killing of tumour cells by macrophages. Nature 236:168–170

Evans R, Alexander P (1976) Mechanisms of extracellular killing of nucleated mammalian cells by macrophages. In: Nelson DS (ed) Immunobiology of the macrophage. Academic, New York, p 535

Fellous M, Kamoun M, Gresser I, Bono R (1979) Enhanced expression of HLA antigens and β_2-microglobulin on interferon-treated human lymphoid cells. Eur J Immunol 9:446–449

Gidlund M, Orn A, Wigzell H, Senik A, Gresser I (1978) Enhanced NK cell activity in mice injected with interferon and interferon inducers. Nature 273:759–761

Gisler RH, Lindahl P, Gresser I (1974) Effects of interferon on antibody synthesis in vitro. J Immunol 113:438–444

Gresser I, Bourali C (1970) Antitumor effects of interferon preparations in mice. J Natl Cancer Inst 45:365–375

Haller O, Hansson M, Kiessling R, Wigzell H (1977) Role of non-conventional natural killer cells in resistance against syngeneic tumour cells in vivo. Nature 270:609–611

Herberman RB, Nunn ME, Lavrin DH (1975) Natural cytotoxic reactivity of mouse lymphoid cells against syngeneic and allogeneic tumors. I. Distribution of reactivity and specificity. Int J Cancer 16:216–229

Herberman RB, Nunn ME, Holden HT, Staal S, Djeu JY (1977) Augmentation of natural cytotoxic reactivity of mouse lymphoid cells against syngeneic and allogeneic target cells. Int J Cancer 19:555–564

Herberman RB, Djeu JY, Kay HD, Ortaldo JR, Riccardi C, Bonnard GD, Holden HT, Fagnani R, Santoni A, Puccetti P (1979) Natural killer cells: characteristics and regulation of activity. Immunol Rev 44:43–70

Herberman RB, Ortaldo JR, Djeu JY, Holden HT, Jett J, Lang NP, Rubinstein M, Pestka S (1980) Role of interferon in regulation of cytotoxicity by natural killer cells and macrophages. Ann NY Acad Sci 350:63–71

Heron I, Berg K (1979) Human leukocyte interferon: analysis of effect on MLC and effector cell generation. Scand J Immunol 9:517–526

Heron I, Berg K, Cantell K (1976) Regulatory effect of interferon on T cells in vitro. J Immunol 117:1370–1373

Heron I, Hokland M, Berg K (1978) Enhanced expression of β_2-microglobulin and HLA antigens on human lymphoid cells by interferon. Proc Natl Acad Sci USA 75:6215–6219

Hewlett G, Opitz HG, Schlumberger HD, Lemke H (1977) Growth regulation of a murine lymphoma cell line by a 2-mercaptoethanol or macrophage-activated serum factor. Eur J Immunol 7:781–785

Horwitz DA, Kight N, Temple A, Allison AC (1979) Spontaneous and induced cytotoxic properties of human adherent mononuclear cells: killing of non-sensitized and antibody-coated non-erythroid cells. Immunology 36:221–228

Huang KY, Donahoe RM, Gordon FB, Dressler HR (1971) Enhancement of phagocytosis by interferon-containing preparations. Infect Immun 4:581–588

Huddlestone JR, Merigan Jr TC, Oldstone MBA (1979) Induction and kinetics of natural killer cells in humans following interferon therapy. Nature 282:417–419

Jett JR, Mantovani A, Herberman RB (1980) Augmentation of human monocyte-mediated cytolysis by interferon. Cell Immunol 54:425–434

Johnson HM, Baron S (1976) The nature of the suppressive effect of interferon and interferon inducers on the in vitro immune response. Cell Immunol 25:106–115

Johnson HM, Bukovic J, Baron S (1975a) Interferon inhibition of the primary in vitro antibody response to a thymus-independent antigen. Cell Immunol 20:104–109

Johnson HM, Bukovic JA, Smith BG (1975b) Inhibitory effect of synthetic polyribonucleotides on the primary in vitro immune response. Proc Soc Exp Biol Med 149:599–603

Johnson HM, Smith BG, Baron S (1975c) Inhibition of the primary in vitro antibody response by interferon preparations. J Immunol 114:403–409

Kärre K, Klein GO, Kiessling R, Klein G, Roder JC (1980) Low natural in vivo resistance to syngeneic leukaemias in natural killer deficient mice. Nature 284:624–626

Keller R (1976a) Cytostatic and cytocidal effects of activated macrophages. In: Nelson DS (ed) Immunobiology of the macrophage. Academic, New York, p 487

Keller R (1976b) Susceptibility of normal and transformed cell lines to cytostatic and cytocidal effects exerted by macrophages. J Natl Cancer Inst 56:369–374

Keller R (1978) Macrophage-mediated natural cytotoxicity against various target cells in vitro. II. Macrophages from rats of different ages. Br J Cancer 37:742–746

Kiessling R, Klein E, Wigzell H (1975) "Natural" killer cells in the mouse. I. Cytotoxic cells with specificity for mouse Moloney leukemia cells. Specificity and distribution according to genotype. Eur J Immunol 5:112–117

Killander D, Lindahl P, Lundin L, Leary P, Gresser I (1976) Relationship between the enhanced expression of histocompatibility antigens on interferon-treated L1210 cells and their position in the cell cycle. Eur J Immunol 6:56–59

Lindahl P, Leary P, Gresser I (1972) Enhancement by interferon of the specific cytotoxicity of sensitized lymphocytes. Proc Natl Acad Sci USA 69:721–725

Lindahl P, Leary P, Gresser I (1974) Enhancement of the expression of histocompatibility antigens of mouse lymphoid cells by interferon in vitro. Eur J Immunol 4:779–794

Lindahl P, Gresser I, Leary P, Tovey M (1976) Interferon treatment of mice: enhanced expression of histocompatibility antigens on lymphoid cells. Proc Natl Acad Sci USA 73:1284–1287

Lindahl-Magnusson P, Leary P, Gresser I (1972) Interferon inhibits DNA synthesis induced in mouse lymphocyte suspensions by phytohaemagglutinin or by allogeneic cells. Nature 237:120–121

Lindahl-Magnusson P, Leary P, Gresser I (1973) Enhancement by interferon of the expression of surface antigens on murine leukemia L1210 cells. Proc Natl Acad Sci USA 70:2785–2788

Lonai P, Steinman L (1977) Physiological regulation of antigen binding to T cells: role of a soluable macrophage factor and of interferon. Proc Natl Acad Sci USA 74:5662–5666

Lucero MA, Fridman WH, Provost MA, Billardon C, Pouillart P, Dumont J, Falcoff E (1981) Effect of various interferons on the spontaneous cytotoxicity exerted by lymphocytes from normal and tumor-bearing patients. Cancer Res 41:294–299

MacFarlan RI, Burns WH, White DO (1977) Two cytotoxic cells in peritoneal cavity of virus-infected mice: antibody-dependent macrophages and nonspecific killer cells. J Immunol 119:1569–1574

Mantovani A (1978) Effects on in vitro tumor growth of murine macrophages isolated from sarcoma lines differing in immunogenicity and metastasizing capacity. Int J Cancer 22:741–746

Mantovani A, Allavena P, Sessa C, Bolis G, Mangioni C (1980a) Natural killer activity of lymphoid cells isolated from human ascitic ovarian tumors. Int J Cancer 25:573–582

Mantovani A, Peri G, Polentarutti N, Allavena P, Bordignon C, Sessa C, Mangioni C (1980 b) Natural cytotoxicity on tumor cells of human monocytes and macrophages. In: Herberman RB (ed) Natural cell-mediated immunity against tumors. Academic, New York, p 1271

Mantovani A, Polentarutti N, Peri G, Bar Shavit Z, Vecchi A, Bolis G, Mangioni C (1980c) Cytotoxicity on tumor cells of peripheral blood monocytes and tumor-associated macrophages in patients with ascites ovarian tumors. J Natl Cancer Inst 64:1307–1315

Masucci MG, Szigeti R, Klein E, Klein G, Gruest J, Montagnier L, Taira H, Hall A, Nagata S, Weissmann C (1980) Effect of interferon-α1 from E. coli on some cell functions. Science 209:1431–1435

Mazzur SR, Paucker K (1967) Studies on the effect of interferon on the formation of antibody in mouse spleen cells. J Immunol 98:689–696

McCoy JL, Herberman RB, Rosenberg EB, Donnelly FC, Levine PH, Alford C (1973) ^{51}Chromium-release assay for cell-mediated cytotoxicity of human leukemia and lymphoid tissue-culture cells. Natl Cancer Inst Monogr 37:59–67

Merigan TC, Chester TJ, Paucker K (1975) Suppression of antibody-producing spleen cells in mice by various interferon preparations versus enhancement by double-stranded RNA. In: Geraldes A (ed) Effects of interferon on cells, viruses, and the immune system, Academic, London, p 347

Minato N, Bloom BR, Jones C, Holland J, Reid LM (1979) Mechanism of rejection of virus persistently infected tumor cells by athymic nude mice. J Exp Med 149:1117–1133

Minato N, Reid L, Cantor H, Lengyel P, Bloom BR (1980) Mode of regulation of natural killer cell activity by interferon. J Exp Med 152:124–137

Miörner H, Landström L, Larner E, Larsson I, Lungren E, Strannegard Ö (1978) Regulation of mitogen-induced lymphocyte DNA synthesis by human interferon of different origins. Cell Immunol 35:15–24

Moore M, Kimber I (1980) Augmentation of human NK and ADCC by interferon. In: Herberman RB (ed) Natural cell-mediated immunity against tumors. Academic, New York, p 569

Ngan J, Lee SHS, Kind LS (1976) Suppressive effect of interferon on ability of mouse spleen cells synthesizing IgE to sensitize rat skin for heterologous adoptive cutaneous anaphylaxis. J Immunol 117:1063–1075

Nunn ME, Djeu JY, Glaser M, Lavrin DH, Herberman RB (1976) Natural cytotoxic reactivity of rat lymphocytes against syngeneic Grossvirus-induced lymphoma. J Natl Cancer Inst 56:393–399

Oehler JR, Lindsay LR, Nunn ME, Herberman RB (1978) Natural cell-mediated cytotoxicity in rats. I. Tissue and stain distribution, and demonstration of a membrane receptor for the Fc portion of IgG. Int J Cancer 21:204–209

Pfizenmaier K, Trostmann H, Röllinghoff M, Wagner H (1975) Temporary presence of self-reactive cytotoxic T lymphocytes during murine lymphocytic choriomeningitis. Nature 258:238–240

Pross HF, Jondal M (1975) Cytotoxic lymphocytes from normal donors: a functional marker of non-T lymphocytes. Clin Exp Immunol 21:226–235

Pross HF, Kerbel RS (1976) An assessment of intratumor phagocytic and surface marker-bearing cells in a series of autochthonous and early passaged chemically induced murine sarcomas. J Natl Cancer Inst 57:1157–1167

Rabinovitch M, Manejias RE, Russo M, Abbey EE (1977) Increased spreading of macrophages from mice treated with interferon inducers. Cell Immunol 29:86–95

Reid L, Jones C, Holland J (1979) Virus carrier state suppresses tumorigenicity of tumor cells in athymic (nude) mice. J Gen Virol 42:609–614

Remington JS, Merigan TC (1970) Synthetic polyanions protect mice against intracellular bacterial infections. Nature 226:361–363

Rinehart JJ, Lange P, Gormus BJ, Kaplan ME (1978) Human monocyte-induced tumor cell cytotoxicity. Blood 52:211–220

Roder JC, Kiessling R, Biberfeld P, Andersson B (1978) Target-effector interaction in the natural killer (NK) cell system. II. The isolation of NK cells and studies on the mechanism of killing. J Immunol 121:2509–2517

Roder JC, Haliotis T, Klein M, Korec S, Jett JR, Ortaldo J, Herberman RB, Katz P, Fauci AS (1980) A new immunodeficiency disorder in humans involving NK cells. Nature 284:553–555

Rosenberg EB, McCoy JL, Green SS, Donnelly FC, Siwarski DF, Levine PH, Herberman RB (1974) Destruction of human lymphoid tissue culture cell lines by human peripheral lymphocytes in ^{51}Cr-release cellular cytotoxicity assay. J Natl Cancer Inst 52:345–352

Rozee KR, Lee SHS, Ngan J (1973) Effect of priming on interferon inhibition of Con A induced spleen cell blastogenesis. Nature 245:16–18

Russell SW, McIntosh AT (1977) Macrophages isolated from regressing moloney sarcomas are more cytotoxic than those recovered from progressing sarcomas. Nature 268:69–71

Schellekens H, Weimar W, Cantell K, Stitz L (1979) Antiviral effect of interferon in vivo may be mediated by the host. Nature 278:742

Schultz RM, Papamatheakis JD, Chirigos MA (1977) Interferon: an inducer of macrophage activation by polyanions. Science 197:674–676

Schultz RM, Pavlidis NA, Stylos WA, Chirigos MA (1978) Regulation of macrophage tumoricidal function: a role for prostaglandins of the E series. Science 202:320–321

Sendo F, Aoki T, Boyse EA, Buato CK (1975) Natural occurrence of lymphocytes showing cytotoxic activity to Balb/c radiation-induced leukemia RLO 1 cells. J Natl Cancer Inst 55:603–609

Senik A, Kolb JP, Örn A, Gidlund M (1980) Study of the mechanism for in vitro activation of mouse NK cells by interferon. Scand J Immunol 12:51–60

Shellam GR (1977) Studies on a Gross-virus-induced lymphoma in rat. V. Natural cytotoxic cells are non-T cells. Int J Cancer 19:225–235

Silva A, Bonavida B, Targan S (1980) Mode of action of interferon-mediated modulation of natural killer cytotoxic activity: recruitment of pre-NK cells and enhanced kinetics of lysis. J Immunol 125:479–484

Smith KA, Cornwell GG, McIntyre OR (1974) The effect of poly I: C and interferon on lymphocyte DNA synthesis. In: Lindahl-Kiessling K, Osoba D (eds) Lymphocyte recognition and effector mechanisms. Academic, New York, p 101

Sonnenfeld G, Mandel AD, Merigan TC (1978) Time and dosage dependence of immunoenhancement by murine type II interferon preparations. Cell Immunol 40:285–293

Stanwick TL, Campbell DE, Nahmias AJ (1980) Spontaneous cytotoxicity mediated by human monocyte-macrophages against human fibroblasts infected with herpes simplex virus-augmentation by interferon. Cell Immunol 53:413–416

Stewart WE II (1981) Non-antiviral actions of interferon. In: Stewart WE II (ed) The interferon system. Springer, Wien New York, p 223

Sykes JA, Maddox IS (1972) Prostaglandin production by experimental tumors and effects of anti-inflammatory compounds. Nature 237:59–63

Szigeti R, Masucci M, Masucci G, Klein E, Klein G (1980) Interferon suppresses antigen- and mitogen-induced leukocyte migration inhibition. Nature 288:594–596

Tagliabue A, Mantovani A, Kilgallen M, Herberman RB, McCoy JL (1979) Natural cytotoxicity of mouse monocytes and macrophages. J Immunol 122:2363–2370

Takasugi M, Mickey MR, Terasaki PI (1973) Reactivity of lymphocytes from normal patients on cultured tumor cells. Cancer Res 33:2898–2902

Talmadge JE, Meyers KM, Prieur DJ, Starkey JR (1980) Role of NK cells in tumour growth and metastasis in beige mice. Nature 284:622–624

Targan S, Dorey F (1980) Interferon activation of "pre-spontaneous killer" (pre-SK) cells and alteration in kinetics of lysis of both "pre-SK" and active SK cells. J Immunol 124:2157–2161

Trinchieri G, Santoli D (1978) Anti-viral activity induced by culturing lymphocytes with tumor-derived or virus-transformed cells – Enhancement of human natural killer cell activity by interferon and antagonistic inhibition of susceptibility of target cells to lysis. J Exp Med 147:1314–1333
Trinchieri G, Santoli D, Koprowski H (1978) Spontaneous cell-mediated cytotoxicity in humans: role of interferon and immunoglobulins. J Immunol 120:1849–1855
Vánky FT, Argov SA, Einhorn SA, Klein E (1980) Role of alloantigens in natural killing. Allogeneic but not autologous tumor biopsy cells are sensitive for interferon-induced cytotoxicity of human blood lymphocytes. J Exp Med 151:1151–1165
Vignaux F, Gresser I (1977) Differential effects of interferon on the expression of H-2 K, H-2 D and Ia antigens on mouse lymphocytes. J Immunol 118:721–723
Virelizier JL, Virelizier AM, Allison AC (1976) Role of circulating interferon in modifications of immune responsiveness by mouse hepatitis virus (MHV-3). J Immunol 117:748–764
Vose BM (1980) Natural killers in human cancer: activity of tumor-infiltrating and draining node lymphocytes. In: Herberman RB (ed) Natural cell-mediated immunity against tumors. Academic, New York, p 1081
Wallen WC, Dean JH, Gauntt C, Lucas DO (1975) Suppression of lymphocyte stimulation in mouse spleen cells by interferon preparations. In: Geraldes A (ed) Effects of interferon on cells, viruses, and the immune system. Academic, London, p 355
Welsh RM (1978) Cytotoxic cells induced during lymphocytic choriomeningitis virus infection of mice. I. Characterization of natural killer cell induction. J Exp Med 148:163–181
Welsh RM, Kiessling RW (1980) Activated natural killer cells induced during the lymphocytic choriomeningitis virus infection in mice. In: Herberman RB (ed) Natural cell-mediated immunity against tumors. Academic, New York, p 671
Welsh RM, Zinkernagel RM (1977) Heterospecific cytotoxic cells early during acute lymphocytic choriomeningitis virus infection. Nature 268:646–648
Wolfe SA, Tracey DE, Henney CS (1976) Induction of "natural killer" cells by BCG. Nature 262:584–586
Zarling JM (1980) Augmentation of human natural killer cell activity by purified interferon and polyribonucleotides. In: Herberman RB (ed) Natural cell-mediated immunity against tumors. Academic, New York, p 687
Zarling JM, Kung PC (1980) Monoclonal antibodies which distinguish between human NK cells and cytotoxic T lymphocytes. Nature 288:394–396
Zarling JM, Tevethia SS (1973) Transplantation immunity to simian virus 40-transformed cells in tumor bearing mice. II. Evidence for macrophage participation at the effector level of tumor cell rejection. J Natl Cancer Inst 50:149–157
Zarling JM, Nowinski RC, Bach FH (1975) Lysis of leukemia cells by spleen cells of normal mice. Proc Natl Acad Sci USA 72:2780–2784
Zarling JM, Sosman J, Eskra L, Borden EC, Horoszewicz JS, Carter WA (1978) Enhancement of T cell cytotoxic responses by purified human fibroblast interferon. J Immunol 121:2002–2004
Zarling JM, Eskra L, Borden E, Horoszewicz J, Carter WA (1979) Activation of human natural killer cells cytotoxic for human leukemia cells by purified interferon. J Immunol 123:63–70
Zarling JM, Schlais J, Eskra L, Greene JJ, Ts'o POP, Carter WA (1980) Augmentation of human natural killer cell activity by polyinosinic acid-polycytidylic acid and its nontoxic mismatched analogues. J Immunol 124:1852–1857
Zarling JM, Bach FH, Kung PC (1981) Sensitization of lymphocytes against pooled allogeneic cells. II. Characterization of effector cells cytotoxic for autologous lymphoblastoid cell lines. J Immunol 125:357–378
Ziegler HW, Kay NE, Zarling JM (1981) Deficiency of natural killer cell activity in patients with chronic lymphocytic leukemia. Int J Cancer 27:321–327
Zinkernagel RM, Doherty PC (1974) Restriction of in vitro T cell mediated cytotoxicity in lymphocytic choriomeningitis within a syngeneic or semi-allogenic system. Nature 248:701–702

CHAPTER 21

Clinical Use of Interferons: Localized Application in Viral Diseases

S. B. GREENBERG and M. W. HARMON

A. Introduction

Since the original reports by ISAACS and LINDENMANN (1957a, b), the use of interferon (IFN) in the prevention and treatment of virus infections has been anticipated. Because of its broad spectrum of antiviral activity, viral infections of the respiratory tract, eye, and skin have been appropriate targets for the potential utilization of IFN. However, only in the past few years have sufficient quantities of IFN been available for clinical evaluation in humans. Thus, there have been few controlled studies with HuIFN, but several anecdotal reports. This chapter will focus on both the basic anatomic and physiologic considerations which pertain to clinical efficacy, and the studies performed to date with locally applied IFN.

B. Respiratory Virus Infections

I. Basic Anatomy and Physiology

Because the nasopharynx is of major importance in the pathogenesis of most respiratory viruses, only the basic anatomy and physiology of the upper airways will be discussed. Anatomically, the beginning of the nasal airway is the anterior nares. The nasal passages are divided by the septum, and the lateral walls are defined by the folds of the turbinates and the meati (PROETZ 1953; NEGUS 1958, PROCTOR et al. 1977; DION et al. 1978). The mucosa contains ciliated epithelium, a rich vasculature, and numerous mucus glands and goblet cells (Fig. 1; BANG 1961; ALI 1965). At the nasopharynx, transition to squamous epithelium is found.

One-half of the total respiratory resistance to airflow is accounted for by the nose. The anterior constriction is the main determinant of resistance to airflow. Nasal vascular congestion responds to autonomic control and changes in ambient air conditions (DRETTNER 1961). Some fluctuation in the patency of one side of the nose in relation to the other has been observed to occur in regular cycles (STOCKSTED 1975; HASEGAWA and KERN 1977).

Most inhaled particles are either large enough (> 5 μm) to be removed in the nose, or small enough (1–2 μm) to be inhaled into the lungs or breathed in and out without deposition (FRY 1970; FRY and BLACK 1973; LARSON et al. 1976). The majority of particles 5–10 μm in size are deposited in the nose with nasal breathing (PATTLE 1961; LANDAHL 1950; LIPPMANN 1970; HOUNAM et al. 1971; HEYDER et al. 1973; ADLER et al. 1973).

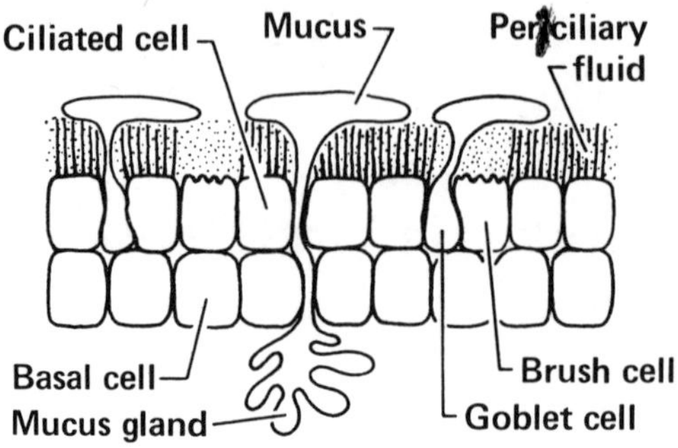

Fig. 1. Schematic representation of human nasal mucosa with the ciliated cells, perciliary fluid, and mucus layer in relation to each other

Most material deposited in the nose is found in the anterior region which contains nonciliated cells. Anatomically, this is near the anterior end of the middle meatus, close to the anterior ethmoid sinuses (NAESSEN 1970). A smaller portion of particles are deposited along the main nasal passage, and are carried backward to the nasopharynx. Others have found two small accumulations of particles in the nasopharynx, one at the terminal points of the mucociliary clearance paths and the other in the crypts of the adenoids (PROCTOR 1977). The exact proportion of particles which penetrate to the lung has yet to be determined, but scans taken after nasal breathing show a heavy concentration in the anterior nares. Thus, it appears that retention time for the majority of the particles in the nose might be prolonged if not for the tendency to sneeze or blow our noses (HOUNAM 1975).

A great deal of work has been performed looking at mucociliary function (LUCAS and DOUGLAS 1933, 1934; WANNER 1977). As early as 1931, HILDING had described the paths of human nasal mucus flow (HILDING 1931, 1932). EWERT (1965) demonstrated the backwards motion of inert dye particles which were placed in the anterior nasal septal mucosa. Others (BANG et al. 1967; BANG and BANG 1977b) have placed colored materials on the anterior nasal mucosa and looked for them in the nasopharynx. A major advance occurred with the development of a new technique by QUINLAN et al. (1969) which could be used in humans to follow the entire path of nasal mucociliary flow. A radioactively tagged particle was placed on the anterior nasal mucosa, with the movement of the particle displayed on an oscilloscope. Using this technique, PROCTOR et al. (1973, 1977) looked at normal nasal mucociliary function in volunteers. Several important observations were made from these studies. First, they found that the average rate of clearance of the single particle was 6 mm/min. It was found that there was consistency in flow rates common to one individual, so that one could characterize certain volunteers as slow or fast movers. The transit time from particle placement to the point at which it was swallowed varied from 4–5 min to over 30 min. Some 20% of their normal volunteers exhibited slow flow (under 3 mm/min). No changes in clearance rates were found when the relative humidity was lowered as low as 10% (ANDERSEN et al. 1971, 1972). Thus, in normal subjects, relative humidity and clean air at 23 °C had no measurable influence on nasal mucociliary function.

In another set of experiments, either cooling or warming the air below or above 23 °C produced some change in nasal mucociliary clearance, usually a slowing. The change which was produced differed from subject to subject and was never very pronounced. In another series of experiments, the same investigators found that sulfur dioxide impairs defense mechanisms in two ways: by slowing nasal mucociliary clearance and by increasing nasal resistance to air flow (ANDERSON et al. 1974). CAMNER et al. (1971) demonstrated that the bronchial clearance rates of monozygotic twins are more similar than those of other pairs of individuals who are not twins. However, in other studies, nasal clearance was found to be less related to genetic factors than bronchial clearance (ANDERSON 1974). Additionally, there was no clear relationship between nasal and bronchial clearance rates.

Mucus secretions of the respiratory tract consist of salts, free protein, carbohydrate-rich glycoproteins, and water (CREETH 1978; PARKE 1978; WIDDICOMBE 1978). The electrolyte content resembles that of serum or bile. Of the 15 or more nonplasma proteins detected in mucus, secretory IgA, lactoferrin, and lysozyme are the most significant. Albumin, IgA, and IgG are the most predominant plasma proteins found in mucus. TAYLOR (1974) demonstrated that capillary loops penetrate the basement membrane of the respiratory epithelium and are found between epithelial cells. Thus, fluid may pass to the surface and thereby maintain the mucus at an optimal dilution.

Despite intensive investigation of both ciliary motion and airway secretions, there is no clear understanding of the mechanisms underlying these basic biologic activities (ISHII 1970; BLAKE and SLEIGHT 1974; ANDERSON 1974; BOAT and KLEINERMAN 1975; FOSTER et al. 1976). PROCTOR (1977) has provided one hypothetical description of mucociliary function. A serous (perciliary) fluid surrounds the cilia (see Fig. 1). The upper layer of fluid moves in the direction of the perciliary fluid, but the layer next to the cell surface remains stationary. Particles are removed with the patches of mucus which are propelled by the tips of the cilia. If a particle penetrates through the periciliary fluid to the cell surface, it may not be cleared at all. Removal of materials not in the upper layers of the perciliary fluids is probably impaired if mucus is absent. Although it is not known if the mucus layer in the nose is continuous, the thickness or viscosity of the mucus is not thought to affect ciliary transport (PROCTOR 1977). What determines whether or not small surface particles penetrate into and through perciliary fluid is not known. For example, little is known about the rate at which soluble materials penetrate to underlying cells, and what factors would influence their movement along the surface.

AOKI and CRAWLEY (1976) studied the distribution and time of removal of human serum albumin $^{99}Tc^{m}$ delivered intranasally to volunteers. Using a gamma camera and an anterior sodium iodide scintillation detector, they found an early fall in activity from the nasal cavity and slower loss of residual material from the anterior segment of the nose. Drops appeared to give a better distribution than a spray, and doses every 20 min gave the best pharmacokinetic response.

The regeneration rate of cells comprising the nasal mucosa has not been completely defined (BANG and BANG 1977b). Although physical trauma, toxic chemicals, bacteria, or viruses may destroy the nasal mucosa, it has been difficult to define the normal rate of mucosal turnover. Several studies have attempted to evaluate mucous membrane regeneration by sequential histologic examination of removed tissue sections (KNOWLTON and MCGREGOR 1928; BOLING 1935; BRETTSCHNEIDER 1958; CONDON 1942, SCHULTZ 1960; HILDING 1965; GRAZIADEI 1970). In humans, several months were needed for complete recovery after surgical removal of the lining of the maxillary sinus (GORHAM and BACHER 1930). However, these studies do not provide a complete understanding of human epithelial cell turnover in the nasopharynx.

The human nasal mucosa and ciliary activity are constantly trying to remove foreign material as quickly as possible. Thus, these normal physiologic mechanisms may be responsible for the apparent difficulty in applying substances locally to the nose. An understanding of the normal nasopharynx may help to define better methods for delivering HuIFN.

II. Intranasally Administered IFN

1. Early Trials

The first clinical trial to prevent respiratory virus infections in humans was performed with monkey IFN which had been produced in monkey kidney cell cultures (Table 1; SCIENTIFIC COMMITTEE ON INTERFERON 1962). The IFN was given as nasal drops or spray to volunteers at the Common Cold Research Unit, Salisbury, England. A low dose (1.5×10^3 U/ml) was given twice daily before and for 2–5 days after virus challenge. The challenge viruses in these experiments, parainfluenza 1 virus, an M strain of rhinovirus, and coxsackievirus A21, were reported to be sensitive in tissue culture to the monkey IFN (SCIENTIFIC COMMITTEE ON INTERFERON 1965). However, no beneficial effect was observed among 38 volunteers who were treated. Another study attempted to prevent a rhinovirus type 2 infection using a total dose of 1.8×10^5 U/ml human leukocyte IFN (HuIFN-α) delivered before and for 2 days after challenge (TYRRELL and REED 1973). Once again, no effect on seroconversion, virus shedding, or symptoms was noted in those volunteers who had received the HuIFN-α.

A few studies in the Russian literature and from elsewhere in Europe suggest that low doses of HuIFN-α prevented or reduced symptomatic influenza and other common respiratory viral infections (SOLOV'EV 1967; SOLOV'EV 1969; IKIC et al. 1975a; ARNAUDOVA 1976; KRASIKOVA et al. 1977; REZNIK et al. 1978). The total dose of HuIFN-α was usually 10^3 U/day; far lower than those reported to be efficacious in later controlled volunteer trials (see Table 1). ARNAUDOVA (1976) reported on a large treatment and prophylaxis study in children with upper respiratory tract infections. The HuIFN-α was given by drops either five times each for 3 days as treatment or three times each day for 3 days in a prophylactic study. Each dose was reported to be 160 U. The severity and duration of disease was altered in both groups. The best effect was found if HuIFN-α was given during the first day of illness. Complications such as bronchopneumonia were reported less often in the treatment groups. These results are similar to the other early published field trials.

In 1973; MERIGAN et al. performed two trials with HuIFN-α in volunteer challenge studies. In one study, influenza B virus was delivered to seronegative recipients who had received 8×10^5 U HuIFN-α or placebo over 16 doses. This dose

Table 1. Intranasal administration of IFN in volunteer studies and field trials

IFN preparation and study design	Disease	Results	References
Monkey IFN; drops or spray; 10^2–10^3 U, placebo-controlled; 38 volunteers	Parainfluenza Rhinovirus Coxsackie A21	No clinical response or antiviral effect	Scientific Committee on Interferon (1965)
HuIFN-α; spray; 10^4 U; 284 volunteers	Influenza H3N2	Clinical protection	SOLOV'EV (1967)
HuIFN-α; spray; 10^3 U given 5–7 days after first use; placebo-controlled; 14,000 subjects	Influenza H3N2	Illness frequency reduced by ~60%	SOLOV'EV (1969)
HuIFN-α; spray; 1.8×10^5 U; placebo-controlled; 9 volunteers	Rhinovirus type 2	No clinical response or antiviral effect	TYRRELL and REED (1973)
HuIFN-α; Spray; 8×10^5 U in 16 doses; placebo-controlled; 22 volunteers	Influenza B	No significant clinical or antiviral effect	MERIGAN et al. (1973)
HuIFN-α; spray; 1.4×10^7 U in 39 doses; placebo-controlled; 32 volunteers	Rhinovirus type 4	Significant reduction in symptoms and virus shedding	MERIGAN et al. (1973)
HuIFN-α; spray; 10^4 U; not placebo-controlled; 118 patients	Influenza H3N2	No difference in illness frequency; faster defervescence	IKIC et al. (1975 a)
HuIFN-α; drops; dose unknown, not placebo-controlled; 198 children	Respiratory viral infections	Reduction in illness frequency	KRASIKOVA et al. (1976)
HuIFN-α; drops; 10^4 each day; concurrent controls; 346 treated children and 522 prophylactically treated children	Respiratory viral infections	Reduction in frequency and severity of illness	ARNAUDOVA (1976)
HuIFN-α; drops; 10^3 U given for 6–12 days; concurrent controls; 774 children	Respiratory viral infections	Illness frequency reduced	REZNIK et al. (1978)
HuIFN-β; drops; total dose unknown; placebo-controlled; 27 volunteers	Rhinovirus type 4	No clinical response or antiviral effect	SCOTT et al. (1980)
HuIFN-α; drops; 5×10^3 U daily for 4 months; 86 volunteers	Influenza H3N2	Reduction in frequency and severity of illness	IMANISHI et al. (1980)
HuIFN-α; drops; 10^4 U every other day; placebo-controlled; 1,137 volunteers	Respiratory viral infections	Reduction in frequency of upper respiratory illnesses	YUNDE et al. (1981)
HuIFN-α; cotton pledget or aerosol; 1–4 × 10^6 U as single or 4 doses; placebo-controlled; 78 volunteers	Rhinovirus type 13	Reduction in illness frequency; antiviral effect only with cotton pledget	GREENBERG et al. (1982)

of HuIFN-α had no effect upon virus shedding, seroconversion, or symptom scores. In the other study, rhinovirus type 4 was administered to volunteers who had received 1.4×10^7 U HuIFN-α or placebo over 39 doses before and after virus challenge. This dose schedule of HuIFN-α resulted in a significant decrease in symptom scores, virus shedding, and seroconversion. No significant side effects were noted in these studies.

2. Recent Trials

Two recent field trials have found a prophylactic effect of low dose HuIFN-α against respiratory viral infections (see Table 1; IMANISHI et al. 1980; YUNDE et al. 1981). IMANISHI et al. (1980) found less fever and fewer symptoms in the HuIFN-α treated group who self-administered 5×10^4 U/ml each day for 4 months. Although there were no differences in serologic responses to the influenza viruses, the group of volunteers who took prophylactic HuIFN-α reported less fever and fewer symptoms compared with a placebo-treated, control group. In a similar study, YUNDE et al. (1981) found a prophylactic effect of HuIFN-α given by spray every other day. The preventive course was for 2–3 months and several trials were performed over a 4-year period. Although HuIFN-α had some clinical effect, the best results were reported when HuIFN-α was given in combination with a traditional Chinese medicine, radix astragali seu Hedysari (RAH). No serology or virus isolations were reported and a clinical diagnosis was made of respiratory virus infection.

A recent attempt to repeat the trial by MERIGAN et al. (1973) using a similar schedule, but with HuIFN-β, was unsuccessful (SCOTT et al. 1980). Although the investigators are not sure as to the reason for the failure to demonstrate efficacy, the instability of the preparation tested may have resulted in the volunteers receiving a lower total dose than had been anticipated. The total dose of HuIFN-β given may have been as low as 6×10^5 U.

3. Transport of Exogenous HuIFN Across the Human Nasal Mucosa

Because of the large dose required for the results of MERIGAN et al. (1973), we have been studying factors which could alter the transport of HuIFN across the nasal mucosa. We have considered three possible explanations for the large in vivo dose requirements of intranasally applied HuIFN. First, the mucus overlying the nasal epithelial cells could contain a substance or substances that inactivate or inhibits the applied HuIFN before it could render the cells resistant to virus challenge. Second, the mucus barrier or rapid clearance mechanisms could prevent the HuIFN from reaching the nasal epithelial cells. Third, the nasal epithelial cells lining the nasal cavity could be intensitive to HuIFN compared with tissue culture cells. We have published a series of experiments which address each of these possibilities (HARMON et al. 1976, 1977, 1980; JOHNSON et al. 1976; GREENBERG et al. 1978).

Previous reports indicated that various body fluids were capable of inhibiting HuIFN (ROSSMAN and VILCEK 1970; CESARIO et al. 1973; CESARIO 1977). To clarify if human nasal secretions could similarly inhibit HuIFN, we investigated the effect of human nasal secretions on the antiviral activity of both HuIFN-α (CANTELL et al. 1974) and HuIFN-β. Nasal secretions from healthy volunteers were mixed with

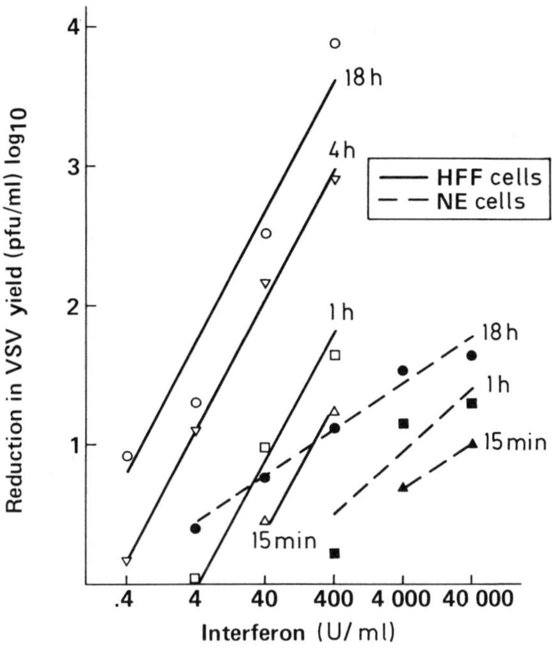

Fig. 2. Comparison of the time and dose–response of IFN in human foreskin fibroblast (HFF) and nasal epithelial (NE) cells challenged with vesicular stomatitis virus (VSV). Times indicated represent the time cells were exposed to IFN at 34 °C. Virus yields were measured 24 h after challenge. HARMON et al. (1980)

low concentrations of HuIFN and tested for antiviral activity in fibroblast cell cultures. Although there was some inhibition of antiviral activity of HuIFN-β at low concentrations (25 U/ml), this inhibition could be overcome at higher concentrations (250 U/ml). HuIFN-α was not significantly affected by the nasal secretions, even at the low concentrations. Thus, inactivation or inhibition by nasal secretions would not explain the in vivo requirement for large doses of HuIFN-α.

If HuIFN-α were rapidly cleared from the nasal cavity, it might not have sufficient time to reach the surface of the nasal epithelial cell. Data obtained in both chimpanzees and humans indicated that significant removal of HuIFN-α from the nose occurs within 1 h and confirms the recovery of low levels of HuIFN-α by MERIGAN et al. (1973). The 5- to 50-fold reduction in recoverable HuIFN-α observed over 60 min suggests that mucociliary clearance mechanisms may be important in determining optimal delivery schedules (JOHNSON et al. 1976).

To investigate the sensitivity of nasal epithelial cells to HuIFN, we developed a human nasal epithelial cell culture system (HARMON et al. 1978, 1980). The cells were scraped from the inferior or middle turbinates of healthy volunteers and placed in culture. The growth of vesicular stomatitis virus (VSV) in HuIFN-treated cells was compared with control, untreated cells as a measure of antiviral activity. Antiviral activity of HuIFN-α and HuIFN-β was found to be both time and concentration dependent in nasal epithelial cells as well as in foreskin fibroblast cells. Rapid onset (15 min to 1 h) of antiviral activity with low concentrations of HuIFN-α was demonstrated (Fig. 2). Thus, these experiments confirm the results of DIANZANI et al. (1978) using an epithelial cell and suggest that the concentration of HuIFN is important in the development of significant antiviral activity. In addition, the nasal epithelial cell may be less sensitive to the action of HuIFN than foreskin fibroblast cells.

A series of experiments was performed to determine if significant antiviral activity could develop in vivo after topical HuIFN-α administration. Adult volunteers had HuIFN-α applied to a small area of nasal mucosa either by nose drops or by a saturated cotton pledget that was left in the nasal cavity for 1 h (GREENBERG et al. 1978). The nasal epithelial cells were scraped from the area of application, as well as from the control, untreated side and challenged with VSV. A cotton pledget saturated with 8×10^4 U HuIFN-α was found to induce antiviral activity in the underlying nasal epithelial cells. However, HuIFN-α delivered by nose drops could induce antiviral activity only when the volunteers were pretreated with oral antihistamines. Because of the atropine-like activity of antihistamines (MELVILLE 1973), decreased mucus production could result in increasing concentrations of HuIFN reaching the cell surface before normal mucociliary clearance mechanisms remove it from the nasal cavity.

In recent studies, we have tested whether low doses of HuIFN-α given prophylactically by cotton pledget or aerosol would be effective against a rhinovirus challenge (GREENBERG et al. 1982). Volunteers for the rhinovirus challenge studies were seronegative for rhinovirus type 13 antibodies. Cotton pledgets were saturated with 0.5 ml phosphate-buffered saline (PBS) containing 5×10^5 U HuIFN-α and placed between the inferior and middle turbinates of each nasal cavity. Untreated (control) volunteers had cotton pledgets saturated with PBS placed similarly on each side. After 1 h, pledgets were removed and, approximately 4 h later, both groups were inoculated with virus.

HuIFN-α or a placebo was administered by aerosol over 1 h. In single-dose experiments, volunteers inhaled the HuIFN-α (1 or 3×10^6 U) or PBS approximately 4 h prior to receiving the virus inoculum. In multiple-dose experiments, volunteers inhaled HuIFN-α (1×10^6 U) or PBS approximately 16 and 4 h prior to and 4 and 16 h following virus inoculation. In the multiple-dose experiment, the total dose of HuIFN-α used was 4×10^6 U. In each study, oral antihistamines were taken approximately 16 and 5 h before rhinovirus challenge by both IFN-treated and control volunteers.

These challenge studies demonstrated a lower frequency of illness in the HuIFN-α-treated volunteers in both the cotton pledget and aerosol studies. An overall 40% reduction in illnesses was documented in the HuIFN-α-treated volunteers. If all trails with both cotton pledget and aerosol were combined, a significant reduction in illness frequency was demonstrated in the HuIFN-α-treated volunteers.

The best results were obtained with the cotton pledgets. Although overall illness frequency was not significantly different, mean symptom scores were significantly reduced in the HuIFN-α-treated group. Virus shedding was significantly reduced on days 2–5, when the distribution of titers was analyzed. However, the total number of isolates was similar. It is of some interest that the pledgets, when assayed for residual HuIFN-α, were found to have ≧90% of the original activity.

Potential explanations for our failure to demonstrate a better preventive effect could include the sensitivity of the challenge virus, the methods of HuIFN-α administration, or the schedule and concentration of HuIFN-α. Rhinovirus type 13, employed in these challenge studies, might be relatively insensitive to HuIFN-α when tested in nasal epithelial cells. Although the challenge virus was sensitive to HuIFN-α in human foreskin fibroblast cell cultures, we could not test its sensitivity in nasal epithelial cells. Several unsuccessful attempts have been made to demonstrate replication of rhinovirus in our nasal epithelial cell cultures. A nasal epithelial cell culture system in which rhinovirus replication is reproducible would be potentially useful, since CAME et al. (1976) have shown that different rhinoviruses may exhibit quite different sensitivities to HuIFN in fibroblast and epithelial cells.

Marked differences in distribution and effectiveness of intranasally applied substances have been described (BUCKNALL 1976; IRAVANI and MELVILLE 1976; PROCTOR 1977; BRAIN and VALBERG 1979). Therefore, the method of HuIFN administration may have contributed to the decreased clinical efficacy. The DeVilbiss No. 40 nebulizer, DeVilbiss Corporation, Somerset, Pennsylvania, was chosen because it generates an aerosol with particle sizes which distribute to both the upper and lower respiratory tracts. Nevertheless, the levels delivered to the nasal mucosa were apparently not sufficient to give significant antiviral protection.

In vivo, we have recovered HuIFN-α from the nasal cavity after removing the cotton pledget and after stopping the aerosol, and approximately 300 U/ml were still present 1 h later. However, the concentration of HuIFN-α actually in contact with the nasal epithelial cell cannot be determined. To increase the fraction of administered HuIFN-α contacting the cell surface, two approaches should be considered: either highly concentrated HuIFN-α delivered intermittently to the nasal mucosa, or prolonged contact with less concentrated preparations.

III. Conclusions

Viral respiratory tract infections continue to be appropriate targets for HuIFN use, but several questions remain to be answered. The dose requirements for significant prophylactic effect differ between the reported volunteer studies and the field trials from eastern Europe, U.S.S.R., China, and Japan. The reasons for the apparently disparate results need further clarification. Since successful prophylaxis will probably require administration on a daily basis, a more intensive evaluation of potential side effects is mandatory. If further studies continue to document a prophylactic effect, then postexposure treatment studies should be initiated. However, it is anticipated that the treatment of respiratory viral infections will not prove to be as efficacious as a prophylactic approach.

C. Ocular Virus Infections

I. Basic Anatomy and Physiology

Since most viral ocular infections involve the cornea or conjunctivae, a brief review of the basic anatomy and physiology of this area would be helpful in analyzing the

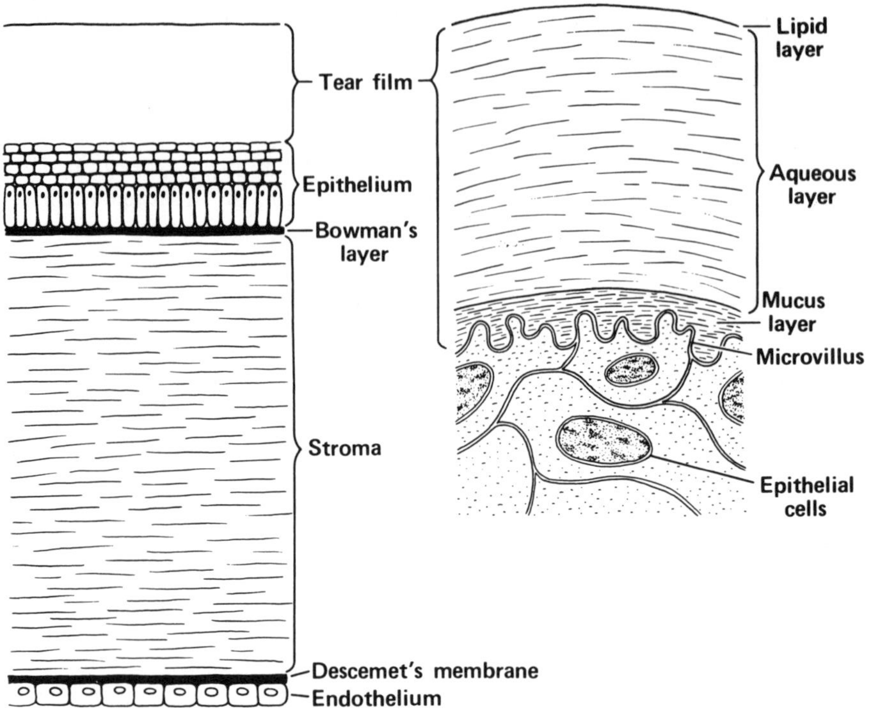

Fig. 3. Schematic representation of human tear film and corneal layers of one eye. Tear film is composed of three layers above the corneal epithelium

clinical trials with topically applied HuIFN. The surface of the eye is covered by a three-layered tear film (Fig. 3). The superficial, oily layer consists mainly of waxy and cholesterol esters and some polar lipids and tends to reduce the rate of evaporation of the underlying tear layer (HOLLY and LEMP 1977). The tear fluid, or aqueous layer, is next and contains inorganic salts, glucose, urea, biopolymers, proteins, and glycoproteins (FORD et al. 1976; HOLLY and LEMP 1977; MILDER 1981). It is secreted by the lacrimal gland and is the thickest layer in the tear film. The deepest stratum of the precorneal tear film is the mucus layer which is elaborated by goblet cells of the conjunctiva and composed of mucoproteins rich in sialomucin. The normal osmotic pressure of tears is equivalent to 0.9%–0.95% NaCl solution (KROGH et al. 1945). Some 25% of tears secreted is lost by evaporation. The remainder leaves the conjunctival sac through the lacrimal–nasal excretory system.

Below the tear film is the cornea which is composed of five discrete layers (Fig. 3; MAURICE 1957). The outermost epithelium consists of five or six layers of cells (JAKUS 1961). Nonkeratinized squamous cells make up the superficial layer. Microvilli have been demonstrated by electron microscopy on the outer membrane of epithelial cells (LEVENSON 1973). Some believe that these microvilli prevent drying of the epithelial cells by trapping tear fluid. The basal layer is composed of columnar cells. Between the columnar epithelial cells and the stroma, a basement membrane (Bowman's layer) has been demonstrated (LA TESSA et al. 1954). Bowman's layer is an acellular, superficial layer found only in primates (WALTMAN 1981). The lower three layers of the cornea are the substantia propria, Descement's membrane, and endothelium. The substantia propria, or stroma, is composed of layers of lamellae and comprises about 90% of the whole cornea. The endothelium is a single layer of cells lining Descement's membrane. Although the cornea is well supplied with sensory nerves, it is avascular. The diseases that commonly affect epithelial structures are accompanied by superficial vascularizations.

The nutrition of the cornea depends on the diffusion of oxygen and glucose and other substances from the surrounding fluids (HARRIS 1960). The transport of drugs across the cornea is determined by the permeability of the corneal layers (COGAN et al. 1944; SADUNAISKY and SPINOWICH 1976). The epithelial and endothelial cell membranes are rich in lipids and, therefore, are more rapidly crossed by lipid-soluble compounds. The stroma is more readily crossed by water-soluble compounds. Substances combining both solubilities will penetrate more freely (SWAN and WHITE 1942). SCHOENWALD and WARD (1978) have demonstrated that the permeation of corticosteroids across excised rabbit corneas was determined by their relative lipid–water solubility. Increased penetration of the applied corticosteroids was found by addition of an acetate group to dexamethasone or prednisone.

Molecular weight and concentration affect the penetration of a drug through the cornea. The permeability of the epithelium is increased if the test solution is hypotonic, i.e., below 0.9%. POTTS (1953) found that 1.35% NaCl damaged the corneal epithelium. However, the pH can be between 4.0 and 10.0 without affecting the permeability of the epithelium (FRIEDENWALD et al. 1944). Agents that reduce surface tension, i.e., wetting agents, increase the permeability of membranes.

II. Intraocularly Administered IFN

1. Early Trials

In early animal trials, IFN was effective against ocular vaccinia infection, but less effective against herpes simplex infection in the rabbit eye (CANTELL and TOMMILA 1960). In the monkey, HuIFN was partially effective in preventing herpetic corneal infection (KAUFMAN et al. 1972), but had no effect on established corneal lesions (NEUMANN-HAEFELIN et al. 1977). A study in rabbits (MCGILL et al. 1977) reported the best results with a single drop of highly concentrated HuIFN administered each day. Antiviral activity followed the first application and was more dependent upon concentration than total number of units administered over a certain time period. This is in agreement with other studies which demonstrated no difference in protective effect with either 2 or 6 drops HuIFN given to monkeys with induced herpes eye infection (SUGAR et al. 1973).

The first report of local IFN administration in human ocular infection came from England and employed monkey IFN in a noncontrolled study (Table 2; JONES et al. 1962). After testing the preparation in the eye of a patient who was to undergo enucleation for a tumor, seven patients with ulcerative vaccinial lesions had the IFN preparation ($\sim 10^3$ U/ml) applied by drops every 30 min along with topical vaccinia convalescent gammaglobulin and oral tetracycline. The observed healing was felt to be due to the IFN. Within 4–24 h after initiating therapy, ulcers began

Table 2. Intraocular administration of IFN

IFN preparation and study design	Disease	Results	References
Monkey IFN; drops every 30 min during the day; uncontrolled; 7 volunteers	Vaccinial keratitis	Improvement	JONES et al. (1962)
Monkey IFN; drops every 1–2 h for 3 days; 2 placebo, 8 treated patients	Herpes keratitis	No effect	PATTERSON et al. (1963)
HuIFN amnion cell-derived; 2 drops every 2 h; nonrandomized controls; 34 patients	Herpes keratitis	Faster healing	TOMMILA (1963)
HuIFN-α; 5–10 × 10^4 U every 4–6 h; 1 renal transplant patient	Herpes keratitis	Rapid healing	KOBZA et al. (1975)
HuIFN-α; 4 × 10^3 U every 2 h for 14 days, no placebo; 28 patients	Adenovirus conjunctivitis	More "effective" response compared with controls	IKIC et al. (1975d)
HuIFN-α; 6 × 10^6 U every 6–8 h; 1 patient	Herpes keratitis	Rapid healing	PALLIN et al. (1976)
HuIFN-α; 2–6 × 10^4 U twice daily; placebo-controlled; 95 patients	Herpes keratitis	No response	KAUFMAN et al. (1976)
HuIFN-α; 7 or 2 × 10^7 U daily for 7 days; placebo-controlled; 55 patients	Herpes keratitis	Improved healing; recurrent rate reduced	JONES et al. (1976b)
HuIFN-α; 6 × 10^4 U every 8 h	Herpes keratitis	No effect on rate of healing	SUNDMACHER et al. (1976a)
HuIFN-α; 3 × 10^6 U every 8 h for 2 days; placebo-controlled; 40 patients	Herpes keratitis	Rapid healing	SUNDMACHER et al. (1976b)
HuIFN-α; 1.1 or 3.3 × 10^7 U; placebo-controlled; 78 patients	Herpes keratitis	Rapid healing	COSTER et al. (1977)
HuIFN-α; 3 × 10^3 U plus secretory IgA; not placebo-controlled; 56 patients	Herpes keratitis	Rapid healing	DE LA PENA et al. (1978)
HuIFN-α and -β; 1 × 10^6 U daily plus debridement; no placebo; 38 patients	Herpes keratitis	No differences in rate of healing between preparations	SUNDMACHER et al. (1978b)
HuIFN-β; 10^5 U/day in divided doses; placebo-controlled; 47 patients	Adenovirus conjunctivitis	More rapid healing; fewer complications	ROMANO et al. (1980)
HuIFN-α; 1.0 × 10^7 U with TFT for 3 days; placebo-controlled; 40 patients	Herpes keratitis	Rapid healing	DE KONING et al. (1982)
HuIFN-α; 1.0 × 10^7 and 3.0 × 10^7 U with TFT; placebo-controlled; 51 patients	Herpes keratitis	Rapid healing	SUNDMACHER et al. (to be published)

to heal and there was no progression of the lesions in any of the patients. Four patients had good healing 1–4 days later. In the three patients who demonstrated a slower response, stromal or extensive ulcerative disease was present. This is the only report of an IFN preparation being studied in vaccinia infection of the eye and most later reports of tropical IFN use were in patients with herpes keratitis.

In 1963, PATTERSON et al. administered monkey IFN, iododeoxyuridine, or placebo to patients with acute ulcerative corneal herpes simplex infections; 2 drops monkey IFN were applied at 1-h intervals during the day and at 2-h intervals at night for 3 days. Healing was demonstrated in more of the IFN- or iododeoxyuridine-treated patients at the end of 3 days than in the placebo-treated patients. However, the differences between controls and IFN-treated patients were not significant.

In the same year, another study reported on the effect of human amniotic cell-derived IFN in the treatment of dendritic keratitis (TOMMILA 1963). The IFN was induced by exposure to ultraviolet-irradiated influenza B virus and had reported a titer of 4–8 U. The treatment schedule for most patients was 2 drops every 2 h until healing began and then every 3 h. The authors concluded that the IFN-treated group began healing several days earlier than a retrospective control group. Differences in severity of the disease and duration of symptoms prior to starting therapy were noted and suggested the need for appropriate controls.

Two case reports of HuIFN-treated patients with herpes keratitis appeared several years later. A renal transplant patient with disseminated cutaneous and ocular herpes simplex infection was treated with HuIFN ($0.5–1 \times 10^5$ U every 6 h for 8 days) (KOBZA et al. 1975). Although the patient had failed to respond to topical iododeoxyuridine, healing occurred and improvement in the corneal opacity was noted on the HuIFN. In a second patient aged 16 months with previous gingivostomatitis, a typical dendritic ulcer was treated with HuIFN-α (6×10^6 U/ml as drops every 8 h for 14 days) (PALLIN et al. 1976). Examination of the cornea after treatment revealed clearing of the stroma.

In 1976, three controlled trials with HuIFN-α in herpes simplex keratitis were published. In an attempt to alter the course of herpes keratitis, 55 patients were treated with HuIFN-α, cautery plus HuIFN-α, or cautery plus placebo (SUNDMACHER et al. 1976a). The dose of HuIFN-α was $3–4 \times 10^4$ U/day in divided doses. The poorest result was found in the group who received HuIFN-α alone. In a subsequent report, SUNDMACHER et al. (1976b) reported on 40 patients treated with higher doses of HuIFN-α. The regimen was 3×10^6 U/ml given as 2 drops twice daily until improvement was detected and then every 3 days until healing occurred. A beneficial result was suggested in that 96% of those receiving HuIFN-α were healed after 3 days compared with 56% of the placebo-treated patients.

In a long-term collaborative trial designed to prevent recurrent herpes simplex keratitis, KAUFMANN et al. (1976) reported no reduction in the incidence of recurrences in an HuIFN-α-treated group compared with placebo-treated controls. The patients were administered HuIFN-α (6.2×10^4 U/ml) or placebo in eyedrops every 12 h at home. A similar study was attempted by JONES et al. (1976a, b) in which HuIFN-α (1.1×10^7 U/ml) or placebo was administered once daily for 7 days. A total of 55 patients were treated and a significant reduction in the number of recurrences was demonstrated in the HuIFN-α-treated group.

One report utilized human interferon (3×10^3 U/ml) and secretory IgA (1.5 mg/ml) in 56 patients with recurrent herpes keratitis (DE LA PENA et al. 1978). This noncontrolled study found reduction in the size of the lesions within 10 days and eventual healing in over 90% of patients. However, there was no apparent effect on the rate of recurrences.

2. Recent Trials

With the availability of higher titered preparations of HuIFN-α, controlled trials were performed against herpes keratitis. COSTER et al. (1977) reported on 78 patients enrolled in a placebo-controlled trial of HuIFN-α in the treatment of dendritic ulcers. In addition to debridement, patients received either 1 drop daily of placebo or HuIFN-α at a concentration of (1.1×10^7 U/ml), of HuIFN-α (3.3×10^7 U/ml). Recurrence rates were significantly reduced in only the patients who received the high dose HuIFN-α.

SUNDMACHER et al. (1976a, b, 1977, 1978a, b, c, 1981) have completed a series of studies in patients with herpetic keratitis. The prophylactic use of a daily application of HuIFN-α (10^6 U/ml) which was found to be effective in the monkey (NEUMANN-HAEFELIN et al. 1977) could not be confirmed in controlled human studies (SUNDMACHER et al. 1977). However, in the past few years, combination therapy with the topical antiherpes agent, trifluorothymidine (TFT) and HuIFN-α have given better results (SUNDMACHER et al. 1981). Although increased healing occurred in patients given 1×10^7 U/ml daily up to the day of fluorescein-negative closure of the corneal epithelium, the best results were found in patients receiving 3×10^7 U/ml daily for up to 3 days beyond the day of fluorescein-negative healing of the epithelium. There was an approximate 50% reduction in healing time of dendritic keratitis by the addition of 3×10^7 U/ml HuIFN-α to the TFT therapy. Similar results were presented in another controlled study in which TFT therapy was compared with TFT plus HuIFN-α given as 1×10^7 U/ml daily (DEKONING et al. 1982). Thus, dendritic keratitis may be one viral disease where exogenous HuIFN should be recommended for treatment (SUNDMACHER et al. 1981).

In a recently published study, ROMANO et al. (1980) found a therapeutic effect of HuIFN-β in patients with epidemic keratoconjunctivitis due to adenovirus type 8. The HuIFN-β was given 8–10 times each day by drops, so that most patients received a total of $1–2 \times 10^6$ U HuIFN-β over 8 days. Compared with the controls, the HuIFN-β-treated patients had a shorter length of disease and fewer complications. One patient who received HuIFN-β had an allergic reaction and in several other cases keratitis punctuata was reported.

III. Conclusions

A beneficial role for the combination therapy of HuIFN with TFT has been reported for herpetic keratitis. These studies suggest that the concentration of HuIFN-α is of major importance in obtaining clinical efficacy. Whether or not HuIFN-α and/or HuIFN-β will be as effective in other ocular virus infections must await confirmation with additional studies. Also the potential usefulness of HuIFN in preventing recurrences of herpetic eye infections must be tested (SCHUSTER et al. 1981).

Table 3. Local administration of IFN in viral skin infections

IFN preparations and study design	Disease	Results	References
Monkey IFN; intradermal injection of 2×10^2 U prior to vaccination; 38 patients	Vaccinia	No vaccinial skin lesions	SCIENTIFIC COMMITTEE ON INTERFERON (1962)
Monkey IFN; subcutaneous; dose unknown; 1 patient	Vaccinia gangrenosa	No response	CONNOLLY et al. (1962)
HuIFN-α; ointment 4×10^3 U/g	Vaccinia/skin lesions	Clinical response	SOOS et al. (1972)
HuIFN-α; ointment 4×10^3 U/g; historical control; 217 patients	HSV-1 Genital herpes Condyloma acuminata	Clinical response	IKIC et al. (1975 a, c, d, e)
HuIFN-β; intradermal 5×10^4 U prior to vaccination; placebo-controlled; 19 patients	Vaccinia	No vaccinial skin lesions	SCOTT et al. (1978)
HuIFN-β; intralesional 3×10^2 U; placebo-controlled; 11 patients	Condyloma acuminata	Minimal reduction in wart growth	SCOTT and CSONKA (1979)

D. Miscellaneous Virus Infections

The first IFN preparations were prepared from embryonic chick cells and when injected into the skin of rabbits, a slight effect on the development of a local vaccinia lesion was found (LINDENMANN et al. 1957). Several years later, preparations of rabbit IFN were tested in a similar way and these were found consistently to inhibit a local smallpox vaccine reaction (ISAACS and WESTWOOD 1959). A double-blind trial with the monkey IFN was initiated to test the effect of this IFN preparation on the development of a smallpox vaccination (Table 3; SCIENTIFIC COMMITTEE ON INTERFERON 1962). Volunteers received 0.1 ml monkey IFN injected intradermally in one site and 0.1 ml control material at another site of the arm. Each site was then challenged with smallpox vaccine and the arms were examined 7 days later by an independent observer. A primary take developed in 37 of the 38 sites pretreated with the control material, but only 14 of the sites treated with monkey IFN had a primary take. In addition, one report in the literature was unsuccessful in treating a complication of smallpox vaccine in 1962. However, the preparation used was of low potency (CONNOLLY et al. 1962). Other recent studies have suggested an effect of injected HuIFN-α and HuIFN-β on vaccinial skin lesions (SOOS et al. 1972; SCOTT et al. 1978).

Treatment of genital warts (condylomata acuminata) by chemical or physical agents has shown variable effectiveness. Two studies have attempted to treat this common viral infection with HuIFN. Both a preliminary noncontrolled study and a double-blind placebo-controlled study, IKIC et al. (1975c, d) found HuIFN given by ointment to be effective in eliminating genital warts in most of the treated women. In another study, HuIFN-β (300 U) was given by injection to the bases of warts in eleven infected male patients, with suggestive evidence that the HuIFN-β did inhibit the growth of the warts (SCOTT and CSONKA 1979). The HuIFN-β was given only once and was associated with some pain from the injection.

In a noncontrolled study, IKIC et al. (1975d) reported on the treatment of labial and genital herpesvirus infections with topically applied HuIFN-α. The HuIFN-α was incorporated into a petrolatum–lanolin ointment at a concentration of 4×10^3 U/g. Each individual was used as a historical control in order to assess the effect of HuIFN-α on the duration of relapse. The patients with the best response had applied the HuIFN-α ointment immediately before the appearance of vesicles. Future controlled studies must confirm these preliminary studies before topically applied HuIFN-α and/or HuIFN-β can be used routinely. In these infections, the method of administration may be crucial to obtaining the optimal responses.

E. Summary

After 20 years of both animal and human studies in the prophylaxis and treatment of viral respiratory, ocular, and skin infections, the hope remains that HuIFN will fulfill its early promise. Although published studies have reported variable results, no significant side effects have been reported with local application of several different preparations. With the advent of unlimited supplies of purified HuIFN, future studies must focus on evaluating the safety, optimal method of administration, and application schedule of these new preparations.

References

Adler KB, Wooten O, Dulfano MJ (1973) Mammalian respiratory mucociliary clearance. Arch Environ Health 27:364–367
Ali MY (1965) Histology of the human nasopharyngeal mucosa. J Anat 99:657–672
Andersen I (1974) A comparison of nasal and tracheobronchial clearance. Arch Environ Health 29:290–293
Andersen I, Lundqvist, Proctor DF (1971) Human nasal mucosal function in a controlled climate. Arch Environ Health 23:408–420
Andersen I, Lundqvist, Proctor DF (1972) Human nasal mucosal function under four controlled humidities. Am Rev Respir Dis 106:439–449
Andersen I, Lundqvist G, Jensen PL, Proctor DF (1974) Human response to controlled levels of sulfur dioxide. Arch Environ Health 28:31–39
Aoki FY, Crawley J (1976) Distribution and removal of human serum albumin-technetium 99m instilled intranasally by drops and spray. Br J Clin Pharm 3:869–878
Arnaoudova V (1976) Treatment and prevention of acute respiratory virus infections in children with leukocytic interferon. Rev Roum Med Virol 27:89–91
Bang BG (1961) The surface pattern of the nasal mucosa and its relation to mucosa and its relation to mucus flow. J Morphol 109:57–72
Bang BG, Mukherjee AL, Bang FB (1967) Human nasal mucus flow rates. John Hopkins Med J 121:38–48
Bang BG, Bang FB (1977a) Nasal mucociliary systems. In: Brian JD, Proctor DF, Reid LM (eds) Respiratory defense mechanisms, vol 5. Dekker, New York, p 405
Bang FB, Bang BG (1977b) Mucous membrane injury and repair. In: Brain JD, Proctor DF, Reid LM (eds) Respiratory defense mechanisms, vol 5. Dekker, New York, p 453
Blake JR, Sleight MA (1974) Mechanics of ciliary locomotion. Biol Rev 49:85–105
Boat TF, Kleinerman JI (1975) Human respiratory tract secretions. 2. Effect of cholinergic and adrenergic agents on in vitro release of protein and mucous glycoprotein. Chest 67 [Suppl]:325
Boling LR (1935) Regeneration of nasal mucosa. Arch Otolaryngol 22:689–724

Brain JD, Valberg PA (1979) Deposition of Aerosol in the respiratory tract. Am Rev Respir Dis 120:1325–1373

Brettschneider H (1958) Electromicroscopic studies of the nasal mucosa. Amt Anz 105:194–204

Bucknall RA (1976) Why aren't antivirals effective when administered intranasally. In: Oxford JS, Williams JD (eds) Chemotherapy and control of influenza. Academic, New York, p 77

Came PE, Schafer TW, Silver GH (1976) Sensitivity of rhinoviruses to human leukocyte and fibroblast interferons. J Infect Dis 133 [Suppl]:A136–139

Camner P, Philipson K, Linnman L (1971) A simple method for nuclidic tagging of monodisperse fluorocarbon resin particles. Int J Appl Radiat Isot 22:731–734

Cantell K, Tommila V (1960) Effect of interferon on experimental vaccinia and herpes-simplex virus infections in rabbits eyes. Lancet 2:682–684

Cantell K, Hirvonen S, Mogensen KE, Pyhala I (1974) Human leukocyte interferon: production, purification, stability, and animal experiments. In: Waymouth C (ed) The production and use of interferon for the treatment and prevention of human virus infections. Tissue Culture Association, Rockville, p 35

Cesario TC (1977) The effect of body fluids on polynucleotide-induced fibroblast interferon and virus-induced leukocyte interferon. Proc Soc Exp Biol Med 155:583–587

Cesario TC, Mandell A, Tilles JG (1973) Inactivation of human interferon by body fluids. Proc Soc Exp Biol Med 144:1030–1032

Cogan D, Hirsch E, Kinsey V (1944) Permeability characteristics of the excised cornea. Arch Ophthalmol 31:408

Condon WB (1942) Regeneration of tracheal and bronchial epithelium. J Thorac Surg 11:333–346

Connolly JH, Dick GWA, Field CMB (1962) A fatal case of progressive vaccinia. Br Med J 1:1315–1317

Coster DJ, Falcon MG, Cantell K, Jones BR (1977) Clinical experience of human leucocyte interferon in the management of herpetic keratitis. Trans Ophthalmol Soc UK 97(2):324–326

Creeth JM (1978) Constituents of mucus and their separation. Br Med Bull 34:17–24

DeKoning EWG, van Bijsterveld OP, Cantell K (1982) Combination therapy for dendritic keratitis with human leucocyte interferon and trifluorothymidine. Br J Ophthalmol 66:509–512

De la Pena NC, Diaz A, Damel A, Bal E, Puricelli L, Ejden J, Lusting ES de (1978) Combined therapy of human interferon (HI) and secretory immunoglobulin (S-IgA) in the treatment of human herpetic keratitis. Biomedicine 28:104–108

Dianzani F, Baron S (1977) The continued presence of interferon is not required for activation of cells by interferon. Proc Soc Exp Biol Med 155:562–566

Dion MC, Jafek BW, Tobin CE (1978) The anatomy of the nose. Arch Otolaryngol 104:145–150

Drettner B (1961) Vascular reactions of the human nasal mucosa on exposure to cold. Acta Otolaryngol Suppl (Stockh) 166:1

Ewert G (1965) On the mucus flow rate in the human nose. Acta Otolaryngol Suppl (Stockh) 200:1–60

Ford LC, DeLange RJ, Petty RW (1976) Identification of a nonlysozymal bacterial factor (beta lysin) in human tears and aqueous humor. Am J Ophthalmol 81:30–33

Foster WM, Bergofsky EH, Bohning DE, Lippmann M, Albert RE (1976) Effect of adrenergic agents and their mode of action on mucociliary clearance in man. J Appl Physiol 41:146–152

Friedenwald J, Hughes W, Hermann H (1944) Acid base tolerance of the cornea. Arch Ophthalmol 31:279

Fry FA (1970) Charge distribution on polystyrene aerosols and deposition in the human nose. J Aerosol Sci 1:135–146

Fry FA, Black A (1973) Regional deposition and clearance of particles in the human nose. J Aerosol Sci 4:113–124

Gorham CB, Bacher JA (1930) Regeneration of the human maxillary antral lining. Arch Otolaryngol 11:763–771

Graziadei PPC (1970) Nasal mucous membranes. Ann Otol 79:422–433

Greenberg SB, Harmon MW, Johnson PE, Couch RB (1978) Antiviral activity of intranasally applied human leukocyte interferon. Antimicrob Agents Chemother 14:596–600

Greenberg SB, Harmon MW, Couch RB, Johnson PE, Wilson SZ, Dacso CC, Bloom K, Quarles J (1982) Prophylactic effect of low doses of human leukocyte interferon against infection with rhinovirus. J Infect Dis 145:542–546

Harmon MW, Greenberg SB, Couch RB (1976) Effect of human nasal secretions on the antiviral activity of human fibroblast and leukocyte interferon. Proc Soc Exp Biol Med 152:598–602

Harmon MW, Greenberg SB, Johnson PE, Couch RB (1977) Human nasal epithelial cell culture system: evaluation of response to human interferons. Infect Immunol 16:480–485

Harmon MW, Greenberg SB, Johnson PE (1980) Rapid onset of the interferon-induced antiviral state in human nasal epithelial and foreskin fibroblast cells. Proc Soc Exp Biol Med 164:146–152

Harris J (1960) Transport of fluid from the cornea. In: Duke-Elder S (ed) Transparency of the cornea. Thomas, Springfield, p 73

Hasegawa M, Kern EB (1977) The human nasal cycle. Mayo Clin Proc 52:27–34

Heyder J, Gebhart G, Heigwer CR, Roth C, Stahlhofen W (1973) Experimental studies of the total disposition of aerosol particles in the human respiratory tract. J Aerosol Sci 4:191–208

Hilding A (1931) Ciliary activity and course of secretion currents of the nose. Proc Mayo Clin 6:285–287

Hilding A (1932) the physiology of drainage of nasal mucus. Arch Otolaryngol 15:92–100

Hilding AC (1965) Regeneration of respiratory epithelium after minimal surface trauma. Ann Otol Rhinol Laryngol 74:903–914

Holly FJ, Lemp MA (1977) Tear physiology and dry eyes. Surv Ophthalmol 22:69–87

Hounam RF, Black A, Walsh M (1971) The deposition of aerosol particles in the nasopharyngeal region of the human respiratory tract. In: Walton WH (ed) Inhaled particles III. Unwin, Old Woking Surrey, p 71

Hounam RF (1975) The removal of particles from the nasopharyngeal (NP) compartment of the respiratory tract by nose blowing and swabbing. Health Phys 28:743–745

Ikic D, Petricevic I, Soldo I, Soos E, Smerdel S, Jusic D (1975a) Treatment with human leukocyte interferon. In: Proceedings of the symposium on clinical use of interferon, Yugoslavia Academy of Sciences and Arts, Zagreb, p 183

Ikic D, Cupak K, Trajer D, Soos E, Jusic D, Smerdel S (1975b) Therapy and prevention of epidemic keratoconjunctivitis with human leukocyte interferon. In: Proceedings of the symposium on clinical use of interferon, Yugoslavia Academy of Sciences and Arts, Zagreb, p 189

Ikic D, Smerdel S, Rajninger-Miholic R, Soos E, Jusic D (1975c) Treatment of labial and genital herpes with human leukocytic interferon. In: Proceedings of the symposium on clinical use of interferon, Yugoslavia Academy of Sciences and Arts, Zagreb, p 195

Ikic D, Orescanin M, Krusic J, Cestar Z (1975d) Preliminary study of the effect of human leukocytic interferon on condylomata acuminata in women. In: Proceedings of the symposium on clinical use of interferon, Yougoslav Academy of Sciences and Arts, Zagreb, p 223

Ikic D, Brnobic A, Jurkovic-Vukelic V, Smerdel S, Jusic D, Soos E (1975e) Therapeutical effect of human leukocyte interferon incorporated into ointment and cream on condylomata acuminata. In: Proceedings of the symposium on clinical use of interferon, Yugoslav Academy of Sciences and Arts, Zagreb, p 235

Imanishi J, Karaki T, Sasaki O, Matsuo A, Oishi K, Pak CB, Kishida T, Toda S, Nagata H (1980) The preventive effect of human interferon-alpha preparation on upper respiratory disease. J Interferon Res 1:169–178

Iravani J, Melville GN (1976) Mucociliary function in the respiratory tract by physico-chemical factors. Pharmacol Ther 2:471–492

Isaacs A, Lindenmann J (1957a) Virus interference. I. The interferon. Proc R Soc Lond [Biol] 147:258–267

Isaacs A, Lindenmann J, Valentine RC (1957b) Virus interference. II. Some properties of interferon. Proc R Soc Lond [Biol] 147:268–273

Isaacs A, Westwood MA (1959) Inhibition by interferon of the growth of vaccinia virus in the rabbit skin. Lancet 2:324–325

Ishii T (1970) The cholinergic innervation of the human nasal mucosa. Pract Otorhinolaryngol 32:153–161

Jakus M (1961) The fine structure of the human cornea. In: Smelser G (ed) The structure of the eye. Academy, New York, p 344

Johnson PE, Greenberg SB, Harmon MW, Alford BR, Couch RB (1976) Recovery of applied human leukocyte interferon from the nasal mucosa of chimpanzees and human leukocyte interferon from the nasal mucosa of chimpanzees and humans. J Clin Microbiol 4:106–107

Jones BR, Galbraith JEK, Al-Hussaini MK (1962) Vaccinial keratitis treated with interferon. Lancet I:875–879

Jones BR, Galbraith JEK, Al-Hussaini MK (1976a) Clinical trials of topical interferon therapy of ulcerative viral keratitis. J Infect Dis 133:169–172

Jones BR, Coster DJ, Falcon MG, Cantell K (1976b) Topical therapy of ulcerative herpetic keratitis with human interferon. Lancet II:128

Kaufman HE, Ellison ED, Centifanto YW (1972) Difference in interferon response from ocular virus infection in rabbits and monkeys. Am J Ophthalmol 74:89–92

Kaufmann HE, Meyer RF, Laibson PR, Waltman SR, Nesburn AB, Shuster JJ (1976) Human leukocyte interferon for the prevention of recurrences of herpetic keratitis. J Infect Dis 133:165–168

Knowlton CD, McGregor GW (1928) How and when the mucous membrane of the maxillary sinus regenerates. Arch Otolaryngol 8:647–656

Kobza K, Emodi G, Just M, Hilti E, Leuenberger A, Binswanger U, Thiel G, Brunner FP (1975) Treatment of herpes infection with human exogenous interferon. Lancet I:1343–1344

Krasikova VA, Poddubnaia AE, Ritova VV, Schastny'i EI, Kuznetsov VP (1977) Interferongenesis and efficacy of refined leukocytic interferon use in acute respiratory viral infections in premature children. Pediatriia 5:42–48

Krogh A, Lund CC, Pedersen-Bjergaard K (1945) The osmotic concentration of human lacrimal fluid. Acta Physiol Scand 10:88–92

Landahl HD (1950) On the removal of air-borne droplets by the human respiratory tract: II. The nasal passages. Bull Math Biophys 12:161–169

Larson EW, Young HW, Walker JS (1976) Aerosol evaluations of the deVilbiss No. 40 and vaponefrin nebulizers. Appl Environ Microbiol 31:150–151

La Tessa A, Teng C, Katrzin H (1954) The histo-chemistry of the basement membrane of the cornea. Am J Ophthalmol 58:171

Levenson JE (1973) The effect of short term drying on the surface ultrastructure of the rabbit cornea: a scanning electron microscopic study. Ann Ophthalmol 5:865

Lindenmann J, Burke DC, Isaacs A (1957) Studies on the production, mode of action and properties of interferon. Br J Exp Path 38:551–562

Lippmann M (1970) Deposition and clearance of inhaled particles in the human nose. Ann Otol Rhinol Laryngol 79:519–529

Lucas AM, Douglas LC (1933) Direction of flow of nasal mucus. Proc Soc Exp Med Biol 31:320–321

Lucas AM, Douglas LC (1934) Principles underlying ciliary activity in the respiratory tract. II. A comparison of nasal clearance in man, monkey and other mammals. Arch Otolaryngol 20:518–541

Maurice D (1957) The structure and transparency of the cornea. J Physiol 136:263–270

McGill JI, Cantell K, Collins P, Finter NB, Laird R, Jones BR (1977) Optimal usage of exogenous human interferon for prevention or therapy of herpetic keratitis. Trans Ophthalmol Soc UK 97(2):324–326
Melville KI (1973) Antihistamine drugs. In: Schachter M (ed) Histamine and antihistamines. Pergamon, Elmsford, p 127 (International encyclopedia of pharmacology and therapeutics, vol 1)
Merigan TC, Hall TS, Reed SE, Tyrrell DAJ (1973) Inhibition of respiratory virus infection by locally applied interferon. Lancet I:563–567
Milder B (1981) The lacrimal apparatus. In: Moses RA (ed) Adler's physiology of the eye. Mosby, St. Louis, p 16
Mishima S, Gasset A, Klyce SD Jr, Baum JL (1966) Determination of tear volume and tear flow. Invest Ophthalmol 5:265–276
Naessen R (1970) The anatomy of drainage of nasal secretions. Acta Otolaryngol 84:326–329
Negus VE (1958) The comparative anatomy and physiology of the nose and paranasal sinuses. Livingstone, Edinburgh
Neumann-Haefelin D, Sundmacher R, Skoda R, Cantell K (1977) Comparative evaluation of human leukocyte and fibroblast interferon in the prevention of herpes simplex virus keratitis in a monkey model. Infect Immunol 17(2):468–470
Pallin O, Lundmark K, Brege KG (1976) Interferon in severe herpes simplex of cornea. Lancet II:1187–1188
Parke DV (1978) Pharmacology of mucus. Br Med Bull 34:89–94
Patterson A, Fox AD, Davies G, MaGurie CH, Sellors PJ, Wright P, Rice NSC, Cobb B, Jones Br (1963) Controlled studies of IDU in the treatment of herpetic keratitis. Ophthalmol Soc UK 83:583–591
Pattle RE (1961) retention of gases and particles in the human nose. In: Davies CN (ed) Inhaled particles and vapours. Pergamon, Oxford, p 302
Potts AM (1953) The nutritional supply of corneal regions in experimental animals II. Am J Ophthalmol 36:127–133
Proctor DF, Andersen I, Lundqvist G (1973) Clearance of inhaled particles from the human nose. Arch Intern Med 131:132–139
Proctor DF, Andersen, Lundqvist G (1977) Nasal Mucociliary Function in Humans. In: Brain JD, Proctor DF, Reid LM (eds) Respiratory defense mechanisms, vol 5. Dekker, New York, p 427
Proetz AW (1953) Essays on the applied physiology of the nose. St. Louis Annals Publishing, St. Louis
Quinlan M, Salman S, Swift DL, Wagner Jr HN, Proctor DF (1969) Measurement of mucociliary function in man. Am Rev Respir Dis 99:3–23
Reznik VI, Shangina DA, Zdanovskaia NI (1978) Trial preventive use of leukocyte interferon in foci of acute respiratory diseases. Vopr Virusol 6:732–734
Romano A, Revel M, Guarari-Rotman D, Blumenthal M, Stein R (1980) Use of human fibroblast-derived (beta) interferon in the treatment of epidemic adenovirus keratoconjunctivitis. J Interferon Res 1:169–178
Rossman TG, Vilcek J (1970) Blocking of interferon action by a component of normal serum. Arch Ges Virusforsch 31:18–23
Sadunaisky JA, Spinowitz B (1976) Drugs affecting the transport and permeability of the corneal epithelium. In: Dikstein S (ed) Drugs and ocular tissues. Karger, Basel, p 57
Saketkhoo K, Yergin BM, Januszkiewicz A, Kovitz K, Sackner MA (1978) The effect of nasal decongestants on nasal mucous velocity. Am Rev Resp Dis 118:251–254
Schastny'i EI, Ritova VV, Krasnikova VA, Feklisova LV, Ulanovskaia TI (1978) Rational approach to the use of exogenous interferon for prevention of respiratory tract infections among children in medical institutions. Vopr Okhr Materin Det 23(1):87–88
Schirmer O (1903) Studien zur Physiologie und Pathologie der Tränenabsonderung und Tränenabfuhr. Albrecht Von Graefes Arch Ophthalmol 56:197–203
Schoenwald R, Ward R (1978) Relationship between steroid permeability across excised rabbit cornea and octanol-water partition coefficients. J Pharm Sci 67:786–791
Schultz EW (1960) Repair of the olfactory mucosa. Am J Pathol 37:1–19

Schuster JJ, Kaufman HE, Nesburn AB (1981) Statistical analysis of recurrence of herpes virus ocular epithelial disease. Am J Ophthalmol 91:328–329
Scientific Committee on Interferon (1962) Effect of interferon on vaccination in volunteers. Lancet I:873–875
Scientific Committee on Interferon (1965) Experiments with interferon in man. Lancet I:505–506
Scott GM, Csonka GW (1979) Effect of injections of small doses of human fibroblast interferon into genital warts. A pilot study. Br J Vener Dis 55(6):442–445
Scott GM, Cartwright T, LeDu G, Dicker D (1978) Effect of human fibroblast interferon on vaccination in volunteers. J Biol Stand 6:73–76
Scott GM, Reed S, Cartwright T, Tyrrell D (1980) Failure of human fibroblast interferon to protect against rhinovirus infection. Arch Virol 65(2):135–139
Solov'ev VD (1967) Some results and prospects in the study of endogenous and exogenous interferon. In: G Rita (ed) The interferons. Academic, New York, p 233
Solov'ev VD (1969) The results of controlled observations on the prophylaxis of influenza with interferon. Bull WHO 41:683–688
Soos E, Ikic D, Jusic D, Smerdel S, Petricevic I, Kunsten D, Soldo I (1972) Treatment of local complications provoked by vaccinia virus with leukocytic interferon. Proc symp on combined vaccines, Yugoslavia Academy Sciences and Arts, Zagreb, pp 179–182
Stocksted P (1952) The physiologic cycle of the nose under normal and pathologic conditions. Acta Otolaryngol (Stockh) 42:175–181
Sugar J, Kaufman HE, Varnell ED (1973) Effect of exogenous interferon on herpetic keratitis in rabbits and monkeys. Invest Ophthalmol 12:378–379
Sundmacher R, Neumann-Haefelin D, Manthey KF, Muller O (1976a) Interferon in treatment of dendritic keratitis in humans: a preliminary report. J Infect Dis 133:160–164
Sundmacher R, Neumann-Haeflin D, Cantell K (1976b) Successful treatment of dendritic keratitis with human leukocyte interferon. Albrecht Von Graefes Arch Klin Exp Ophthalmol 201:39–45
Sundmacher R, Neumann-Haefelin D, Manthey KF (1977) Human-interferon therapy in dendritic keratitis. Ber Zusammenkunft Dtsch Ophthalmol Ges 74:615–618
Sundmacher R, Cantell K, Haug P, Neumann-Haefelin D (1978a) Role of debridement and interferon in the treatment of dendritic keratitis. Albrecht Von Graefes Arch Klin Exp Ophthalmol 207:77–82
Sundmacher R, Cantell K, Skoda R, Hallermann C, Neumann-Haefelin D (1978b) Human leukocyte and fibroblast interferon in a combination therapy of dendritic keratitis. Albrecht Von Graefes Arch Klin Exp Ophthalmol 208:229–233
Sundmacher R, Cantell K, Haug P, Neumann-Haefelin D (1978c) Interferon prophylaxis of dendritic keratitis recurrence during local steroid therapy. Ber Zusammenkunft Dtsch Ophthalmol Ges 75:344–346
Sundmacher R, Cantell K, Neumann-Haefelin D (1981) Evaluation of interferon in ocular viral diseases. In: Schellekens H, Maeyer E de, Galasso G (eds) The biology of the interferon system. Interferon meeting, 21–24 April 1981. Elsevier/North Holland, Amsterdam
Swan K, White N (1942) Corneal permeability: factors affecting penetration of drugs into the cornea. Am J Ophthalmol 25:1043
Taylor M (1974) The origin and functions of nasal mucus. Laryngoscope 84:612–621
Tommila V (1963) Treatment of dendritic keratitis with interferon. Acta Ophthalmol 41:478–482
Tyrrell DAJ, Reed SE (1973) Some possible practical implications of interferon and interference. In: Brown W, Unger J (eds) Non-specific factors influencing host resistance. Karger, Basel, p 438
Waltman SR (1981) The cornea. In: Moses RA (ed) Adler's physiology of the eye. Mosby, St. Louis, p 38
Wanner A (1977) Clinical aspects of mucociliary transport. Am Rev Resp Dis 116:73–125
Widdicombe JG (1978) Control of secretion of tracheobronchial mucus. Br Med Bul 34:57–61
Yunde H, Guoliang M, Shuhua W, Yuying L, Hantang L (1981) Effect of radix astragali seu hedysari on the interferon system. Chinese Med J 94:35–40

CHAPTER 22

Clinical Use of Interferons: Systemic Administration in Viral Diseases

J. A. ARMSTRONG

A. Introduction

Systemic application of interferon to viral infections in humans was most recently reviewed by BILLIAU and DE SOMER (1980) and up-to-date accounts of ongoing activities in this area have been provided by DUNNICK and GALASSO (1979, 1980). Early clinical trials of interferon were discouraging. For instance, a double-blind controlled trial of monkey interferon against common cold virus infections in volunteers showed no evidence of antiviral effect (SCIENTIFIC COMMITTEE ON INTERFERON 1965). However, the doses of interferon used, approximately 10^4 U per patient, have since been shown to be quite insufficient. A new era in application of interferon began with the development of methods to produce human leukocyte interferon on a large scale. CANTELL (1977) pioneered these efforts and much of the leukocyte interferon used in the clinical trials to be discussed here was produced in Helsinki under his direction.

In most acute virus infections the interferon-sensitive step, that is, virus replication, is of relatively short duration and is rapidly terminated by the specific immune response. Such infections would seem to require the prophylactic use of interferon for best effect. However there exists a number of viral infections which can be characterized as persistent, chronic, or recurrent and in which the phase of virus replication is accessible to chemotherapy. It is such infections that have been the target of many of the more recent clinical trials. Prominent among these are infections caused by the five human herpesviruses. These viruses include herpes simplex virus type 1, (HSV-1) characteristic of cold sores and other herpes occurring above the waist, herpes simplex virus type 2, (HSV-2) usually involved in genital infections, cytomegalovirus (CMV), the varicella zoster virus (VZV), and the Epstein–Barr virus (EBV), the most frequent cause of infectious mononucleosis. Other targets of recent trials have included hepatitis B, papillomata, presumably due to papovavirus infection and various virus infections, particularly those occurring in the immunocompromised patient.

B. Herpesviruses

I. Herpes Simplex Viruses

Although the sensitivity of HSV to interferon is still under active investigation, there is sufficient data in the literature (RASMUSSEN and FARLEY 1975; LAZAR et al. 1980; IMANISHI et al. 1980) to suggest that sensitivity is adequate to justify clinical trials. Many of these trials have been directed at herpes keratitis, and are discussed elsewhere in this volume, but studies directed against herpes simplex infections in other sites have also been undertaken. Two of these have been generally directed at infections in renal transplant recipients. Such patients, immunosuppressed for graft survival, are subject to numerous virus infections, particularly those due to the herpesviruses which may be latent in the patient at the time of transplantation. WEIMAR et al. (1978) reported that human fibroblast interferon (IFN-β) was administered to 8 of 16 patients in a double-blind study. The patients received 3×10^6 U intramuscularly twice weekly for 3 months starting 1–2 h prior to transplantation. They were followed clinically and serologically for evidence of virus infections, including those due to HSV. Although four of eight patients receiving placebo had evidence of infections and only one patient receiving interferon was infected during the study period, the small numbers of patients involved preclude any conclusions. This is one of the few studies in which fibroblast interferon was used. No side effects were seen, but although no interferon levels were measured, experience of others suggests that serum interferon would not have been detectable.

In a study reported by CHEESEMAN et al. (1979), 41 renal transplant recipients were followed for a minimum of 8 months or until death or retransplantation, with a median follow-up time of 17 months. Some 21 patients received interferon in a double-blind study design; 30 patients had antibody to herpes simplex virus before transplantation and 19 developed a serologic response during the study period while 24 excreted HSV in throat washings. About one-half of the seropositive patients developed lesions. Interferon treatment had no apparent effect on any of these parameters. The patients in this study received 3×10^6 U leukocyte interferon for 15 doses given twice weekly starting at the time of transplantation. Both of the studies probably involved only reactivated herpes infection. CHEESEMAN et al. (1979) observed infection only in patients with herpes antibody at the time of transplantation. WEIMAR et al. (1978), on the other hand, do not report antibody studies.

A more predictable model of reactivated HSV infection was utilized by PAZIN et al. (1979). It had been observed that patients undergoing microneurosurgical decompression of the trigeminal sensory root for the treatment of trigeminal neuralgia had a high frequency of reactivated herpes infection a few days following surgery (PAZIN et al. 1978). Of those patients with a positive history of cold sores, 60% reactivated. Although the disease was not generally severe, the model is exceptionally advantageous for the study of prophylactic or therapeutic antiviral agents. The time of stimulus to reactivation, that is, the surgery, is precisely known and the onset of disease, which may be characterized by viral shedding in the oropharynx as well as lesions on the face, occurs 1–4 days after the stimulus. Patients received interferon or placebo according to a randomization schedule and the study was double-blind. Human leukocyte interferon, 7×10^4 Ukg^{-1} day^{-1}, was administered in divided intramuscular doses in the morning and evening for 5 days, beginning on the day before operation. Patients were interviewed and examined daily for cutaneous or intraoral herpetic lesions and viral throat wash cultures were obtained daily after the operation for 6–8 days. In order to maximize the proportion of patients expected to have disease, only those with positive histories of herpes labialis were enrolled.

PAZIN et al. (1979) report that 9 of 19 patients receiving interferon and 15 of 18 patients receiving placebo reactivated during the study period as manifested by herpetic lesions or virus in the throat wash. Since this reduction in proportion was shown to be statistically significant, this phase of the study was terminated. The most significant effect of interferon was reduction in frequency and duration of virus shedding in the oropharynx. Whereas 42% of 127 cultures from placebo-treated patients were positive for HSV, only 9% of 134 were positive in the interferon-treated group. Interferon treatment commenced 1 day prior to the reactivating stimulus of surgery and was continued for 5 days; this trial should be considered, at least in part, prophylactic. In order to discover in which stage of the reactivation process interferon is effective the trial is being continued and preliminary results indicate that interferon given before surgery is ineffective (M. HO, G.J. PAZIN and J.A. ARMSTRONG 1983, unpublished work). The same group of investigators have initiated a double-blind study of the effect of interferon on genital herpes infection in women. Subjects are enrolled within 72 h of the initial episode of genital herpes and receive 10 doses of approximately 3×10^6 U human leukocyte interferon over 14 days. It is hoped that the establishment of latent recurrent genital herpes infection as well as the course of primary disease may be modified by this protocol.

II. Cytomegalovirus

Although CMV is more resistant to interferon than other viruses (GLASGOW et al. 1967), the chronic or recurrent nature of the infection has prompted several investigators to initiate clinical trials. ARVIN et al. (1976) treated 5 patients with neonatal CMV infection using IFN-α, 1.7–3.5×10^5 Ukg^{-1}, intramuscularly for 7–14 days. Transient suppression of viruria was observed in one infant. EMÖDI et al. (1976) report that they suppressed viruria in three of four infants with congenital CMV infection and in two of five with acquired infections by administering leukocyte interferon (5×10^5–10^6 Uday^{-1}). WEIMAR et al. (1978, 1979b) and CHEESEMAN et al. (1979) as already mentioned, conducted double-blind trials of interferon in renal transplant recipients. These studies were particularly focused on CMV infection which occurs with high frequency in this group. WEIMAR et al. (1978, 1979b) detected CMV infection in four of eight patients, in both the interferon-treated and placebo-treated groups. They showed no ameliorating effect. On the other hand, CHEESEMAN et al. (1979) report that human leukocyte interferon, 3×10^6 U intramuscularly twice weekly for 15 doses gave some evidence of efficacy. Virus excretion was not prevented, but it was delayed in onset from 4.2 weeks after surgery in controls to 7.2 weeks in the treated group. O'Reilly et al. (1976) treated 2 patients who developed CMV infection following allogeneic bone marrow transplantation. In one patient, the authors believed that significant clinical improvement accompanied by a disappearance of viremia may have been associated with the interferon treatment. MEYERS et al. (1980) treated eight patients after bone marrow transplantation. All patients had biopsy-proven CMV pneumonia and received 2–5 doses of 2×10^4–6.4×10^5 U kg^{-1} day^{-1} leukocyte interferon. There was no evidence of therapeutic efficacy. Overall, trials of interferon on CMV infections in humans have not been encouraging to date.

III. Varicella Zoster Virus

Although normally self limiting, infections with VZV, like those caused by CMV are of special importance in the immunocompromised host. EMÖDI et al. (1975 b) administered human leukocyte interferon in daily doses of 10^6 U for 5–8 days to 37 patients with herpes zoster. This was not a randomized double-blind study, but after the first ten patients, every third received placebo material. It is the impression of EMÖDI et al. that the duration of pain was shortened and the development of crust formation was enhanced by interferon treatment.

A double-blind study of human leukocyte interferon in the treatment of herpes zoster in cancer patients was undertaken by MERIGAN et al. (1978). The study was carried out in three phases. The first 30 patients were randomized into a placebo group and a group receiving a relatively unpurified human leukocyte preparation at a rate of 4.2×10^4 U kg^{-1} day^{-1} for 8 days or until no new lesions appeared. The second 30 patients were randomized similarly into placebo and treated groups, but the interferon was used was more purified and could be given at 1.7×10^5 Ukg^{-1} day^{-1}. In the third phase of the study, the purified interferon preparation was used at 5.5×10^5 Ukg^{-1} day^{-1} in a double-blind manner as described. Thus, a total of 45 patients received interferon at three dose levels and 45 patients received placebo material. Lymphoma was the most common underlying disease in all three groups of patients. The highest dose of interferon significantly slowed the progression of zoster in the primary dermatome involved and decreased the number of days of new vesicle formation. Pain and the severity of postherpetic neuralgia were also diminished at the two highest dosage levels. Visceral complications occurred in 6 placebo-treated patients and only one interferon-treated patient. Herpes zoster is due to reactivation of previously acquired VZV infection. Primary varicella, a benign disease in the healthy child, may occur in the immunosuppressed host where it can be associated with visceral dissemination and death. With this in mind, ARVIN et al. (1978) treated 18 patients, who developed varicella while under chemotherapy for malignancy, with human leukocyte interferon in a randomized double-blind, placebo-controlled trial. Patients were enrolled within 48 h of the appearance of the exanthem and were given human leukocyte interferon, 4.2×10^4 Ukg^{-1}, every 12 h until no progression of infection had been observed for 24 h. The mean duration of therapy was 6.4 days. Four patients received a further purified preparation at 2.55×10^5 Ukg^{-1}. Complications of varicella occurred in six of nine placebo-treated patients but in only two of nine interferon recipients. The duration of the period of new vesicle formation was not significantly reduced. Although iododeoxyuridine or cytosine arabinoside was also administered to some of the patients, these drugs were not given until visceral involvement was seen and have not affected the parameters used to assess interferon response. Thus interferon, in well-tolerated doses, has shown modest effect against VZV infections.

IV. Epstein–Barr Virus

CHEESEMAN et al. (1980 b) report the results of a placebo-controlled trial of human leukocyte interferon on EBV excretion and antibody in 41 renal transplant recipients. Of these, 23 received antithymocyte serum which increased the frequency of oropharyngeal shedding. In this subgroup, interferon appeared to reduce the proportion of patients in which shedding was observed; 10 of 12 interferon-treated patients and 5 of 11 placebo-treated patients were observed to shed EBV in the oropharynx. When antithymocyte serum was not given, the overall rate of excretion of virus was only 33% and was not altered by interferon treatment. The 21 patients received 3×10^6 U interferon intramuscularly twice a week, beginning just before renal transplantation and continuing for a total of 15 doses; 20 patients received placebo. Interferon had no apparent effect on changes in EBV-specific antibody titers. All patients were seropositive for this virus on entry into the study. Therefore, no effect on primary disease could be investigated.

V. Summary of Herpesvirus Infections

Clinical trials have been carried out or are in progress in patients with infections caused by all five human herpesviruses. No significant effect has been seen with fibroblast interferon administered systemically, but leukocyte interferon has been shown to ameliorate infections caused by EBV, CMV, VZV, and HSV-1. In most cases, the effects have been modest. No evidence has been given to show that latent virus infections can be eradicated. Perhaps the most striking effect was seen in herpes labialis following neurosurgery (PAZIN et al. 1979), where a marked reduction in frequency of reactivation and particularly in oropharyngeal virus excretion was described.

C. Hepatitis B Virus Infection

Chronic active hepatitis due to hepatitis B virus is an unusual example of a disease in which virus replication is prolonged. It should therefore represent an appropriate target for interferon therapy. On the other hand, the lack of a cell culture system for the cultivation of this agent has precluded definite knowledge concerning sensitivity to interferon, although experiments in chimpanzees with an interferon inducer have suggested that it is quite susceptible (PURCELL et al. 1976). GREENBERG et al. (1976) treated four chronic active hepatitis patients with leukocyte interferon at doses between 6×10^3 and 17×10^4 U kg^{-1} day^{-1}. Three of the patients had circulating Dane particle markers. The Dane particle is believed to be the virion and the markers include DNA polymerase activity, HB_cAg and Dane particle-associated DNA. The HB_eAg, usually detected as a soluble antigen as well as the HB_sAg may also be part of the Dane particle, but they are predominantly found circulating independently. The Dane particle markers fell in response to interferon treatment, but after short courses of up to 10 days, rapidly returned to pretreatment levels. However there was evidence that prolonged treatment for at least 1 month resulted in prolonged depression of the markers. Circulating HB_sAg was more resistant to interferon. Long-term treatment resulted in a slight reduction in circulating antigen in one patient, a striking reduction in one other, and no change in two patients. No significant changes in liver function were observed. WEIMAR et al. (1980) administered IFN-α to 8 of 16 chronic active hepatitis patients enrolled in a double-blind, placebo-controlled study. They received 12×10^6 U daily for 1 week. The dose was then halved weekly until discontinuation after week 6 in order to find the optimal dose for long-term therapy. HB_cAg-specific DNA polymerase activity fell during the first 2 days of therapy in six of eight patients. No further changes were observed in DNA polymerase and no significant changes were seen in serum levels of HB_sAg or HB_eAg. Frequency of HB_cAg-positive liver cell nuclei was not decreased. It is noteworthy that one patient receiving placebo became negative for DNA polymerase during treatment. The authors concluded that IFN-α, as presently administered, was not clinically useful in HBV-induced chronic active hepatitis.

There have also been a number of pilot studies with fibroblast interferon (IFN-β). Desmyter et al. (1976) gave IFN-β to a single patient with chronic active hepatitis. A treatment course consisted of seven doses of 10^7 U injected intramuscularly every alternate day. No changes in circulating antigens were demonstrated, but a reduction in the frequency of HB_sAg and HB_cAg in liver hepatocytes was demonstrated by fluorescent antibody staining of biopsy specimens. Weimar et al. (1977), using IFN-β from the same source (Billiau et al. 1979b), treated five patients and observed an equal number of controls concurrently. No placebo was administered. Although DNA polymerase activity, HB_eAg, HB_sAg, and liver enzymes were followed, no effect was observed on any indicators of virus activity in the interferon-treated patients, although one control patient showed a striking decline in DNA polymerase activity. Dolan et al. (1979) reported on a single patient with chronic hepatitis. Interferon treatment, 10^6 $Uday^{-1}$ intramuscularla for 82 days was said to result in a decrease of HB_sAg and disappearance of the Dane particle markers. Iwarson et al. (1980) report similar results in a patient receiving 3×10^6 $Uday^{-1}$ for 10 days. Kingham et al. (1977) report two patients treated with IFN-β, 10^7 U daily for 2 weeks. Although no detectable effect on antigenemia was noted, anti-HB_cAg antibodies and DNA-binding antibodies declined during the treatment. The significance of this observation is obscure. It may perhaps be accounted for by the immunomodulatory activities of interferon which Carter et al. (1980) have suggested may be important for the putative effect of interferon in hepatitis infection. Billiau et al. (1979b) have summarized data on nine patients with chronic active hepatitis who were treated with fibroblast and in some cases leukocyte interferons. These may include patients already mentioned (Weimar et al. 1976; Desmyter et al. 1976). Reduction in circulating DNA polymerase, transaminases, and a decline in HB_cAg in hepatocytes was observed in seven of the patients. In addition, six patients with acute or fulminating hepatitis were treated. No effects could be documented. Weimar et al. (1979a) compared the effect of IFN-β with that of IFN-α in six patients treated sequentially with these materials. Fibroblast interferon induced a fall in serum transaminase activities in all patients, whereas IFN-α caused a decline in HBV-specific serum DNA polymerase activity. The investigators suggested that IFN-α and IFN-β may differ fundamentally in their mode of action against HBV.

In summary, one may say that studies on the chemotherapy of chronic active hepatitis with interferon are encouraging, but unsatisfactory. In only two studies (Weimar et al. 1977, 1980) was any effort made to provide satisfactory controls. In these trials, no clinically significant favorable outcome was reported. There is no doubt that conduct of a satisfactory clinical trial in a disease where parameters of infection fluctuate over time is going to be extremely difficult. The difficulty is compounded where the disease is so uncommon that any one center usually has only a few cases available.

D. Other Virus Infections

When CHEESEMAN and her colleagues followed renal transplant recipients receiving human leukocyte interferon (Sect. B; CHEESEMAN et al. 1979, 1980 b), they also examined parameters of BK papovavirus infection (CHEESEMAN et al. 1980 a). In a randomized double-blind study, 21 patients received 3×10^6 U interferon intramuscularly twice a week, beginning just before renal transplantation and continued for 15 doses. A group of 20 patients received placebo; 4 interferon-treated and 4 placebo-treated patients underwent seroconversion and 3 patients, all in the interferon group, excreted BK virus in the urine. The authors conclude that no significant effect could be demonstrated. In vitro experiments showed that significant inhibition of BK virus by interferon could only be demonstrated when the interferon was continuously present in the culture medium.

INGIMARSSON et al. (1980) have taken the opportunity to study acute infections in patients receiving leukocyte interferon for the adjuvant therapy of osteosarcoma. Clearly, not all such infections would be viral in origin, but most of the symptoms such as coryza, cough, fever, and sore throat, on which the study is based are compatible with viral disease. The patients received daily intramuscular injections of 3×10^6 U interferon for 1 month and the same dose was given thrice weekly for the next 17 months. Two control groups were used; 19 age-matched controls and a gross control group of 54 relatives from the same households as the patients. Both frequency and duration of infections and symptoms were statistically significantly less in the interferon-treated group.

Chronic persistent infections such as subacute sclerosing panencephalitis (SSPE) and congenital rubella syndrome have been treated with systemic interferon in a small number of patients. BEHAN (1981) reports on three patients with SSPE who were given daily injections with 3×10^6 U interferon intramuscularly. Two children received 25 and 90 injections. The third patient received 20 injections as well as an additional 12×10^6 U intrathecally over 3 days. Unfortunately, no benefits were seen. Congential rubella syndrome was treated with interferon by LARSSON et al. (1976). The patients received 3×10^6 U interferon daily for 2 weeks and during this period there was a regression of cutaneous symptoms which continued to complete healing within 2 months. Viremia disappeared, but excretion of rubella virus in the urine continued and serum antirubella IgM was present throughout as an indication of the persistent viral infection.

Seven cases of juvenile laryngeal papillomatosis, a condition associated with a papovavirus, have been treated with IFN-α (HAGLUND et al. 1981). The regimen, three weekly doses of 3×10^6 U, was reduced to 1–2 doses per week in 3 patients. Treatment was intermittent, lasting from 2 to more than 3 years. On most occasions the papillomata regressed during treatment although concomitant surgery was often required. Frequently the disease recurred after cessation of interferon administration, but again regressed when treatment was reinstituted. The authors conclude that IFN-α can favorably affect the clinical course of the disease.

Many of the trials described are simply case reports. Therefore the recent controlled trials of systemic therapy or prophylaxis are summarized in Table 1. Only three controlled trials of IFN-β (fibroblast origin interferon) have been identified. No favorable effect was seen and we may have to conclude that this interferon will not be useful if administered systemically, perhaps because of its rapid clearance

Table 1. Recent controlled trials of systemic interferon therapy/prophylaxis

Patient group (number)[a]	Study design (Interferon used)[b]	Virus involved	Result	References
Renal transplant recipients (21 IFN + 20 P = 41)	Double-blind with placebo (IFN-α)	CMV HSV EBV BKV	Favorable No effect Favorable No effect	Cheeseman et al. (1979) Cheeseman et al. (1979) Cheeseman et al. (1980 a) Cheeseman et al. (1980 b)
Renal transplant recipients (9 IFN + 9 P = 18)	Double-blind with placebo (IFN-β)	Various: CMV, HSV, VZV, influenza, rubella, RSV[c], etc.	No effect	Weimar et al. (1978) Weimar et al. (1979 b)
Neurosurgery for tic douloureux (19 IFN + 18 P = 37)	Double-blind with placebo (IFN-α)	HSV	Favorable	Pazin et al. (1979)
Varicella in children with cancer (9 IFN + 9 P = 18)	Double-blind with placebo (IFN-α)	VZV	Inconclusive	Arvin et al. (1978)
Zoster in cancer patients (45 IFN + 45 P = 90)	Double-blind with placebo (IFN-α)	VZV	Favorable with high dose	Merigan et al. (1978)
Zoster in adults (29 IFN + 9 P = 38)	Placebo-controlled (IFN-α)	VZV	Favorable	Emödi et al. (1975 b)
Chronic active hepatitis (5 IFN + 5 C = 10)	Concurrent controls (IFN-β)	Hepatitis virus B	No effect	Weimar et al. (1977)
Osteosarcoma patients (19 IFN + 73 C = 92)	Concurrent matched and gross controls (IFN-α)	Acute infections	Favorable	Ingimarsson et al. (1980)
Chronic active hepatitis (8 IFN + 8 P = 16)	Double-blind with placebo (IFN-β)	Hepatitis virus B	Reduced DNAP[d] activity	Weimar et al. (1980)

[a] IFN patients receiving interferon; P patients receiving placebo; C other controls. The last number is total patients enrolled
[b] IFN-α human leukocyte interferon; IFN-β human fibroblast interferon
[c] RSV respiratory syncytial virus
[d] DNAP DNA polymerase

from the vascular space as discussed in Sect. E.I. However, IFN-α, of leucocyte origin, has been shown to be effective in controlled trials against four herpesviruses: CMV, EBV, HSV, and VZV, although in no case was the effect truly dramatic.

To round out our view of the antiviral spectrum of interferon, it is worth briefly mentioning some significant trials of locally applied interferon. In perhaps the first trial in which realistically high doses of interferon were given, MERIGAN et al. (1973) reported that 1 day of prophylaxis and 3 days of treatment resulted in statistically significant prevention of clinical symptoms of viral shedding in volunteers challenged with rhinovirus type 4. A single prophylactic dose of intranasal interferon only slightly delayed the onset of influenza B infection, which is of interest since SOLOV'EV (1969) had previously reported that small doses of interferon (about 256 U) would, if administered repeatedly, have significant prophylactic effect on influenza infection. Even smaller intranasal doses, given repeatedly, (about 32 U) were reported to be effective in aborting outbreaks of respiratory disease in a study of 774 children in 24 institutions (REZNIK et al. 1978). IKIC et al. (1975f) treated 39 influenza patients by inhalation of 10^4 U leukocyte interferon and reported significant prophylaxis when these patients were compared with 64 untreated controls. Local treatment with IFN-α has also been claimed to prevent and aid healing of epidemic keratoconjunctivitis due to adenovirus (IKIC et al. 1975c). Local leukocyte interferon has also been used for the treatment of complications due to smallpox vaccination (IKIC et al. 1975e) and condyloma acuminata presumably due to a papovavirus (IKIC et al. 1975a, b, d).

In contrast to the favorable results found with IFN-α in treatment of experimental rhinovirus infection, it has recently been reported by SCOTT et al. (1980) that fibroblast interferon (IFN-β) was inactive under essentially the same conditions. A group of 15 patients treated with interferon received 10^7 U/day intranasally, divided into three doses, 9 a.m., 2 p.m., and 7 p.m., for 5 days, beginning the day prior to challenge; 14 patients received placebo. No effect on clinical course or virus titers in nasal washings was observed.

Fibroblast interferon has also been used locally by SCOTT and CSONKA (1979) in the treatment of genital warts. Small doses of IFN-β (300 U) or placebo were injected into matched warts in each of 11 patients. Analysis of changes in size suggested that growth of the warts was inhibited by interferon. Recently, HO et al. (1981) and PAZIN et al. (1981) showed regression (decrease in size) of warts by intralesional injection of IFN-α. Some warts regressed entirely after treatment. The effect was shown to be dose responsive in a double-blind experiment in which a series of matched warts in a single patient were injected with placebo or graded doses of IFN-α. The lowest dose at which regression was shown was 1.2×10^6 U injected over 15.5 weeks. Intramuscular administration of IFN-α had little effect on size of the warts.

E. Pharmacokinetics and Toxicology of Systemically Administered Interferon

These topics have been recently reviewed by MERIGAN (1977) and GREENBERG et al. (1980).

Table 2. Serum interferon levels after intramuscular injection of leukocyte interferon (IFN-α)

Dose	Time after injection (h)	Serum level[a] (U/ml)	References
7–10 × 10^4 U/kg	3–9	40–60	CANTELL et al. (1974)
	20	< 20–20	
3 × 10^6 U/48 h	4–12	17–200	CHEESEMAN et al. (1979)
	18–24	15–20	
	> 24	None	
3.5 × 10^4 U/kg/12 h	1	32	PAZIN et al. (1979)
	12–24[b]	16–32	
	48	8 (= background level)	
4 × 10^4 U/kg/24 h	4	< 30	MEYERS et al. (1980)
8 × 10^4 U/kg/24 h	4	103	
1.6 × 10^5 U/kg/24 h	4	184	
3.2 × 10^5 U/kg/24 h	4	257	
6.4 × 10^5 U/kg/24 h	4	768	
8.5 × 10^4 U/kg/12 h	2–6	22	ARVIN et al. (1976)
9 × 10^4 U/kg/12 h	2–6	50	
1.75 × 10^5 U/kg/12 h	2–6	303	
10^6 U/24 h	0.5	10–50	EMÖDI et al. (1975a)
	2	10–100+	
	6	10–100+	
		< 10–10	
4.2 × 10^4 U/kg/day	4.6	52	MERIGAN et al. (1978)
1.7 × 10^5 U/kg/day	4.6	238	
5.1 × 10^5 U/kg/day	4.6	455	

[a] Mean or range
[b] After 5 days treatment

I. Pharmacokinetics

Much of our knowledge of the pharmacokinetics of interferon has come from studies carried out in conjunction with antiviral or antitumor trials (CANTELL et al. 1974; JORDAN et al. 1974; EMÖDI et al. 1975a, b; MERIGAN 1977). From these studies it appears that there are three definable kinetic phases after intravenous injection of leukocyte interferon. The initial phase, lasting about 1 h, is characterized by a half-life of about 15 min. There is a second clearance phase with a half-life of 2–4 h and a third phase characterized by a 24–48 h half-life. Peak serum titers of 800 U/ml were observed after the intravenous infusion of 60 × 10^6 U over 5 h (EMÖDI et al. 1975a).

Some representative examples of serum interferon levels obtained after intramuscular injection of IFN-α are shown in Table 2. At commonly used doses, interferon titers of less than 100 U/ml are generally seen in the serum. They are well maintained and with very large doses, high concentrations may be achieved. For instance, JORDAN et al. (1974) administered three doses of 80×10^6 U intramuscularly at 24-h intervals, peak titers were seen several hours after injection and ranged from 200 to 400 U. Interferon was still readily detectable 48 h after the last injection. Thus, sufficient data is available to enable one to devise a dose regimen leading to a predictable serum level (CANTELL et al. 1974). However, there is little data relating serum levels to prophylactic or therapeutic efficacy. It has been shown in the rabbit (FERNIE 1976) that intravenously administered interferon rapidly leaves the vascular space and that by 30 min after injection, the concentration of interferon, as measured by antiviral activity, was higher in the major organs than in the blood. If human interferon is distributed similarly, substantial levels may be present in some organs. However interferon does not effectively cross the blood–brain barrier. For instance, JORDAN et al. (1974) were unable to detect interferon in the cerebrospinal fluid of a patient with a serum titer of 278 U/ml. Therefore interferon has been administered intrathecally on a number of occasions (MERIGAN 1977; DE CLERCQ et al. 1975; BEHAN 1981) in order to maintain levels in the central nervous system. It is reasonable to ask whether maintenance of specified levels of interferon has any particular therapeutic significance. Interferon-treated cells can maintain the antiviral state hours or days following contact with interferon, although the establishment of optimal antiviral activity may take several hours of contact between the interferon and the cell in vitro. In any case, there is no reason to assume that interferon must be continuously present in order to maintain the antiviral state.

The pharmacokinetics of fibroblast interferon (IFN-β) are not as well described, largely because appreciable serum levels are hard to attain. For instance, EDY et al. (1978) found no interferon in the serum of individuals who had received 3×10^6 U IFN-β intramuscularly. Even when 1.8×10^7 U were given, interferon was detectable in the blood of only one of the five patients.

II. Toxicology

The most common side effect of interferon administration is fever, which has been noted by almost all investigators in a proportion of patients (see, for instance, PAZIN et al. 1974; JORDAN et al. 1974; EMÖDI et al. 1975a). The peak temperature is usually seen 2–6 h after the initial dose of interferon and tends to decrease with repeated injections (MERIGAN 1977). A hypotensive episode was described in one patient who received a rapid intravenous injection of human leukocyte interferon (STRANDER et al. 1973). Another commonly observed side effect is reversible repression of hemopoietic activity. MERIGAN et al. (1978), GREENBERG et al. (1976), CHEESEMAN et al. (1979), and PAZIN et al. (1979) all describe transient leukopenia with or without thrombocytopenia and depression of reticulocytes. In no cases were these changes irreversible. In neonates treated with human leukocyte interferon for symptomatic CMV infection, decrease in weight gain as well as fever was observed (ARVIN et al. 1976). Fluid intake and weight gain were restored with cessation of treatment. Lassitude and malaise are often reported and it has been suggested that ambulatory dosage should not exceed 1.7×10^5 U kg^{-1} day^{-1} (MERIGAN 1977). Serum transaminases have also been found to be elevated after interferon treatment (PAZIN et al. 1979; ARVIN et al. 1976). Minimal alopecia was reported in 6 of 37 cancer patients treated with 3–9 $\times 10^6$ U/day IFN-α (GUTTERMAN et al. 1978). Fibroblast interferon displays toxicology similar to that of IFN-α. BILLIAU et al. (1979a) described fever, delayed skin reactivity, lymphopenia, and cutaneous allergy following intramuscular injection. The allergic reaction was almost certainly due to bovine serum components which were present in the preparation and to which several patients developed antibodies.

It has never been clear to what extent the side effects of interferon are an intrinsic property of the molecule and to what extent they are due to impurities present in the preparations that have been most widely used to date (INGIMARSSON et al. 1979). SCOTT et al. (1981) recently compared the toxicity of partially purified IFN-α, a material frequently used in previous clinical trials, with the toxicity of a preparation purified by two passages through a monoclonal antibody column. The latter preparation had a specific activity of 2.5×10^8 U per milligram protein and was approximately 170 times as pure as the partially purified material. Six female and three male volunteers received one injections of each preparation as well as an injection of the human serum albumin which was used as a stabilizing vehicle. The mean intramuscular doses were 1.3×10^6 and 1.12×10^6 U per meter^2 body surface area for the partially and highly purified preparations, respectively. The acute effects of the interferon preparations on pulse rate, fever, and white blood cell counts were extremely similar. Generalized symptoms such as headache, malaise, chills, and fatigue, were also the same. Intradermal injection of the two preparations showed no difference in late (4–8 h) skin inflammatory reactions. It must be concluded that the acute side effects of IFN-α are an intrinsic property of the molecule and furthermore, that these side effects may be sufficient to limit the systemic use of large amounts of IFN-α to nontrivial conditions.

References

Arvin AM, Yeager AS, Merigan TC (1976) Effect of leukocyte interferon on urinary excretion of cytomegalovirus by infants. J Infect Dis 133:205–210

Arvin AM, Feldman S, Merigan TC (1978) Human leukocyte interferon in the treatment of children with cancer: a preliminary controlled trial. Antimicrob Agents Chemother 13:605–607

Behan PO (1981) Interferon in treatment of subacute sclerosing panencephalitis. Lancet 1:1059–1060

Billiau A, De Somer P (1980) Clinical use of interferon in viral infections. In: Stringfellow DA (ed) Interferon and interferon inducers. Dekker, New York, pp 113–144

Billiau A, De Somer P, Edy VG, De Clerq E, Heremans H (1979a) Human fibroblast interferon for clinical trials pharmacokinetics and tolerability in experimental animals and humans. Antimicrob Agents Chemother 16:56–63

Billiau A, Edy VG, De Somer P (1979b) The clinical use of fibroblast interferon. In: Chandra P (ed) Antiviral mechanisms in the control of neoplasia. Plenum, New York, pp 675–696

Cantell K (1977) Prospects for the clinical use of exogenous interferon. Med Biol 55:69–73

Cantell K, Pyhala L, Strander H (1974) Circulating human interferon after intramuscular injection into animals and man. J Gen Virol 22:453–455

Carter WA, Dolen JG, Leong SS, Horoszewicz JS (1980) Interferon and hepatitis infection: current results and possible amplification of the therapeutic response. In: Interferon: Khan A, Hill NO, Dorn GL (eds) Properties and clinical uses. Leland Fikes Foundation, Dallas, pp 693–699

Cheeseman SH, Black PH, Rubin RH, Cantell K, Hirsch MS (1980a) Interferon and BK papovavirus – clinical and laboratory studies. J Infect Dis 141:157–161

Cheeseman SH, Henle W, Rubin RH, Tolkoff-Rubin NE, Cosimi B, Cantell K, Winkle S, Herrin JT, Black PH, Russell PS, Hirsch MS (1980 b) Epstein-Barr virus infection in renal transplant recipients. Ann Int Med 93:39–42

Cheeseman SH, Rubin RH, Stewart JA, Tolkoff-Rubin NE, Cosimi AB, Cantell K, Gilbert J, Winkle S, Herrin JT, Black PH, Russell PS, Hirsch MS (1979) Controlled clinical trial of prophylactic human leukocyte interferon in renal transplantation. N Engl J Med 300:1345–1349

De Clercq E, Edy VG, De Vlieger H, Eeckels R, Desmyter J (1975) Intrathecal administration of interferon in neonatal herpes. J Ped 86:736–738

Desmyter J, De Groote J, Desmet VJ, Billiau A, Ray MB, Bradburne AF, Edy VG, De Somer P (1976) Administration of human fibroblast interferon in chronic hepatitis-B infection. Lancet 2:645–647

Dolen JG, Carter WA, Horoszewicz JS, Vladutiu AO, Leibowitz AI, Nolan JP (1979) Fibroblast interferon treatment of a patient with chronic active hepatitis. Increased number of circulating T lymphocytes and elimination of rosette-inhibitory factor. Am J Med 67:127–131

Dunnick JK, Galasso GJ (1979) Clinical trials with exogenous interferon: summary of a meeting. J Infect Dis 139:109–123

Dunnick JK, Galasso GJ (1980) Update on clinical trials with exogenous interferon. J Infect Dis 142: 293–299

Edy VG, Billiau A, De Somer P (1978) Non-appearance of injected fibroblast interferon in circulation. Lancet 1:451–452

Emödi G, Just M, Hernandez R, Hirt HR (1975 a) Circulating interferon in man after administration of exogenous human leukocyte interferon. J Natl Cancer Inst 54:1045–1049

Emödi G, Rufli T, Just M, Hernandez R (1975 b) Human interferon therapy for herpes zoster in adults. Scand J Infect Dis 7:1–5

Emödi G, O'Reilly R, Muller A, Everson LK, Biswanger U, Just M (1976) Effect of human exogenous leukocyte interferon in cytomegalovirus infections. J Infect Dis 133:199–204

Fernie BF (1976) A comparison between the tissue distribution and blood clearance of rabbit interferon and iodinated ovalbumin after intravenous injection into the rabbit. Dissertation, University of Pittsburgh

Glasgow LA, Hanshaw JB, Merigan TC, Petralli JK (1967) Interferon and cytomegalovirus in vivo and in vitro. Soc Exp Biol Med 125:843–849

Greenberg SB, Harmon MW, Couch RB (1980) Exogenous interferon: stability and pharmacokinetics. In: Stringfellow DA (ed) Interferon and interferon inducers. Dekker, New York, pp 57–87

Greenberg HB, Pollard RB, Lutwick LI, Gregory PB, Robinson WS, Merigan TC (1976) Effect of human leukocyte interferon on hepatitis B virus infection in patients with chronic active hepatitis. N Engl J Med 295:517–522

Gutterman JU, Blumenschein GR, Alexanian R, Yap HY, Buzdar AU, Cabanillas F, Hortobagyi GN, Hersh EM, Rasmussen SL, Harmon M, Kramer M, Pestka S (1980) Leukocyte interferon-induced tumor regression in human metastatic breast cancer, multiple myeloma, and malignant lymphoma. Ann Intern Med 93:399–406

Haglund S, Lundquist P, Cantell K, Strander H (1981) Interferon therapy in juvenile laryngeal papillomatosis. Arch Otolaryngol 107:327–332

Ho M, Pazin GJ, White LT, Haverkos H, Wechsler RL, Breinig MK, Cantell K, Armstrong JA (1981) Intralesional treatment of warts with interferon-α and its long-term effect on NK cell activity. In: DeMaeyer E, Galasso G, Schellekens H (eds) The biology of the interferon system. Elsevier/North-Holland, Amsterdam, pp 361–365

Ikic D, Bosnic N, Smerdel S, Jusic D, Soos E, Delimar N (1975 a) Double blind clinical study with human leukocyte interferon in the therapy of condylomata acuminata. In: Ikic D (ed) Proc symp clinical use of interferon. Yugoslav Acad Sci Arts, Zagreb, pp 229–233

Ikic D, Brnobic A, Jurkovic-Vukelic V, Smerdel S, Jusic D, Soos E (1975 b) Therapeutical effect of human leukocyte interferon incorporated into ointment and cream on condylomata acuminata. In: Ikic D (ed) Proc symp clinical use of interferon. Yugoslav Acad Sci Arts, Zagreb, pp 235–238

Ikic D, Cupak K, Trajer D, Soos E, Jusic D, Smerdel S (1975c) Therapy and prevention of epidemic keraconjunctivitis with human leukocyte interferon. In: Ikic D (ed) Proc symp clinical use of interferon. Yugoslav Acad Sci Arts, Zagreb, pp 189–194

Ikic D, Orescanin M, Krusic J, Cestar Z, Alac Z, Soos E, Jusic D, Smerdel S (1975d) Preliminary study of the effect of human leukocytic interferon on condylomata acuminata in women. In: Ikic D (ed) Proc symp clinical use of interferon. Yugoslav Acad Sci Arts, Zagreb, pp 223–227

Ikic D, Petricevic I, Cupak K, Trajer D, Soldo I, Soos E, Jusic D, Smerdel S (1975e) Human leukocytic interferon treatment of complications due to vaccination against smallpox. In: Ikic D (ed) Proc symp clinical use of interferon. Yugoslav Acad Sci Arts, Zagreb, pp 207–212

Ikic D, Petricevic I, Soldo I, Soos E, Smerdel S, Jusic D (1975f) Treatment of influenza with human leukocytic interferon. In: Ikic D (ed) Proc symp clinical use of interferon. Yugoslav Acad Sci Arts, Zagreb, pp 183–187

Imanishi J, Matsubara M, Kishida T, Ozaki Y, Kurimura T (1980) Comparative studies on the inhibitory effects of interferon on various strains of herpes simplex viruses in vitro. Biken J 23:107–111

Ingimarsson S, Cantell K, Strander H (1979) Side effects of long-term treatment with human leukocyte interferon. J Infect Dis 140:560–563

Ingimarsson S, Cantel K, Strander H (1980) Acute infections in patients receiving interferon. In: Khan A, Hill NO, Dorn GL (eds) Interferon: Properties and clinical uses. Leland Fikes Foundation, Dallas, pp 633–644

Iwarson S, Norkrans G, Hagberg R, Nordenfelt E (1980) Interferon treatment in acute hepatitis B infection with prolonged course. Scand J Infect Dis 12:233–234

Jordan GW, Fried RP, Merigan TC (1974) Administration of human leukocyte interferon in herpes zoster. I. Safety, circulating antiviral activity, and host responses to infection. J Infect Dis 130:56–62

Kingham JGC, Ganguly NK, Shaari ZD, Holgate ST, McGuire MJ, Mendelson R, Cartwright T, Scott GM, Richards BM, Wright R (1977) Treatment of HBsAg-positive chronic active hepatitis with human fibroblast interferon. Gut 18:A952

Larsson A, Forsgren M, Hard AF, Segerstad S, Strander H, Cantell K (1976) Administration of interferon to an infant with congenital rubella syndrome involving persistent viremia and cutaneous vasculitis. Acta Paediatr Scand 65:105–110

Lazar R, Breinig MK, Armstrong JA, Ho M (1980) Response of cloned progeny of clinical isolates of herpes simplex virus to human leukocyte interferon. Infect Immun 28:708–712

Merigan TC (1977) Pharmacokinetics and side effects of interferon in man. In: Baron S, Dianzani F (eds) The interferon system: a current review to 1978. University of Texas, Medical Branch, Austin, pp 541–547

Merigan TC, Reed SE, Hall TS, Tyrell DAJ (1973) Inhibition of respiratory virus infection by locally applied interferon. Lancet 1:563–567

Merigan TC, Rand KH, Pollard RB, Abdallah PS, Jordan GW, Fried RP (1978) Human leukocyte interferon for the treatment of herpes zoster in patients with cancer. N Eng J Med 298:981–987

Meyers JD, McGruffin RW, Neiman PE, Singer JW, Thomas ED (1980) Toxicity and efficacy of human leukocyte interferon for treatment of cytomegalovirus pneumonia after marrow transplantation. J Infect Dis 141:555–562

O'Reilly RJ, Everson LK, Emödi G, Hansen J, Smithwick EM, Grimes E, Pahwa Rajandra Pahwa S, Schwartz S, Armstrong D, Siegal FP, Gupta S, Dupont B, Good RA (1976) Effects of exogenous interferon in cytomegalovirus infections complicating bone marrow transplantation. Clin Immun 6:51–61

Pazin GJ, Armstrong JA, Lam MT, Tarr GC, Jannetta PJ, Ho M (1979) Prevention of reactivated herpes simplex infection by human leukocyte interferon after operation on the trigeminal root. N Eng J Med 301:225–230

Pazin GJ, Ho M, Haverkos JA, Armstrong JA, Breinig MC, Wechsler HL, Arvin A, Merigan TC, Cantell K (1981) Effects of interferon-alpha on human warts. J Interferon Res 2:235–243
Purcell RH, Gerin JL, London WT, Wagner J, McAuliffe VJ, Popper H, Palmer AE, Lvovsky E, Kaplan PM, Wong DC, Levy HB (1976) Modification of chronic hepatitis-B virus infection in chimpanzees by administration of an interferon inducer. Lancet 2:757–761
Rasmussen L, Farley LB (1975) Inhibition of herpesvirus hominis replication by human interferon. Infect Immun 12:104–108
Reznik VI, Shangina DA, Zdanovskaya NI (1978) Prophylaxis with leukocyte interferon in foci of acute respiratory diseases. Vopr Virusol 0:732–734
Scientific Committee on Interferon (1965) A report to the medical research council. Experiments with interferon in man. Lancet 1:505–506
Scott GM, Csonka GW (1979) Effect of injections of small doses of human fibroblast interferon into genital warts a pilot study. Br J Vener Dis 55:442–445
Scott GM, Reed S, Cartwright T, Tyrrell D (1980) Failure of human fibroblast interferon to protect against rhinovirus infection. Arch Virol 65:135–140
Scott GM, Secher DS, Flowers D, Bate J, Cantell K, Tyrrell DA (1981) Toxicity of interferon. Br Med J 282:1345–1348
Solov'ev VD (1969) The results of controlled observations on the prophylaxis of influenza with interferon. Bull WHO 41:683–688
Strander H, Cantell K, Carlström G, Jakobsson PA (1973) Clinical and laboratory investigations on man: systemic administration of potent interferon to man. J Natl Cancer Inst 51:733–742
Weimar W, Heijtink RA, Schalm SW, Van Blankenstein M, Schellekens H, Masurel N, Edy VG, Billiau A, De Somer P (1977) Fibroblast interferon in HBsAg-positive chronic active hepatitis. Lancet 2:1282
Weimar W, Schellekens H, Lameijer LDF, Masurel N, Edy VG, Billiau A, De Somer P (1978) Double-blind study of interferon administration in renal transplant recipients. Eur J Clin Invest 8:255–258
Weimar W, Heijtink RA, Schalm SW, Schellekens H (1979 a) Differential effects in HBsAg positive chronic active hepatitis. Eur J Clin Invest 9:151–154
Weimar W, Lameijer LDF, Edy VG, Schellekens H (1979 b) Prophylactic use of interferon in renal allograft recipients. Transplant Proc 11:69–70
Weimar W Heijtink RA, Ten Kate FJP, Schalm SW, Masurel N, Schellekens H, Cantell K (1980) Double-blind study of leukocyte interferon administration in chronic hepatitis B surface antigen positive hepatitis. Lancet 1:336–338

CHAPTER 23

Clinical Use of Interferons: Central Nervous System Disorders

A.M. SALAZAR, C.J. GIBBS, JR., D.C. GAJDUSEK, and R.A. SMITH

A. Introduction

Interest in the experimental treatment of central nervous system (CNS) disorders has been stimulated by the introduction of interferon (IFN) into clinical use. Presently incurable viral diseases of the brain such as subacute sclerosing panencephalitis (SSPE) and progressive multifocal leukoencephalopathy (PML), and neurologic diseases with putative viral etiologies (multiple sclerosis and amyotrophic lateral sclerosis) are potential treatment targets. However, treatment of neurologic diseases with IFN presents special drug delivery problems because the brain and spinal cord are isolated from the systemic circulation by the blood–brain barrier. To date, experimental treatment of neurologically ill patients with IFN has been limited. Well-designed clinical trials will need to be based on knowledge of the pharmacokinetics and tolerance of IFN in both animals and humans, and a number of variables must be considered. In in vitro studies, viruses such as herpesviruses and papovaviruses demonstrate variable susceptibility to IFN and it is to be expected that IFNs will behave differently in different patient populations. The production by cloned cell lines of a variety of cloned IFNs, each of which may have unique properties, will further complicate therapy.

B. Pharmacology

I. Pharmacokinetics

While recoverable levels of the different types of IFN in body fluids after administration do not necessarily correlate with in vivo activity and some authors prefer to measure overall therapeutic response, pharmacokinetic studies are nevertheless usually essential to proper therapeutic trials. The route of administration of IFN has a significant effect on its distribution (CANTELL and PHYALA 1973). A single bolus of human leukocyte IFN administered by the intravenous (i.v.) route is rapidly cleared from the circulation, whereas after intramuscular (i.m.) injection, serum levels can be detected for a prolonged period. CANTELL et al. (1974) found that leukocyte IFN given i.m. in a dose of 3×10^6 U/kg will maintain a serum level of about 100 U/ml for 12 h, suggesting that i.m. IFN is pooled within muscle and then slowly released into the circulation. However, the blood–cerebrospinal fluid (CSF) barrier prevents systemically administered IFN from reaching the CNS. When high CSF levels of IFN are induced by use of poly(I)·poly(C) or after intracerebral inoculation of virus, serum IFN remains low. HABIF et al. (1975) in-

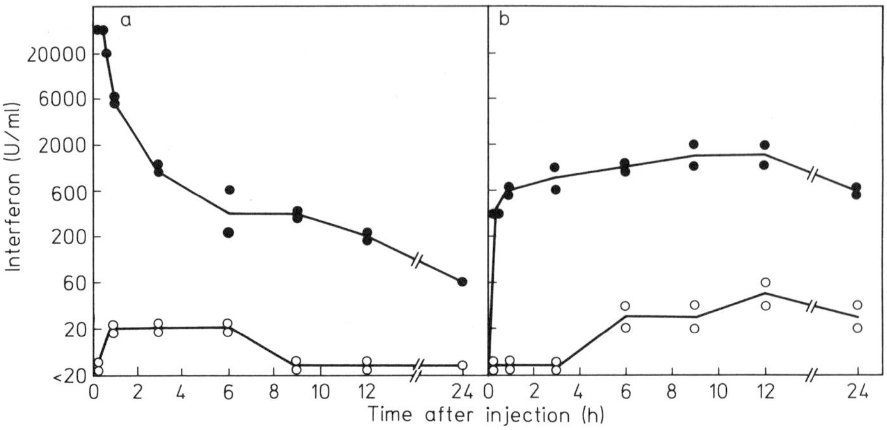

Fig. 1a, b. IFN level in serum (*full circles*) and CSF (*open circles*) of monkeys at different times after i.v. (**a**) or i.m. (**b**) injection of 30×10^7 U concentrated human leukocyte IFN. HABIF et al. (1975)

jected 3×10^6 U IFN i.v. or i.m. into stump-tailed monkeys and simultaneously measured serum and CSF levels of IFN. After i.v. injection, up to 20 U/ml were detected for 6 h, but slightly higher levels (up to 60 U/ml) were detected 6–24 h after i.m. injection (Fig. 1). It was also concluded from these studies that after steady state serum levels are reached there is about a 30-fold difference between IFN levels in serum and CSF. JABLECKI et al. (1981) determined simultaneous serum and CSF IFN levels after subcutaneous (s.c.) or i.v. injection of $3–6 \times 10^6$ U IFN-α using amyotrophic lateral sclerosis (ALS) patients as experimental subjects. CSF titers of IFN were low after s.c. administration of 6×10^6 U (5–10 U were detectable 8–24 h after injection; Fig. 2). After i.v. infusion of 6×10^6 U over 1 min, a small CSF IFN peak was seen, again delayed. Conversely, HABIF et al. (1975) demonstrated that high levels of CSF IFN were maintained for a prolonged period after intrathecal injection of relatively small amounts of IFN into primates (Fig. 3). Similar results were obtained by HO et al. (1974) in rabbits (Fig. 4) and HILFENHAUS et al. (1981) in monkeys.

Very little information is available regarding the fate of IFN injected intraventricularly in humans or other primates (CAMINITI 1980). BROWN et al. (1975) have described an antagonist to IFN in primate brain in vitro. BILLIAU (1981) killed rhesus monkeys 3 h after intralumbar administration of IFN-β, and was able to recover IFN from the surface of the cortex, but not from the deeper layers; no results were reported after intraventricular administration. D. POPLACK et al. (1981, unpublished work) titered serum and CSF IFN after injection of IFN-α intraventricularly in rhesus monkeys. This route of administration was chosen because it was expected to provide better perfusion of the brain than the lumbar route; drugs injected into the lumbar sac leak into the epidural space, pool caudally and normally fail to enter the ventricles when they ascend rostrally. In contrast, because of the dynamics of the normal CSF circulation, IFN injected into a ventricle would be expected to be widely distributed, even to the lumbar region. In normal rhesus

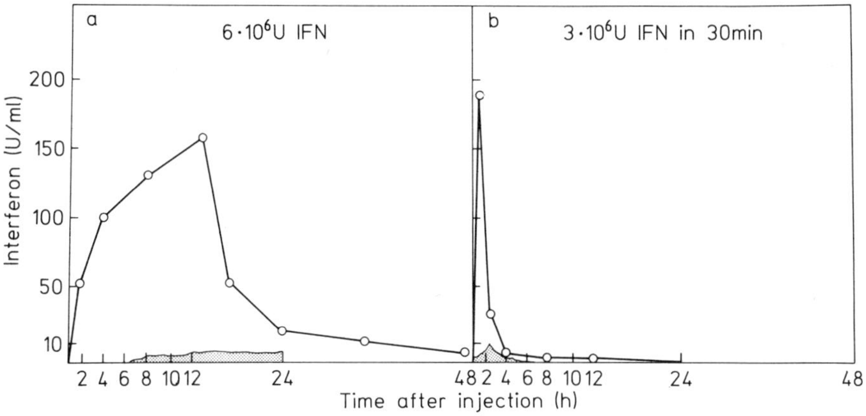

Fig. 2a, b. IFN levels in serum (*circles*) and CFS (*stippled area*) in human after s.c. (**a**) or i.v. (**b**) administration of leukocyte IFN. JABLECKI et al. (1981)

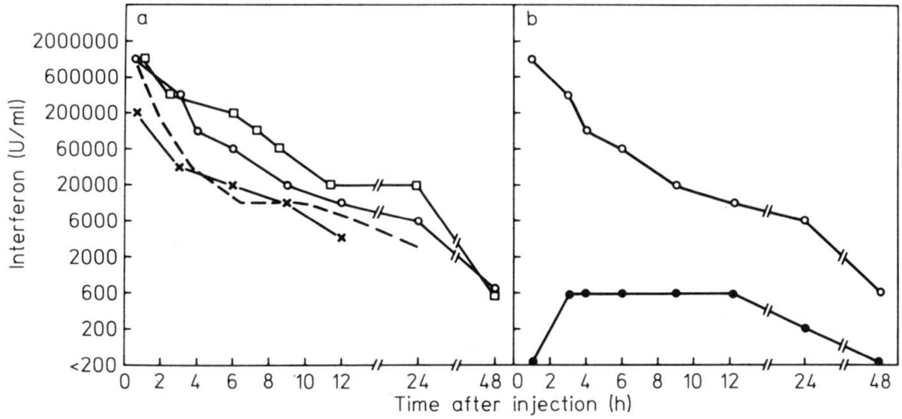

Fig. 3a, b. IFN levels in CSF and serum of monkeys at different times after injection of human leukocyte IFN into cerebrospinal canal. **a** IFN in CSF after injection of: 3×10^6 U (*circles*); 10^7 U (*squares*); or 10^6 U (*crosses*). The blood clearance rate (*broken line*) after i.v. injection of IFN is inserted for comparison of slopes only. The curve is taken from Fig. 1a, which gives the actual IFN titers; **b** IFN in CSF (*open circles*) and serum (*full circles*) after injection of 10^7 U. HABIF et al. (1975)

monkeys, high IFN levels can be obtained after intraventricular injection of 100,000 U IFN. Similar results in humans have been obtained after administration of up to 10^6 U intraventricularly via an Ommaya CSF reservoir; 2 h after injection, the level of IFN was 3,500 U/ml and serial sampling demonstrated a half-life of 2 h (R. SMITH et al. 1981, unpublished work).

II. Tolerance

In the clinical setting, intrathecal IFN has been relatively well tolerated. Malaise and fever have been common side effects on systemic administration, but these ef-

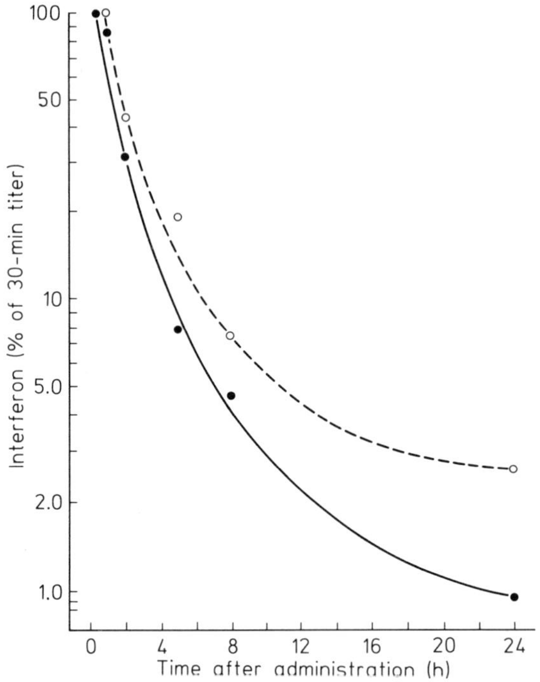

Fig. 4. IFN in the CSF space. IFN was injected into the cisterna magna or into a ventricle, and its disappearance was followed by analysis of CSF samples obtained through a cisternal catheter. Kinetics of disappearance of ^{131}I after intracisternal (*full circles*) and intraventricular (*open circles*) injection. HO et al. (1974)

fects usually diminish with repeated administration. Potential side effects suggested by reports of IFN enhancement of neuronal excitability in vitro have not been noted in vivo (CAVET and GRESSER 1979). HABIF et al. (1975) noted fever 5–8 h after administration of intracisternal IFN to monkeys with the response varying in individual animals (38.5°–40.5 °C). A.M. SALAZAR, H. AMYX, and C.J. GIBBS (1982, unpublished work) similarly studied the tolerance of intracisternal IFN in normal rhesus monkeys. No clinical signs of toxicity were seen at doses of 40,000–200,000 U IFN-α or IFN-β. At the lowest dose of IFN-α, CSF remained normal, but at higher doses a mild CSF pleocytosis was elicited (mostly lymphocytes) and there was a modest increase in CSF protein. Some lots of IFN-β evoked a more pronounced transient polymorphonuclear pleocytosis which diminished on repeated administration, but another lot purified by a more advanced process did not, suggesting that some IFNs may be better tolerated than others and that differences in manufacture and purification play a significant role in tolerance (Table 1). Use of more highly purified preparations should resolve this question.

To date only a few patients have been treated with intrathecal IFN, and most have been restricted to the intralumbar route. DECLERCQ et al. (1975) gave 600,000 U IFN intrathecally (up to twice a day) to a neonate with herpes encephalitis; 2–4 h after injection temperatures ranged from 36°–38.5 °C, and after 4 days of treat-

Table 1. Intrathecal IFN in rhesus monkeys

Dose (U)	CSF analysis (Cells per milliliter/milligram protein) Time (h)			
	0	5	24	48
IFN-α				
4×10^4	0/20	0/20	0/20	0/20
1×10^5	0/20	0/40	0/20	300/40 [a]
2×10^5	0/40	0/60	0/60	400/60 [a]
IFN-β [b]				
2×10^5	0/80	5,400/300 [c]	5,700/140 [c]	900/ [c]
2×10^5	900/	2,800/160		
2×10^5	850/140	1,800/260 [c]		
2×10^5	0/80	500/80 [c]		
2×10^5	0/80	1,600/100 [c]		

[a] Predominantly lymphocytes
[b] IFN-β figures represent weekly and biweekly sequential injections
[c] Predominantly polys

ment a mononuclear CSF pleocytosis was noted (211 white blood cells). MERIGAN (1977), reporting the postmortem findings in two additional cases of neonatal herpes encephalitis treated with intrathecal therapy (50,000 U/day), found no evidence for meningeal inflammation at the site of inoculation. One patient with Creutzfeldt–Jakob disease (VERVERKEN et al. 1979), and three rabies suspects (C. CHANY 1980, personal communication) treated with up to 2×10^6 U intrathecal IFN daily for 2 weeks tolerated treatment without serious sequelae. Malaise and fever were noted at the onset, but these symptoms became less apparent within a few days. Five patients with meningeal leukemia received over 10^6 U IFN-β without ill effects (MISSET et al. 1981). After installation of an Ommaya reservoir R. SMITH et al. (1981, unpublished work) injected up to 10^6 U IFN-α into the right lateral ventricle of an ALS patient. For 6 h the patient remained normal, but thereafter she developed a fever (up to 39 °C), frontal headache, and nausea. The headache was identical to that after systemic administration of 6×10^6 U IFN, and although its character was suggestive of a migrainous etiology, ergotamine tartrate failed to abort it. Mild CSF pleocytosis was noted, but protein remained normal and the patient did not develop signs of meningeal irritation. After weekly injection of 250,000 U for 5 weeks, another patient remained asymptomatic, but on biweekly treatments he developed mild pleocytosis, anorexia, and fatigue. These symptoms resolved over 5 days and the CSF cell count returned to normal. Their experience suggests that purified IFN-α may cause mild, reversible meningeal irritation after repeated intrathecal injection. Similarly, L.G. SALFORD et al. (1981, unpublished work) have administered 4×10^6 U IFN-α daily intratumor to five brain tumor patients for 1 month, again without intolerable ill effects.

Finally, in a therapeutic trial for multiple sclerosis (see Sect. C.II.1), JACOBS et al. (1981a, b) have administered $1–2\times10^6$ U IFN-β intrathecally to ten patients. Each patient received 10^6 U per meter^2 of body surface via the lumbar route twice a week for 4 weeks, then once a month for 5 months. Side effects included transient fever, headache, myalgias, and malaise, but in no case were these severe enough to necessitate cessation of therapy. A moderate increase in CSF protein was seen along with a variable sterile pleocytosis of 35–1,750 white cells at the end of 1 month of treatment, but this had cleared at 6 months. CSF glucose remained normal. There was no clustering of maximum pleocytosis at any stage of therapy, no relation of the degree of pleocytosis to signs of systemic toxicity, and no relation of the degree of systemic toxicity to any particular stage of the therapy. (Other findings are discussed in Sect. C.II.1.)

C. Clinical Use

I. Viral Diseases of the Central Nervous System

1. Rabies

The variable efficacy of postexposure rabies prophylaxis with vaccination and hyperimmune serum regimens, coupled with the prolonged nature and morbidity of these regimens, has prompted a search for new methods of treatment in this disease. Variations in efficacy of various vaccines have been related by some authors (STEWART and SULKIN 1966; WIKTOR et al. 1976; BAER and CLEARY 1972; BAER 1977; NOZAKI 1975) to their ability to induce IFN production independent of vaccine potency, suggesting that the IFN system is crucial in the host's defense against rabies virus. Rabies virus itself is only a modest inducer of IFN in mice and hamsters (STEWART 1979) and a number of in vitro and in vivo studies indicate that the exogenous addition or superinduction of this agent may be useful in both the prophylaxis and treatment of rabies.

Therapeutic trials in animals have been mostly prophylactic. FENJE and POSTIC (1970) showed that rabbits could be protected from rabies by injection of poly(I) · poly(C) 24 h before or after exposure to rabies virus; it was presumed that protection occurred through induction of endogenous IFN. JANIS and HABEL (1972) and BAER et al. (1977) also found injections of poly(I) · poly(C) or of IFN-α combined with vaccine to be most effective when injected i.m. at the site of viral inoculation, confirming the notion that the rabies virus appears to be localized to the initial site of inoculation for much of its incubation period before migrating up the nerves into the CNS (KAPLAN et al. 1962). The protective effect in monkeys was most dramatic when the combined treatment was started 6 h after inoculation, while a delay of treatment onset to 24 h resulted in 50% mortality. On the other hand, the addition of PICLC or IFN does not appear to interfere with the production of antibody induced by a single potent dose of human diploid cell (HDC) vaccine (BAER et al. 1977).

HILFENHAUS et al. (1977) demonstrated the efficacy of human IFN-α alone in the treatment of monkeys inoculated with rabies, particularly when used both i.m. and intrathecally. In these and other experiments, IFN-α was administered every other day, beginning 24 h after inoculation and was continued as long as 2 weeks. In a control group, one in ten animals survived after virus inoculation, whereas under optimum treatment conditions with both i.m. and intrathecal IFN eight in ten animals survived. Good protection was demonstrated even when the onset of treatment was delayed as long as 11 days (MAJER et al. 1977). Antibody titers were only modest in the surviving animals, especially those treated i.m., again suggesting that the combination of IFN therapy with active immunization could have been even more effective in prophylaxis. VODOPIJA et al. (1981) treated several nonimmunized patients bitten by proven rabid animals, using HDC vaccine and 2×10^6 U IFN-α i.m. Vaccine was repeated after 3, 7, 14, 30, and 90 days. None of the patients has developed disease after 12–19 months.

The treatment of rabies after the onset of clinical symptoms poses a much more difficult problem. In spite of the fulminant clinical course of this illness, indicating severe neuronal dysfunction, the pathologic changes in cases dying early are relatively mild, suggesting that CNS damage is not necessarily irreversible even after the onset of clinical symptoms, and that vigorous treatment is not necessarily futile (STEWART 1979). At least one case of rabies has survived without sequelae after vigorous supportive therapy (HATTWICK et al. 1972). MAJER et al. (1977) were unable to reverse the disease in cynomolgus monkeys with i.m. and intrathecal IFN begun after the onset of symptoms, possibly in part because of the difficulties involved in the intensive supportive care required by such animals. Relatively crude preparations of IFN-α have been used intrathecally in France to treat three patients with terminal rabies, again without clear success (C. CHANY 1980, personal communication). In summary, however, the animal data available to date suggest that the intraventricular use of the newer, more highly purified IFN preparations, combined with vigorous supportive therapy, may still offer the best hope in the clinical management of rabies. Likewise, the use of either IFN or its inducers, in conjunction with potent HDC vaccines, promises to improve and simplify the prophylactic management of this dread disease.

2. Herpesviruses

a) Herpes Zoster

While herpesviruses have been reported to be only moderately sensitive to IFNs in vitro and levels of circulating IFN are low in patients with herpes zoster, high titers may be present in the vesicles as the disease runs its course (MERIGAN et al. 1978), suggesting that IFN may be involved in the healing of herpetic eruptions. Based on this rationale, MERIGAN et al. performed a placebo-controlled, randomized double-blind study of the effect of IFN on the evolution of herpes zoster among immunosuppressed patients with cancer; early treatment seemed to limit cutaneous and visceral spread and may have decreased the incidence of postherpetic neuralgia. Other clinical studies have similarly demonstrated a benficial effect in systemic herpes zoster infections (STRANDER et al. 1973; JORDAN 1974; EMODI et al. 1975; ANONYMOUS 1980; CATALANO and BARON 1970; KERN and GLASGOW 1977; KOBZE et al. 1975).

b) Herpes Simplex

OVERALL et al. (1981) have demonstrated high titers of IFN-α in acute herpes simplex vesicles, and various studies have also demonstrated an effect of IFN preparations against genital and labial herpes as well as in herpetic keratitis. PAZIN et al. (1979) treated 19 patients with trigeminal neuralgia with IFN-α (70,000 U kg^{-1} day^{-1} for 5 days prior to surgery) and noted a decrease in the recurrence rate of herpes labialis as well as a significant decrease in virus shedding. Similarly, IKIC et al. (1975) achieved resolution of herpetic lesions using an IFN ointment applied topically. These studies are reviewed in greater detail by STEWART (1979) and YABROV (1980).

Herpes simplex encephalitis, on the other hand, is a much more serious and usually fatal condition, and even those patients who survive as a result of treatment with adenine arabinoside are commonly burdened with permanent neurologic disability. Early in the course of herpes encephalitis IFN-α can be found in relatively low titers in the spinal fluid (but not in the serum), whereas they become undetectable after about day 10 of the infection (HILFENHAUS and ACKERMANN 1981; LEBON et al. 1979; LEGASPI et al. 1980). The last mentioned authors also detected IFN in temporal lobe brain biopsy specimens obtained between the days 3 and 10 of illness. From these and other studies it would appear that the herpes simplex virus is able to induce only a relatively weak IFN response in the CSF, and that the addition of exogenous IFN may be helpful in this disease.

IFN as well as several IFN inducers have been shown by various workers to have a beneficial effect in experimental herpes infections in mice, but the few reported trials in humans have been disappointing. BELLANTI et al. (1971) treated a child with herpes encephalitis by i.v. poly(I) · poly(C) with no beneficial effects, and SKURKOVICH (1981) reported treating a boy with herpes encephalitis by IFN-rich plasma; the child recovered (YABROV 1980). DECLERCQ et al. (1975) used a crude preparation of IFN-α (600,000 U intrathecally in eight doses over 6 days) in an infant with terminal neonatal herpes. Although the patient died of his illness, there was no overt toxicity with this route of administration, and relatively high IFN levels were maintained in the lumbar fluid with little or no spillover into the serum. MERIGAN (1977) also reported treating two patients with advanced neonatal herpes by 50,000 U IFN-α intrathecally without success.

In summary, while some experimental data suggest that IFN administered early intrathecally (or perhaps intraventricularly) could be useful in herpetic encephalitis, the few human trials to date have been disappointing. The potential use of IFN for this disease must be considered in the context of the demonstrated (albeit only partial) usefulness of adenine arabinoside and of the newer antiherpetic drugs such as acycloguanine (acyclovir), trisodium phosphonoformate, and bromovinyldeoxyuridine (BVDU) (DECLERCQ 1981). Recent in vitro experiments also suggest that combination of IFN with such antiviral drugs may be beneficial (LERNER and BAILEY 1981).

c) Cytomegalovirus

As with the other herpesviruses, cytomegalovirus (CMV) is only moderately sensitive to IFN in vitro, and results of both animal and human clinical trials have been equivocal. EMODI et al. (1976) observed that lymphocytes of infants with CMV produced less IFN than normal subjects, and he subsequently reported inhibition of viruria after treatment with IFN-α in nine patients with either congenital or acquired CMV infection, although viremia persisted (EMODI et al. 1976).

Other authors have reported similar results, even with IFN-α in high doses; but generally there was no alteration in the course of the disease and viruria returned after cessation of treatment (ARVIN et al. 1976; O'REILLY et al. 1976; MERIGAN et al. 1977). CHEESEMAN et al. (1977, 1979), in a controlled study, confirmed that prophylactic IFN will decrease viremia and shedding in renal transplant patients, but with no change in mortality; that study is now expanding (HIRSH et al. 1981). Again, the apparent usefulness of other antiherpetic drugs such as phosphonoacetic acid and acyloguanine must be considered in such studies in the future.

3. Arbovirus Encephalitis (Togaviruses)

As a group, most arboviruses have proven to be quite sensitive to the effects of IFN and IFN inducers in vitro, but in general this sensitivity does not correlate with virulence (HALLUM et al. 1970; LUBY et al. 1975; LUBINIECKI et al. 1974a, b; STEPHEN 1977). LUBY et al. (1969, 1971) determined viral and IFN titers in serum, spinal fluid, and various brain areas of patients dying of St. Louis encephalitis (SLE) and Western equine encephalitis (WEE) and found them to be highest in the basal ganglia of the patient with WEE. IFN was found in certain other brain areas and in spinal fluid, but not in serum, suggesting that it was produced in specific areas of the brain. The localized IFN titers did not necessarily correlate with local viral titers and were much higher in the patient dying of WEE than in a patient dying in a comparable stage of SLE, again indicating that there is not always a direct relation between IFN levels and either virulence or virus titers (ANONYMOUS 1969).

In vivo experiments likewise confirm the potential value of IFN, although generally only when given before or shortly after exposure to the virus. Venezuelan equine encephalitis (VEE) virus infections have been succesfully prevented in mice and monkeys by systemic tilorone or PICLC (KUEHNE et al. 1977; STEPHEN et al. 1979). STEPHEN et al. (1979) noted a delay and decrease in viremia after treatment of VEE-infected monkeys with PICLC and, although some of their treated monkeys succumbed to what they felt were problems in handling, they concluded that IFN altered the pathogenesis of VEE favorably.

Japanese encephalitis (JE) virus infections in mice and hamsters were prevented, sometimes markedly, by both IFN and the IFN inducers PICLC and carboxymethylacridanone when given prophylactically (SINGH and POSTIC 1970; LIU 1978; TAYLOR et al. 1980). PICLC reduced mortality by 50% and prolonged survival in monkeys treated 8–24 h after intranasal infection with a lethal dose of JE virus (WORTHINGTON et al. 1973; HARRINGTON et al. 1977).

Tickborne encephalitis (TBE) was successfully prevented in mice by the use of the IFN inducer tilorone with or without poly(I)·poly(C) 24 h prior to virus challenge (HOFMAN and KUNZ 1972), and with the IFN inducer RFf2 combined with vaccine (DAVIDOVA et al. 1979). Russian investigators have also reported modification of TBE in monkeys treated i.v. with PICLC 6 h before inoculation intracerebrally with a lethal dose of virus. Four of six treated animals survived (two without sequelae), whereas all four controls died (BURGASOVA et al. 1977).

PRANGE and WISMANN (1981) recently reported improvement in three encephalitis patients treated with intrathecal IFN (one herpes zoster and two undiagnosed). Although we know of no formal human trials of IFN or IFN inducers in the arbovirus (togavirus) encephalitides, studies have demonstrated both in vitro and in vivo sensitivity of many of these viruses. Trials in humans, particularly after the onset of symptoms, would most likely require high doses administered intrathecally. Intraventricular administration of the drug to clinically ill animals would help to clarify this question.

4. Slow Virus Diseases (Conventional Viruses)

The "slow" viral infections of the nervous system include those caused by altered or defective forms of conventional viruses such as measles and herpes (usually involving an active host immune response with inflammation) and those caused by unconventional agents such as kuru, scrapie, and Creutzfeldt–Jakob disease (which result in little or no immune reponse or inflammation). Among the former, perhaps the most interesting include subacute sclerosing panencephalitis (SSPE), progressive rubella panencephalitis (PRP), progressive multifocal leukoencephalopathy (PML), and possibly Reye's syndrome. (Some authors would also include multiple sclerosis, but this will be discussed under a separate heading.)

a) Subacute Sclerosing Panencephalitis

A number of studies have demonstrated the etiologic relationship of the measles virus to SSPE (ZEMAN and KOLAR 1968; LENNETTE et al. 1968; CONNOLLY et al. 1967; FREEMAN et al. 1967) and a decreased incidence of the disease in the United States has been noted since the introduction of the measles vaccine (JABBOUR et al. 1972). Studies of the potential therapeutic uses of IFNs in SSPE have been disappointing. JONCAS et al. (1976) found high IFN levels in the CSF of 3 of 8 patients with SSPE and only 4 of 64 diseased controls, but they found no correlation between IFN levels and other disease parameters such as CSF cell count, protein, and measles titers; the findings suggested to them that IFN would not be helpful.

FREEMAN (1968) and LEAVITT et al. (1971) reported using the IFN inducer pyran copolymer combined with dibromdesoxyuridine in three SSPE patients with only very transient improvement in one (accompanied by induction of a hemolytic–uremic syndrome). CHANY (1981) briefly reported combined IFN and isoprinosine treatment of three SSPE patients in Paris with complete recovery in one patient treated early in the disease and failure in a second. GUGGENHEIM and BARON (1977) treated seven cases of SSPE by i.v. poly(I)·poly(C) with no improvement in any case, although the levels of IFN induced were only modest. Finally, BEHAN (1981) treated three SSPE patients using 3×10^6 U daily i.m. for 20–90 days. One patient also received 12×10^6 U intrathecally over 3 days, but there was no clinical benefit in any case. The authors concluded that partly purified IFN-α was of no value in SSPE.

In an unsuccessful attempt to treat the related condition PRP with isoprinosine, WOLINSKI et al. (1979) also noticed increasing levels of serum IFN throughout the course of illness in two patients, along with a factor that inhibited IFN production in normal donor lymphocytes. They suggested a role for such an inhibitor in the early stages of PRP.

b) Reye's Syndrome

Reye's syndrome is an acute encephalopathy in children, associated with fatty degeneration of the liver, which has been linked with viral infections, especially influenza B, although the exact etiology and pathogenesis of the disease remains controversial (REYE et al. 1963; GLICK et al. 1970; SHANNON et al. 1975). ISAACS et al. (1966) described an IFN inhibitor in influenza B-infected cells (CHANY and BRAILOWSKY 1967), and ROZEE et al. (1979) have linked Reye's syndrome to a combination of certain viral infections and exposure to emulsifiers in pesticide sprays. They demonstrated an effect of polyoxyethylene ether polymers on the antiviral state induced by IFN and were able to develop an animal model of Reye's syndrome. Exogenous IFN reduced the mortality in this model. GUGGENHEIM and BARON (1977) treated seven cases of Reye's syndrome with poly(I)·poly(C) i.v. in doses of 0.1–1.0 mg/kg. In spite of induction of only relatively low levels of IFN, four of seven patients recovered completely and one recovered with sequelae. Further trials in this disease have not been reported, but may be worth pursuing.

c) Progressive Multifocal Leukoencephalopathy

PML is a progressive demyelinating disease described by ASTROM et al. in 1958 and occurring in association with carcinomatosis, lymphomas, leukemia, sarcoidosis, and other debilitating conditions. Papovaviruses were first demonstrated by electron microscopy in 1964 in brain from a patient dying of PML, and were subsequently isolated from brain material (ZuRHEIN and CHOU 1965; ZuRHEIN 1969; PADGET et al. 1971; WEINER et al. 1972, 1973; NARAYAN et al. 1973).

Although there are no published trials of IFN in this disease, the IFN sensitivity of SV40 virus in vitro has been demonstrated (TODARO and BARON 1965; OXMAN and TAKEMOTO 1970; YAKOBSON et al. 1977; HAJNICK and BOREKY 1979; TEVETHIA et al. 1979; KINGSMAN and SAMUEL 1980). Poly(I)·poly(C) has likewise been demonstrated to inhibit SV40 viral oncogenesis in rats (VANDEPUTTE et al. 1970). CHEESEMAN et al. (1980) studied the effects of IFN-α on excretion of the related BK papovavirus in renal transplant patients and demonstrated no effect, but the relevance of these findings to treatment of PML remains unclear. Therapeutic trials in this rare condition would most likely require intraventricular IFN administration.

5. Slow Virus Diseases (Unconventional Viruses)

This group of chronic CNS degenerative diseases includes mink encephalopathy as well as scrapie in sheep and kuru and Creutzfeldt–Jakob disease in humans (GAJDUSEK 1966; GIBBS 1968, 1971). While the "viruses" responsible for these conditions have not been identified, they are transmissible through intracerebral inoculation of infected brain tissues into various species (including primates, rodents, goats, and cats) and can reach titres of 10^7 LD_{50} per gram brain tissue. The virus is resistant to a variety of inactivating procedures including heat (80 °C), freezing, formalin, ethanol, ionizing and ultraviolet radiation, and a variety of proteases and nucleases.

Attempts to ameliorate the course of scrapie and Creutzfeldt–Jakob disease have been generally unsuccessful. KATZ and KOPROWSKI (1968) found that the scrapie agent neither induces IFN in infected animals nor prevents IFN production in response to other stimuli. GRESSER and PATTISON (1968) and FIELD et al. (1969) failed to modify the course of disease in intracerebrally inoculated mice treated with either IFN or the IFN inducer statolon. WORTHINGTON et al. (1972) repeated these experiments using long-term administration of poly(I) · poly(C) in mice challenged peripherally with low doses of the scrapie agent and again failed to show a beneficial effect. The IFN response to poly(I) · poly(C) in infected animals however, was not impaired. A similar experiment using intracerebrally administered PICLC in mice infected with Creutzfeldt–Jakob disease, has shown only equivocal benefit (A.M. SALAZAR, H. AMYX, and C.J. GIBBS 1980, unpublished work).

More recently, A.M. SALAZAR, H. AMYX, and C.J. GIBBS (1981, unpublished work) have administered IFN-α, IFN-β, or PICLC intracisternally and intraventricularly to eight monkeys clinically ill with either kuru, Creutzfeldt–Jakob disease, or scrapie. Some animals received biweekly injections for as long as 2 months, but in no case was the disease ameliorated. In some animals, the disease appeared to accelerate, but this is often seen in response to the stress of repeated handling. There are only three such therapeutic attempts reported in humans. KOVANEN et al. (1980) used 3×10^6 U IFN-α daily s.c. in two patients with Creutzfeldt–Jakob disease for 4 and 13 months, with no influence on the course of the disease. They suggested that intrathecal administration might be worthwhile. VERVERKEN et al. (1979), however, reported treating a case of Creutzfeldt–Jakob disease this way with repeated injections of 10^6 U IFN-β intrathecally. The clinical course of the disease as well as the pathology at autopsy were unaltered. In summary, the evidence available to date indicates that IFNs alone are not likely to be useful in Creutzfeldt–Jakob disease. Combination therapy with other agents, however, remains to be explored.

II. Dysimmune Neurologic Diseases

1. Multiple Sclerosis

A combination of viral and immunologic factors has long been suspected in the etiology of this disease (LISAK 1980). Several virally induced animal models of demyelination have been described, (MARTIN and NATHANANSON 1979; WEINER and STAHLMAN 1978) and in some patients, multiple sclerosis has been linked with exposure to a specific virus (ADAMS and IMAGOWA 1962; COOK et al. 1978; HAASE et al. 1981). Immunologic abnormalities include the presence of demyelinating serum factors (BORNSTEIN and APPEL 1965), elevation of immunoglobulins and immune complexes in the CSF (TOURTELLOTTE 1969; TACHOVSKY et al. 1976; MASSON 1979; W.C. WALLEN 1981, personal communication), and fluctuations in cellular immune regulation (LISAK 1980; DENMAN 1980; ARNASON and WAXMAN 1980).

Variations in suppresor T-cell activity in the course of multiple sclerosis have been noticed by several authors, with a decrease shortly before or in the early phases of an exacerbation (ANTEL et al. 1978, 1979, 1981; HUDDLESTONE and OLDSTONE 1979; WALLEN et al. 1981; PATY et al. 1981). The suppressor cell population however, may actually be increased during periods of remission and appears to be largely composed of TG cells, which bear surface receptors for the Fc portion of IgG and will bind circulating immune complexes (MORETTA et al. 1977, 1978; SANTOLI et al. 1978; HUDDLESTONE and OLDSTONE 1979). It has been found that some of these cells are less responsive to the natural cytotoxic enhancing properties of IFN during an acute exacerbation, possibly because of masking of IFN surface receptors by bound immune complexes in the early phases of the exacerbation (TACHOVSKY et al. 1976; ZARLING et al. 1978; W.C. WALLEN 1981, personal communication; FRIDMAN et al. 1981). Such cells from multiple sclerosis patients may also produce less IFN than controls when confronted with certain viral antigens or poly(I)·poly(C) (NEIGHBOUR et al. 1979, 1981; BENCZUR et al. 1980; SANTOLI 1981). IFN, in turn, has been implicated as a possible mediator of the immunosuppressive action of suppressor T-lymphocytes (NOTKINS 1975; DEMAYER et al. 1975; NEIGHBOUR et al. 1979; EPSTEIN 1977; JOHNSON et al. 1977; MIORNER et al. 1978; KADISH et al. 1980; BALKWILL et al. 1981; SONNENFELD et al. 1977); while under other circumstances it may be immunoenhancing (EPSTEIN 1977; GRESSER et al. 1979; DEMAYER 1981; SKURKOVITCH 1981). The roles of host and virus genetics, IFN type, timing, and dosage, as well as the stage of disease in these apparently paradoxical actions remain to be explored.

IFN levels in the blood and CSF of multiple sclerosis patients have been studied by various authors, but results have been difficult to interpret because some studies have not specified the stage of the disease, and it is sometimes difficult to obtain spinal fluid just before or very early in an exacerbation. As early as 1968, SIBLEY and TOURTELLOTTE found IFN activity in 19% of fresh frozen multiple sclerosis brain autopsy specimens, more so in specimens which were less active pathologically. In 1971, HAAHR reported finding IFN in the CSF of two multiple sclerosis patients, but E. KUWERT and H. LEVY (1979, unpublished work) failed to confirm this. LUBIKOVA et al. (1979) reported finding CSF IFN in only 8 of 49 patients, while DEGRE et al. (1976) reported IFN in the CSF of almost one-half of their 36 patients. More recently W.C. WALLEN (1981, personal communication) has found IFN in the CSF of patients in the active phase of the disease, but not during remission. These findings again suggest that IFN fluctuates with disease activity and may play a role in the exacerbation – remission cycle of multiple sclerosis patients.

It can be postulated that a "rechallenge" by a viral antigen early in an exacerbation could lead to formation of immune complexes which would modify IFN sensitivity and/or production in a certain population of "presensitized" suppressor T-cells. This could then lead to a decrease in suppressor activity which could set the stage for increased antibody production, cell-mediated attack on oligodendrocytes previously labeled by viral antigen (WISNIEWSKI 1977), and demyelination. Such demyelination would be maximal in those portions of the myelin sheath closest to the circulation (perivenular) or the CSF. The inflammatory response and increased antigen release (TRAUGOTT and RAINE 1981; PANITCH et al. 1978; COHEN et al. 1976; WHITTAKER et al. 1980) resulting from these events would be expected to result in formation not only of IgG (TOURTELLOTTE 1969), but of large amounts of IFN-γ as well, which could then help reestablish suppressor activity and induce remission (HAAHR 1971; DEGRE et al. 1976; W.C. WALLEN et al. 1981, personal communication; EPSTEIN 1977; HOOKS et al. 1980; JACOBS et al. 1981, 1982). Early addition of exogenous IFN in such a model would be expected to accelerate the onset of remission and minimize CNS damage (Fig. 5). Alternatively, IFN might also play a role in the phenomenon of viral persistence (MINATO 1980; SEKELLICK and MARCUS 1980), or in normalizing altered target cell surface receptors.

Experimental trials until recently have been small and have involved the systemic use of IFN or its inducers. FOG (1980) used IFN-α in dose of $2.5–5 \times 10^6$ U/day i.m.

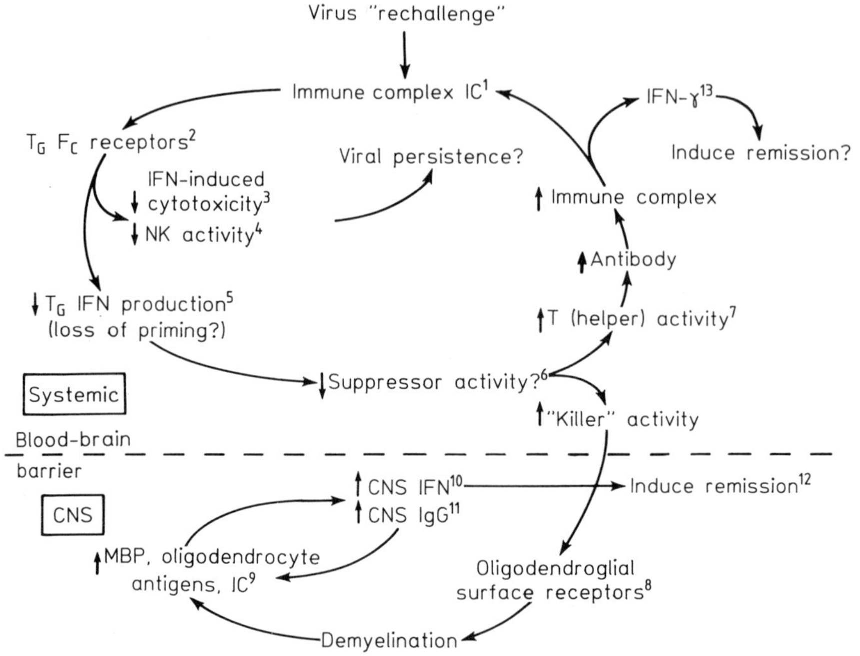

Fig. 5. Simplified hypothetical sequence of events in a multiple sclerosis exacerbation. See text for explanation. Abbreviations: IC immune complex; MBP myelin basic protein; NK natural killer; T_G T-suppressor lymphocyte.

References:

1 TACHOVSKY et al. (1976), W.C. WALLEN (1981, personal communication)
2 MORETTA et al. (1977), SANTOLI et al. (1978), HUDDLESTONE and OLDSTONE (1979), W.C. WALLEN (1981, personal communication)
3 W.C. WALLEN (1981, personal communication)
4 BENCZUR et al. (1980)
5 NEIGHBOUR et al. (1979, 1981), BENCZUR et al. (1980)
6 NOTKINS (1975), ANTEL et al. (1978, 1979), NEIGHBOR et al. (1979), W.C. WALLEN et al. (1981, personal communication), BALKWILL et al. (1981), DEMAYER (1976, 1981)
7 ANTEL et al. (1978), MORETTA et al. (1978)
8 WISNIEWSKI (1977), MANCONI et al. (1978)
9 COHEN et al. (1976), WHITTAKER et al. (1980)
10 DEGRE et al. (1976), W.C. WALLEN (1981, personal communication), EPSTEIN (1977, 1981), HOOKS et al. (1980)
11 TOURTELLOTTE (1969), ABRAMSKY et al. (1977), TRAUGOTT et al. (1981), PANITCH et al. (1978)
12 JACOBS et al. (1981, 1982)
13 HOOKS et al. (1980), SKURKOVICH (1981)

for as long as 15 months with no alteration in the progress of the disease. He postulated that the principal problem was failure of IFN delivery across the blood–brain barrier. VERVERKEN et al. (1979) used 0.05×10^6 U/kg IFN-β every other day intramuscularly to treat three patients with progressive multiple sclerosis, again with negative results. They also postulated that intrathecal IFN could be useful in this disease. Results from a larger, double-blind cooperative study using high doses of IFN-α i.m. in active multiple sclerosis patients are not yet available (T.C. MERIGAN et al. 1981, personal communication). BORNSTEIN et al. (1980) have reported improvement in 4 of 16 patients in an open pilot study using the synthetic polypeptide copolymer I i.m., but they have not related this improvement to the possible IFN-inducing properties of this agent. Finally, SALAZAR et al. (1981) have reported improvement in a young man with subacute postinfections demyelinating encephalomyelitis after i.v. treatment with the synthetic inducer PICLC. Improvement was most marked in those neurologic functions affected by an exacerbation which had occurred 1.5 months before treatment.

In a recently completed randomized trial of intrathecal purified IFN-β in patients with active disease, JACOBS et al. (1981, 1982) chose 20 patients with active multiple sclerosis (disease duration 12–255 months). Ten were treated with up to 2×10^6 U intralumbar twice a week for 4 weeks, then once a month for the next 5 months (i.e., for a total treatment period of 6 months). Ten disease controls were continued on routine therapy, including adrenocorticotropic hormone in some. At the end of an 18-month observation period, there was a slight worsening in the exacerbation rate among controls (0.71–0.92 exacerbations per year). Neurologic status in one was better, in four unchanged, and in five worse. IFN recipients, on the other hand, whose pretreatment exacerbation rates had been somewhat worse than in controls (1.8 per year), remained almost exacerbation free (only three exacerbations in two patients, posttreatment rate 0.2 per year). One of these latter patients showed an abrupt termination of her exacerbation 1 day after retreatment with 10^6 U intralumbar IFN. The neurologic status of treated patients was better in five, unchanged in four, and worse in one. Side effects (reported earlier in this section) included transient fever, headache, and CSF pleocytosis, but were tolerable and never necessitated cessation of therapy (JACOBS et al. 1981, 1982).

In summary, several lines of investigation suggest that IFN may be involved in the pathogenesis of multiple sclerosis and specifically in the dynamics of the exacerbation–remission cycle. Some clinical investigators have observed improvement in multiple sclerosis patients undergoing treatment with IFN, particularly during an exacerbation. However, in light of the variable nature of this disease and the long list of previous "cures" ending in disappointment, these results must be interpreted with caution, and further trials are indicated. The effect of IFNs on long-standing neurologic residuals of previous exacerbations also remains to be explored.

2. Recurrent Dysimmune Polyneuropathy (Landry–Guillain–Barré Syndrome)

While many peripheral neuropathies are not related to viral or dysimmune disease, a large proportion of patients usually given a diagnosis of Landry–Guillain–Barré ascending paralysis do fall in this category (IQBAL et al. 1981; DALAKAS and ENGEL 1981). Many of these patients develop their symptoms shortly after a minor viral infection, and follow a monophasic course, but others can develop a chronic, relapsing–remitting disease with demyelination and have been considered to suffer from a peripheral counterpart to multiple sclerosis.

ENGEL et al. (1978) treated one such patient (who had failed to respond to immunosuppresants and corticosteroids) using PICLC 100 μg/kg i.v. once a week. The patient, who had been ill and practically wheelchair-ridden for 14 years, showed a marked step of improvement about 48 h after each dose, and, after seven weekly treatments was able to walk 6 miles and lift heavy objects. His improvement has been sustained over the last 3 years with periodic retreatments. These studies have been extended to include nine other patients with chronic dysimmune neuropathies; very encouraging results have been noted in most (ENGEL et al. 1981). PICLC in these and one other patient has induced serum IFN levels of 100–500 U/ml, as well a rapid and marked, but very transient decrease in circulating T-lymphocytes and an increase in macrophages. The relation of these changes to the clinical improvements noted is not known (SALAZAR et al. 1981). While the patients studied to date have suffered chronic forms of this condition, results have been so encouraging that this drug or exogenous IFNs alone should probably also be considered in the treatment of the more common, severe, acute monophasic forms of the Landry–Guillain–Barré syndrome.

III. Degenerative Diseases of the Central Nervous System

1. Amyotrophic Lateral Sclerosis

ALS is a progressive neurologic condition in which both upper and lower motor neurons degenerate, leading to profound weakness, amyotrophy, and death in 1–4 years. Although the basic cause of this disease has not been totally elucidated, a viral etiology has been postulated since the earliest descriptions of the disease by Charcot, and there are several indirect lines of evidence to suggest a slow or persistent viral infection in at least some cases of motor neuron disease.

That certain viruses can selectively attack the motor neurons has been conclusively demonstrated by our experience with anterior poliomyelitis, and the delayed, postpolio form of motor neuron disease may be due to a chronic, persistent form of the virus (CAMPBELL et al. 1969; MULDER et al. 1972). In addition, other chronic postinfectious conditions such as those following TBE, Vilyuisk encephalomyelitis in Russia, and postencephalitic parkinsonism in western Europe all include amyotrophic cases (PETROV 1970; GAIDUSEK 1982; MUELLER and SCHALTENBRAND 1979; GREENFIELD et al. 1954). Some cases with the amyotrophic form of Creutzfeldt–Jakob disease, a rare presenile dementia of proven "slow viral" etiology, combine the clinical features of both ALS and Creutzfeldt–Jakob disease; and it appears that this may represent a transitional condition between the two. More recently, an imperfect animal model of motor neuron disease has been developed using murine retrovirus in wild mice (GARDNER et al. 1973). IFN itself was not detected in the spinal cord tissue of two ALS patients (JOHNSON 1976).

In summary, although conventional virologic techniques, including electron microscopy, immunologic survey, transmission experiments, and newer DNA hybridization techniques, have not definitively detected a virus, there is good indirect evidence to suggest an unconventional very slow or persistent viral infection as the etiology of at least some cases of ALS. Antiviral therapeutic agents still seem to be one of the most promising modes of therapy (SERVER and WOLINSKI 1982). In the absence of a good animal model for the human disease, most such drug trials have been on ALS patients themselves; unfortunately, these have been unsuccessful (FESTOFF and CRIGGER 1980).

To our knowledge, there have been only three reported trials of IFN in ALS patients. OLSON et al. (1978) used the IFN inducer tilorone (1 g/week) in 16 ALS cases in a double-blind, placebo-controlled study with no benefit after 4 months of therapy. W.K. ENGEL and H.B. LEVY (1977, unpublished work) used 50–270 m/kg PICLC i.v. in several patients, and RISSANEN et al. (1980) treated two ALS patients with 3×10^6 U/day s.c. IFN-α for up to 3 months. No beneficial effect was noted in either trial.

However, in view of the known impermeability of the blood–brain barrier to IFNs (especially in the absence of any inflammation), these trials cannot be considered definitive, and intralumbar or intraventricular therapy, alone or in combination with other agents, still appears to be worth pursuing; two such pilot trials are currently in progress in the United States. Given the probable variety of etiologies in the motor neuron diseases, one could hope for a response only in a certain portion of cases at best.

2. Alzheimer's Presenile Dementia

The Clinical and pathologic similarities between Alzheimer's disease and Creutzfeldt–Jakob disease (MASTERS et al. 1981; SALAZAR et al. 1982), as well as the reported transmission of a spongiform encephalopathy to primates from brain tissues of a patient with Alzheimer's disease (in the laboratory of D.C. GAJDUSEK and C.J. GIBBS) have fueled speculation about a possible viral etiology in this disease (REWCASTLE 1978). However, GOUDSMIT et al. (1980) have recently reviewed the subject with a detailed analysis of 50 other such transmission experiments in the same laboratory, and have concluded that an infectious etiology has not yet been demonstrated with any degree of certainty. No trials of IFN in Alzheimer's disease have been reported. In any case, the potential use of IFN in this disease must be considered in light of the negative results reported in the treatment of other slow virus diseases such as scrapie and Creutzfeldt–Jakob disease.

IV. Neoplasms of the Central Nervous System

The use of interferons in the treatment of CNS tumors has been limited, mostly because of the impermeability of the blood–brain barrier to the drug. In neoplasms that are very sensitive to IFN, or when there is marked disruption the blood–brain barrier (as in the neovascularity surrounding many malignant brain tumors) sufficient penetration of the drug after i.v. administration can be expected, but in most situations, intraventricular or intrathecal administration may be more advantageous.

BROSTRÖM et al. (1980) reported development of cerebral metastases in a young boy with osteosarcoma who had otherwise responded for 5 years to i.m. IFN-α. They concluded that the relapse was probably due to the impermeability of the blood–brain barrier. TREUNER et al. (1980), however, reported dramatic regression of a nasopharyngeal carcinoma with cerebral extension in a young boy treated with 4×10^6 U IFN-β i.v. and topically. Furthur trials are in progress, but have not been reported (NIETHAMMER and TREUNER 1981; CANTELL et al. 1981).

BILLIAU and DESOMMER (1980) treated a child with neuroblastoma unsuccessfully using 1.7×10^6 U IFN-β repeatedly, but SAITO (1981) reported in vitro sensitivity of a neuroblastoma cell line to IFN. A large study on 26 neuroblastoma patients is now in progress in Germany (NIETHAMMER and TREUNER 1981).

Meningeal leukemia has been treated with IFN unsuccessfully by several investigators. However, MISSET et al. (1981) reported using 1.3×10^6 U IFN-β intrathecally daily or every other day in five patients with meningeal relapse of acute lymphoid leukemia or leukemic lymphosarcoma and obtained complete remission in one patient after 11 injections. LUNDBLAD and LUNDGREN (1981) and COOK et al. (1983) reported in vitro inhibition of a glioma cell line by IFN-β, but L.G. SALFORD et al. (1981, unpublished work) treated five patients with malignant gliomas with 4×10^6 U IFN-α i.m. and intratumor via a CSF reservoir daily with no clinical improvement. At least three of their patients have died, but postmortem examination showed encapsulation of the tumor. NAKAMURA et al. (1982) have used the inducer PICLC in seven patients, with improvement in two. Trials of IFN-β in gliomas are currently in progress in Japan (SANO et al. 1983) and the United States.

In summary, only a few isolated attempts at IFN therapy have been reported in nervous system neoplasms. While most have been disappointing, encouraging results with invasive nasopharyngeal carcinoma indicate the need for furthur trials. Negative results with systemic therapy must be evaluated in light of the known impermeability of the intact blood–brain barrier to IFNs.

D. Conclusions

Although it may be premature to assign a place to IFNs (alone or in combination with other drugs) in the expanding treatment armamentarium of neurologists and related specialists, the excitement generated by the introduction of IFN into clinical use is likely to be well founded. The prophylactic management of rabies, the treatment of multiple sclerosis and related dysimmune conditions including certain chronic polyneuropathies, and the treatment of some CNS neoplasms are particularly promising areas. Selective use of particular IFN species now available through genetic engineering may be of value, especially in the dysimmune CNS diseases. The growing availability of purified IFNs, coupled with the repeated demonstration of their relative safety after intralumbar and intraventricular administration paves the way for further clinical trials, and ensures that many of the questions posed in this brief review will soon be answered.

Acknowledgments. Dr. SMITH gratefully acknowledges support of his work by a grant from the Thagard Oil Corporation and the Muscular Dystrophy Association of America. We also thank Dr. MARIE CLAUDE MOREAU-DUBOIS, and Dr. KARI CANTELL for their help and advice.

References

Abramsky O, Lisak RP, Silberberg DH et al. (1977) Antibodies to oligodendroglia in a patient with multiple sclerosis. N Engl J Med 297:1207–1211

Adams JM, Imagawa DT (1962) Measles antibodies in multiple sclerosis. Pro Soc Exp Biol Med 111:562–566

Anonymous (1969) St Louis Encephalitis. Lancet 11:1346

Anonymous (1980) Antiviral treatment of varicella zooster and herpes simplex. Lancet i:1337

Antel JP, Weinrich M, Arnason BGW (1978) Mitogen responsiveness and suppressor cell function in multiple sclerosis – influence of age and disease activity. Neurology 28:999–1003
Antel JP, Arnason BGW, Medof ME (1979) Suppressor cell functions in multiple sclerosis-correlation with clinical disease activity. Ann Neurol 5:338–342
Antel JP, Oger J, Arnason BGW (1981) Differences between antibody induced modulation of supressor cells and suppressor cell changes in multiple sclerosis. Ann Neurol 10(1):92
Arnason BGW, Waksman BH (1980) Immunoregulation in multiple sclerosis. Ann Neurol 8(3):237–240
Arvin AM, Yeager AS, Merigan TC (1976) Effect of leucocyte interferon on urinary excretion of Cytomegalovirus by infants. J Inf Dis 133:A205–212
Astrom KE, Mancall EL, Richardson EP (1958) Progressive multifocal leucoencephalopathy. Brain 81:93
Baer GM (1977) Antiviral action of interferon in animal systems-effect of interferon on rabies infections of animals. Tex Rep Biol Med 35:461
Baer GM, Cleary WFA (1972) A model in mice for the pathogenesis and treatment of rabies. J Infect Dis 520–528
Baer GM, Shaddock JH, Moore VA, Yage PA, Baron SS, Levy HB (1977) Successful prophylaxis against rabies in mice and rhesus monkeys – the interferon system and vaccine. J Infect Dis 136:286–294
Balkwill FR, Fitzharris P, Knight RA (1981) The role of interferons in effector T-cell generation. Antiviral Res Abstr 1(1):52
Behan P (1981) Interferon in treatment of subacute sclerosing panencephalitis. Lancet i:1059
Bellanti JA, Catalano LWd, Chambers RW (1971) Herpes simplex encephalitis. J Pediatr 78:136
Benczur M, Petranyi Gy, Palffy Gy, Varga M, Talas M, Motsy B, Foldes I, Hollan SR (1980) Dysfunction of natural killer cells in multiple sclerosis – a possible pathogenetic factor. Clin Exp Immunol 39:657–662
Billiau A (1981) Interferon therapy-pharmacokinetic and pharmacological aspects. Arch Virol 67:121–133
Billiau A, DeSommer P (1980) Clinical use of interferons in viral infections. In: Stringfellow D (ed) Interferon and interferon inducers. Decker, New York, chap 5
Bornstein MD, Appel SH (1965) Tissue culture studies of demyelination. Ann NY Acad Sci 122:280–286
Bornstein MB, Miller D, Teitlebaum D, Arnon R, Sela M (1980) Treatment of multiple sclerosis with a synthetic polypeptide – preliminary results. Ann Neurol 8(1):117
Brostrom A, Snorri I, Strander H, Soderberg (1980) Adjuvant interferon treatment and the late development of cerebral metastases in a patient with osteosarcoma. Acta Orthop Scand 51:589–594
Brown P, Sarragne C, Chany C, Gibbs CJ Jr, Gajdusek DC (1975) Tissue antagonists of interferon in primate brain. In: Geraldes A (ed) Effects of interferon on cells, viruses, and the immune system. Academic, London, pp 337–343
Burgasova MP, Andzhaparidze OG, Bektemirov TA, Bogomolova NN, Boriskin IS (1977) Effect of a poly I–poly C complex with poly-L-lysine on experimental tick-borne encephalitis. Vopr Virusol 4:438–441
Campbell AMG, Williams ER, Pearce J (1969) Late motor neuron degeneration following poliomyelitis. Neurology 19:1101–1106
Caminiti B (1980) Interferon and inducers of interferon – a bibliography of in vivo and in vitro studies with nonhuman primates. Primate Information Center. University of Washington, Seattle
Cantell K, Phyala L (1973) Circulating interferon in rabbits after administration of interferon by different routes. J Gen Virol 20:97
Cantell K, Phyala L, Strander H (1974) Circulating human interferon after intramuscular injection in animals and man. J Gen Virol 25:453
Cantell K, DeThe G, Gresser I, Huang WH, Klein G, Strander H, Zeng Y (1981) Plans for an interferon trial on patients with nasopharyngeal carcinoma in the People's Republic of China. Antiviral Res Abstr, 1(1):38

Catalano LW, Baron S (1970) Protection against herpes virus and encephalomyocarditis virus encephalitis with a double-stranded RNA inducer of interferon. Proc Soc Exp Biol Med 133:684–687

Cavet MC, Gresser I (1979) IFN enhances the excitability of cultured neurones. Nature 278:559–560

Chany C (1981) Perspectives in virology XI. Liss, New York, p 266 (discussion)

Cheeseman SH, Rinaldo Jr CR, Hirsch MS (1977) Use of interferon in cytomegalovirus infections in man. Tex Rep Biol Med 35:523

Cheeseman SH, Rubin RH, Stewart JA, Tolkoff-Rubin N, Cosimi AB, Cantell K, Gilbert J, Winkle S, Herrin JT, Black PH, Russell PS, Hirsh MS (1979) Controlled clinical trial of prophylactic human-leucocyte interferon in renal transplantation. N Engl J Med 300:1345–1349

Cheeseman SH, Black PH, Rubin RH, Cantell K, Hirsh MS (1980) Interferon and BK papovavirus-clinical and laboratory studies. J Infect Dis 141(2):157–161

Cohen SR, Hendon RM, McKhann GM (1976) Myelin basic protein in cerebrospinal fluid as an indicator of active demyelination. Arch Neurol 33:384

Connolly JH, Allen IV, Hurwitz LJ, Miller JH (1967) Measles virus antibody and antigen in subacute sclerosing panencephalitis. Lancet 1:542

Cook AW, Carter WA, Nidzgorski F, Akatar L (1983) Human brain tumor derived cell lives: growth rate reduced by human fibroblast interferon. Science 219:881–883

Cook SD, Menomna J, Dowling PC (1978) Serologic abnormalities in multiple sclerosis. Neurology 28(2):129–131

Dalakas MC, Engel WK (1981) Chronic relapsing (dysimmune) polyneuropathy-pathogenesis and treatment. Ann Neurol 9(suppl):134–145

Davydova AA, Shubladze AZ, Nusik NN, Bukata LA, Barinsky IF (1979) Experimental study of Viremia in Immune Host in Tick-Borne Encephalitis. Vopro Virusol 2:176–179

DeClercq E (1981) Antiviral potentials of interferon as opposed to other antiviral agents. Antiviral Res (Abstr) 1(1):32

DeClercq E, Edy VG, DeVlieger H, Eeckels R, Desmyter J (1975) Intrathecal administration of interferon in neonatal herpes. J Pediatr 86:736

Degre M, Dahl H, Janduik B (1976) Interferon in the serum and cerebrospinal fluid in patients with multiple sclerosis and other neurological disorders. Acta Neurol Scand 53:152–160

DeMayer E (1976) Interferon and delayed-type hypersensitivity to a viral antigen. J Infect Dis 133(Suppl):A63

DeMayer E (1981) Interferon and the immune system-an overview. Antiviral Res (Abstr) 1(1):17

DeMayer E, DeMayer JG, Vandeputte M (1975) Inhibition by interferon of delayedtype hypersensitivity in the mouse. Proc Nat Acad Sci USA 72(5):1753–1757

Denman AM (1980) Virus-Lymphocyte interactions and demyelinating disease. In: Boese A (ed) Search for the cause of multiple sclerosis and other chronic diseases of the nervous system. Verlag Chemie, Weinheim, 163

Emodi G, Rufli T, Just M, Hernandez R (1975) Human interferon therapy for herpes zoster in adults. Scand J Infect Dis 7:1–5

Emodi G, O'Reilly R, Muller A, Everson LK, Binswanger M (1976) Just: effect of human exogenous leukocyte interferon in cytomegalovirus infections. J Infect Dis 133:199–204

Engel WK, Cuneo RA, Levy HB (1978) Polyinosinic-polycytidylic acid treatment of neuropathy. Lancet i:503–504

Engel WK, Bernad PG, Levy HB (1981) Polyinosinic-polycytidylic acid poly L Lysine (Poly ICLC): a new anti-dysimmune effect remarkably beneficial in neuropathies. Neurology 311(2):154

Epstein L (1977) The effects of interferons on the immune response in vitro and in vivo. In: Stewart WE II (ed) Interferons and their actions, CRC, Cleveland, chap 6

Epstein LB, Cox DR, Lucas DO, Weil J, Epstein CJ (1981) The biology and properties of interferon-gamma – an overview. Antiviral Res (Abstr) 1(1):21

Fenje P, Postic B (1970) Protection of rabbits against experimental rabies by poly I poly C. Nature 226:171–172

Festoff BW, Crigger NJ (1980) Therapeutic trials in amyotrophic lateral sclerosis – a review. In: Mulder DW (ed) The diagnosis and treatment of amyotrophic lateral sclerosis. Houghton Mifflin, Boston, chap 22

Field EJ, Joyce G, Keith A (1969) Failure of interferon to modify scrapie in the mouse. J Gen Virol 5:149–150

Fog T (1980) Interferon treatment of multiple sclerosis patients – a pilot study. In: Boese A (ed) Search for the cause of multiple sclerosis and other chronic diseases of the nervous system. Verlag Chemie, Weinheim, p 490

Freeman JM (1968) Treatment of subacute sclerosing panencephalitis with 5-bromo-2-deoxyuridine and pyran copolymer. Neurology 18 (part 2):176

Freeman JM, Magoffin RL, Lennett EH, Herndon RM (1967) Additional evidence of the relation between subacute inclusion body encephalitis and measles virus. Lancet 1:980

Fridman WH, Vignaux F, Aguet M, Gresser I (1981) Interferon enhances "in vitro" and "in vivo" expression of Fc-gamma receptors – a possible mechanism for immunoenhanced effects of interferon. Antiviral Res (Abstr) 1(1):18

Gajdusek DC (1982) Foci of motor neuron disease in high incidence in isolated populations of East Asia and the Western Pacific. In: Rowland LP (ed) Human motor neuron diseases. Raven, New York, pp 363–394

Gajdusek DC, Gibbs CJ Jr, Alpers M (1966) Experimental transmission of a kuru-like syndrome to chimpanzees. Nature 209:794–796

Gardner MB, Henderson BE, Officer JE, Rongey RW, Parker JC, Oliver C, Este JD, Huebner RJ (1973) A spontaneous lower motor neuron disease apparently caused by indigenous type-c RNA virus in wild mice. J Natl Cancer Inst 51:1243–1254

Gibbs CJ Jr, Gajdusek DC (1971) Transmission and characterization of the agents of spongiform virus encephalopathies, kuru, Creutzfeldt-Jakob disease, scrapie and mink encephalopathy. In: Rowland LP (ed) Immunological disorders of the nervous system, vol XLIX. Williams and Wilkins, Baltimore, pp 383–410

Gibbs CJ Jr, Gajdusek DC, Asher DM, Alpers MP, Beck E, Daniel PM, Matthews WB (1968) Creutzfeldt-Jakob disease (subacute spongiform encephalopathy): Transmission to the chimpanzee. Science 161:388–389

Goudsmit J, Morrow CH, Asher DM, Yanagihara RT, Masters CL, Gibbs CJ, Gajdusek DC (1980) Evidence for and against the transmissibility of Alzheimer Disease. Neurology 30:945–950

Glick TH, Likosky WH, Levitt WH, Mellin LP, Reynolds DW (1970) Reyes syndrome – an epidemiologic approach. Pediatrics 46:371

Greenfield JG et al. (1954) Postencephalitic parkinsonism with amyotrophy. J Neurol NeuroSurg Psychiatry 17:50–57

Gresser I, Pattison IH (1968) An attempt to modify scrapie in mice by the administration of interferon. J Gen Virol 3:295–297

Gresser I, DeMaeyer JG, Tovey MC, DeMaeyer E (1979) Electrophoretically pure mouse interferon exerts multiple biologic effects. Proc Natl Acad Sci USA 76:5308–5312

Guggenheim MA, Baron S (1977) Clinical studies of an interferon inducer, polyriboinosinic-polyribocytidylic acid (Poly(I) Poly(C)) in children. J Infect Dis 136:50

Haahr S (1971) Virus inhibiting activity in the cerebro-spinal fluid from patients with acute and chronic neurological diseases. Acta Pathol Microbiol Scand 79:606–608

Haase AT, Ventura T, Gibbs CJ, Jr, Tourtellotte WW (1981) Measles virus nucleotide sequences: detection by hybridization in situ. Science 212:672–674

Habif DV, Lipton R, Cantell K (1975) Interferon crosses blood brain barrier in monkeys. Proc Soc Exp Biol Med 149:287–293

Hajnick AV, Boreck YL (1979) Antiviral and anticellular effects of interferon on the mouse embryonic cells transformed by viruses and/or chemical carcinogen. Acta Biol Med Ger 38(5–6):821–827

Hallum JV, Thacore HR, Younger JS (1970) Factors affecting the sensitivity of different viruses to interferon. J Virol 6:156–162

Harrington DG, Hilmas DE, Elwell MR, Whitmore RE, Stephen EL (1977) Intranasal infection of monkeys with Japanese encephalitis virus: clinical response and treatment with a nuclease-resistant derivate of Poly(I)–Poly(C). Am J Trop Med Hyg 26:1191–1194
Hattwich MAW, Weiss TT, Stechschuft CJ, Baer GM, Gregg MB (1972) Recovery from rabies a case report. Ann Intern Med 76:931–942
Hilfenhaus J, Ackermann R (1981) Endogenous interferon in the cerebrospinal fluid of herpes encephalitis patients (41047). Soc Exp Biol Med 166:205–209
Hilfenhaus J, Weinmann E, Majer M, Barth R, Jaeger O (1977) Administration of human interferon to rabies virus-infected monkeys after exposure. J Inf Dis 135:846
Hilfenhaus J, Damm H, Hofstaetter T, Mauler R, Ronneberger H, Weinmann E (1981) Pharmakokinetics of Human IFN beta in monkeys. J Interferon Res 1:427–436
Hirsh MS, Rubin RH, Cheeseman SH, Schooley RT (1981) Prophylactic interferon alpha in renal transplant recipients. Antiviral Res (Abstr) 1(1):29
Ho M, Nash C, Morgan CW, Armstrong JA, Carroll RG, Postic B (1974) Interferon administered in the cerebrospinal space and its effect on rabies in rabbits. Infect Immunol 9:286–293
Hofmann H, Kunz C (1972) The protective effect of the interferon inducers tilorone hydrochloride and poly I:C on experimental tick-borne encephalitis in mice. Arch Virol 37:262–266
Hooks JJ, Moutsopoulos HM, Notkins AL (1980) The role of interferon in immediate hypersensitivity and autoimmune diseases. Ann NY Acad Sci 350:21–32
Huddlestone JR, Oldstone MBA (1979) T Suppressor (Tg) lymphocytes fluctuate in parallel with changes in the clinical course of patients with multiple sclerosis. J Immunol 123:1615–1618
Ikic D, Smerdel S, Rajninger-Miholic M, Soos E, Justic D (1975) Treatment of labial and genital herpes with human leucocyte interferon. Proc symp clin use of interferon, Yugoslav Acad Sci Arts, Zagreb, pp 195–202
Iqbal A, Oger JJF, Arnason GBW (1981) Cell mediated immunity in idiopathic polyneuritis. Ann Neurol 9(suppl):65–69
Isaacs A, Rotem Z, Fantes KH (1966) An inhibitor of the production of interferon ("blocker"). J Virol 29:248–254
Jabbour JT, Duenas DA, Sever JL, Kres HM, Horta-Barbosa L (1972) Epidemiology of subacute sclerosing panencephalitis (SSPE). JAMA 220:959–962
Jablecki C, Cantell K, Connor J, Kingsbury D, Hamburger R, Westall F, Smith R (1981) Experimental treatment of ALS with interferon; pharmacokinetic studies. Ann Neurol 10(1):82
Jacobs L, O'Malley J, Freeman J, Ekes R (1981) Intrathecal interferon reduces exacerbations of multiple sclerosis. Science 214:1026–1028
Jacobs L, O'Malley J, Freeman A, Murawski J, Ekes R (1982) Intrathecal interferon in multiple sclerosis. Arch Neurol 39:609–615
Janis B, Habel K (1972) Rabies in rabbits and mice: protective effect of polyribocytidylic acid. J Infect Dis 125:345–353
Johnson HM (1978) Differentiation of the immunosuppressive and antiviral effects of interferon. Cell Immunol 36:220–230
Johnson RT (1976) Virologic studies of ALS: an overview. In: Andrews JM, Johnson RT, Brazier MAB (eds) Amyotrophic lateral sclerosis: recent research trends. Academic, New York, pp 173–178
Johnson HM, Stanton GJ, Baron S (1977) Relative ability of mitogens to stimulate production of interferon by lymphoid cells and to induce suppression of the in vitro immune response. Proc Soc Exp Biol Med 154:138–141
Jordan GW, Fried RP, Merigan TC (1974) Administration of human leukocyte interferon in herpes zoster. I. Safety, circulating antiviral activity, and host responses to infection. J Inf Dis 130(1):541
Joncas JH, Robillard LR, Boureault A, Leyritz M, McLaughlin BJM (1976) Interferon in serum and cerebrospinal fluid in subacute sclerosing panencephalitis. J Can Med Assn 115:309

Kadish AS, Tansey FA, Yu GSM, Doyle AT, Bloom BR (1980) Interferon as a mediator of human lymphocyte suppression. J Exp Med 151:637–650
Kaplan MM, Cohen C, Koprowski H, Dean D, Ferrigan L (1962) Studies on the local treatment of wounds for the prevention of rabies. Bull WHO 26:765–775
Katz M, Koprowski H (1968) Failure to demonstrate a relationship between scrapie and production of interferon in mice. Nature 219:639–640
Kern ER, Glasgow LA (1977) Effect of interferon on systemic herpesvirus infections. Tex Rep Biol Med 35:472
Kingsman SM, Samuel CE (1980) Mechanism of interferon action. Interferon-mediated inhibition of simian virus-40 early RNA accumulation. Virology 101(2):458–465
Kobze K, Emodi G, Just M, Hilti E, Leuenberger A, Binswanger U, Theil G, Bunner F (1975) Treatment of herpes infection with human exogenous interferon. Lancet I:1343–1344
Kovanen J, Haltia M, Cantell K (1980) Failure of interferon to modify Creutzfeldt-Jakob disease. Br Med J 29 March p 902
Krim M (1977) Prophylaxis and therapy with interferons. In: Stewart WE II (ed) Interferons and their actions. CRC, Cleveland
Kuehne RW, Pannier WL, Stephen EL (1977) Evaluation of various analogues of tilorone hydrochloride against Venezuelan equine encephalitis virus in mice. Antimicrob Agents Chemother 11:92–97
Leavitt T, Merigan TC, Freeman JM (1971) Hemolytic-Uremic-Like syndrome following polycarboxylate interferon induction. Treatment of Dawson's inclusion-body encephalitis. Am J Dis Child 121:43
Lebon P, Ponsot G, Aicardi J, Goutieres F, Arthuis M (1979) Early intrethecal synthesis of interferon in herpes encephalitis. Biom 31:267–271
Legaspi RC, Gatmaitan B, Bailey EJ, Lerner AM (1980) Interferon in biopsy and autopsy specimens of brain – its presence in herpes simplex virus encephalitis. Arch Neurol 37:76–79
Lennette EH, Magoffin RL, Freeman JM (1968) Immunologic evidence of measles virus as an etiological agent in subacute sclerosing panencephalitis. Neurology 18(1):2
Lerner AM, Bailey EJ (1981) In vitro susceptibility studies of antiviral agents in combination versus HSV-1 and HSV-2: Ara A, Ara Hx and interferon in several tissue cultures. In: Nahmias AJ, Dowdle WR, Schinazi RF (eds) The human herpesviruses. Elsevier, New York, p 670
Lisak RP (1980) Multiple sclerosis: evidence for immunopathogenesis. Neurology 30:99–105
Liu JL (1978) Effects of mouse serum interferon and interferon inducers on dengue and Japanese Encephalitis virus infections in weanling mice. Kobe J Med Sci 24:153–163
Lubiniecki AS, Armstrong JA, Ho M (1974a) Eastern equine encephalitis virus quantitative study of the effects of interferon on virus replication. Arch Virol 45:52–64
Lubiniecki AS, Armstrong JA, Ho M (1974b) The pattern of virus-specific peptide synthesis in rabbit cells infected with eastern equine encephalitis virus and its response to interferon (37944). Soc Exp Bio Med 145:1014–1017
Lubikova H, Brever S, Kocisova M (1979) Assay of interferon and viral antibodies in the cerebrospinal fluid in clinical neurology and psychiatry. Acta Biol Med Germ 38:879–893
Luby JP (1975) Sensitivities of neurotopic arboviruses to human interferon. J Inf Dis 132:361
Luby JP, Stewart WE II, Sulkin E, Sanford JP (1969) Interferon in human infections with St. Louis encephalitis virus. Ann Intern Med 71:703–709
Luby JP, Sanders CV, Sulkin SE (1971) Interferon assays and quantitative virus determinations in a fatal infection in man with western equine encephalomyelitis virus. J Trop Med Hyg 20:765
Lundblad D, Lundgren E (1981) Block of a glioma cell line in the DNA-replicative stage of the cell cycle by interferon. Antiviral Res (abstr) 1(1):55

Majer M, Weinman N, Hilfenhaus J (1977) The role of interferon in the prevention and treatment of rabies. Symp on prep stand clin use of interferon, Zagreb, Yugoslav Acad Sci Arts

Manconi PE, Zaccheo D, Bugiani O et al. (1978) Surface markers on lymphocytes from human cerebrospinal fluid-predominance of T-lymphocytes bearing receptors for the FC segment of IgG. Eur Neurol 17:87–91

Martin JR, Nathananson N (1979) Animal models of virus-induced demyelination. In: Zimmerman HM (ed) Progress in neuropathology, vol 4. Raven, New York, pp 27–50

Masson PL (1979) Humoral immunity in neurological disease. In: Karcher D, Lowenthal A (eds) Circulating immune complexes in neurological disorder. Plenum, New York, p 361

Masters C, Gajdusek DC, Gibbs CJ (1981) The familial occurrence of Creutzfeldt-Jakob disease and Alzheimers disease. Brain 104:535–558

Merigan TC (1977) Pharmacokinetics and side effects of interferon in man. Tex Rep Biol Med 35:541

Merigan TC, Rand KH, Pollard RB, Abdallash PS, Jordan GW, Fried RP (1978) Human leukocyte interferon for the treatment of herpes zoster in patients with cancer. N Engl J Med 298:981–987

Minato N, Reid L, Neighbor A, Bloom BR, Holland J (1980) IFN, NK cells and persistent virus infection. Ann NY Acad Sci 350:42–52

Miorner H, Landstrom LE, Larner E, Larsson I, Lundgen E, Strannegard O (1978) Regulation of mitogen-induced lymphocyte DNA synthesis by human interferon of different origins. Vir Imm 35:15–24

Misset JL, Mathe G, Horosewicz JS (1981) Intrathecal IFN in meningeal leukemia. N Engl J Med 305:1283–1284

Moretta L, Webb SR, Grossi CE, Lydyard PM, Cooper MD (1977) Functional analysis of two human T-cell subpopulations – help and suppression of B cell responses by T cells bearing receptors for IgM or IgG. J Exp Med 146:184

Moretta L, Ferrarini L, Cooper MD (1978) Characteristics of human T cell subpopulations as defined by specific receptors for immunoglobulins. Contem Top Immunobiol 8:19–53

Mueller WK, Schaltenbrand G (1975) Attempts to reproduce ALS in laboratory animals by inoculation of Schu virus isolated from a patient with apparent ALS. J Neurol 220:1–19

Mulder DW, Rosenbaum RA, Layton DD Jr (1972) Late progression of poliomylitis or forme fruste amyotrophic lateral sclerosis. Mayo Clin Proc 47:756–761

Nakamura O, Shitara N, Matsutani M, Takakura K, Machida H (1982) Phase I–II trials of Poly(ICLC) in malignant brain tumor patients. J Interferon Res 2:1–4

Narayan O, Penney JB Jr, Johnson RT, Herdon RM, Wiener LP (1973) Etiology of progressive multifocal leukoencephalopathy. Identification of papovavirus. N Engl J Med 289:1278–1282

Neighbour PA, Bloom BR (1979) Absence of virus-induced lymphocyte suppression and interferon production in multiple sclerosis. Proc Natl Acad Sci USA 76:476–480

Neighbour PA, Aaron EM, Bloom BR (1981) Interferon responses of leukocytes in multiple sclerosis. Neurology 31:561–566

Niethammer D, Treuner J (1981) The use of IFN-B as an antitumor agent in children. Antiviral Res Abstr 1:(1)35

Notkins AL (1975) Interferon as a mediator of cellular immunity in viral infections. In: Notkins AL (ed) Viral immunology and immunopathology. Academic, New York, p 149

Nozaki J, Atanasiu P (1975) Evaluation of interferon induced by rabies vaccines. Ann Microbiol 126(3):381–388

Olson WH, Simons JA, Halaas GW (1978) Therapeutic trial of tilorone in ALS: lack of benefit in a double-blind, placebo-controlled study. Neurology 28:1293–1295

O'Reilly RJ, Evrson LK, Emodi G, Hansen J, Smithwich EM, Grimes E, Pahwa S, Pahwa R, Schwartz S, Armstrong D, Siegal FP, Gupta S, DuPont B, Good RA (1976) Effect of exogenous interferon in cytomegalovirus infection complicating bone marrow transplantation. Clin Immunol Immunopath 6:51–58

Overall JC Jr, Spruance SL, Green JA (1981) Viral-induced leukocyte interferon in vesicle fluid from lesions of recurrent herpes labialis. J Inf Dis 143:543–547
Oxman MN, Takemoto KK (1970) Comparative interferon sensitivity of SV40 and polyoma virus. J Inf Dis 141:429–442
Padgett BL, Zu Rhein GM, Walker DL, Eckroade RJ, Dessel BH (1971) Cultivation of papova-like virus from human brain which progressive multifocal leukoencephalopathy. Lancet 1:1257–1260
Panitch HS, Hafler DA, Johnson KP (1978) Antibodies to myelin basic protein in multiple sclerosis: Clinical correlations. Neurology 28:394
Paty DW, Kastrukoff LF, Hiob L (1981) Chronic progressive multiple sclerosis has low suppressor cell levels. Ann Neurol 10:97
Pazin GJ, Armstrong JA, Lam MT, Tarr GC, Janetta PJ (1979) Prevention of reactivated herpes simplex infection by human leucocyte interferon after operation on the trigeminal root. N Engl J Med 301:225
Petrov PA (1970) V. Vilyuisk encephalitis in Yakut Republic (USSR). Am J Trop Med Hyg 19:146–150
Prange H, Wismann H (1981) Intrathecal use of interferon in encephalitis. N Eng J Med 305:1283–1284
Rewcastle NB, Gibbs CJ Jr, Gajdusek DC (1978) Transmission of familial Alzheimer's disease to primates. J Neur Exp Neurol 37:679
Reye RDK, Morgan G, Baral J (1963) Encephalopathy and fatty degeneration of the viscera, a disease entity in childhood. Lancet ii:749
Rissanen A, Palo J, Myllyla G, Cantell K (1980) Interferon therapy for ALS. Ann Neur 7(4)
Rozee KR, Lee SHS, Laltoo M, Crocker JFS (1979) A mouse model of reyes syndrome: The effect of emulsifiers (polyoxyethylene ether polymers) on the interferon response. In: Khan A, Hill NO, Dorn GL (eds) Interferon properties and clinical uses. Leland Fikes Foundation, Dallas, p 279
Rozee KR, Lee SH, Crocker JF, Digout AS, Arcinue E (1982) Is a compromised IFN response an etiologic factor in Reyés syndrome? Can Med Assoc J 126:798–802
Saito H (1981) Effect of interferon on induction of morphological differentiations in mouse neuroblastoma clone NB41A3 line cells. Antiviral Res (Abstr) 1:(1)54
Salazar AM, Engel WK, Levy HB (1981) Poly ICLC in the treatment of postinfectious demyelinating encephalomyelitis. Arch Neurol 38:382–383
Salazar AM, Brown P, Gajdusek DC, Gibbs CJ (to be published) Alzheimer's disease-relation to Creutzfeldt-Jakob disease and other slow virus infections. In: Reisberg B (ed) Textbook of Alzheimer's disease and senile dementia. Free Press, New York
Sano K, Masakatsu N, Takakura K (1982) Effects of HUIFN-β on gliomas. 3rd international conference for interferon research. Miami, November 1982
Santoli D, Moretta L, Lisak R, Gilden D, Koprowski H (1978) Imbalances in T cell subpopulations in multiple sclerosis patients. J Immunol 120:1369–1371
Santoli D, Hall W, Kastrukoff L, Lisak RP, Perussia B, Trinchieri G, Koprowski H (1981) Cytotoxic activity and interferon production by lymphocytes from patients with multiple sclerosis. J Immunol 126:1274
Sekellick MJ, Marcus PI (1980) The IFN system as a regulator of persistent infection. Ann NY Acad Sci 350:545–557
Server AC, Wolinski JS (1982) Approaches to antiviral therapy. In: Rowland LP (ed) Pathogenesis of motor neuron diseases. Raven, New York, pp 519–546
Shannon DC, DeLong R, Bercu G, Glick T, Herin JT, Moylan FMB, Todres ID (1975) Studies on the pathophysiology of encephalopathy in Reyes syndrome: Hyperammonemia in Reyes syndrome. Pediatrics 56:999–1004
Sibley WA, Tourtellotte WW (1968) Interferon assay of multiple sclerosis tissue. Trans Am Neurol Assoc 93:124–127
Singh B, Postic B (1970) Enhanced resistance of mice to virulent Japanese B encephalitis virus following inactivated vaccine and Poly I:C. J Infect Dis 122:339
Skurkovich SV (1981) The possible role of interferon inhibitor in the formation of remission in autoimmune diseases and allergy of immediate type (AI and AD IT) – hypothesis. Antiviral Res (Abstr) 1:(1)65

Sonnenfeld G, Mandel AD, Merigan TC (1977) The immunosuppressive effect of type II mouse interferon preparations on antibody production. Cell Immunol 34:193–206
Stephen EL, Scott SK, Eddy GA, Levy HB (1977) Effect of interferon on togavirus and arenavirus infections of animals. Tex Rep Biol Med 35:449–453
Stephen EL, Hilmas DE, Levy HD, Spertzel RO (1979) Protective and toxic effects of a nuclease-resistant derivative of polyriboinosinic-polyribocytidylic acid on Venezuelan equine encephalomyelitis virus in rhesus monkeys. J Infect Dis 139(3):267–272
Stewart WE II (1979) The interferon system. Springer, Wien New York
Stewart WE II, Sulkin SE (1966) Interferon production in hamsters experimentally infected with rabies virus. Proc Soc Exp Biol Med 123:650–653
Stewart WE II, Sulkin E (1968) Evaluating the role of interferon in rabies infection. Bacteriol Proceedings V:23
Strander H, Cantell K, Carlstrom G, Jakobson PA (1973) Clinical and laboratory investigations on man – systemic administration of potent interferon to man. J Natl Cancer Inst 51:733–739
Tachovsky TG, Lisak RP, Koprowski H et al. (1976) Circulating immune complexes in multiple sclerosis and other neurological diseases. Lancet 2:997–999
Taylor JL, Schoenherr C, Grossberg SE (1980) Protection against Japanese encephalitis virus in mice and hamsters by treatment with carboxymethylacridanone, a potent interferon inducer. J Infect Dis 142(3):394
Tevethia SS, Greenfield RS, Rieder V, Tevethia MJ (1979) Biology of SV40 transplantation antigen (TrAg). Inhibition by human interferon of expression of SV40 TrAg in SV40 infected monkey cells. Virology 95(2):587–592
Todaro GJ, Baron S (1965) The role of interferon in the inhibition of SV-40 transformation of mouse cell line 3T3. Proc Natl Acad Sci USA 54:752
Tourtellotte WW (1969) Cerebrospinal fluid immunoglobulins and the central nervous system as an immunologic organ particularly in multiple sclerosis and subacute sclerosing panencephalitis. In: Rowland LP (ed) Immunological disorders of the nervous system. Williams and Wilkins, New York, chap 8
Traugott U, Raine C (1981) Antioligodendrocyte antibodies in cerebrospinal fluid of multiple sclerosis and other neurologic diseases. Neurology 31:695
Treuner J, Niethammer D, Dannecker G, Hagmann R, Neef V, Hofscheider PH (1980) Successful treatment of nasopharyngeal carcinoma with interferon. Lancet i:817–818
Vandeputte M, Datta SK, Billiau A, DeSomer P (1970) The effect of Poly I:C on polyoma oncogenesis in rats. Eur J Cancer 6:323
Ververken H, Carton H, Billiau A (1979) Intrathecal administration of interferon in MS patients? In: Karcher S, Lowenthal A, Strosberg A (eds) Humoral immunity in neurological diseases. Plenum, New York, p 625
Vodopija I, Smerdel S, Bakalaic Z, Svjetlicic M, Ljubicic M (1981) Treatment of persons exposed to rabies with human diploid cell strain rabies vaccine and human leucocyte interferon. Antiviral Res (Abstr) 1(1):32
Wallen WC, Houff SA, Iivanainen M, Calabrese VP, Devries GH (1981 a) Suppressor cell activity in multiple sclerosis. Neurology 31:668
Weiner LP, Stohlman SA (1978) Viral models of demyelination. Neurology 28(2):129–131
Weiner LP, Herndon RM, Narayan O, Johnson RT, Shah K, Rubinstein LJ, Preziosi TJ, Conley FK (1972) Isolation of virus relate to SV40 from patient with progressive multifocal leukoencephalopathy. N Engl J Med 286:385–390
Weiner LP, Narayan O, Penney JB, Herndon RM, Feringa ER, Tourtellotte WW, Johnson RT (1973) Papovavirus of JC type in progressive multifocal leukoencephalopathy. Arch Neurol 29(1):1–3
Whittaker JN, Lisak RP, Bashir RM, Fitch OH, Seyer JM, Krance R, Lawrence JA, Chien LT, O'Sullivan P (1980) Immunoreactive myelin basic protein in the cerebrospinal fluid in neurologic disorders. Ann Neurol 7:58–64
Wiktor TJ, Koprowski H, Mitchell JR, Merigan TC (1976) Role of interferon in prophylaxis of rabies after exposure. J Inf Dis 133(Suppl):A260
Wisniewski HM (1977) Immunopathology of demyelination in autoimmune disease and virus infections. Br Med Bull 33:54–59

Wolinski JS, Dau PC, Buimovici-Klein E, Mednick J, Berg BO, Lang PB, Cooper LZ (1979) Progressive rubella panencephalitis: immunovirological studies and results of isoprinosine therapy. Clin Exp Immunol 35:397–404
Worthington M (1972) Interferon system in mice infected with the scrapie agent. Infect Immun 6(4):643–645
Worthington M, Levy H, Rice J (1973) Late therapy of an arbovirus encephalitis in mice with interferon and interferon stimulators. Proc Soc Exp Biol Med 143:638
Yabrov AA (1980) Interferon and nonspecific resistance. Human Sciences, New York
Yakobson E, Revel M, Winocour E (1977) Inhibition of SV40 replication by interferon treatment late in the lytic cycle. Virology 80(1):225–228
Zarling JM, Sosman J, Eskra L, Borden EC, Horoszewicz JS, Carter WA (1978) Enhancement of T-cell cytotoxic responses by purified human fibroblast interferon. J Immunol 121:2002
Zeman W, Kolar O (1968) Reflection on the etiology and pathogenesis of subacut sclerosing panencephalitis. Neurology 18(2):1
Zu Rhein GM (1969) Association of papova-virions with a human demyelinating disease(-progressive multifocal leucoencephalopathy). Prog Med Virol 11:185–247
Zu Rhein GM, Chou S (1965) Particles resembling papova viruses in human cerebral demyelinating diseases. Science 148:1477

CHAPTER 24

Clinical Investigation of Interferons: Status Summary and Prospects for the Future

J.U. GUTTERMAN

A. Introduction

The clinical investigation of the interferons has opened the door to an exciting new era in cancer research. Although the interferons are often touted as "immunologic agents," (and they do indeed have an important effect on various aspects of the immune system) it is critically important to focus on the profound changes directly induced by them on the biochemical and biologic behavior of tumor cells. So, since a variety of effects – including those on the immune system – are brought about by interferons, they should most accurately be considered biologic agents in the treatment of cancer. In this chapter, no attempt will be made to give an exhaustive summary of every published paper. Key references, however, will be noted.

Interferon was discovered as an antiviral agent in 1957. The way for the study of interferons in cancer was paved by the report of PAUCKER et al. (1962). In what is now regarded as the first major study in this area, it was shown that interferons had important antiproliferative activities. Further knowledge evolved slowly, however. In critically important studies GRESSER (1977) demonstrated that interferon was able to impede tumor growth in laboratory mice. STRANDER and his co-workers in Stockholm suggested that partially pure leukocyte interferon could delay the recurrence of osteogenic sarcoma in patients who had received definitive surgery and radiotherapy (STRANDER 1977). This was one of the first hints of the clinical potential of interferon in cancer patients, although a small number of patients with malignancy had previously been treated with very crude preparations of leukocyte interferon with questionable, but positive results.

B. Leukocyte Interferon (IFN-α)

While further clinical investigation in cancer was, for the most part, delayed by the tremendous scarcity of impure leukocyte interferon and the inordinate expense involved in producing such material for in-depth clinical studies, a few important pharmacologic studies were carried out. Studies with leukocyte interferon were conducted by STRANDER, CANTELL, and their associates (STRANDER et al. 1973) as well as other workers (JORDAN et al. 1974). These clinical investigations demonstrated that partially pure leukocyte interferon could safely be administered to patients by the intramuscular route, and that blood levels sufficent to suppress the growth in vitro of tumor cells were achievable. Additional commentary on the pharmacologic behavior of interferon will be made elsewhere in this book.

In 1978, MERIGAN and his group of scientists at Stanford and our group at M.D. Anderson observed that partially pure leukocyte interferon produced by

CANTELL and his co-workers at the Finnish Red Cross was capable of inducing regression of established tumor in patients with advanced malignancy (MERIGAN et al. 1978; GUTTERMAN et al. 1980). These observations, along with those published by STRANDER, led to a large grant from the American Cancer Society for further clinical research studies and brought increased awareness of, and enthusiasm for, the potential of interferon for cancer research. MERIGAN reported that three patients with nodular poorly differentiated lymphocytic lymphoma achieved partial remissions when treated with 10×10^6 U leukocyte interferon for 30 days.

MERIGAN'S results were similar to ours. We observed patients with advanced metastatic breast cancer achieve partial remissions. In the initial report, 7 of 17 patients treated with 3×10^6 U/day by the intramuscular route achieved substantial tumor regression, primarily in soft tissue regions. We achieved nearly the same results in patients with a B-cell neoplasm (nodular poorly differentiated leukemia) with a similar dose schedule. Both groups achieved little response with a less-differentiated lymphocytic tumor, histocytic lymphoma. Finally, multiple myeloma, also a B-cell neoplasm, was observed to be sensitive to leukocyte interferon by both the Swedish and our group (MELLESTEDT et al. 1979). Patients with advanced multiple myeloma achieved substantial regression in serum paraproteins, and/or secretion of abnormal light chains in the urine.

In the beginning these results were somewhat surprising, for experiments in tumor-bearing animals had never demonstrated regression in established metastases (GRESSER and TOVEY 1978). The minimum doses of interferon necessary for an antitumor effect in mice were considerably larger than those being given in the clinic. (Of course, it may not be possible to equate a unit of mouse interferon to a unit of human interferon in a meaningful fashion.) In addition, most of the preclinical studies had been carried out with fibroblast interferon (which may have contained small amounts of leukocyte interferon), but these early tumor regression experiments in the clinic were carried out with leukocyte interferon. The kinetics and biologic behavior of most of the murine tumor models, which have been important in the development of many anticancer chemotherapeutic drugs, may not necessarily be appropriate for the evaluation of biologic agents which work by mechanisms different from chemotherapy.

During the 3 years since these initial results with leukocyte interferon were reported, there has been increasing availability of partially pure leukocyte and fibroblast interferon for clinical studies of patients with varying malignancies. What follows is a brief review of these results, and subsequent to this is an outline of the more recent work with recombinant DNA-derived interferons. This chapter will conclude with a discussion of the many exciting laboratory and clinical studies that are now being carried out with newer preparations of interferon.

I. Malignant Lymphoma

MERIGAN'S group has published an updated analysis of results in nodular poorly differentiated lymphocytic lymphoma (LOUIE et al. 1981). Of 11 patients, 5 demonstrated sustained objective responses to partially pure leukocyte interferon. Some patients with Hodgkin's disease and chronic lymphocytic leukemia have also been reported to benefit from this material (GUTTERMAN et al. 1980; STRANDER et al. 1978; KRIM 1980; MATHE et al. 1981).

II. Acute Leukemias

There have been a few reports of transient benefical effects in patients with acute lymphocytic and acute myeloblastic leukemia. One of the first studies of the use of exogenous interferon to treat human cancer was reported by FALCOFF et al. (1966). They treated 18 patients with acute leukemia with very low doses of crude human leukocyte interferon and concluded it was well tolerated and appeared to increase survival time. The study was not controlled and no statistically significant results were reported.

HILL et al. (1979) reported on the treatment of patients with acute leukemia with buffy-coat-derived interferon. Five patients with acute lymphocytic leukemia (ALL), three with acute myelogenous leukemia (AML), and one with chronic myeloid leukemia (CML) in blast crisis received very high doses of $0.5–2.0 \times 10^6$ U/kg body weight for up to 2 months. One patient received 5×10^6 U/kg for 8 days and one received 10×10^6 U/kg on each of 2 days, 1 week apart. Interferon was given by intravenous bolus in divided doses. All five ALL patients receiving high doses of interferon responded with partial clearing of the leukemic blasts from the peripheral blood and bone marrow, as did two of the AML patients and the one patient in blast crisis of CML. Because of limited supplies, no patient could be maintained on interferon, and remissions did not prove durable after discontinuation of therapy.

III. Multiple Myeloma

More recent extensions of patients series with multiple myeloma suggest that the true response rate may be of the order of 25%–30%. The trials sponsored by the American Cancer Society confirmed the activity of interferon in multiple myeloma. Thus, OSSERMAN et al. (1981) using 3×10^6 U/day intramuscularly reported tumor response in 4 of 21 patients.

The suggestion that patients with IgA type myeloma may be more sensitive to partially pure leukocyte interferon has been made (H. STRANDER 1982, personal communication). In a study conducted to ascertain the effectiveness of fibroblast interferon, two patients who failed to respond to fibroblast interferon subsequently received leukocyte interferon. One of these patients showed a transient reduction in Bence Jones proteinuria (BILLIAU et al. 1981 b).

IV. Breast Cancer

In addition to the results of the studies conducted at M.D. Anderson, the American Cancer Society recently reported that, of 23 evaluable patients with metastatic breast cancer in a multiinstitutional study, there were 5 partial remissions and 4 improvements (BORDEN et al. 1982). Stable or progressive disease occurred in 14 of these patients. There was no correlation of response to estrogen receptor status, disease-free interval, or dose escalation to 9×10^6 U.

V. Other Tumors

A variety of other tumors have been assessed in pilot studies. These include malignant melanoma (KROWN et al. 1981), squamous and adenocarcinoma of the lung, brain tumors, colon and prostate cancer, etc. With the exception of those patients with lung cancer (STRANDER 1981), there have been anecdotal responses in many of these tumors.

Through the persistent work of FINTER and FANTES in the United Kingdom, a highly purified form of leukocyte interferon (IFN-α) has been developed for clinical studies. They used the Namalwa Burkitt's lymphoma cell line to produce large amounts of "lymphoblastoid interferon". This material contains at least eight of the species of leukocyte interferon (see Sect. D). Phase I studies demonstrated that this interferon is biologically and clinically active. Antitumor effects have been reported in a variety of human malignancies (PRIESTMAN 1980). Large doses of this material have been administered by the intravenous route as well (ROHATINER et al. 1982).

C. Fibroblast Interferon (IFN-β)

Clinical investigation of partially pure fibroblast interferon, although on the increase, has not progressed as rapidly as that of leukocyte interferon (STRANDER 1981). There have been several tumor types in which individual patients have achieved tumor regression. These include patients with breast cancer (POUILLART et al. 1982) both in Europe and Japan, nasopharyngeal carcinoma, and medulloblastoma. The response in patients with nasopharyngeal carcinoma (TREUNER et al. 1980) is particularly important, for this tumor has been associated with a possible viral etiology.

The pharmacologic behavior of this glycosylated molecule is quite different from that observed with leukocyte interferon. Following an intramuscular inoculation, low levels of interferon activity are detectable in the serum (BILLIAU 1981 a). Substantial amounts of fibroblast interferon, on the other hand, can be measured in the serum following intravenous administration. While large scale production of leukocyte interferon is now possible – due largely to the work of CANTELL – the large scale production of partially pure fibroblast interferon has not progressed as rapidly.

In contrast to the potential efficacy in solid tumors in a few patients, most patients with hematopoietic tumors have not, apparently, responded to fibroblast interferon (BILLIAU 1981 b). Lymphomas, myelomas, and perhaps other hematologic tumors may, therefore, be more sensitive to leukocyte interferon. Only further clinical evaluation will be able to verify this. There is some published evidence for tissue specificity for the interferons. STRANDER and co-workers first suggested that osteosarcoma cells were more sensitive in vitro to fibroblast than to leukocyte interferon. In contrast, lymphoma cells appeared more sensitive to leukocyte interferon than to fibroblast interferon (EINHORN and STRANDER 1977).

Although most of the interest has been focused on the use of interferon by systemic administration, positive results with topical treatment of localized tumors have been reported. As a result, intratumoral inoculation of leukocyte and fibroblast interferon has been associated with regression of local tumor. IKIC et al. (1981) have shown that topical treatment of several tumors, including breast cancer and cervical carcinoma, can produce responses to a very crude preparation of leukocyte interferon.

Other workers have achieved similar results with fibroblast interferon (STRANDER 1981).

D. Recombinant DNA-Derived Interferon

With the successful insertion of a gene for leukocyte interferon into *Escherichia coli* (NAGATA et al. 1980), there has been extraordinarily rapid development of recombinant DNA technology in the production of interferon in the last 2 years (GOEDDEL et al. 1980). Thus in 1982, numerous species of leukocyte interferon, and a single species of fibroblast interferon, have all been produced by recombinant DNA technology. In addition to this, IFN-γ has been expressed in *E. coli* (see Chaps. 7 and 22). A great deal is now known about the nucleotide and amino acid sequences of various interferons. Biosynthesis of interferons and their subsequent purification have increased the speed and depth with which clinical research can now be accomplished.

One of the remarkable facts of gene splicing has been the demonstration that leukocyte interferon is a multigene family. The previous clinical studies with leukocyte interferon had, therefore, been carried out with heterogeneous preparations. But there is now a plethora of interferons available for clinical investigation, and among the things to be investigated is the evaluation of human lymphoblastoid interferon, which can be produced on an industrial scale and purified by immunoaffinity chromatography.

The first clinical investigation of a recombinant leukocyte interferon species was reported recently (GUTTERMAN et al. 1982). A collaborative study by the University of Texas, M.D. Anderson Hospital and Tumor Institute, Stanford University, and Hoffmann La Roche, Inc. reported on the pharmacokinetics, single dose tolerance, and biologic activity of increasing doses of a single species of leukocyte interferon, the so-called IFLrA or IFN-α_2.

In this study, 16 patients with disseminated cancer received escalating intramuscular injections of IFLrA in doses ranging from 3 to 198×10^6 U. At the two lowest doses of 3 and 9×10^6 U, there was a crossover evaluation between IFLrA and partially pure leukocyte (IF-C) interferon prepared in Finland. The pharmacokinetics were studied by measuring serum levels of interferon by a modified cytopathic effect bioassay as well as an enzyme immunoassay. In general, the maximum observed serum concentration increased with increasing doses. The half-life ranged from 6 to 8 h regardless of the dose. And also in general, the mean serum concentrations of IFLrA and IF-C were similar. The clinical side effects of pure interferon were nearly identical to those described for naturally occurring partially purified interferon. These included fever, chills, myalgias, headache, fatigue, and reversible leukopenia and granulocytopenia. Minimal and rare abnormalities in liver or renal chemistry were noted. Eight patients noted transient and minimal numbness of the hands and/or feet. This was reversible in all cases. Three patients developed low titers of IgG antibody to IFLrA, although no clinical symptoms were noted. Of 16 patients, 7 demonstrated objective evidence of tumor regression during the study. Pure IFLrA was well absorbed after intramuscular administration, achieving appropriate serum concentrations with safety and tolerance at least as good as partially purified interferon. It appears to be a biologically active compound with effects on normal and neoplastic cells.

There were many scientific questions associated with the initial clinical study of so-called biosynthetic interferon. The first was whether or not an interferon protein devoid of carbohydrate would exhibit the same pharmacologic and biologic properties as the naturally occurring interferon. It is now known that most of the major leukocyte species are devoid of carbohydrate, and so, in retrospect, it was not surprising that the pharmacologic profile was similar to that achieved with heterogeneous preparations of leukocyte interferon (RUBINSTEIN et al. 1981). Based on studies carried out in monkeys, we had anticipated that IFLrA would not induce fever and perhaps many of the other side reactions seen with the crude preparations. We were wrong. Based on this study, as well as that carried out by SCOTT et al. (1981) with a purified preparation of buffy-coat-derived leukocyte interferon, most if not all the "toxic" side effects are due to the interferon molecule itself. It appears from the work of SCHELLEKENS et al. (1981) that tests in monkeys cannot be used to predict whether or not a particular human leukocyte interferon preparation will be pyrogenic.

The single IFLrA or IFN-α_2 species seems to retain important biologic properties of the multispecies preparations, including antiviral, antiproliferative, and immunomodulating activity (GOEDDEL et al. 1980; GUTTERMAN et al. 1982; EVINGER et al. 1981). Also, in the human studies, important effects on the hematopoietic system as well as tumor regression have been reported and confirmed (GUTTERMAN et al. 1982).

Subsequent phase I studies have now been completed and phase II efficacy studies in many tumors are now being conducted with the IFLrA or IFN-α_2. It seems that lymphomas may be as sensitive to IFLrA as to crude interferon. It is not clear at this point, however, whether other tumors such as breast cancer will be as sensitive to this particular species. It would not be surprising if some of the tumors known to be sensitive to the heterogeneous leukocyte interferon proved to be less sensitive to a single species. Recently, IFLrD (IFN-α_1) has also been introduced into clinical studies. It is anticipated that clinical studies with recombinant DNA-derived fibroblast interferon and IFN-γ will be initiated during 1983.

As of 1983, there is an increasing availability of all three major classes of interferon. Clinical phase I pharmacologic studies with partially pure immune interferon (IFN-γ) have recently been initiated at M.D. Anderson and the National Cancer Institute. Although the results of those studies have not been reported, they will serve as an important framework for subsequent studies with recombinant DNA-derived IFN-γ.

E. General Comments About Studies to Date and Future Directions

It is clear that patients with a variety of malignancies respond to differing doses of varying interferon preparations. Some patients have remained in partial or complete remission for 4 years or longer (GUTTERMAN and QUESADA 1982). With standard chemotherapy or hormonal therapy, such responses (i.e., well-documented *regression* of measurable tumor) are the hallmark of a potentially active approach to cancer therapy. Although most of the responses reported with single types of interferon in patients with advanced metastatic diseases have been less than complete remissions (i.e., complete clinical disappearance of tumor), there have been individual patients in whom this has occurred.

Not surprisingly, many patients treated with interferons have failed to respond. A common denominator for the lack of response or, for that matter, a positive response, has not been identified. Until large amounts of pure interferons became available, adequate dose–response studies could not be conducted in a sufficient number of patients. Therefore, the true efficacy of any particular form of interferon on any particular form of cancer could not be ascertained. Such studies in these areas are now under way. It should, however, be emphasized that, even with effective cancer chemotherapy, complete remissions for new drugs during phase I and phase II studies are not common. Only with the use of combinations of agents (i.e., combination chemotherapy) have significant numbers of complete remissions for a variety of cancers been reported. Of course, long-term studies to assess the effect on survival with so-called adjuvant studies have not been undertaken.

It should be pointed out at this juncture that most of the tumors reported to respond to interferon are frequently treated fairly effectively with chemotherapy. But patients with advanced breast cancer, nodular poorly differentiated lymphocytic lymphoma, multiple myeloma, for example, are rarely cured by chemotherapy. Thus, the need for developing new, original, and scientifically sound approaches to treatment is obvious. Recently, a human cancer that has proved to be unresponsive to most systemic therapy, metastatic renal cell carcinoma, has proven to be usually sensitive to partially pure human leukocyte interferon (QUESADA et al. 1983). Of 19 patients in one study at M.D. Anderson, 7 achieved at least a partial remission. These results have been confirmed by the UCLA urology group.

It has been my distinct impression from both our own experience and from reviewing the literature (EPSTEIN and MARCUS 1981) that the most sensitive tumors to leukocyte interferon are well-differentiated tumors that tend to be slowly growing, such as renal tumors, NPDL, or chronic myelogenous leukemia. Rapidly growing tumors, which tend to be more poorly differentiated (and are usually sensitive to chemotherapy) such as AML and histocytic lymphomas, tend to be resistant to interferon. Thus, the interferons will probably be active in several human tumors that respond poorly to chemotherapy. The reasons for the greater sensitivity of well-differentiated tumors are not clear, but they probably include the presence of a cell surface receptor for interferon, kinetic characteristics of the tumor, etc. It should also be kept in mind that the interferons might directly influence the differentiation of a tumor (KEAY and GROSSBERG 1980).

How will patients with different tumors be selected for treatment with the various interferons that will eventually be available? It will be nearly impossible to study each of the many species of leukocyte interferon adequately in the clinic. What is needed are preclinical methods to determine the biologic differences among these various gene products and to determine individual sensitivity of a particular patient's tumor to interferon (EPSTEIN and MARCUS 1981). One possible approach is the binding of these pure interferon proteins to cell surface receptors (ZOON et al. 1982). We now know that interferons bind to such cell surface receptors. The evidence to date suggests that leukocyte and fibroblast (type I) interferons bind to one receptor, and immune interferon or IFN-γ (type 2) binds to a separate receptor (BRANCA and BAGLIONI 1981). Although it is likely that the various leukocyte interferon species bind to the same receptor, the avidity of each species for the receptor may vary, depending on the tissue or tumor type.

It is not clear what in vitro biologic or biochemical parameter (or parameters) will predict that a tumor will prove to be sensitive to interferon in vivo. For example, there can be a disparity among the antiviral, antiproliferative, and antiretroviral activity (which probably measures changes at the membrane) of a particular interferon preparation. It certainly does not make sense to continue assessing only antiviral activity of an interferon preparation for anticancer work, but what should we measure? Recently, NASO et al. (1982) and CZARNIECKI et al. (1981) have suggested assessing the effect of interferons on retrovirus production.

It is also clear that measuring the ability of an interferon protein to induce 2′,5′-oligo(A) polymerase (also referred to as synthetase) or one of the protein kinases known to be affected by interferon does not necessarily correlate with antigrowth activity (FRIEDMAN 1981). Cancer is a heterogeneous disease, and only certain fractions of a given tumor population may be sensitive to interferon (LOETEM and SACHS 1978). Development of resistance to interferon has now been reported by several groups. LIN et al. (1982) suggested that the occurrence of a resistant phenotype was a nonrandom event. Resistant cells retained sensitivity to double-stranded RNA. Thus, the use of combination therapy will be important to deal with various clonal populations as well as to help prevent the development of resistant populations of cells.

The question which remains to be answered is: where will interferon research studies go from here? With the enormity of the work which still needs to be done, there are many directions in which interferon studies can go. One such example is the need to integrate the interferons into the mainstream of cancer therapy, for example, chemotherapy. It appears from preclinical investigation that chemotherapy and interferons may, at the very least, be additive in their effects against growing tumor cells. But the effects of interferon on drug-metabolizing enzymes must be considered before designing combination studies (SONNENFELD et al. 1980). Unfortunately, lack of support for the production of mouse interferon has precluded research on some of the types of studies with chemotherapy in preclinical models. But with the recent availability of a hybrid molecule consisting of two cloned leukocyte-derived interferon proteins which is active on mouse tissues (STREULI et al. 1981), these and other areas may soon be explored. Similar studies may soon be commenced in the hairless mouse as well.

The elucidation of the biochemical pathways of interferon's antiproliferative activities may be quite important for further clinical studies. For example, it is known that interferon inhibits the enzyme ornithine decarboxylase (ODC), an important enzyme in the polyamine pathway (TAYLOR-PAPADIMITRIOU 1980). With the recent availability of an irreversible inhibitor of the ODC enzyme, i.e., α-difluoromethylornithine (DFMO) (PRAKASH et al. 1980), interesting studies combining interferon and specific enzyme inhibitors are now possible. Besides the use of interferons alone or in combination with conventional therapy in patients with metastatic disease, it is plain that the use of these biologic agents in patients with minimal disease allows for exciting applications of these materials. One of the major limitations of current chemotherapeutic treatments is the failure to eliminate all neoplastic cells and to prevent recurrences or metastases in patients. But since the chemotherapeutic drugs and interferons have completely different mechanisms, the interferons may be quite important in eliminating the slowly growing tumor population (cells in G0 or G1 phases) (HOROSZEWICZ et al. 1979; CREASEY et al. 1980); chemotherapy tends rather to eliminate rapidly proliferating cells. Interferon may also reduce the opportunity for the emergence of clones resistant to drugs, and it may also be effective against cells that have already developed drug resistance. Because of the different mechanisms of action, interferons may be more effective in early than in late disease. Still, the recent report that interferons may increase the metastatic potential in vitro – at least in a single cell line of Ewing's sarcoma – should be kept in mind (SIEGAL et al. 1982).

Using interferons together is an interesting possibility for combination therapy. The possibility that two forms of interferon may be additive or synergistic has been suggested (FLEISCHMAN et al. 1980). This possibility arises from work which shows that IFN-γ can potentiate the antiviral, antitumor activity of type 1 interferons in the mouse and against human cells in vitro. It should also be remembered that immune interferon may have different efficiencies as antiviral and antiproliferative agents (RUBIN and GUPTA 1980).

Careful attention to the interactions of interferons and various growth and transforming substances, which are becoming more widely recognized, need to be investigated (TAYLOR-PAPADIMITRIOU 1980). For example, interferon inhibits the biologic effects of epidermal growth factor (LIN et al. 1980). The biochemical mechanisms for this inhibition have not been explained to my knowledge. The reports that interferon can induce phenotypic reversion of transformed cells (BROUTY-BOYE et al. 1981 a) and induce profound biochemical changes at the cell membrane and within the cytoskeleton are of great interest (BROUTY-BOYE et al. 1981 b). There is increasing evidence that the protein products of oncogenes, many of which are protein kinases which phosphorylate tyrosine residues, have major biologic effects on the cytoskeleton of cells. With the report that interferon may affect actin cables and vinculum, and the increasing evidence of the interaction of oncogene products and these cytoskeletal structures, might it be that interferons are affecting the functions of various oncogene products? Could there be specificity for these oncogene products? With the powerful gene splicing technology it is possible, in theory, to generate molecules that may have specificity for different tissues or different abnormal proteins responsible for neoplastic transformation.

In addition to the direct action of interferon on the tumor cell, the immunomodulatory effects may play a key role in the clinical antitumor effects reported (HERBERMAN et al. 1981). However, the monitoring of the function of specialized cells such as the natural killer cells, or macrophages, is unlikely to offer much insight for clinical studies. Although natural killer activity can be activated in patients receiving various interferon preparations, these changes are not necessarily consistent and suppression of activity has been reported. This may be desirable if interferon is changing the distribution of certain lymphocyte subpopulations from the circulation into the tissues (GRESSER 1981; REID et al. 1981). Activation of specialized cytotoxic cells may be most important when the interferons are studied in early stages of malignancy, before widespread metastases have developed. It is conceivable that they could be used in combination with monoclonal antibodies which might allow for more specific homing in of the monoclonal antibodies and increase their therapeutic efficacy.

We are somewhat ignorant of the best way to give interferon to patients, i.e., the optimal dose, route, and schedule. Although the belief that "more is better" is common, and massive doses of leukocyte and lymphoblastoid interferons have been given, it is not clear whether these very large doses (sometimes quantities as great as 0.5 mg pure interferon have been administered in a single dose) are superior to low doses. It is also not clear whether it is preferable to give interferon daily or intermittently. According to one point of view, giving large doses of a hormonal substance on a daily continuous basis would be less preferable than intermittent use, since receptors undergo modification (or downregulation) when continually exposed to large doses of a hormone.

Key biochemical events necessary to exert an antiproliferative effect may be inhibited by continuous exposure to interferon. The toxicity of large doses of pure leukocyte interferon can be formidable; severe fatigue, weight loss, anorexia, and other gastrointestinal symptoms might preclude the administration of such doses of interferon to many patients for any length of time, i.e., more than 2 weeks. When these factors are taken into account, it appears that intermittent pulsing schedules such as were developed for corticosteroids in the treatment of certain malignancies might be a preferable schedule and should be studied. Certainly, many studies employing interferon every second or third day are now under way. It is clear that daily doses of interferon are not required to induce important antitumor effects. It really should be emphasized here that this writer is not advocating that "high" doses (more than 30×10^7 U) are less effective than "low" doses ($3–10 \times 10^6$ U) for cancer. It is likely that each tumor will display a unique sensitivity pattern to interferon, i.e., some patients responding at low doses and some requiring larger doses for benefit.

The precise mechanism of myelosuppression is yet another area in need of investigation. Interferon-induced changes in lymphocyte distribution patterns in the body have been reported in animals (GRESSER et al. 1981), and the leukocyte interferons are known to suppress the white cell and granulocyte counts. In the clinical studies carried out at M.D. Anderson in breast cancer patients, and more recently in renal cell carcinoma patients, there has been an interesting correlation between the suppression of tumor growth and the suppression of the white blood cell and granulocyte counts. Whether this represents an intrinsic genetic sensitivity of normal and tumor cells to interferon in a particular patient, or indicates a biologic effect on differentiation in vivo is unclear (VERMA et al. 1979).

Interesting biologic effects can occur with fever which may affect key functions of tumor cells, but the precise role or necessity of temperature elevation in the clinical use of interferons has not been well studied (BOCCI 1980). Elevated temperatures can potentiate several biologic effects of interferons in vitro (DELBRUCK et al. 1980; YERUSHALMI et al. 1982); it is unclear as to whether the fever is an important component of the antitumor activity of interferon. While we are unsure of the cause of the febrile response, it is thought that it may result from induction of prostaglandins (YARON et al. 1977), but the role of prostaglandins in human cancer is also unclear. For example, the inhibition of prostaglandin synthetase (fatty acid cyclooxygenase) may interfere with the antiviral activity of interferons (POTTAHIL et al. 1980).

The other toxicities of interferon may also be quite important in ongoing research. The "fatigue syndrome" may be associated with important central nervous system effects, and this in particular deserves careful study. It is known that interferons in vitro, and now in vivo, can induce lupus-like inclusions in cells in vitro and in vivo (RICH 1981; RICH et al. 1983). With the recent report of circulating acid-labile IFN-α in patients with systemic lupus erythematosis and perhaps other autoimmune conditions (PREBLE et al. 1982), important pathologic consequences of administering large doses of interferon must be taken into account. The induction of antibodies to interferon, both by the natural fibroblast (VALLBRACHT et al. 1981) and leukocyte (TROWN et al. 1983), as well as by the recombinant DNA-derived molecules have been reported (GUTTERMAN et al. 1982). Autoantibodies to leukocyte interferon have also been reported (TROWN et al. 1983).

Infections are a common cause of death in patients with a variety of malignancies, including Kaposi's sarcoma in the immunocompromised host. STRANDER's early observations that interferons offered protection against viral infections need verification (INGIMARSSON 1980). Since interferons may also have bacteriostatic effects, the influence of interferons on other bacterial infections needs to be evaluated carefully. It is conceivable that high doses may inhibit antibacterial mechanisms.

More work in the area of cancer prevention is required. Prevention should be given special consideration in high-risk groups or premalignant cases. Certain benign cases such as juvenile laryngeal papilloma and other forms of warts respond to systemic interferon (HAGLUND et al. 1981). One patient who had both benign laryngeal papilloma and an associated malignant squamous carcinoma of the lung showed an interesting differential effect. There was complete resolution of the premalignant lesion, but no effect on the malignant lesion.

F. Conclusion

Our understanding of malignancy has increased tremendously during the last 5 years. With the advent of recombinant DNA technology, monoclonal antibodies, and other advances in biochemistry and cell biology and immunology, an improved understanding of cancer has occurred. It is anticipated that these insights will be increased over the coming years. The roles of cancer genes, their gene products, and growth factors and transforming substances are becoming prominent in the therapeutic strategy against human malignancies. Central to this, I think, will be the role of the interferons, the first natural cell-regulatory molecules that are clearly active in human cancer. Thus, the in-depth studies of the interrelationships of interferons with a variety of growth factors and transforming substances need to be evaluated. Although truly little of how interferons cause a regression of human cancer is understood at this time, the basic and clinical understandings of interferons are expected to progress rapidly within several years. It is my prediction that these powerful molecules will be looked upon as prototypical substances in the eventual biologic control and cure of malignancy.

Acknowledgments. This research was supported by Hoffmann La Roche, Inc. and grants from the Alfred and Mary Lasker Foundation, the Enid Haupt Foundation, the Interferon Foundation, and the James E. Lyon Medical Foundation. Research conducted in part by the Clayton Foundation for Research and the James E. Lyon Foundation. DR. GUTTERMAN is a Senior Clayton Foundation investigator.

References

Billiau A (1981a) Interferon therapy: pharmacokinetic and pharmacological aspects, brief review. Arch Virol 67:121–133

Billiau A (1981b) The clinical value of interferons as antitumor agents. Eur J Cancer Clin Oncol 17:949–967

Billiau A, Bloemmen J, Bogaerts M, Claeyes H, Van Damme J, De Ley M, De Somer P, Drochmans A, Heremans H, Kreil A, Schetz J, Tricot C, Vermylen C, Verwilghen R, Waer M (1981) Interferon therapy in multiple myeloma: failure of human fibroblast interferon administration to affect the course of light chain disease. Eur J Cancer Clin Oncol 17:875–882

Borden E, Holland J, Dao T, Gutterman JU, Wiener L, Chang YC, Patel J (1982) Leukocyte-derived interferon (alpha) in human breast carcinoma. The American Cancer Society phase II trial. Ann Intern Med 97:1–6

Branca A, Baglioni C (1981) Evidence that types I and II interferons have different receptors. Nature 294:768–770

Brouty-Boye D, Gresser I (1981) Reversibility of the transformed and neoplastic phenotype. I. Progressive reversion of the phenotype of X-ray-transformed C3H/10T ½ cells under prolonged treatment with interferon. Int J Cancer 28:165–174

Brouty-Boye D, Cheng YS, Chen L (1981) Association of phenotypic reversion of transformed cells induced by interferon with morphological and biochemical changes in the cytoskeleton. Cancer Res 41:4174–4184

Bocci V (1980) Possible causes of fever after interferon administration. Biomedicine 32:159–162

Creasey AA, Bartholomew JC, Merigan TC (1980) Role of G_0–G_1 arrest in the inhibition of tumor cell growth by interferon. Proc Natl Acad Sci USA 77:1471–1475

Czarniecki CW, Sreevalsan T, Friedman R, Panet A (1981) Dissociation of interferon effects on murine leukemia virus and emcephalomyocarditis virus replication in mouse cells. J Virol 37:827–831

Delbruck HG, Allouche M, Jasmin C (1980) Influence of increased temperature on the inhibition of rat osteosarcoma cell multiplication "in vitro" by interferon. Biomedicine 33:239–241

Einhorn S, Strander M (1977) Is interferon tissue-specific? Effect of human leukocyte and fibroblast interferons on the growth of lymphoblastoid and osteosarcoma cell lines. J Gen Virol 35:573–577

Epstein L, Marcus S (1981) Review of experience with interferon and drug sensitivity testing of ovarian carcinoma in semisolid agar culture. Cancer Chemother Pharmacol 6:273–277

Evinger M, Maeda S, Pestka S (1981) Recombinant human leukocyte interferon produced in bacteria has antiproliferative activity. J Biol Chem 256:2113–2114

Falcoff E, Falcoff R, Fournier F, Chany D (1966) Production en masse purification partielle et caracterisation d'un interferon destiné à des essais therapeutiques humans. Ann Inst Pasteur III: 562

Friedman RM (1981) Interferons, a primer. Academic, New York

Fleischman WR Jr, Kleyn KM, Baron S (1980) Potentiation of antitumor effect of virus-induced interferon by mouse immune interferon preparations. J Natl Cancer Inst 65:963–

Goeddel DV, Yelverton E, Ullrich A, Heymeker HL, Miozzari G, Holmes W, Seeburg TD, Dull T, May L, Stebbing N, Crea R, Maeda S, McCandliss R, Sloma A, Tabor JM, Gross M, Familletti P, Pestka S (1980) Human leukocyte interferon produced by E. coli is biologically active. Nature 287:411–467

Gresser I (1977) Antitumor effects of interferon. In: Becker F (ed). Cancer, a comprehensive treatise, vol 5. Chemotherapy. Plenum, New York
Gresser I, Tovey M (1978) Antitumor effects of interferon. Biochem Biophys Acta 516:231–247
Gresser I, Guy-Grand D, Maury C, Maunoury MT (1981) Interferon induced peripheral lymphadenopathy in mice. J Immunol 127:1569–1575
Gutterman J, Blumenschein GR, Alexanian R, Yap HY, Buzdar AU, Cabanillas F, Hortobagyi GN, Hersh EM, Rasmussen SL, Harmon M, Kramer M, Pestka S (1980) Leukocyte interferon-induced tumor regression in human metastatic breast cancer, multiple myeloma and malignant lymphoma. Ann Intern Med 93:300–406
Gutterman JU, Fein S, Quesada J, Horning S, Levine J, Alexanian R, Bernhardt L, Kramer M, Spiegel H, Colburn W, Trown P, Merigan T, Dziewanowski Z (1982) Recombinant leukocyte a interferon: Pharmacokinetics, single-dose tolerance, and biologic effects in cancer patients. Ann Intern Med 96:549–556
Gutterman J, Queseda J (1982) Clinical investigation of partially pure and DNA derived interferon in human cancer. In: The interferon system: a review to 1982. Part II. Tex Rep Biol Med 41:626–633
Haglund S, Lundquist PG, Cantell K, Strander H (1981) Interferon therapy in juvenile laryngeal papillomatosis. Arch Otolaryngol 107:327–332
Herberman R, Ortaldo JR, Rubinstein M, Pestka S (1981) Augmentation of natural and antibody-dependent cell-mediated cytotoxicity by pure human leukocyte interferon. J Clin Immunol 1:149–153
Hill NO, Loeb E, Pardue AS, Dorn GL, Kahn A, Hill JM (1979) Human leukocyte interferon responsiveness of acute leukemia. J Clin Hematol Oncol 9:137–149
Horoszewicz JS, Leg SS, Carter WA (1979) Noncycling tumor cells are sensitive targets for the antiproliferative activity of human interferon. Science 207:1091–1093
Ikic D, Kirhmajer V, Maricic Z, Jusic D, Krusic J, Knezevic M, Rode B, Soos E (1981) Application of human leukocyte interferon in patients with carcinoma of the uterine cervix. Lancet 1:1027–1030
Ingimarsson S, Carlstrom G, Cantell K, Strander H (1980) Virus infections and recurrence of osteosarcoma in patients receiving human leukocyte interferon. Int J Cancer 26:395–399
Jordan GW, Fried RP, Merigan T (1974) Administration of human leukocyte interferon in herpes zoster. I. Safety, circulation antiviral activity and host responses to infection. J Infect Dis 133:56–62
Keay S, Grossberg SE (1980) Interferon inhibits the conversion of 3T3-L1 mouse fibroblast into adipocytes. Proc Natl Acad Sci USA 77:4099–4103
Krim M (1980) Towards tumor therapy with interferons. Part II. Interferons: in vivo effects. Blood 55:875–884
Krown S, Burk M, Kirkwood J, Kerr D, Nordlund J, Morton D, Oestgen H (1981) The American Cancer Society clinical trial of human leukocyte interferon in malignant melanoma: preliminary results. In: De Maeyer E, Galasso G, Schellekens H (eds) The biology of the interferon system. Elsevier/North-Holland Biomedical, Amsterdam, pp 397–400
Lin SL, Ts'o P, Hollenberg MD (1980) The effects of interferon on epidermal growth factor action. Biochem Biophys Res Comm 96:168–174
Lin S, Greene J, Ts'o P, Carter W (1982) Sensitivity and resistance of human tumor cells to interferon and $rI_n \cdot rC_n$. Nature 297:417–419
Lotem J, Sachs L (1978) Genetic dissociation of different cellular effects of interferon on myeloid leukemic cells. Int J Cancer 22:214–220
Louie AC, Gallager JG, Sikora K, Levy R, Rosenberg SA (1981) Follow-up observations on the effect of human leukocyte interferon in non-hodgkins lymphoma. Blood 58:712–
Mathe G, Goutner A, Gastiaburu J, De Vassal F, Misset JL (1981) A phase I–II trial of treatment of chronic lymphatic leukemia by human leukocyte interferon. In: De Maeyer E, Galasso G, Schellekens H (eds) The biology of the interferon system. Elsevier/North-Holland Biomedical, Amsterdam

Mellestedt H, Ahre A, Bjorkolm M, Johansson B, Ahre A, Holm G, Strander H (1979) Interferon therapy in myelomatosis. Lancet 1:245–279

Merigan T, Sikora K, Breeden JH, Levy R, Rosenberg SA (1978) Preliminary observations on the effect of human leukocyte interferon in non-hodgkins lymphoma. N Engl Med 299:1449–1453

Nagata S, Taira H, Hall A, Johnsrud L, Streuli M, Escodi J, Boll W, Cantell K, Weissmann C (1980) Synthesis in E. coli of a polypeptide with human leukocyte interferon activity. Nature 284:316–320

Naso RB, Wu YH, Edbauer CA (1982) Antiretroviral effect of interferon: proposed mechanism. J Interferon Res 2:75–96

Osserman EF, Sherman WH, Alexanian R, Gutterman JU, Humphrey RL (1981) Human leukocyte interferon (HuαIFN) in multiple myeloma (MM): the American Cancer Society sponsored trial. In: De Maeyer E, Gallasso G, Schellekens H (eds) The biology of the interferon system. Elsevier/North-Holland Biomedical, Amsterdam

Paucker K, Cantell K, Henle W (1962) Quantitative studies viral interference in suspended L. cells. III. Effect of interfering viruses and interferon on the growth rate of cells. Virology 17:324

Pottahil R, Chandrabose K, Cuatrecasas P, Lang DJ (1980) Establishment of the Interferon-mediated antiviral state: role of fatty acid cyclooxygenase. Proc Natl Acad Sci USA 77:5437–5440

Pouillart P, Palangie T, Jouve M, Garcia-Giralt E, Fridman W, Magdelena H, Falcoff E, Billiau A (1982) Administration of fibroblast interferon to patients with advanced breast cancer: possible effects on skin metastases and on hormone receptors. Eur J Cancer Clin Oncol 18:929–937

Prakash N, Schecter P, Mamont P, Grove J, Koch-Weser J, Sjoerdsma A (1980) Inhibition of EMT6 tumor growth by interference with polyamine biosynthesis; effects of α-difluoromethyl-ornithine, an irreversible inhibitor or ornithine decarboxylase. Life Sci 26:131–194

Preble OT, Black R, Friedman R, Klippel J, Vilcek J (1982) Systemic Lupus erythematosus: presence in human serum of unusual acid-labile leukocyte interferon. Science 215:429–431

Priestman TJ (1980) Initial evaluation of human lymphoblastoid interferon in patients with advanced malignant disease. Lancet 2:133–

Quesada J, Swanson D, Trindade A, Gutterman JU (1983) Renal cell carcinoma: antitumor effects of leukocyte interferon. Cancer Res 43:940–947

Reid LM, Minato N, Gresser I, Holland J, Kadish A, Bloom BR (1981) Influence of anti-mouse interferon serum on the growth and metastasis of virus persistently-infected tumor cells and of human prostatic tumors in athymic nude mice. Proc Natl Acad Sci USA 78:1171–1175

Rich SA (1981) Human lupus inclusions and interferon. Science 213:772–775

Rich SA, Owens TR, Bartholomew LE, Gutterman JU (1983) Immune interferon does not stimulate formation of alpha and beta interferon induced human lupus-type inclusions. Lancet i:127–128

Rohatiner A, Balkwill FR, Griffin DB, Malpas JS, Lister TA (1982) A phase I study of human lymphoblastoid interferon administered by continuous infusion. Cancer Chemother 9:97–102

Rubin BY, Gupta SL (1980) Differential efficacies of human type I and type II interferons as antiviral and antiproliferative agents. Proc Natl Acad Sci USA 77:5928–5932

Rubinstein M, Levy W, Moschera J et al. (1981) Human leukocytes interferon: isolation and characterization of several molecular forms. Arch Biochem Biophys 210:307–318

Schellekens H, De Reus A, Bolhuis R, Fountoulakis M, Schein C, Escodi J, Nagata S, Weissman C (1981) Comparison of the antiviral efficiency in rhesus monkeys of human interferon-α 2 from E. coli. Nature 292:775–776

Scott GM, Secher DS, Flowers D, Bate J, Cantell K, Tyrrell DAJ (1981) Toxicity of interferon. Br Med J 282:1345–1348

Siegal GP, Thorgeirsson UP, Russo R, Wallace D, Liotta L, Berger S (1982) Interferon enhancement of the invasive capacity of Ewing sarcoma cells in vitro. Proc Natl Acad Sci USA 79:4064–4068

Sonnenfeld G, Harned C, Thaniyavarn S, Huff T, Mandel AD, Nerland DE (1980) Type II interferon induction and passive transfer depress and the murine cytochrome P-450 drug metabolism system. Antimicrob Agents Chemother 17:969–972

Strander H (1977) Interferons: anti-neoplastic drugs? Blut 35:277–288

Strander H (1978) Anti-tumor effects of interferon and its possible use as an anti-neoplastic agent in man. The interferon system: a current review to 1978

Strander H (1981) Clinical trials conducted with interferon on tumor patients in Europe. In: De Maeyer E, Galasso G, Schellekens H (eds) The biology of the interferon system. Elsevier/North-Holland Biomedical, Amsterdam, pp 383–390

Strander H, Cantell K, Carlston G, Jakobsson P (1973) Clinical and laboratory investigations of man: systemic administration of potent interferon to man. J Natl Cancer Inst 51:733–742

Streuli M, Hall A, Boll W, Stewart II WE, Nagata S, Weissman C (1981) Target cell specificity of 2 species of human interferon-α produced in Escherichia coli of hybrid molecules derived from them. Proc Natl Acad Sci USA 78:2949–2952

Taylor-Papadimitriou J (1980) Effects of interferon on cell growth and function. In: *Interferon 1980* I. Gresser, ed. 2:13 London: Academic Press

Treuner J, Neithammer D, Dannecker G, Hagmann R, Neef V, Hofschneider PH (1980) Successful treatment of nasopharyngeal carcinoma with interferon. Lancet 1:817–818

Trown PW, Kramer MJ, Dennin Jr RA, Connell EV, Palleroni AV, Quesada JR, Gutterman JU (1983) Antibodies to natural recombinant human leukocyte interferons (HuIFN-α s) in cancer patients. Lancet i:81–83

Vallbracht A, Treuner J, Flehmig B, Joester KE, Niethammer D (1981) Interferon-neutralizing antibodies in a patient treated with human fibroblast interferon. Nature 289:496–497

Verma D, Spitzer G, Gutterman J, Zander A, McCredie K, Dicke K (1979) Human leukocyte interferon preparation blocks granulopoietic differentiation. Blood 54:1423–1427

Yaron M, Yaron I, Gurari-Rotman D, Revel M, Lindner HR, Zor U (1977) Stimulation of prostaglandin E. production in cultured human fibroblasts by poly I·C and human interferon. Nature 257:457–459

Yerushalmi A, Tovey M, Gresser I (1982) Antitumor effect of combined interferon and hyperthermia in mice (41367). Proc Soc Exp Biol Med 169:413–415

Zoon K, Zur Nedden D, Arnheiter H (1982) Specific binding of human α interferon to a high affinity cell surface binding site on bovine kidney cells. J Biol Chem 257:4695–4697

CHAPTER 25

Utilization of Stabilized Forms of Polynucleotides

H.B. LEVY and F.L. RILEY

A. Introduction

Within a few years after the description of interferon by ISAACS and LINDENMANN (1957), it was recognized that interferon potentially was a broad-spectrum antiviral agent of possibly high value in clinical medicine. However, the difficulty of preparing enough interferon, either nonhuman or human, prevented the adequate testing of this potentiality. Serious efforts were made to find nonreplicating agents that would cause the host to synthesize its own interferon in large quantity. While a number of compounds were found that are capable of causing mice, and possibly humans, to make interferon, they either induced too small amounts or were too toxic (MERIGAN 1973). FIELD et al. (1967) reported that a number of natural and synthetic double-stranded (ds) RNAs are capable of inducing interferon. In particular, the dsRNA polyinosinic·polycytidylic acid (poly(I)·poly(C)) was highly effective in rodents as an interferon inducer (FIELD et al. 1967), as an antiviral agent (PARKS and BARON 1968; WORTHINGTON et al. 1973) and as an antitumor agent (ZELEZINCK and BHUYAN 1969; LEVY et al. 1969).

Preclinical toxicity studies led to phase I trials in cancer patients in two studies (ROBINSON et al. 1976; YOUNG 1971). Toxicity was very mild, but there were only very low levels of interferon induced, and no antitumor action was found. In monkeys and in chimpanzees, no interferon was induced by poly(I)·poly(C) (H.B. LEVY and C.J. GIBBS 1972, unpublished work).

Like most dsRNAs, poly(I)·poly(C) is pyrogenic in rabbits. Figure 1 shows the fever response curve of a rabbit injected with poly(I)·poly(C). If poly(I)·poly(C) is incubated with human serum (or ribonuclease), the ability of the compound to elicit fever in rabbits is lost, as shown in Fig. 2. Associated with this loss of pyrogenicity is a loss of interferon-inducing capacity (NORDLUND et al. 1970). The dsRNA is hydrolyzed to smaller oligonucleotides, including acid-soluble products.

The ability to hydrolyze poly(I)·poly(C) is much greater in human serum than in mouse serum. In general, animal species that have high hydrolytic capacity are poor responders to poly(I)·poly(C), and good responders have low hydrolytic capacity. While these observations are consistent with the idea that there is a cause-and-effect relationship between hydrolytic capacity and interferon production, they certainly do not establish such a cause-and-effect relationship. One of the points that will be emphasized in this chapter deals with the frequency with which hydrolysis resistance of a polynucleotide is associated with its ability to induce interferon in primates.

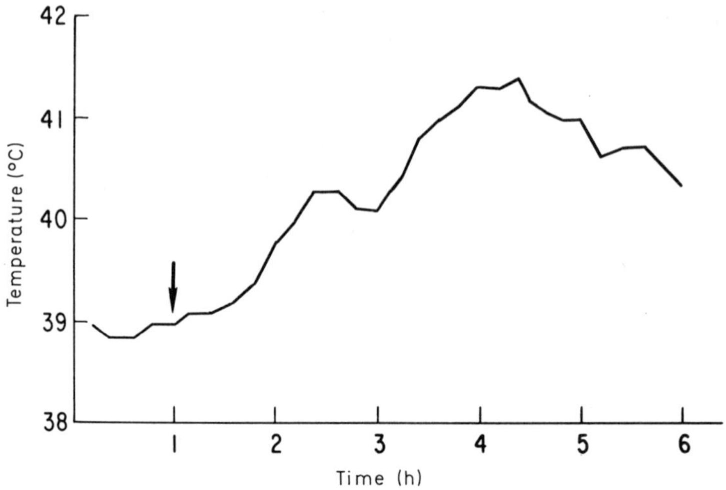

Fig. 1. Fever response in rabbits (mean of three) after intravenous injection (*arrow*) of 30 μg poly(I)·poly(C) in 0.17 ml 0.15 *M* pyrogen-free saline

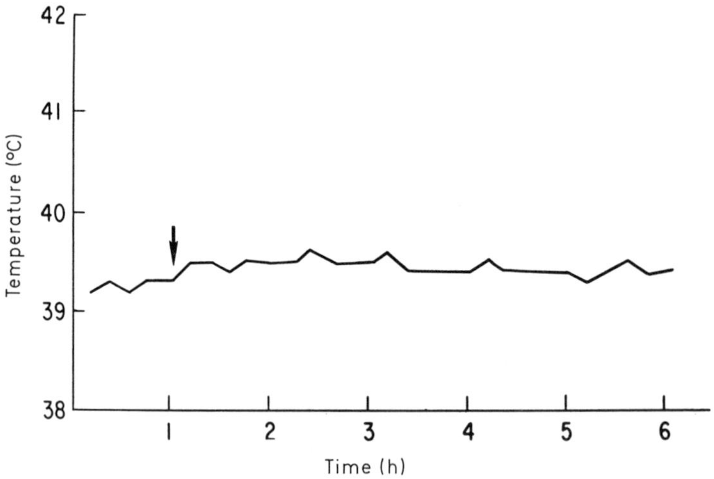

Fig. 2. Fever response in rabbits (mean of three) after intravenous injection of 30 μg poly(I)·poly(C) in 0.15 ml 0.15 *M* pyrogen-free saline that had been treated with 20 μg/ml pancreatic ribonuclease plus 30 U/ml T_1 ribonuclease

In general, two approaches have been used to prepare polynucleotide inducers that are at least partially protected from hydrolysis. One involves making the dsRNA from modified nucleotides with the hope that such a dsRNA will be more resistant to hydrolysis. The other is to complex the dsRNA with another substance with the same goal in mind. Examples of both approaches follow.

B. Thiolated Derivatives

There is a group of sulfur-containing dsRNAs that are more resistant to hydrolysis than is plain poly(I)·poly(C). They are of two types. One has the sulfur as a side chain in the pyrimidine ring, and the other has the sulfur substituting for one of the oxygens in the phosphate backbone, yielding thiophosphate groups. The general conclusion from these studies is that such substitution does not appear to offer any significant clinical advantage over nonthiolated compounds. Thioketo substitution in the 2 position in uracil or cytosine in poly(U) or poly(C) greatly increased the resistance to hydrolysis of the dsRNA made by subsequent complexing with poly(A) or poly(I), respectively. In general, thioketo substitution also raised the thermal denaturation or "melting" temperature T_m over that of the unsubstituted polynucleotide (REUSS et al. 1976). There was, however, no regular alteration in the amount of interferon induced as a result of such changes. There were both increases and decreases, depending on: (1) the test system used, tissue culture cells in vitro or rabbit or dogs in vivo; and (2) the particular chemical complexes studied.

In a somewhat related study, poly(C) with 1%–10% of the poly(C) substituted by 5-mercaptocytosine was prepared and annealed with poly(I). In general, the larger the amount of substituted base, the lower was the T_m. Also, in general, the poorer was the interferon induction in tissue culture. On hydrolysis with ribonuclease, the thiolated compounds yielded larger fragments (O'MALLEY et al. 1975).

Somewhat more encouraging results were obtained at first with compounds in which each phosphate was replaced by a thiophosphate. Such thiophosphate derivatives were 0.1–0.01 as sensitive to hydrolysis by various enzymes and were significantly better as interferon inducers both in tissue culture and in rabbits than were the unsubstituted compounds (DECLERCQ et al. 1969). Later studies, however, showed that greater in vivo toxicity of the thiophosphates minimized any potential clinical advantage they might have offered (T.C. MERIGAN, personal communication). There are several difficulties inherent in all the studies with sulfur-containing polynucleotides. It is apparent that many specific structural factors are important in determining whether a given compound will induce interferon in any test system. When one substitutes a sulfur for an oxygen, one changes the chemical specificity as well as resistance to hydrolysis and T_m. It is not easy to distinguish which of these factors may be responsible for any increase or decrease in the interferon-inducing capacity of the modified complexes. In addition, increased resistance to hydrolysis becomes important from a clinical viewpoint only when dealing with certain animal species, particularly primates. Primate sera have a relatively high hydrolytic capacity for dsRNA. Poly(I)·poly(C) is a good interferon inducer in rodents, but not in primates – see Sect. F. In none of the studies on the sulfur-containing analogs was in vivo interferon-inducing capacity in primates tested.

C. DEAE-Dextran

A different approach to enhancing the action of dsRNA was taken by DIANZANI et al. (1968). It had previously been observed that treatment of cells with polybasic substances, such as diethylaminoethyl (DEAE)-dextran enhanced the infectivity of viral RNA, presumably by facilitating the uptake of the infectious RNA. Working on the hypothesis that cellular uptake of poly(I)·poly(C) is necessary for it to be effective as an interferon inducer, DIANZANI et al. treated mouse L-cells with 10 μg/ml poly(I)·poly(C) with and without 400 μg/ml DEAE-dextran added immediately prior to the inducer. The L-cells did not respond to 10 μg/ml plain poly(I)·poly(C), but those cultures that had DEAE-dextran in addition to the poly(I)·poly(C) yielded 300 U/ml interferon. The mechanism of this enhancement, however, appears to be complicated. One can prepare a complex of poly(I)·poly(C) with DEAE-dextran simply by mixing the two in proper proportions. Such a complex is more resistant to hydrolysis by RNase than is plain poly(I)·poly(C). When this dextran complex is administered to mice it elicits ten times more serum interferon than does poly(I)·poly(C). It is also more effective in L-cells than is the uncomplexed dsRNA.

On the basis of these data, it would appear that the enhanced resistance to hydrolysis may play an important role in increasing the effectiveness of poly(I)·poly(C) as an inducer. However, treatment of L-cells with DEAE-dextran before adding the stabilized inducer leads to still higher effectiveness. That the L-cell membranes are modified by treatment with DEAE-dextran is indicated because such treated cells are extremely resistant to swelling by water, and to disruption with a Dounce homogenizer (H.B. LEVY, F.L. RILEY, and DIANZANI 1976, unpublished work). It could indeed be that the DEAE-dextran-treated cell does allow uptake of the inducer, but it could also be that DEAE-dextran is bound at the surface of the cell and gives additional protection against nucleases on the cell membrane. Dextran sulfate, an anionic polymer that rapidly combines with DEAE-dextran, a cationic polymer, very rapidly removes the enhancing action of DEAE-dextran on the cell. However, this observation does not sharply distinguish between the two possible explanations – enhanced uptake or increased resistance to hydrolysis.

A number of basic substances in addition to DEAE-dextran, including neomycin, protamine, histone, and methylated albumin all have been shown to enhance the action of poly(I)·poly(C) in tissue culture and in some instances in mice (BILLIAU et al. 1970). One problem with all these preparations, however, is that they are very insoluble ($\leqq 10^{-5}$ *M*), and yield precipitates at higher concentrations. Not surprisingly, such complexes act as better antiviral agents than uncomplexed poly(I)·poly(C), both in tissue culture and in mice. They have not been studied for toxic effects, nor have they been tested in primates.

D. Liposomes

A procedure which augments the induction of interferon by poly(I)·poly(C) is the inclusion of the dsRNA into liposomes (STRAUB et al. 1974). Both negatively and positively charged liposomes were toxic to L-cells and, therefore, their effectiveness could not be determined. However, when given to mice, both types increased interferon production by poly(I)·poly(C) by 5- to 15-fold, with positive liposomes being somewhat more effective than negative ones. Radioactive tracing techniques revealed that both the lipid and their poly(I)·poly(C) component were rapidly cleared from the bloodstream and were concentrated in the liver. The rate of degradation to acid-soluble components of poly(I)·poly(C) in liposomes was slower than that of unprotected poly(I)·poly(C). The increased inducing activity, therefore, might have been due to increased cellular uptake as well as greater resistance to hydrolyses. No studies of in vivo toxicity were reported, nor were there reports of studies in primates.

E. Stabilization with Polylysine

RICE et al. (1970) showed that the addition of poly-D-lysine ($\sim 10^5$ daltons) to poly(I)·poly(C) (6 *S*) increased the interferon-inducing capacity in mice by about 5- to 10-fold. However, the poly-D-lysine complex with this low molecular weight poly(I)·poly(C) was not significantly better than plain poly(I)·poly(C) made with 9 *S* homopolymers. When poly-D-lysine was added to 9 *S* poly(I)·poly(C), a precipitate was formed at all concentrations greater than about 10^{-5} *M*.

Some 8 years before the role of dsRNA in interferon induction was appreciated, FELSENFELD and HUANG (1959) described the formation of a stable complex between a dsRNA (A+U) and polylysine. TSUBOI et al. (1966) later studied extensively the interaction of poly-L-lysine with poly(I)·poly(C). These latter studies were done at low ionic concentrations and at very low concentrations of poly(I)·–poly(C) ($\sim 5.0 \times 10^{-5}$ *M*) and poly-L-lysine ($\sim 2.25 \times 10^{-5}$ *M*). The complex was formed at room temperature. The poly-L-lysine used in these complexes was of a high molecular weight (60–90,000). These investigators reported the binding reaction of poly-L-lysine to polynucleotide to be quantitative, irreversible, and with a definite stoichiometric ratio. The poly-L-lysine: poly(I)·poly(C) ratio at these concentrations was 0.5 NH_2: 1 PO_4. The thermal denaturation profile of this complex was found to be a one-step transition with a T_m at about 89 °C in a solvent which contained 0.05 *M* NaCl+0.001 *M* Na citrate ($\sim 0.3 \times$ standard saline–citrate). Complexes formed between poly(I)·poly(C) and poly-L-lysine with less poly-L-lysine than the 0.5 NH_2: 1:üPO_4 ratio gave two-step thermal denaturation profiles with T_m at 57° and 89 °C. The lower temperature T_m indicated that there was still free poly(I)·poly(C).

TSUBOI et al. (1966) also proposed a model for the poly(I)·poly(C)–poly-L-lysine complex. Knowing that in the A form of poly(I)·poly(C), the translation distance along the helix axis per nucleotide pair is 3.0 Å, they concluded that poly-L-lysine would probably wind around the double-helical poly(I)·poly(C) core in a helix fully extended with a long pitch at about 28° to the helix axis of poly(I)·poly(C).

It is of interest to note that the model proposed by these authors for poly-L-lysine–DNA complex is quite different from the RNA–poly-L-lysine model described. They concluded that a molecular model similar to that of deoxyribonucleoprotamine proposed by WILKINS (1956) would be acceptable for the poly-L-lysine–DNA complex. In this model, an almost fully extended polypeptide chain also winds helically around the double-stranded polynucleotide chains. Unlike the RNA model, however, the pitch of the polypeptide helix is the same as that of the polynucleotide helices. This model requires one amino acid residue per nucleotide residue, i.e., NH_2: PO_4 = 1: 1, as is experimentally observed. On the other hand, this model would not be acceptable for poly(I)·poly(C)–poly-L-lysine complex, where NH_2: PO_4 ratio is 0.5: 1.

Additional studies were later done by HAYNES et al. (1970) on complexes of DNA, RNA and synthetic polynucleotides (A+U) and (I+C), with poly-L-lysine

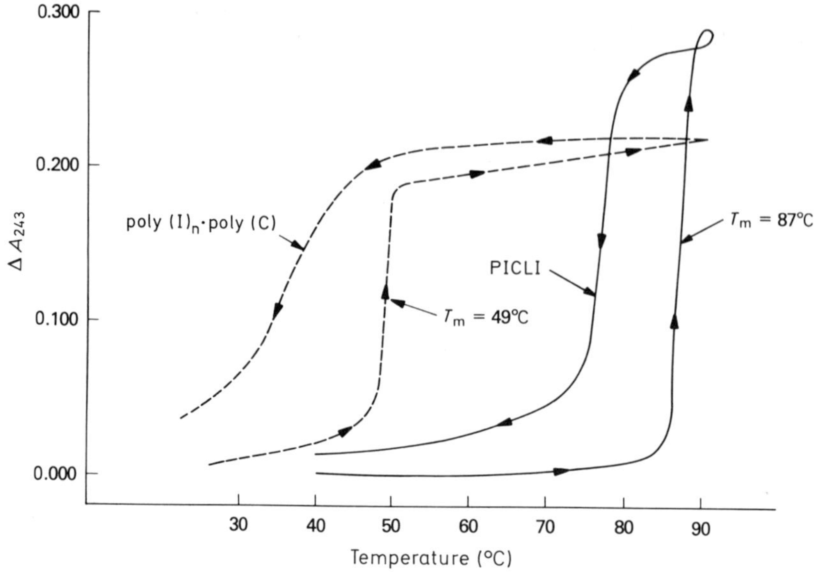

Fig. 3. Thermal denaturation of poly(I)·poly(C) and the poly-L-lysine complex of poly(I)·–poly(C) (PICLC). The compounds, at a poly(I)·poly(C) concentration of 50 µg/ml in 0.1 × standard saline–citrate, were heated to the indicated temperatures (T_m) in a recording spectrophotometer set at 243 n

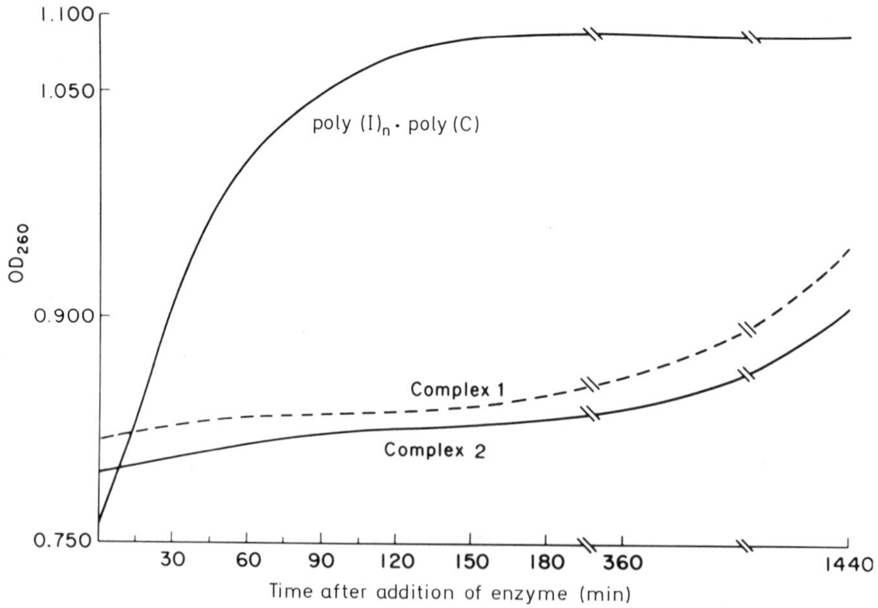

ig. 4. Hydrolysis by ribonuclease of PICLC complex compared with poly(I)·poly(C). Hy-rolysis of poly(I)·poly(C) and two different lots of poly-L-lysine complex by pancreatic Nase. The complexes, at a poly(I)·poly(C) concentration of 50 µg/ml in 0.15 *M* NaCl and .001 *M* phosphate buffer (pH 7.2), were exposed to pancreatic RNase/5 µg/ml at room emperature (about 25 °C). Optical density readings (260 nm) were taken at 10-min intervals

prepared at high salt concentrations. They reported that the complexes containing DNA and the synthetic polynucleotides show anomalous circular dichroism, with greatly enhanced rotational strength, and an inversion of sign in DNA and poly(A+U). DNA remained in the B form, as determined by X-ray diffraction, and there was no evidence of any large degree of distortion of the helix. The poly(A+U) complex, it was determined, was evidently in the three-stranded form.

These data were obtained in solutions approximately 10^{-5} *M*, or a few μg/ml. When attempts were made to prepare solutions of higher concentrations, a heavy gummy precipitate was obtained. However, if one first forms a complex between polylysine and carboxymethylcellulose and then adds poly(I)·poly(C), a soluble material is obtained. This material, poly(ICLC), or PICLC for short, is thermodynamically more stable than poly(I)·poly(C), as shown in thermal denaturation studies (Fig. 3). These studies were done in 0.1 × standard saline–citrate, as PICLC did not "melt" below 100 °C in standard saline–citrate. The new compound is more resistant to hydrolysis by human sera or RNase than is poly(I)·poly(C) (Fig. 4). PICLC induces 5–10 times more interferon in mice than does poly(I)·poly(C) (LEVY et al. 1975 a). It is also of interest to note that it has been reported that single-stranded poly(I) or poly(C) complexed with polylysine and carboxymethylcellulose act as antiviral agents in mice, but do not induce the formation of serum interferon (STEBBING and DAWSON 1979). The mechanism of this action is obscure.

F. PICLC in Monkeys

The important difference between poly(I)·poly(C) and PICLC is that the latter is able to induce significant quantities of interferon in primates. Figure 5 shows representative interferon induction kinetics in two rhesus monkeys. In studies designed to determine the lethal dose of PICLC in monkeys (20–40 mg/kg), up to 200,000 U interferon per milliliter serum were found.

G. Importance of Size of Components of PICLC

It has been shown by several groups that the molecular size of poly(I) and poly(C) in poly(I)·poly(C) is one of the determinants of the degree of effectiveness as an interferon inducer, with the larger homopolymers giving rise to somewhat better inducers in mice. A more striking dependence on size of homopolymers and of poly-L-lysine is seen in PICLC as it relates to ability to induce interferon in monkeys. A series of PICLC preparations were made using poly-L-lysine of molecular weight 27,00 in a complex with polynucleotides of either 4, 6, or 9 *S* (LEVY et al. 1981). Table 1 shows the differences among these three preparations. For convenience, these complexes are referred to as 4, 6, and 9 *S* PICLC.

It can be seen that as the size of the dsRNA increases so does the T_m, from about 84 °C for 4 *S* to 88.5 °C for the 9 *S* complex. The resistance to hydrolysis by RNase A is also increased as the size is increased. The 4 *S* complex is nearly totally hydrolysed by RNase, whereas the 9 *S* complex is only hydrolysed by about 7.8% (increase in A_{260}). The interferon-inducing capacity can be seen to increase significantly as the size of the molecule increases. 4 *S* PICLC induces very little interferon in monkeys whereas 9 *S* PICLC induced more than 1,000 U.

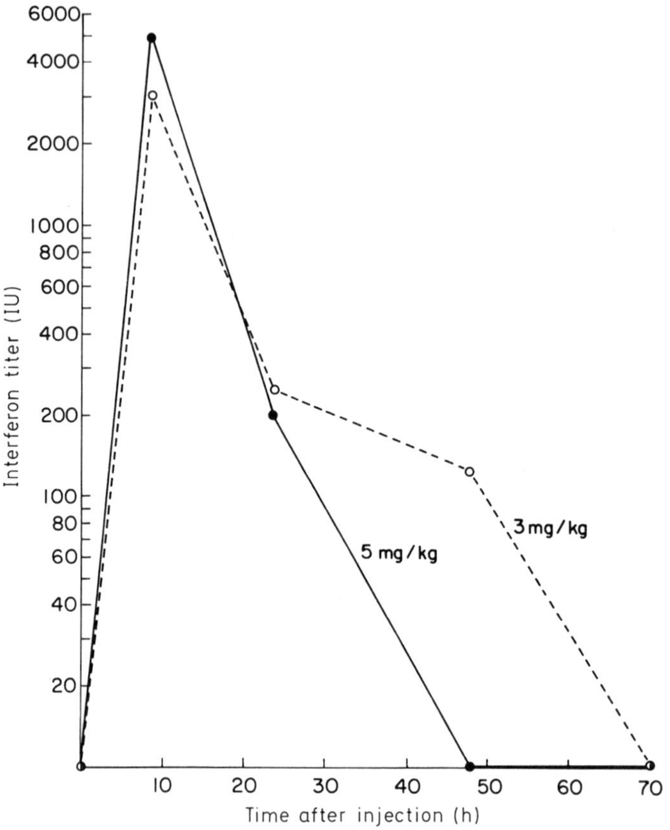

Fig. 5. Kinetics of induction of serum interferon in rhesus monkeys by intravenous administration of 3 or 5 mg/kg PICLC (one monkey per dose)

In another set of experiments, 9 *S* homopolynucleotides were used to formulate complexes with poly-L-lysines of various sizes (LEVY et al. 1981). The results are seen in Table 2. As illustrated, increasing the size of poly-L-lysine increased the resistance of the complex to hydrolysis by RNase A. More importantly again, however, was the fact that as the size of the poly-L-lysine increased so did the interferon-inducing capacity of the complex. The complex containing 2,000 daltons polylysine induced only about 10 U interferon in monkeys, whereas the complex with 27,000 daltons poly-L-lysine induced more than 1,000 U. Not shown is the observation that increased size of poly-L-lysine had only a slight effect on the T_m of the complexes. They all "melted" at about 88 °C.

Thus, in both series of complexes the ability to induce interferon in primates runs parallel to the ability to resist hydrolysis. It is not unreasonable to consider that PICLC in primates is like poly(I)·poly(C) in rodents, with PICLC being effective in primates because of its ability to resist the increased hydrolytic activity of primate serum. All the subsequent studies presented here were done with PICLC made with 9 *S* poly(I)·poly(C), and 27,000 daltons polylysine.

Table 1. Correlation between homopolymer size, hydrolysis, and interferon induction in monkeys by PICLC

S values of poly(I) and poly(C) in PICLC[b]	Hydrolysis of PICLC[a] (%)	T_m	Peak serum interferon levels ($\log_{10}$ U/ml)
9	7.8	88.5	3.2
6	39.0	86.0	1.75
4	100.0	84.0	0.3

[a] Hydrolysis of poly(I)·poly(C) considered as 100%, RNase 20 μg/ml, 1 h, 25 °C
[b] Poly-L-lysine used was of molecular weight 27,000

Table 2. Correlation between molecular weight of poly-L-lysine, hydrolysis, and interferon induction in monkeys by PICLC[a]

Molecular weight of poly-L-lysine	Hydrolysis of PICLC[b]	Peak serum interferon levels ($\log_{10}$ U/ml)
27,000	7.8	3.2
17,000	11.4	2.0
3,400	27.2	1.4
2,000	61.6	1.2

[a] Homopolynucleotides were about 9 *S*
[b] Hydrolysis of poly(I)·poly(C) taken as 100%, RNase 20 μg/ml, 1 h, 25 °C

H. Antiviral Studies in Monkeys

Levels of drug of 1–3 mg/kg have proven effective in controlling a number of viral diseases in monkeys. Rabies remains a serious problem in many countries, particularly where relatively crude antiserum and vaccine are used. Frequent and painful injections are required. Allergic encephalitis is a sequela of importance. The combination of one dose of PICLC and one or two doses of vaccine have proven efficacious in postexposure prophylaxis of street rabies infection in monkeys (BAER et al. 1977). Table 3 summarizes some results. Studies in monkeys are necessarily restricted to small numbers of animals. In order to achieve statistically significant results, a very large challenge of virus must be used to ensure death of all the control monkeys. With this unnaturally high infection, treatment must begin within 48 h of infection. With mice, larger numbers of animals can be used, and a less severe challenge of virus is possible. Under these conditions, treatment can be delayed for up to 1 week after infection. Table 4 gives a list of virus infections in monkeys that have been treated systemically with PICLC. With the exception of Bolivian hemorrhagic fever and Tacaribe virus, all have benefited.

PICLC induces the formation of adequate levels of interferon in chimpanzees (PURCELL et al. 1976). There is a model of chronic hepatitis B in young chimpan-

Table 3. Effect of PICLC and human diploid cell vaccine 48 h after rabies infection in rhesus monkeys[a]

	Number dead
Untreated	8/8
Vaccine	5/8
Vaccine + PICLC	0/8

[a] This experiment was done twice with similar results

Table 4. Virus diseases of animals treated with PICLC

Disease	Animal	Results	References
Simian hemorrhagic fever	Monkey	Complete protection if given before virus, none if given after virus	LEVY et al. (1975b)
Venezuelan equine encephalitis	Monkey	With nonlethal virus challenge, PICLC reduced viremia by 50%	STEPHEN et al. (1979)
Yellow fever	Monkey	75% protection up to 8 h after challenge	STEPHEN et al. (1977b)
Japanese encephalitis	Monkey	50% protection up to 24 h after challenge	HARRINGTON et al. (1977)
Tacaribe	Mice	No effect of PICLC	E. L. STEPHEN (1977, unpublished work)
Rabies	Monkey and mouse	See text	BAER et al. (1977)
Hepatitis	Chimpanzee	See text	PURCELL et al. (1976)
Machupo	Monkey	Possible worsening of disease	G. A. EDDY (1978, unpublished work)
Tickborne encephalitis	Monkey	Strong beneficial effect	BURGASOVA et al. (1977)
Vaccinia	Monkey	Strong beneficial effect	ANDZHAPARIDZE et al. (1977)
Vaccinia skin lesions	Rabbit (topical treatment)	Spread of lesions stopped	LEVY et al. (1978)

zees. When chimpanzees were injected with PICLC at 1 mg/kg body weight, they produced up to 750 U interferon per milliliter serum. When hepatitis B carriers were treated with PICLC, evidence of the virus disappeared during the treatment, but reappeared 16 weeks after treatment was terminated (Fig. 6). Whether or not really prolonged treatment would have a more permanent effect has not been determined.

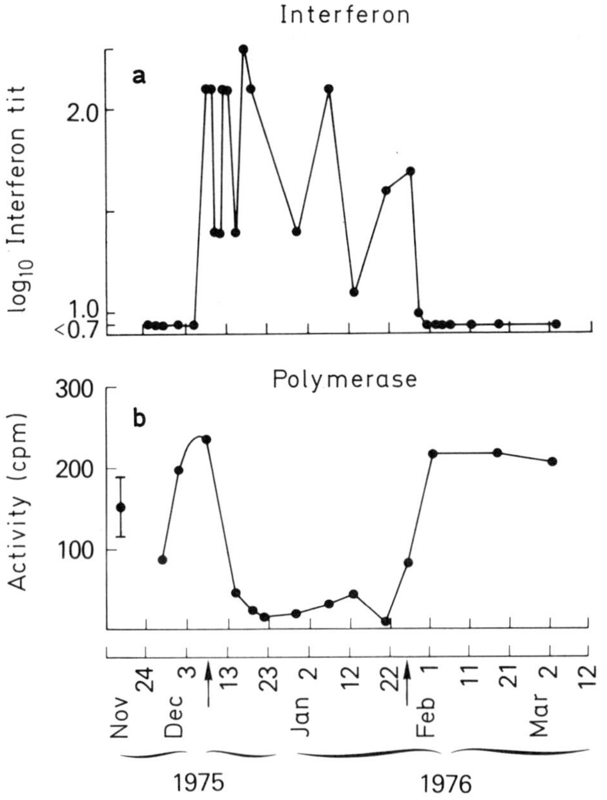

Fig. 6a, b. Treatment of chronic hepatitis in young chimpanzees with poly(I)·poly(C). Interferon titer (**a**) and virus-associated polymerase activity (**b**) are shown. The beginning and end of the treatment period are indicated by *arrows* on the abscissa. The *circle* and *bar* on the graph of DNA polymerase response indicate the mean (±1 standard deviation) of polymerase activity detected in six serum samples obtained during the 5 weeks immediately preceding the experiment

J. Adjuvant Actions

PICLC has proven to be a good immune adjuvant in primates. When used in conjunction with a number of weak vaccines, the action of the vaccine has been strongly augmented. Among the vaccines are those to Venezuelan equine encephalomyelitis virus (HARRINGTON et al. 1979), swine influenza virus (STEPHEN et al. 1977a), Japanese encephalitis virus (D.G. HARRINGTON 1978, unpublished work), an envelope antigen to herpesvirus (KLEIN et al. 1981), *Hemophilus influenzae* (LEVY et al. 1980) and Rift Valley fever virus (J. MOE 1978, unpublished work).

Monovalent influenza virus subunit vaccine, designated A/swine X-53, prepared from ANJ/76 (New Jersey, swine) is only moderately to weakly effective when given as a single dose to young people. When the vaccine was given to monkeys with and without one dose of PICLC, HAI antibody titers in the serum of those receiving the adjuvant were detectable earlier and rose to higher levels than

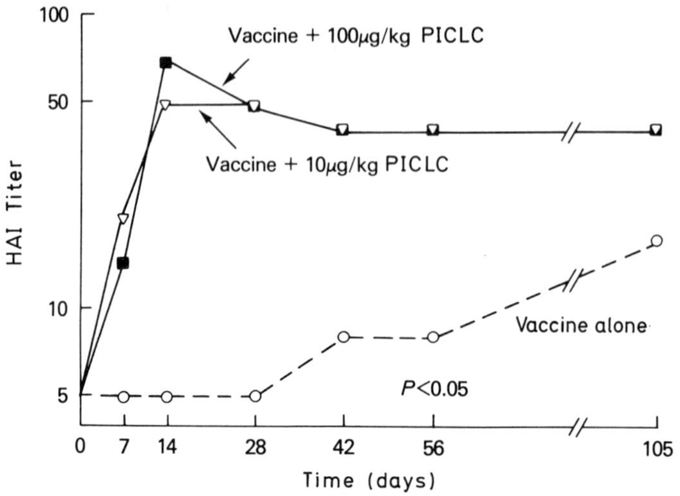

Fig. 7. Effect of one injection of PICLC on antibody production by rhesus monkeys in response to a subunit vaccine to swine influenza (four monkeys per group). *Asterisks* indicate $P<0.05$

in monkeys receiving vaccine alone. Four monkeys were used per group, each receiving 200 chick cell agglutinating units. Figure 7 shows results with monkeys receiving as little as 10 μg drug per kilogram body weight, an amount that would induce no interferon and is associated with no detected physiologic or pathologic changes (STEPHEN et al. 1977 a).

Analogous results were obtained in monkeys with inactivated Venezuelan equine encephalomyelitis virus vaccine (HARRINGTON et al. 1979). Figure 8 shows some of the data. It can be seen that antibody levels in serum were boosted about 40-fold after primary immunization when one compares levels attained after administration of vaccine along with PICLC with that attained with vaccine alone, and perhaps 200-fold after a secondary immunization. There was no alteration in the progression of IgM and IgG development. At the peak of antibody levels, most of the antibody was IgG. Polylysine complexed to carboxymethylcellulose, without poly(I)·poly(C), had no adjuvant action.

A polysaccharide vaccine made from *H. influenzae* is a poor vaccine in very young children, where the disease threat is maximum. The vaccine is also poor in young monkeys. Table 5 shows this. The data presented are normalized values obtained by radioimmune assays done by Dr. Porter Anderson (LEVY et al. 1980). The value of 100 was assigned in each case to the amount of radioactivity found using the serum obtained prior to immunization. The vaccine alone caused a minimum boost, but when given with PICLC there was a more pronounced boost.

Polyadenylic·polyuridylic acid complexed to carboxymethylcellulose and polylysine was not so effective as PICLC. PICLC is not a universal adjuvant. With albumin and pneumococcal polysaccharide antigen, there was inhibition of antibody production (H.B. LEVY 1980, unpublished work).

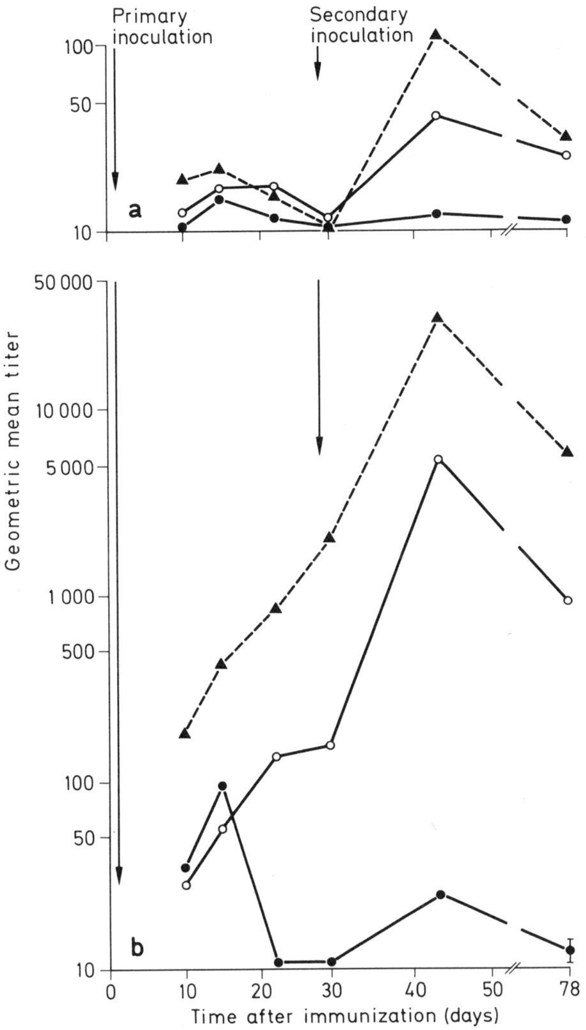

Fig. 8a, b. Serum neutralizing antibody response by immunoglobulin class of rhesus monkeys inoculated on days 0 and 28 with (**a**) inactivated Venezuelan equine encephalitis virus vaccine ($N=4$), or (*b*) vaccine combined with 200 µg/kg PICLC ($N=4$), Symbols: *triangles* whole serum antibody titers; *circles* antibody from IgG fraction; *squares* antibody from IgM fractions

K. Studies in Humans

LEVINE et al. (1979) reported on a phase I study to determine what levels of drug would be acceptable and what levels of interferon could be induced in terminal cancer patients. Doses of PICLC ranging from 0.5 to 24 mg/m^2 were administered according to the following regimen. One injection of the drug at the lowest level was given, and the patient observed for a period of 1 week. Then 14 daily doses were given. At least three patients were treated at each drug level before going on to the

Table 5. Effect of low doses of PICLC on antibody production by rhesus monkeys in response to a polysaccharide vaccine for *Hemophilus influenzae* [a]

Treatment	Pretreatment	Day 7	Day 14	Day 20	Day 28	Day 34	Day 42
Vaccine	100	590	348	286	225	187	113
Vaccine +PICLC, 0.3 mg/kg	100	5,643	5,040	3,340	2,063	2,162	780
Vaccine +PICLC, 0.03 mg/kg	100	6,589	3,904	1,884	1,132	839	721

[a] Numbers represent the amount of radioactivity in the immune precipitate obtained from sera at the indicated time, normalized to the amount of radioactivity present in the precipitate from the pretreatment sera = 100

Table 6. Mean peak serum interferon titers after treatment with PICLC

Dose levels (mg/m^2)	Interferon titer (IU/ml)[a]
0.5	15 (0–25)[b]
2.5	15 (0–25)
7.5	198 (25–250)
12.0	1,940 (200–5,000)
18.0	4,473 (600–15,000)
27.0	5,820 (2,000–10,143)

[a] Assay was done in HFS4 cells, using vesicular stomatitis virus as challenge and cytopathic effect as endpoint (IU); 8-h sample following first dose; ≧3 trials at each level

[b] Numbers in parentheses indicate range

Table 7. Mean peak cerebrospinal fluid interferon titers after treatment with PICLC

Dose level (mg/m^2)	IU/ml [a]
0.5	5 (0–10)[b]
12.0	34 (5–63)
18.0	55 (0–115)
27.0	515 (79–1,000)

[a] Assay was done in HFS4 cells, using vesicular stomatitis virus as challenge and cytopathic effect as endpoint (IU); 8-h sample following first dose; ≧3 trials at each level

[b] Numbers in parentheses indicate range

next higher level. Twenty-five patients with a wide variety of terminal cancers were studied. All had become refractory to other therapy. Peak serum interferon levels were usually found 8 h after injection. Table 6 shows the mean peak serum interferon level found for each of the drug levels. At 18 and 27 mg/m^2, levels of serum interferon up to 15,000 U were found, but because of the toxicity noted, those doses were not considered acceptable. At 12 mg/m^2, the highest tolerated dose, peak serum interferon levels of about 2,000 U were achieved. At the higher levels of drug, significant levels of interferon were found in the cerebrospinal fluid (Table 7).

There were a number of toxic manifestations associated with administration of the drug in this study. They are summarized in Table 8. Fever was always seen, although the degree tended to decrease with repeated administration. Fever, myalgia, and leukopenia are reminiscent of what is seen with administration of exoge-

Table 8. PICLC toxicity

Manifestation	No./total
Fever	25/25 (100)[a]
Nausea	11/25 (44)
Thrombocytopenia and leukopenia	17/25 (68)
Hypotension[b]	7/25 (28)
Syndrome of erythema, polyarthralgia, and polymyalgia[b]	4/25 (16)
Renal failure[b]	1/25 (4)
Trial aborted[c]	5/25 (20)

[a] Numbers in parentheses indicate percentage of total
[b] Related to dose level and/or magnitude of interferon induction
[c] 3 hypotension; 1 renal failure (27 mg/m^2); 1 serum sickness (?). Maximum tolerated dose 12 mg/m^2

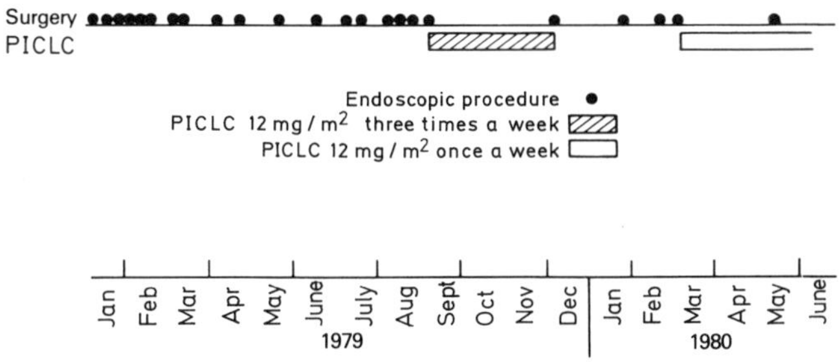

Fig. 9. Effect of PICLC on frequency of surgical intervention in juvenile laryngopapilloma in a child. Each *circle* represents a surgical intervention

nous interferon. Hypotension is sometimes seen and appears to be dose related. Variations from this pattern of toxicity have been seen in some of the other clinical studies and will be mentioned later.

The Children's Hospital Cancer Testing Group (B. LAMPKIN and H.B. LEVY 1980–1982, unpublished work) has looked at the effect of PICLC on far advanced cases of the null type of acute lymphoblastic leukemia in children. No remissions have been induced, although antileukemic effects, as evidenced by a marked decrease in the absolute number of lymphoblasts in the blood of four patients and in the bone marrow of at least one. These children were very ill and showed toxicity at lower levels of drug than seen in the study by LEVINE. Similarly, a phase I toxicity study by KROWN et al. (1980) at the Sloan-Kettering Institute, New York, on patients with a wide variety of malignancies also revealed toxicity at lower levels of drug than reported by LEVINE.

In contrast, in studies done by B. LEVENTHAL, J. WHIZNANT, and H.B. LEVY (1978–1980, unpublished work) at Johns Hopkins and the University of North Carolina on healthy children with juvenile laryngopapilloma, toxicities were less than those seen by LEVINE. Fever, mild myalgia, and occasional rises in liver en-

Table 9. Effect of PICLC on refractory multiple myeloma in humans

M component type	Comments
Kappa light chains	67% decrease in Bence Jones protein (BJ) excretion, plus correction of hypercalcemia and disease stabilization with first period of treatment; 44% decrease in BJ excretion when PICLC restarted 2 months later; normocalcemic for 5 months
IgG kappa	M component decrease from 5.2–3.9 g; improved bone pain and performance status (became ambulatory) for 2–3 months
IgG lambda	Trial stopped because of toxicity (malignant hypertension)
IgM kappa	Plasmapheresis requirement decreased from every 14 days to every 28 days
IgG kappa	Stable disease parameters for 2 months
Lambda light chains	Died 1 week after initiation of PICLC
IgG kappa	50% decrease in serum IgG M component, plus symptomatic benefit

Table 10. Types of neurologic disease treated with PICLC

Eight patients with dysimmune neurologic diseases refractory to high prolonged doses of prednisone plus azathioprene or cyclophosphamide have shown moderate to dramatic improvement. These include:
Chronic dyschwannian neuropathy;
Chronic dysneuronal neuropathy;
Chronic myopathy (polymyositis);
Acute dysneuronal neuropathy;
Post infectious demyelinating encephalomyelitis, involving cerebellum, cerebrum, and brain stem

zymes were seen. These patients also were able to tolerate even higher levels of drug than did the patients seen by LEVINE. There was also marked improvement in the clinical condition of all seven patients. A typical course is seen in Fig. 9. Each circle represents a surgical intervention. It can be seen that surgery was required less and less frequently after treatment with PICLC began. The regimen for these patients consisted of initiation at 4 mg/m^2 and working up to 12 or even 15 mg/m^2 over several weeks.

Less dramatic, but of some interest, were the results obtained by DURIE and SALMON on patients with multiple myeloma (B. DURIE, S. SALMON, and H.B. LEVY, unpublished work), summarized in Table 9. These were patients who had become refractory to all other therapy. There was subjective and objective improvement in these people, but only of a modest degree. They received about 4–6 mg/m^2 of the drug, once or twice a week, and produced interferon levels ranging from 100 to 1,000 U per milliliter serum. Their toxic manifestations consisted of fever, some transient leukopenia, no hypotension, but one incident of hypertension, and transient but sometimes severe myalgia.

Encouraging results have been seen in patients with paralytic neurologic diseases. Eight patients have been treated so far, as summarized in Table 10. These patients were all severely or totally paralyzed. They all were benefited by PICLC treatment to the point where they were able to approximate a normal life (ENGEL et al. 1978; SALAZAR et al. 1981). The first seven cases involved peripheral nerve neuropathies; the last one was a central nervous system neuropathy resembling an acute phase of multiple sclerosis. The patient was completely paralzyed and unresponsive to other therapy. Two days following each weekly treatment with PICLC, there was a definite increase in muscular strength. After 9 months of therapy, he was dismissed and was able to walk with a cane for balance.

L. Comparison of Interferon Inducers with Exogenous Interferon

There are some advantages offered by exogenous interferon and some by inducers of interferon. The inducers are relatively cheap, available in unlimited quantity, very stable, and capable of inducing higher levels of serum interferon than are currently attainable by administration of exogenous interferon. PICLC is an immune adjuvant; interferon generally does not appear to be so. That can be an advantage or a disadvantage for PICLC, depending on the circumstances. On the other hand, interferon inducers require response on the part of the host to produce interferon. If, for some reason, the host is not able to respond, then little or no interferon will be made. Also, while the general nature of the toxicity of interferon and PICLC appear to be qualitatively similar, it may be that the inducer causes more intense side reactions, possibly because of the higher levels of interferon made. Finally, the human race has been exposed to interferon since its beginning. The inducers to some extent represent an unknown.

References

Andzhaparidze DG, Bektemirov TA, Burgasova MP (1977) The effect of poly(I)-poly(C) complex with poly-L-lysine on the course of vaccina infection monkeys. Vopr Virusol 3:339–343

Baer GM, Shaddock JH, Moore SA, Yager PA, Baron SS, Levy HB (1977) Successful prophylaxis against rabies in mice and rhesus monkeys: the interferon system and vaccine. J Infect Dis 136:286–291

Billiau F, Buckler C, Dianzani F, Uhlendorf C, Baron S (1970) Influence of basic substances on the induction of the interferon mechanism. Ann NY Acad Sci 178:657–667

Burgasova MP, Andzhaparidze DG, Bektemirov TA, Bogomolova NN, Yu SB (1977) Influence of poly(I)-poly(C) complex with poly-L-lysine on experimental tick-borne encephalitis. Vopr Virusol 4:438–441

DeClercq E, Eckstein F, Merigan TC (1969) Interferon induction increased through chemical modification of a synthetic polyribonucleotide. Science 163:1137–1139

Dianzani F, Cantagalli P, Gagnoni S, Rita G (1968) Effect of DEAE-Dextran on production of interferon induced by synthetic double-stranded RNA in L-cell cultures. Proc Soc Exp Biol Med 128:708–710

Engel WK, Cuneo RA, Levy HB (1978) Poly ICLC treatment of neuropathy. Lancet 1:503–504

Felsenfeld G, Huang S (1959) The interaction of polynucleotides with cations. Biochem Biophys Acta 34:234–242

Field AK, Tytell AA, Lampson GP, Hilleman MR (1967) Inducers of interferon and host resistance. II. Multistranded synthetic polynucleotide complexes. Proc Natl Acad Sci USA 58:1004–1010

Harrington DG, Hilmas DE, Elwell MR, Whitmore RE, Stephen EL (1977) Intranasal infection of monkeys with Japanese encephalitis virus: clinical response and treatment with a nuclease resistant derivative of poly(I)·poly C. Am J Trop Med Hyg 26:1191–1198

Harrington DG, Crabbs CL, Hilmas DE, Brown JR, Higbee GA, Cole FE Jr, Levy HB (1979) Adjuvant effects of low doses of a nuclease-resistant derivative of polyinosinic-polyribocytidylic acid on antibody responses of monkeys to inactivated Venezuelan equine encephalomyelitis virus vaccine. Infect Immun 24:160–166

Haynes M, Garrett RA, Gratzer WB (1970) Structures of nucleic acid-poly base complexes. Biochemistry 9:4410–4416

Isaacs A, Lindenmann J (1957) Virus interference. I. The interferon. Proc R Soc Lond [Biol] 147:258–268

Klein RJ, Buimovici-Klein E, Moser H, Moucha R, Hilfenhaus J (1981) Efficacy of a virion envelope herpes simplex virus vaccine against experimental skin infection in hairless mice. Arch Virol 68:73–80

Krown S, Oettgen H, Stewart W, Levy HB (1980) Phase I trial of poly ICLC in cancer patients. In: Chirigos M (ed) Proceedings of symposium on biological modifiers in treatment of cancer, March, 1980. Raven, New York

Levine AS, Sivalich M, Wiernick PH, Levy HB (1979) Initial clinical trials in cancer patients of polyriboinosinic-polyribocytidylic acid stabilized with poly-L-lysine, in carboxymethylcellulose [poly(ICLC)], a highly effective interferon inducer. Cancer Res 39:1645–1650

Levy HB, Lvovsky E (1978) Topical treatment of vaccinia virus infection with an interferon inducer in rabbits. J Infect Dis 137:78–81

Levy HB, Law LN, Rabson AS (1969) Inhibition of tumor growth by polyinosinic-polycytidylic acid. Proc Natl Acad Sci USA 62:357–361

Levy HB, Baer C, Baron S, Buckler CE, Gibbs CJ, Iadarola MJ, London WT, Rice J (1975 a) A modified polyriboinosinic-polyribocytidylic acid complex that induces interferon in primates. J Infect Dis 132:434–439

Levy HB, London W, Fuccillo DA, Baron S, Rice J (1975 b) Prophylactic control of simian hemorrhagic fever in monkeys by an interferon inducer, polyriboinosinic-polyribocytidylic acid poly-L-lysine. J Infect Dis 133:A 256–A 259

Levy HB, Lvovsky E, Riley FL, Harrington D, Anderson A, Moe J, Hilfenhaus J, Stephen E (1980) Immune modulating effects of poly(ICLC). Ann NY Acad Sci 350:33–41

Levy HB, Riley FL, Lvovsky E, Stephen E (1981) Interferon induction in primates by poly ICLC. Effect of component size. Infect Immun 34:416–421

Merigan TC (1973) Non-viral substances which induce interferons. In: Finter N (ed) Interferon and interferon inducers. North-Holland/American Elsevier, New York, p 45

Nordlund JJ, Wolff SM, Levy HB (1970) Inhibition of biologic activity of poly I·poly C by human plasma. Proc Soc Exp Biol Med 133:439–444

O'Malley JA, Ho YK, Chakrabarti P, DiBerardino L, Chandra P, Orinda DAO, Byrd DM, Bardos TJ, Carter WA (1975) Antiviral activity of partially thiolated polynucleotides. Mol Pharmacol 11:61–69

Parks JH, Baron S (1968) Herpetic keratoconjunctivitis: therapy with synthetic double-stranded RNA. Science 162:811–813

Purcell RH, London WT, McAuliffe VJ, Palmer AE, Kaplan PM, Gerin JL, Wagner J, Popper H, Lvovsky E, Wong DC, Levy HB (1976) Modification of chronic hepatitis-B virus infection in chimpanzees by administration of an interferon inducer. Lancet 2:757–761

Reuss K, Scheit KH, Saiko O (1976) Induction of interferon by polyribonucleotides containing thiopyrinidines. Nucleic Acids Res 3:2861–2875

Rice JM, Turner W, Chirigos MA, Rice NR (1970) Enhancement by poly-D-lysine of Poly I:C induced interferon production in mice. Appl Microbiol 19:867–869

Robinson RA, DeVita VT, Levy HB, Baron S, Hubbard SP, Levine AS (1976) A phase I-II trial of multiple dose polyriboinosinic-polyribocytidylic acid in patients with leukemia or solid tumors. J Natl Cancer Inst 57:599–602

Salazar AM, Engel WK, Levy HB (1981) Poly(ICLC) in the treatment of postinfectious demyelinating encephalomeningitis. Arch Neurol 38:382–384
Stebbing N, Dawson KM (1979) The formation of complexes between polynucleotides, carboxymethylcellulose and polylysine which are anti-viral in mice without inducing interferon. Mol Pharmacol 16:313–323
Stephen EL, Hilmas DE, Mangiofico JA, Levy HB (1977a) Swine influenza virus vaccine: potentiation of antibody responses in rhesus monkeys. Science 197:1289–1290
Stephen EL, Sammons ML, Pannier WL, Baron S, Spertzel PO, Levy HB (1977b) Effect of a nuclease resistant derivative of polyinosinic-polycytidylic acid complex on yellow fever in rhesus monkeys. J Infect Dis 136:122–126
Stephen EL, Hilmas DE, Levy HB, Spertzel RO (1979) Protective and toxic effects of a nuclease resistant derivative of poly I·poly C on Venezuelan equine encephalitis virus in rhesus monkeys. J Infect Dis 139:267–271
Straub SX, Garry RF, Magee WE (1974) Interferon induction by poly(I):poly(C) enclosed in phospholipid particles. Infect Immun 10:783–792
Tsuboi M, Matsuo K, Ts'o OP (1966) Interaction of poly-L-lysine and nucleic acids. J Mol Biol 15:256–267
Wilkins MHF (1956) Physical studies of the molecular structure of deoxyribose nucleic acid and nucleoprotein. Cold Spring Harbor Symp Quant Biol 21:75–90
Worthington M, Levy H, Rice J (1973) Late therapy of an arbovirus encephalitis in mice with interferon and interferon stimulators. Proc Soc Exp Biol Med 143:638–643
Young CW (1971) Interferon induction in cancer with some observations on the clinical effects of poly I·poly C. Med Clin North Am 55:721–728
Zeleznick LD, Bhuyan BK (1969) Treatment of leukemic (L-1210) mice with double-stranded polyribonucleotides. Proc Soc Exp Biol Med 130:126–128

CHAPTER 26

Therapeutic Applications of Double-Stranded RNAs

J.J. GREENE, P.O.P. TS'O, D.R. STRAYER, and W.A. CARTER

A. Introduction

Double-stranded (ds)RNAs are extremely potent biologic modifiers, capable of exerting a profound influence on cells at nanomolar concentrations. The modulating effects of dsRNA are comprised of a broad spectrum of actions within which the induction of interferon (IFN) synthesis is but one component (CARTER and DECLERCQ 1974). In fact, the effects attributed to dsRNA are so diverse as to include those which are considered beneficial such as its immunoadjuvant effect as well as those which are considered toxic, such as its pyrogenic effect.

The prospects for the clinical application of dsRNA were originally founded on its property to induce IFN synthesis. Consequently, most if not all the pioneering studies on the clinical potential of dsRNA have used the synthetic compound poly(I)·poly(C) which is among the most effective inducers of IFN synthesis. It is now recognized that the efficacy of dsRNA, and poly(I)·poly(C) in particular, as chemotherapeutic agents is greatly influenced by its other biologic actions. While some of these other effects can enhance the clinical usefulness of dsRNAs, others restrict it.

Studies using poly(I)·poly(C) as the prototype dsRNA have revealed certain requirements in structure and in extent of persistence for dsRNA in the induction of IFN synthesis (Chap. 11). Similar, but not identical requirements exist for poly(I)·poly(C) in the induction of many of the other biologic effects. Modifications designed to effect specific changes in the structural characteristics of poly(I)·poly(C) can alter its therapeutic effectiveness.

This chapter focuses on the variety of biologic actions elicited by dsRNA and their significance to the clinical utilization of dsRNA. Discussed herein are the principles by which the spectrum of actions produced by dsRNA can be modulated. Application of these principles has resulted in the development of mismatched analogs of poly(I)·poly(C) for which their beneficial effects have been dissociated from much of their deleterious effects. In particular, the mismatched analog poly(I)·poly(C_{12}U) can be shown to have preserved IFN induction ability across a wide set of test systems while being much reduced in its capacity in triggering toxic responses. Owing to the low toxicity of these inducers, they are especially suited for clinical use.

B. Spectrum of Actions Produced by dsRNA

The diversity of molecular and cellular responses elicited by dsRNA is illustrated in Fig. 1. These effects can be either the direct result of dsRNA or the indirect con-

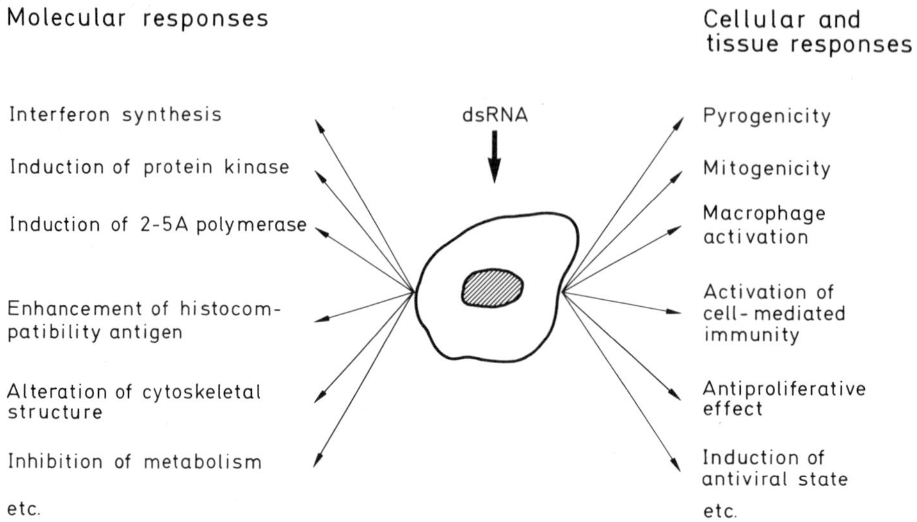

Fig. 1. Representation of the variety of biologic effects elicited by dsRNA. These effects are discussed in the text

sequence of a primary action produced by dsRNA. Distinguishing between direct and indirect effects can be especially difficult since IFN is almost invariably produced in response to dsRNA. IFN itself is responsible for a wide variety of actions and some of these may overlap with those produced directly by dsRNA. Each of these effects is ultimately the result of one or more cellular interactions of dsRNA with cells. Not all of these effects, however, are discernible at the cellular level. Indeed, some become evident only at the level of the organism. Among the best characterized actions of dsRNA are the following:

I. Effects on Humoral Immune Response

Double-stranded RNAs have both an enhancing and suppressive effect on humoral immunity. Their in vivo adjuvant effects have been demonstrated in a number of animal systems, but primarily in the mouse (TURNER et al. 1970; CHESTER et al. 1971; BRAUN et al. 1971; SCHMIDTKE and JOHNSON 1971; CONE and JOHNSON 1971; COLLAVO 1972; MORAHAN et al. 1972a, b). CONE and JOHNSON (1971) showed that, in the mouse, the dsRNA adjuvant effect requires the presence of T-lymphocytes. In addition, the adjuvant action of dsRNA is stringently dependent upon maintenance of a double-stranded structure. SCHMIDTKE and JOHNSON (1971) showed that alteration of the poly(A)·poly(U) complex by chemical modification, heat denaturation, or ribonuclease digestion greatly reduced its enhancing effect on antibody synthesis. In this study, the single strands, poly(A) or poly(U), had no adjuvant activity. The size of the dsRNA complex is another determinant of its adjuvant action. MORAHAN et al. (1972b) determined that the minimum size of poly(I)·poly(C) needed to enhance antibody formation was greater than that required for IFN induction.

Whether dsRNA enhances or suppresses the antibody response is dependent on the dose of dsRNA as well as upon the temporal relationship between the introduction of dsRNA and antigen. The optimal dose for poly(I)·poly(C) to enhance the antibody response in the mouse is 10–1,000 μg when given either intraperitoneally or intravenously. Doses in excess of 1,000 μg result in suppression of the humoral response (BRAUN et al. 1971; BRAUN and ISHIZUKA 1971). When dsRNA is given to animals before the introduction of antigen, there is suppression of the humoral response; but when given after the antigen, there is enhancement (CHESTER et al. 1971; COLLAVO 1972; SCHMIDTKE and JOHNSON 1971).

Many aspects of the in vivo humoral response to dsRNA are reflected in the murine spleen cultures, including both the enhancing (BRAUN and ISHIZUKA 1971; ISHIZUKA et al. 1971; CONE and MARCHALONIS 1972) and suppressive (JOHNSON et al. 1975) effects of dsRNA. Moreover, the dsRNA dose dependency and the temporal relationship between dsRNA and antigen, similar to those observed in vivo, are also observed in this in vitro system. Studies using spleen culture derived from normal mice and containing functional B- and T-lymphocytes and those derived from athymic hairless mice which lack T-lymphocytes have shown that the in vitro dsRNA-induced antibody response requires the presence of T-cells (CONE and MARCHALONIS 1972; JOHNSON et al. 1975). The T-cell-dependent immunosuppressive effect observed by JOHNSON et al. (1975) could be largely neutralized by anti-IFN globulin (JOHNSON and BARON 1976). This finding suggests that at least some of the humoral modulary effects of dsRNA are mediated by IFN. An interesting application of dsRNA's adjuvant action has been reported by LEVY et al. (1980). These investigators greatly increased immunization of monkeys with vaccines that are normally only weakly effective by administering the vaccine with poly(I)·poly(C) which was stabilized with poly-L-lysine and carboxymethylcellulose.

II. Effects on Cell-Mediated Immune Response

Along with its effects on humoral response, dsRNA has also been shown to affect the cell-mediated immune response. Poly(I)·poly(C) has been employed in studies with mice to determine its effect on the graft-versus-host reaction. These studies have shown that poly(I)·poly(C) can temporarily enhance the rejection of spleen cells (CANTOR et al. 1970) or tail skin (TURNER et al. 1970) grafted to isogeneic recipients. Optimal enhancement of the graft-versus-host reaction occurred at poly(I)·poly(C) doses that were tenfold higher than that required for maximal enhancement of the humoral response (TURNER et al. 1970). This action of poly(I)·poly(C) is unlikely to be mediated by IFN since IFN has only suppressive effects on graft-versus-host response (HIRSCH et al. 1973; DEMAEYER and DEMAEYER-GUIGNARD 1977).

Macrophage activity is affected by dsRNA. Poly(I)·poly(C) can enhance macrophage activity in vivo (SCHULTZ et al. 1976) as well as in vitro (SCHULTZ et al. 1977a). The in vitro effect was dose dependent and required greater than 24 h exposure to poly(I)·poly(C). The reticuloendothelial system is also affected by poly(I)·poly(C). While MORAHAN et al. (1972a) did not observe a significant change in the uptake of sheep red blood cells after administration of poly(I)

·poly(C) at 1 mg/kg, CHESTER et al. (1971) noted a biphasic effect on carbon clearance when higher doses (5 mg/kg) were used. There was a decrease in the clearance rate if poly(I)·poly(C) was administered before the injection of carbon, but there was an increase in the rate if poly(I)·poly(C) was given after the carbon injection.

Natural killer (NK) cell activity is another aspect of the cell-mediated response affected by dsRNA. Poly(I)·poly(C) and other dsRNAs have been shown to enhance NK activity in animals (COOK 1980 a, b), as well as in humans (HERBERMAN et al. 1979; ZARLING et al. 1980). Since IFN can produce many of the same effects as dsRNA on NK and macrophage activity, it is unlikely that these actions of dsRNA are entirely due to the direct effect of dsRNA (SCHULTZ et al. 1977 b).

III. Effects on the Hematopoietic System

Poly(I)·poly(C) has been shown to produce lymphopenia and thrombocytopenia in animals (DEGRE 1973; CARTER et al. 1976) and in humans (see Sect. C.II). Moreover, poly(I)·poly(C) can inhibit the proliferation of pluripotent stem cells in mice (MCNEIL et al. 1972; GIDALI et al. 1981). The effects of poly(I)·poly(C) on the hematopoietic system are not entirely inhibitory. TOMIDA et al. (1980) reported the inhibition by poly(I)·poly(C) of leukemogenicity of myeloid leukemia cells injected into syngeneic SL mice. This inhibition, however, was the result of normal differentiation induced in the leukemia cells by poly(I)·poly(C). In one case, a mismatched analog of poly(I)·poly(C), poly(I)·poly(C_{12}U) induced the differentiation of leukemia cells in a patient suffering from chronic myelogenous leukemia in blast crisis (STRAYER et al. 1981). Treatment with poly(I)·poly(C_{12}U) effected a dramatic improvement in the condition of this patient which is likely to be related to the differentiation – promoting activity of the RNA.

IV. Mitogenic and Toxic Effects on Cells

Murine T- and B-lymphocytes (RUHL et al. 1974; DIAMANTSTEIN et al. 1974; JOHNSON and HAN 1974; DIAMANTSTEIN and BLITSTEIN-WILLINGER 1975) and human spleen cells (O'MALLEY et al. 1979) exhibit a mitogenic response when exposed to dsRNA. Poly(I)·poly(C) has been reported to have a mitogenic effect on human fibroblasts in culture at very low concentrations (1–10 µg/ml) while at higher concentrations it is inhibitory (BARRACK and HOLLENBERG 1981). More frequently, dsRNA has only an inhibitory effect on the growth of human fibroblasts (O'MALLEY et al. 1979) and other mammalian cells (CORDELL-STEWART and TAYLOR 1971). Some components of this inhibitory effect are likely to be independent of IFN since growth inhibition is observed, even in presence of neutralizing amounts of antibody to IFN (J.J. GREENE 1982, unpublished work). However, IFN and dsRNA together have a synergistic anticellular effect. STEWART et al. (1973) showed that cytotoxicity occurs only if IFN and dsRNA are both present. EMENY and MORGAN (1979) have reported that for many but not all cell cultures, the anticellular effect was more pronounced with IFN and dsRNA together than with either compound alone. The structural requirements for the synergistic effect of dsRNA are similar to those for IFN induction. It is likely that the cytotoxic synergism between IFN and dsRNA is related to the role of dsRNA as a cofactor in the IFN-induced enzymic systems, particularly those which inhibit protein synthesis. This action of dsRNA is discussed in Chap. 8.

Poly(I)·poly(C) has an antitumor effect on transplantable tumors. DeClercq (1977) found that poly(I)·poly(C) arrested the growth of L-cells in hairless mice. Exogenous IFN failed to duplicate these effects. To demonstrate further the independence of this action from IFN, DeClercq et al. (1978) studied the effects of poly(I)·poly(C) and IFN on the growth of human HT-1080 fibrosarcoma and A-375 melanoma cells in hairless mice. In this xenogeneic system, only mouse IFN can be produced by poly(I)·poly(C) treatment. They found that poly(I)·poly(C) inhibited both tumors while human and mouse IFNs had no effect. Other antitumor effects are discussed in Sects. C.I and C.II.

V. Pyrogenic Effect

Pyrogenicity was among the first biologic effects observed for dsRNA (Merigan and Regelson 1967). It is also one of the most sensitive responses to dsRNA with nanogram amounts being effective in increasing body temperature in rabbits (Ts'o et al. 1976) and microgram quantities in humans (Sect. C.II). Recent experiments involving digestion of poly(I)·poly(C) with ribonuclease demonstrated that enzymic hydrolysis of poly(C) coincides with the loss of pyrogenicity (J.J. Greene, P.O.P. Ts'o, and W.A. Carter 1982, unpublished work). This experiment reveals that the double-stranded poly(I)·poly(C) is intrinsically pyrogenic.

VI. Other Effects

Double-stranded RNA can exert a myriad of other effects among which are intrinsic interference (not mediated by IFN) with viral replication (Kjeldsberg and Flikke 1971), stimulation of hyaluronic acid (Yaron et al. 1976, 1978) and prostaglandin E synthesis (Yaron et al. 1977, 1978) in synovial fibroblasts. The inflammatory process is affected in a complex manner by dsRNA since poly(I)·poly(C) has been reported both to induce acute joint inflammation (Yaron et al. 1979) and inhibit the acute inflammatory response (Koltai and Mecs 1973). The extent to which induced IFN mediates the effects of dsRNA in modulating the inflammation process and its effects on synovial fibroblasts remains to be investigated.

One expression of the antitumor effect poly(I)·poly(C) is its ability to prevent malignant transformation in vitro of murine M 2 fibroblasts by the chemical carcinogens, *N*-methyl-*N'*-nitro-*N*-nitrosoguanidine (MNNG) and 7,12-dimethylbenz-[a]anthracene (Marquardt 1973). Mouse IFN had no effect on transformation; this observation suggests that the inhibitory effect of poly(I)·poly(C) is not mediated by IFN. An interesting aspect of this action of poly(I)·poly(C) is that it can inhibit malignant transformation by MNNG without affecting the mutagenic action of MNNG as measured by the yield of 8-azaguanine and ouabain resistance mutants (Marquardt 1981).

C. Poly(I)·poly(C): Antiviral and Antitumor Activities and Toxicity

I. Animal Studies

The antiviral and antitumor properties of poly(I)·poly(C) have been extensively studied in a number of different animal systems (STEWART 1979). The antiviral studies (Table 1 A) all demonstrated that poly(I)·poly(C) is an effective prophylaxis against infection by a variety of nononcogenic viruses. In the case of oncogenic viruses, the majority of the studies observed inhibition of oncogenesis by both DNA and RNA tumor viruses, but a small number of studies have reported enhancement of oncogenesis. Its effectiveness in moderating the course of established, symptomatic disease was less conclusive. For some of these viruses studied, however, clinical manifestation of the disease usually occurs after virus replication has been naturally arrested. Therefore, treatment with poly(I)·poly(C) is not expected to ameliorate the symptoms of disease caused by these viruses.

Poly(I)·poly(C) is effective in inhibiting transplantable tumors in animals (Table 1 B). The growth of B16 malignant melanoma cells in mice was arrested by poly(I)·poly(C) (BART and KOPF 1969) and, in some cases, apparent cures were observed (BART et al. 1971). Injections of poly(I)·poly(C) induced the regression of reticulum cell sarcoma (LEVY et al. 1969; LEVY et al. 1970) and inhibited L 929 tumors (DECLERCQ 1977) in mice. The primary antitumor action of poly(I)·poly(C) in these studies is likely to be the induction of IFN synthesis since correlation between serum IFN levels and tumor inhibition was observed at least in certain cases (BART et al. 1973). Immunostimulation appears less likely since poly(I)·poly(C) was also effective in thymectomized, irradiated, leukopenic mice (BART et al. 1975). Although in the study by DECLERCQ (1977), the poly(I)·poly(C) inhibition of L 929 tumors in athymic mice could not be duplicated by the injection of exogenous IFN, suggesting that a non-IFN, nonthymic activity was responsible. This observation could be the result of intrinsic antiproliferative action of poly(I)·poly(C) (GREENE et al., to be published). However, GRESSER et al. (1978) demonstrated that injection of anti-IFN antibodies into mice together with poly(I)·poly(C) eliminated its antitumor effect.

Poly(I)·poly(C) has also been shown to inhibit chemical and radiation-induced neoplasias. Formation of tumors in mice following injections of 9,10-dimethylbenzanthracene (GELBOIN and LEVY 1970) or methylcholanthrene (ELGIO and DEGRE 1973) was inhibited by injections of poly(I)·poly(C). Inhibition of chemically induced tumors is dependent upon injection of the RNA at an early stage in the tumorigenesis process (ELGIO and DEGRE 1973). One study reported an enhancement by poly(I)·poly(C) of thymic lymphomas induced by dimethylbenzanthracene (BALL and MCCARTER 1971). The induction of primary neoplasia by X-irradiation has been reported to be both inhibited (BALL and MCCARTER 1971) and increased (LIEBERMAN et al. 1971) by poly(I)·poly(C).

A variety of toxic side effects produced by poly(I)·poly(C) became apparent during the therapeutic evaluation of poly(I)·poly(C) in animals. Among the toxic responses observed are: pyrogenicity in rabbits (LINDSAY et al. 1969; HILLEMAN 1970; PHILIPS et al. 1971); diminution of hematopoietic stem cells in mice and rats (PHILIPS et al. 1971); stimulation of autoimmune disease in mice (STEINBERG et al. 1969); and lymphopenia, thrombocytopenia, anemia, splenomegaly, and thymic

Table 1. Therapeutic application of poly(I) · poly(C) in animals

Disease model	References	Remarks
A. Antiviral studies		
Influenza	NEMES et al. (1969) LINDH et al. (1969)	Effective only when administered prior to viral challenge; intranasal route most effective
Vaccinia	LINDH et al. (1969) NEMES et al. (1969)	Marked prophylactic effect
Herpes encephalitis	LINDH et al. (1969) CATALANO and BARON (1970) CATALANO et al. (1972)	Effective in mice when given within 4 days of infection
Rabies	FENJE and POSTIC (1970) JANIS and HABEL (1972) HARMON and JANIS (1975)	Effective in rabbit and mice when administered at 6, 7, 8 h after infection
Arboviral encephalitis	POSTIC and SATHER (1970) WORTHINGTON and BARON (1971)	Effective in mice when given within 3 days of infection
Enteroviral encephalitis	LINDH et al. (1969) NEMES et al. (1969) GRESSER et al. (1969) CATALANO and BARON (1970)	Delay in mortality and increase in survival observed in mice
Rhabdoviral neuritis	RICHMOND and HAMILTON (1969) DECLERCQ and MERIGAN (1969) DECLERCQ et al. (1970) DECLERCQ and DESOMER (1971) DECLERCQ (1972)	Complete prophylaxis observed when given prior to infection; reduction in severity of disease when given after infection
B. Antitumor studies		
MSV-induced sarcoma	RHIM et al. (1969) BARON et al. (1970) KENDE and GLYNN (1971) WEINSTEIN et al. (1971) DECLERCQ and MERIGAN (1971) RHIM and HUEBNER (1971) SLAMON (1973, 1975)	Generally effective in inhibiting tumor induction in mice; action appears to be independent of IFN and is highly dependent on age and strain of mice; under some conditions, may stimulate tumor formation
Adenovirus-induced tumors	LARSON et al. (1969a)	Effective, especially when given prior to infection; more effective in female than in male mice
SV40-induced, and transplanted tumors	LARSON et al. (1970)	Little or no effect

Table 1 (continued)

Disease model	References	Remarks
Polyoma-induced tumor	VANDEPUTTE et al. (1970)	Inhibited oncogenesis in mice
RSV-induced sarcoma	NEMES et al. (1969)	Only minor inhibition of tumor formation
FLV-induced leukemia	LARSON et al. (1969 b)	Significant antitumor effect, but strongly influenced by timing of treatment
Erythroblastosis	SLAMON (1973)	Protection only if given prior to infection
B16 transplanted melanomas	BART and KOPF (1969) BART et al. (1971)	Inhibited growth
L929 transplanted tumors	DECLERCQ (1977)	Inhibited growth
Carcinogen-induced tumors	GELBOIN and LEVY (1978)	Inhibits tumor formation
X-ray-induced tumors	BALL and MCCARTER (1971) LIEBERMAN et al. (1971)	Can be either inhibited or increased

Abbreviations: *FLV*, Friend leukemia virus; *MSV*, murine sarcoma virus; *RSV*, Rous sarcoma virus; *SV*, simian virus

atrophy in mice (CARTER et al. 1976). Many of these effects are reminiscent of those produced by endotoxin (STEWART 1979) and are premonitory for the application of poly(I)·poly(C) in humans.

II. Human Studies

Clinical trials of poly(I)·poly(C) in humans have revealed that it can have a beneficial effect on the course of some, but not all viral diseases (Table 2A). The first human application of poly(I)·poly(C) was for the treatment of herpes keratitis. When poly(I)·poly(C) was applied as eyedrops at a concentration of 1 mg/μl, IFN was produced (CENTIFANTO et al. 1970) and beneficial effects were noted (GUERRA et al. 1970; GALIN et al. 1976).

With the success of poly(I)·poly(C) in treating herpes keratitis, considerable interest arose about its use as a prophylaxis against upper respiratory infection. Therefore, poly(I)·poly(C) was given intranasally to determine its effect against challenge by rhinoviruses and influenza viruses (HILL et al. 1971, 1972). These studies showed that poly(I)·poly(C) was ineffective in reducing the incidence of infection or of virus shedding in the regimen adopted, but it did appear to reduce the severity of the symptoms.

FREEMAN et al. (1977) treated 24 cancer patients suffering from herpes simplex or varicella zoster with intravenous injections of poly(I)·poly(C) at dosages of 3–12 mg/kg. Three of the patients had prolonged progress of their viral disease after receiving poly(I)·poly(C), but for the others there was a suggestion that poly(I)

Table 2. Therapeutic application of poly(I) · poly(C) in humans

Disease model	References	Remarks
A. Antiviral studies		
Herpes keratitis	CENTIFANTO et al. (1970) GUERRA et al. (1970) GALIN et al. (1976)	Local application by eyedrops; definite improvement of condition
Herpes simplex and varicella zoster	FREEMAN et al. (1977)	Intravenous administration; some reduction in the duration of the disease
Varicella zoster	FREEMAN et al. (1981)	Aborted development of overt disease
Rhinoviral and influenza viral infections	HILL et al. (1971, 1972)	Nasal spray application; no reduction in incidence, but reduction in the severity of the symptoms
Reye's syndrome, polio, rubella, subacute sclerosing panencephalitis	GUGGENHEIM and BARON (1977)	No beneficial effect
Amyotropic lateral sclerosis	ENGEL et al. (1978)	Intravenous administration of PICLC; no improvement
Chronic neuropathy	ENGEL et al. (1978)	Intravenous administration of PICLC; dramatic improvement
Demyelinating encephalomyelitis	SALAZAR et al. (1981)	Intravenous administration of PICLC; dramatic improvement
B. Antitumor studies		
Acute lymphoblastic leukemia	MATHE et al. (1970)	Remission observed in 5 of 15 patients
Various malignancies	DEVITA et al. (1970)	Phase I study only
Various malignancies	YOUNG (1971)	Phase I study; no antitumor activity evident
Various malignancies	FIELD et al. (1971)	Phase I study
Acute leukemia/solid tumors	CORNELL et al. (1976)	Phase I study
Acute myelogenous leukemia	MCINTYRE et al. (1977)	Increased duration of remission
Various malignancies with concomitant herpes infections	FREEMAN et al. (1977)	Primarily phase I study
Leukemia/solid tumors	ROBINSON et al. (1976)	Possible arrest of tumors in some cases, but no effect on leukemia
Acute leukemia/solid tumors	LEVINE et al. (1979)	PICLC used; phase I study; 2 of 25 patients responded

·poly(C) reduced the duration of the infection. In a follow-up study, poly(I)·poly(C) was administered intravenously to six children with cancer who were exposed to varicella zoster (FREEMAN et al. 1981). This treatment was successful in aborting the development of overt disease. However, from the number of patients studied, it was not possible to assess the significance of these results.

GUGGENHEIM and BARON (1977) conducted a study in which 15 children with a variety of neurologic disorders of likely viral etiology were treated with 0.1–1.0 mg/kg poly(I)·poly(C) injected intravenously. In spite of the fact that 8–500 U/ml serum IFN was detected after injection, no beneficial effect of the treatment was observed. However, ENGEL et al. (1978) obtained a remarkable remission when he treated one patient suffering from chronic neuropathy with poly(I)·poly(C), stabilized with poly-L-lysine and carboxymethylcellulose. This material also produced a dramatic improvement in the condition of one patient with demyelinating encephalomyelitis (SALAZAR et al. 1981), but had no beneficial effect on two patients with amyotropic lateral sclerosis.

The efficacy of poly(I)·poly(C) for the treatment of human malignancies has yet to be fully evaluated, but from the studies to date, it does appear to have a marginal antitumor activity. Although many studies have been reported in which poly(I)·poly(C) was administered to cancer patients (Table 2B), almost all of these were phase I studies designed to establish dosage and evaluate toxicity. Little emphasis was placed on treatment of the disease so that in these studies only one dose of poly(I)·poly(C) was usually given and the condition of the patient monitored for only a short period of time. Some beneficial effects have, however, been reported. MATHE (1970) using poly(I)·poly(C) (1 mg m^{-2} day^{-1}) achieved remission in 5 of 15 acute lymphoblastic leukemic patients who began treatment with fewer than 50% blast cells in their marrow. MCINTYRE et al. (1977) treated acute myelogenous leukemia patients in remission with single intravenous doses of 6–8 mg poly(I)·poly(C)/kg and found that this treatment increased the length of remission. In a multiple dose study, poly(I)·poly(C) was administered in doses of 0.3–75 mg/m^2 to 26 patients with solid tumors and 11 patients with leukemias (ROBINSON et al. 1976). Of the patients with solid tumors treated with poly(I)·poly(C), 9 did not have any progress of their disease during treatment, but all 11 of the leukemia patients showed signs of progressive disease in spite of treatment. LEVINE et al. (1979) treated 19 patients with solid tumors and 6 patients with acute leukemia with poly(I)·poly(C) stabilized with poly-L-lysine and carboxymethylcellulose (PICLC). Over a 6-week period of observation, 23 of 25 patients demonstrated progressive disease. One adult with acute undifferentiated leukemia achieved partial remission and one child with acute lymphoblastic leukemia achieved complete remission. However, since these patients who responded were previously under other chemotherapy, the effect of this prior therapy on the remissions cannot be delineated.

In *all* studies in which poly(I)·poly(C) was administered parentally, toxic side effects were encountered. The toxic effects (shown in order of prevalence) include: fever, leukopenia, and thrombocytopenia, hypertension/hypotension, coagulation abnormalities, elevation of liver enzymes (serum glutamicoxaloacetic and glutamicpyruvic transaminases), decrease in renal function, and hypersensitivity. These side effects were sufficiently severe to have discouraged many of the initial investigators from proceeding to a phase II study.

D. Modulating the Spectrum of Activities Triggered by dsRNA

It is now axiomatic that in order for dsRNA to induce IFN synthesis, it must fulfill certain structural requirements. The triggering of other responses by dsRNA is likely to be governed by similar, but not necessarily identical requirements. Such is, indeed, the case for the activation by dsRNA of 2,5-oligoadenylate synthetase (also referred to as 2–5 A polymerase) and IFN-induced phosphokinase. Activation of the phosphokinase involves the recognition of a much larger region of poly(I)·poly(C) structure than either the activation of the polymerase or the induction of IFN syntheses (MINKS et al. 1980). Therefore, it is conceivable for dsRNA to induce IFN synthesis and activate the polymerase without activating the phosphokinase. This situation illustrates the modulation of cellular processes by dsRNA at two levels of discrimination: (1) by inducing IFN synthesis, dsRNA can affect the levels of the intracellular enzymes, 2–5 A polymerase and protein kinase; and (2) by acting as a cofactor, dsRNA can impose control on the activation of these enzymes. Another factor directly affecting the response to dsRNA is the temporal requirement for the exposure to dsRNA. This concerns the time required for the dsRNA to trigger a specific response. In the case of IFN induction, this time constant is very short; of the order of a few minutes at 37 °C (PITHA et al. 1972).

In general, the biologic responses to dsRNA can be classified into two broad categories from the standpoint of therapeutic treatment: the desirable effects such as the antiviral and antineoplastic effects, and the undesirable effects of toxicity. Differences in the structural and/or temporal requirements of the desirable and undesirable responses provide the basis for designing a polynucleotide duplex of greater therapeutic efficacy than poly(I)·poly(C) (Fig. 2). The shorteness of the time constant for IFN induction, which means that dsRNA needs to persist for only a short time to induce IFN synthesis, suggests that the temporal requirement can best be exploited to increase efficacy.

Following this approach, the poly(I)·poly(C) complex was interrupted by the introduction of unpaired bases (uracil or guanine) into the poly(C) strand (CARTER et al. 1972). The resultant analogs contained mismatched regions which increased their susceptibilities to nuclease degradation. Therefore, the effective half-lives of the mismatched analogs are less than that of their parent compound (CARTER et al. 1972, 1976). The therapeutic effectiveness of these analogs are described in Sect. E.

Another, divergent application of this approach is exemplified by complexing poly(I)·poly(C) with poly-L-lysine and carboxymethylcellulose (PICLC, RICE et al. 1970, 1971; LEVY et al. 1975). Human plasma contains a particularly high nucleolytic activity, capable of degrading poly(I)·poly(C) with a half-life of 6 min (DECLERCQ 1979). Complexation with poly-L-lysine and carboxymethylcellulose alters the temporal characteristics of poly(I)·poly(C) so that it becomes more resistant to nuclease, and, hence, has a longer half-life under clinical conditions. The rationale here is that by virtue of its longer persistence in blood, smaller amounts of PICLC are needed to attain the same IFN titers as poly(I)·poly(C) (LEVY 1980). Studies in cats (STRINGFELLOW and WEED 1980), primates (PURCELL et al. 1976), and in humans indicate that this is indeed the case. A detailed discussion of this analog is presented in Chap. 25 of this volume.

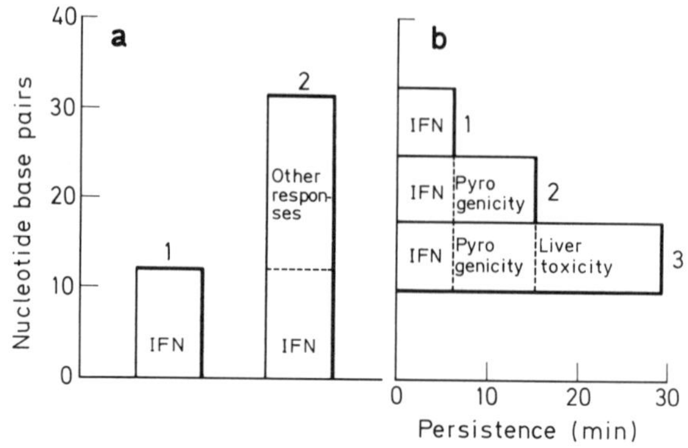

Fig. 2a, b. Hypothetical representation of situations where the structural and temporal requirements for dsRNA in inducing IFN need not overlap with requirements for inducing the toxic responses. **a** structural requirement for dsRNA in the minimum number of ribosyl base pairs necessary for the induction of IFN synthesis and other responses. This requirement for IFN synthesis is met when the dsRNA contains at least 12 ribosyl base pairs (box 1). Other responses including toxic responses may be induced if the dsRNA contains *more* than 12 ribosyl base pairs. If the requirement for a toxic response is greater than 12 base pairs, as illustrated in box 2, then dsRNA can be constructed which is capable of inducing IFN synthesis without that particular toxic effect; **b** temporal requirement for dsRNA to persist to induce IFN synthesis and toxic responses. This requirement for IFN synthesis is known to be less than 5 min. If, for illustrative purposes, the temporal requirements for dsRNA to induce pyrogenicity and liver toxicity are shown to be 5 and 15 min, respectively, then a dsRNA which persists for greater than 15 min (box 3) will induce both pyrogenicity and liver toxicity in addition to IFN synthesis. Persistence for less than 15 min results in pyrogenicity and IFN production, but not liver toxicity (box 2). Complete separation of IFN induction from pyrogenicity and liver toxicity occurs if the dsRNA persists for less than 5 min (box 1)

E. Poly(I)·poly(C_{12}U): An Interferon Inducer with Few Toxic Responses

This mismatched analogs of poly(I)·poly(C) containing U or G interspersed into the poly(C) strand, retained their ability to induce IFN synthesis, provided that the frequency of random insertions was not greater than 1 residue in 12 (CARTER et al. 1972). IFN induction under these conditions is retained since the mismatched analogs would preserve at least 0.5–1 helical turn of perfectly base paired dsRNA – a structural prerequisite for the "triggering" of IFN synthesis (GREENE et al. 1978).

Studies of two of the mismatched analogs poly(I)·poly(C_{12}U) and poly(I)-poly(C_{29}G) in rabbit, mouse, and human in vitro systems have shown these analogs to be less toxic than poly(I)·poly(C). In rabbits, both mismatched duplexes were as effective as poly(I)·poly(C) in inducing IFN synthesis (Ts'o et al. 1976) but, as shown in Fig. 3, were considerably less antigenic and pyrogenic than poly(I)-poly(C) (CARTER et al. 1976). Repeated administration of the mismatched analogs to mice resulted in less toxicity than poly(I)·poly(C) to critically sensitive organs, including bone marrow elements, liver cells, thymocytes, and splenocytes while be-

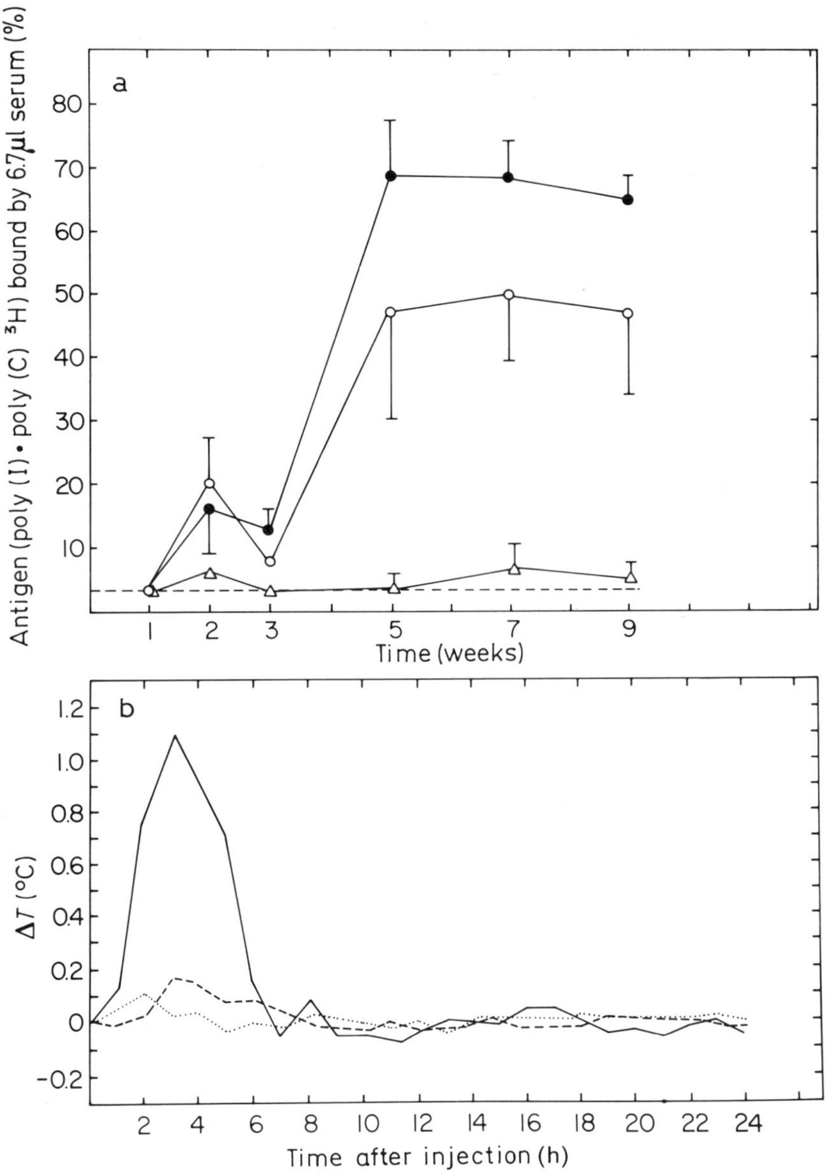

Fig. 3. a Differential production of antibody against dsRNA by repeated administration of poly(I)·poly(C) and its mismatched analogs in rabbits. Each point represents the mean of four or five sera ± standard error (*vertical bars*). No significant statistical differences were seen until 3 weeks, poly(I)·poly(C), poly(I)·poly($C_{12}U$), ($P<0.01$); at 5 weeks, poly(I)·poly(C), poly(I)·poly($C_{29}G$), poly(I)·poly($C_{12}U$), ($P<0.05$); at 7 weeks, poly(I)·poly(C), poly(I)·poly($C_{29}G$), poly(I)·poly($C_{12}U$), ($P<0.01$); at 9 weeks, poly(I)·poly(C), poly(I)·poly($C_{29}G$), poly(I)·poly($C_{12}U$), ($P<0.01$). *Full circles* poly(I)·poly(C); *open circles* poly(I)·poly($C_{29}G$); *triangles* poly(I)·poly($C_{12}U$); *broken line* normal rabbit serum. **b** Temperature in rabbits after 1.0 μg/kg intravenous doses of polynucleotide duplexes. Each curve is the average of four animals. *Full line* poly(I)·poly(C); *broken line* poly(I)·poly($C_{12}U$); *dotted line* poly(I)·poly($C_{29}G$)

Table 3. Effect of mispairing bases on the spectrum of biologic effects in humans

Biologic response	Poly(I) · poly(C)	Poly(I) · poly(C_{12}U)
Interferon induction [a] (in vitro)	10	10
Interferon induction (in vivo)	+	+
Immunosurveillance [a] (NK cell activation, in vitro)	10	9
Mitogenicity [a] (splenocytes, in vitro)	10	2
Activation of 2–5A polymerase and protein kinase	N.D. [c]	+
Pyrogenicity [b]	+	+
Liver toxicity	+	–
Bone marrow toxicity	+	–
Coagulopathy	+	–
Hypertension/hypotension	+	–

[a] Rank order of dsRNA where 10 indicates "most effect" and 1 indicates "little or no effect"
[b] Comparative studies on the pyrogenicity of poly(I) · poly(C) and poly(I) · poly(C_{12}U) have not yet been done. Based on the limited number of patients studied to date (STRAYER et al. 1981), the pyrogenicity resulting from poly(I) · poly(C_{12}U) may be less severe than that resulting from poly(I) · poly(C)
[c] N.D. = "not done"

ing as effective in protecting against a variety of lethal viral challenges (CARTER et al. 1976; Ts'o et al. 1976). When toxicity was evaluated on a variety of human tissue culture cells, the mismatched compounds did not detrimentally affect human cell functions (O'MALLEY et al. 1979). Moreover, the mismatched analogs were nearly as effective as the parent compound poly(I)·poly(C) in the activation of NK cells (ZARLING et al. 1980) and are capable of activating the human IFN-induced enzymes 2–5A polymerase and protein phosphokinase (MINKS et al. 1979; C. BAGLIONI 1981, personal communication).

On the basis of the reduced toxicity demonstrated in these preclinical studies, poly(I)·poly(C_{12}U) was selected for phase I–II study in human cancer patients. Preliminary results (STRAYER et al. 1981) indicate that poly(I)·poly(C_{12}U) can have a positive, beneficial effect on the course of several malignant diseases such as chronic myelogenous leukemia (blast crisis) and multiple myeloma while being devoid of many toxic effects normally associated with poly(I)·poly(C). Poly(I)·poly(C_{12}) has also been shown to induce detectable levels of serum IFN, and to stimulate 2–5 A polymerase in vivo (J.J. GREENE et al. 1982, unpublished work; C. BAGLIONI et al. 1982, unpublished work). Table 3 demonstrates some of the comparative differences in the spectrum of biologic activities of poly(I)·poly(C) and poly(I)·poly(C_{12}U) in humans. Clearly, the mismatched analog has a higher therapeutic ratio.

F. Conclusions

Double-stranded RNAs exert a wide diversity of biologic effects which are evident at both the cellular and organism levels. Some of these effects have clearly contributed to producing the positive therapeutic responses observed with poly(I)·poly(C) in animals and in humans. Nonetheless, the clinical promise of poly(I)·poly(C) has not yet been totally fulfilled. This is primarily due to two obstacles: (1) toxic side effects produced by poly(I)·poly(C); and (2) hyporeactivity, whereby animals progressively lose their ability to respond to successive administrations of poly(I)·poly(C) (DeClercq 1972; Stewart 1979; Stringfellow 1980). Fortunately, these obstacles are not insurmountable. The toxic response, like IFN induction, is determined by certain structural and temporal requirements for the RNA. As described here, the requirements for IFN induction and toxicity are not identical. Thus, the mismatched complex poly(I)·poly(C_{12}U) can induce the IFN system while circumventing many of the toxic effects. The hyporeactive state can be reduced or eliminated by the administration of prostaglandins together with dsRNA (Stringfellow 1973) and possibly by modifying the structure of the dsRNA (O'Malley et al. 1975). It is conceivable that hyporeactivity can be overcome by altering the temporal characteristics of the dsRNA as well.

For clinical applications, synthetic dsRNA has certain advantages over the use of exogenous IFN. First, dsRNA possesses the potential for generating multiple species of IFNs. This property would remove the possible necessity of targeting a specific type or subtype of IFN to a particular cell type. Second, dsRNA has the known ability to activate the intracellular mediators which are synthesized after exposure to IFN. Third, synthetic dsRNA can be specifically modified to alter its structural and temporal characteristics so that only selective components within its spectrum of biologic effects will be exploited. Fourth, dsRNA in combination with IFN can override acquired cellular resistance to IFN alone (Lin et al., to be published). Finally, the biologic effects of dsRNA are not identical to those of IFN and in certain cases, dsRNA may act more effectively than IFN as therapeutic agents. In light of these considerations and of the diverse and pronounced effects produced by dsRNA, it is not overoptimistic to expect that synthetic dsRNA can have significant therapeutic utility, either alone or in combination with IFN. However, the full potential of the clinical application of dsRNA will not be fully realized without significant basic studies on this very interesting molecule.

References

Ball JK, McCarter JA (1971) Effect of polyinosinic-polycytidylic acid on induction of primary or transplanted tumors by chemical carcinogens or irradiation. J Natl Cancer Inst 46:1009–1011

Baron S, DuBuy H, Buckler CE, Johnson ML, Park J, Billiau A, Sarma P, Huebner RJ (1970) Induction of interferon and viral resistance in animals by polynucleotides. Ann NY Acad Sci 173:568–572

Barrack ER, Hollenberg MD (1981) Mitogenesis on normal human fibroblasts by polyinosinic·polycytidylic acid and other synthetic polymers: enhancement of action by glucocorticoids. J Cell Physiol 108:445–454

Bart RS, Kopf AW (1969) Inhibition of the growth of murine malignant melanoma with synthetic double-stranded ribonucleic acid. Nature 224:372–373
Bart RS, Kopf AW, Silagi S (1971) Inhibition of the growth of murine malignant melanoma by polyinosinic·polycytidylic acid. J Invest Dermatol 56:33–38
Bart RS, Kopf AW, Vilcek J, Lam S (1973) Role of interferon in the antimelanoma effects of poly(I)·poly(C) and Newcastle disease virus. Nature 245:229–230
Bart RS, Lam S, Cooper JS, Kopf AW (1975) Retention of antimelanoma effect of polyinosinic-polycytidylic acid in neonatally thymectomized, irradiated, leukopenic mice. J Invest Dermatol 65:285–288
Braun W, Ishizuka M (1971) Antibody formation: reduced response after administration of excessive amounts of non-specific stimulators. Proc Natl Acad Sci USA 68:1114–1116
Braun W, Ishizuka M, Yajima Y, Webb D, Winchurch R (1971) Spectrum and mode of action of poly A: U in the stimulation of immune responses. In: Beers R, Braun AG (eds) Biological effects of polynucleotide. Springer, Berlin Heidelberg New York
Cantor H, Asofsky R, Levy HB (1970) The effect of polyinosinic-polycytidylic acid upon graft-vs-host activity in BALB/c mice. J Immunol 104:1035–1038
Carter WA, DeClercq E (1974) Viral infection and host defense. Science 186:1172–1178
Carter WA, Pitha PM, Marshall LW, Tazawa I, Tazawa S, Ts'o POP (1972) Structural requirements of the $rI_n{\cdot}rC_n$ complex for induction of human interferon. J Mol Biol 70:567–587
Carter WA, O'Malley JA, Beeson M, Cunnington P, Kelvin A, Vere-Hodge A, Alderfer JL, Ts'o, POP (1976) An integrated and comparative study of the antiviral effects and other biological properties of the polyinosinic·polycytidylic acid duplex and its mismatched analogues. III. Chronic effects and immunological features. Mol Pharmacol 12:440–453
Catalano LW, Baron S (1970) Protection against herpes virus and encephalomyocarditis virus encephalitis with a double-stranded RNA inducer of interferon. Proc Soc Exp Biol Med 133:684–688
Catalano LW, London WT, Rices JM, Sever JL (1972) Prophylactic and therapeutic use of poly I·poly C (poly-D-lysine) against herpes virus encephalitis in mice. Proc Soc Exp Biol Med 140:66–71
Centifanto YM, Goorha RM, Kaufman HE (1970) Interferon induction in rabbit and human tears. Am J Ophthalmol 60:1006–1010
Champney KJ, Levine DP, Levy HB, Lerner AM (1979) Modified polyriboinosinic-polyribocytidylic acid complex: sustained interferonemia and its physiological associates in humans. Infect Immun 25:831–837
Chester TJ, DeClercq E, Merigan TC (1971) Effect of separate and combined injections of poly rI: poly RC and enditoxin on reticuloendothelial activity, interferon, and antibody production in the mouse. Infect Immun 3:516–520
Collavo D (1972) Immune reactivity following poly I·poly C treatment in mice. Nature 237:154–156
Cone RE, Johnson AG (1971) Regulation of the immune system by synthetic polynucleotides. III. Action on antigen-reactive cells of thymic origin. J Exp Med 133:665
Cone RE, Marchalonis JJ (1972) Adjuvant action of poly AU on T cell during the primary immune response in vitro. Aust J Exp Biol Med Sci 50:69–77
Cook RM (1980a) Spontaneous cytotoxicity of murine cells treated with the interferon inducers BRL 5907 and BRL 10739. Immunology 39:151–157
Cook RM (1980b) Immunoregulatory activity of double-stranded RNA (BRL 5907): characterization of murine effector cells. J Reticuloendothel Soc 27:495–505
Cordell-Stewart B, Taylor MW (1971) Effect of double-stranded viral RNA on mammalian cells in culture. Proc Natl Acad Sci USA 68:1326–1330
Cornell CJ, Smith KA, Cornwell III GG, Burke GP, McIntyre OR (1976) Systemic effects of intravenous polyriboinosinic-polyribocytidylic acid in man. J Natl Cancer Inst 57:1211–1216
DeClercq E (1972) Hyporeactivity to interferon production by dsRNA associated with hyporeactivity to antiviral protection and hyporeactivity to toxicity. Proc Soc Exp Biol Med 141:340–345

DeClercq E (1974) Synthetic interferon inducers. Top Curr Chem 52:173–208
DeClercq E (1977) Effect of mouse interferon and polyriboinosinic acid·polyribocytidylic acid on L-cell tumor growth in nude mice. Cancer Res 37:1502–1506
DeClercq E (1979) Degradation of poly(inosinic acid)·poly(cytidylic acid) $[(I)_n \cdot (C)_n]$ by human plasma. Eur J Biochem 93:165–172
DeClercq E, Desomer P (1971) Comparative study of the efficacy of different forms of interferon therapy in the treatment of mice challenged intranasally with VSV. Proc Soc Exp Biol Med 138:301–307
DeClercq E, Merigan TC (1969) Local and systemic protection by synthetic polyanionic interferon inducers in mice against vesicular stomatitis virus. J Gen Virol 5:359–367
DeClercq E, Merigan TC (1971) Moloney sarcoma virus-induced tumors in mice: Inhibition or stimulation of (poly I)·(poly C). Proc Soc Exp Biol Med 137:590–594
DeClercq E, Nuwer MR, Merigan TC (1970) The role of interferon on the protective effect of synthetic double-stranded polyribonucleotide against intranasal vesicular stomatitis virus challenge in mice. J Clin Invest 49:1565–1577
DeClercq E, Georgiades J, Edy VG, Sobis H (1978) Effect of human and mouse interferon and of polyriboinosinic acid·polyribocytidylic acid on the growth of human fibrosarcoma and melanoma tumors in nude mice. Eur J Cancer 14:1273–1282
Degre M (1973) Influence of polyinosinic: polycytidylic acid on correlating white blood cells in mice. Proc Soc Exp Biol Med 14:1087–1091
DeMaeyer E, DeMaeyer-Guignard J (1977) Effect of interferon on cell-mediated immunity. Tex Rep Biol Med 35:370–374
DeVita V, Canellas G, Carbone P, Baron S, Levy H, Gralnick H (1970) Clinical trials with the interferon inducer polyinosinic-polycytidylic acid. Proc Am Assoc Cancer Res 11:21
Diamantstein T, Blitstein-Willinger E (1975) Relationship between biological activities of polymer. I. Immunogenicity, C3 activation, mitogenicity for B cells and adjuvant properties. Immunology 29:1087–1092
Diamantstein T, Blitstein-Willinger E, Schulz G (1974) Polyanions and lipopolysaccharide act on different subpopulations of B cells. Nature 250:596–597
Elgio K, Degre M (1973) Polyinosinic-polycytidylic acid in two-stage carcinogenesis. Effect on epidermal growth parameters and interferon induction in treated mice. J Natl Cancer Inst 51:171–177
Emeny JM, Morgan MJ (1979) Susceptibility of various cells treated with interferon to the toxic effects of poly(rI)·poly(rC) treatment. J Gen Virol 43:253–255
Engel WK, Cuneo R, Levy HB (1978) Treatment of neuropathy with stabilized polyinosinic-polycytidylic acid. Lancet 1:503–504
Fenje P, Postic B (1970) Protection of rabbits against experimental rabies by poly I·poly C. Nature 226:171–172
Field AK, Young CW, Krakoff IH, Tytell AA, Lampson GP, Nemes MM, Hilleman MR (1971) Induction of interferon in human subjects by poly I: C. Proc Soc Exp Biol Med 136:1180–1186
Freeman AD, Al-Bussam N, O'Malley JA, Stutzman L, Bjornsson S, Carter WA (1977) Pharmacologic effects of polyinosinic·polycytidylic acid in man. J Med Virol 1:79–93
Freeman AI, Bogger-Goren S, Brecher ML, O'Malley JA (1981) Prevention of varicella zoster (VZ) with poly(I)·poly(C) given during the incubation period. J Interferon Res 1:457–462
Galin MA, Chowchuveck E, Kronenberg B (1976) Therapeutic use of inducers of interferon on herpes simplex keratitis in humans. Ann Ophthalmol 8:72–76
Gelboin HV, Levy HB (1970) Polyinosinic-polycytidylic acid inhibits chemically induced tumorigenesis in mouse skin. Science 167:205–207
Gidali J, Feher I, Talas M (1981) Proliferation inhibition of murine pluripotent haemopoietic stem cells by interferon or poly I: C. Cell Tissue Kinet 14:1–7
Greene JJ, Alderfer JL, Tazawa I, Tazawa S, Ts'o POP, O'Malley JA, Carter WA (1978) Interferon induction and its dependence on the primary and secondary structure of poly(inosinic acid)·poly(cytidylic acid). Biochemistry 17:4214–4220

Greene JJ, Lin SL, Ts'o POP, Carter WA (to be published) Distinct antiproliferative actions of interferon and dsRNA
Gresser I, Fontaine-Brouty-Boye D, Bouralio C, Thomas MT (1969) A comparison of the efficacy of endogenous, exogenous and combined endogenous-exogenous interferon in the treatment of mice infected with encephalomyocarditis virus. Proc Soc Exp Biol Med 130:236–241
Gresser I, Maury C, Bandu MT, Tovey M, Maunoway MT (1978) Role of endogenous interferon in the antitumor effect of poly I·C and statolon as demonstrated by the use of anti-mouse interferon serum. J Natl Cancer Inst 21:72–77
Guerra R, Frezzotti R, Bonanni R, Dianzani F, Rita G (1970) A preliminary study on treatment of human herpes simplex keratitis with an interferon inducer. Ann NY Acad Sci 173:823–826
Guggenheim MA, Baron S (1977) Clinical studies of an interferon inducer, poly I·poly C in children. J Infect Dis 136:50–58
Harmon MW, Janis B (1975) Therapy of murine rabies after exposure: efficacy of polyinosinic-polycytidylic acid alone and in combination with three rabies vaccines. J Infect Dis 132:241–247
Herberman RB, Ortaldo J, Bonnard G (1979) Augmentation by interferon of human natural and antibody dependent cell mediated cytotoxicity. Nature 277:221–223
Hill DA, Baron S, Levy HB, Bellianti J, Buckler CE, Cannellos G, Carbone P, Canock RM, Devita V, Guggenheim MA, Homan E, Kapikian AZ, Kirschstein RL, Mills J, Perkins JC, Van Kirk JE, Worthington M (1971) Clinical studies of induction of interferon by polyinosinic-polycytidylic acid. In: Pollard M (ed) Perspectives in virology, vol 7. Academic, New York
Hill DA, Baron S, Perkins JC, Worthington M, Van Kirk JE, Mills J, Kapikian AZ, Chanock RH (1972) Evaluation of an interferon inducer in viral respiratory disease. JAMA 219:1179–1184
Hilleman MR (1970) Prospects for the use of double-stranded ribonucleic acid (poly I:C) inducers in man. J Infect Dis 121:196–211
Hirsch MS, Ellis DA, Proffitt MR, Black PH, Chirigos MA (1973) Effects of interferon on leukemia virus activation in graft-vs-host disease. Nature 244:102–103
Ishizuka M, Braun W, Matsumoto T (1971) Cyclic AMP and immune responses: I. Influence of poly A:U and cAMP on antibody formation in vitro. J Immunol 107:1027–1035
Janis B, Habel K (1972) Rabies in rabbits and mice: protective effect of polyriboinosinic-polyribocytidylic acid. J Infect Dis 125:345–353
Johnson HM, Baron S (1976) The nature of the suppressive effect of interferon and interferon inducers on the in vitro immune response. Cell Immunol 25:106–109
Johnson AG, Han IH (1974) Mitogenic activity of polynucleotides on thymus-influenced lymphocytes. In: Braun W, Lichenstein LM, Pasker CW (eds) Cyclic AMP, cell growth, and the immune response. Springer, Berlin Heidelberg New York, pp 77–83
Johnson HM, Bukovic JA, Smith BG (1975) Inhibitory effect of synthetic polyribonucleotides on the primary in vitro immune response. Proc Soc Exp Biol Med 149:599–603
Kende M, Glynn JP (1971) Modification of the response of autochthonous Moloney sarcoma virus-induced tumors to poly·IC by DEAE-dx. Chemotherapy 16:281–284
Kjeldsberg E, Flikke M (1971) Antiviral activity of polyinosinic-polycytidylic acid in the absence of cell controlled RNA synthesis. J Gen Virol 10:147–154
Koltai M, Mecs E (1973) Inhibition of the acute inflammatory response by interferon inducers. Nature 242:525–526
Larson VM, Clark WR, Hilleman MR (1969a) Influence of synthetic (poly-I·C.) and viral double-stranded ribonucleic acids on adenovirus 12 oncogenesis in hamsters. Proc Soc Exp Biol Med 131:1002–1008
Larson VM, Clark WR, Dagle GE, Hilleman MR (1969b) Influence of synthetic double-stranded ribonucleic acid, poly I:C on Friend leukemia in mice. Proc Soc Exp Biol Med 132:602–607
Larson VM, Panteleakis PN, Hilleman MR (1970) Influence of synthetic double-stranded ribonucleic acid (polyIC) on SV40 viral oncogenesis and transplant tumor in hamsters. Proc Soc Exp Biol Med 133:14–20

Levine AJ, Sivulich JM, Wiernik PH, Levy HB (1979) Initial clinical trials in cancer patients of polyriboinisinic-polyribocytidylic acid stabilized with poly-L-lysine and carboxymethycellulose [poly(ICLC)], highly effective interferon inducer. Cancer Res 39:1645–1650

Levy HB (1980) Induction of interferon by polynucleotides. In: Stringfellow DA (ed) Interferon and interferon inducers-clinical applications. Dekker, New York, pp 167–186

Levy HB, Law LW, Rabson AS (1969) Inhibition of tumor growth by polyinosinic acid-polycytidylic acid. Proc Nat Acad Sci USA 62:357–359

Levy HB, Asofsky R, Riley F, Garapin A, Cantor H, Adamson R (1970) The mechanism of the antitumor action of poly I·poly C. Ann NY Acad Sci 173:640–659

Levy HB, Baer G, Baron S, Buckler CE, Gibbs MJ, Iadarda MJ, London WT, Rice JA (1975) Modified polyriboinosinic: polyribocytidylic acid complex that induces interferon in primates. J Infect Dis 132:434–439

Levy HB, Lvovsky E, Riley F, Harrington D, Anderson A, Moe J, Hilfenhaus J, Stephen E (1980) Immune modulating effects of poly ICLC. Ann NY Acad Sci 33–41

Lieberman M, Merigan TC, Kaplan HS (1971) Inhibition of radiogenic lymphoma development in mice with interferon. Proc Soc Exp Biol Med 138:575–578

Lin SL, Greene JJ, Ts'o POP, Carter WA (1982) Sensitivity and resistance of human tumor cells to interferon and $rI_n \cdot rC_n$ action. Nature 297:417–419

Lindh HF, Lindsay HL, Mayberry BR, Forbes M (1969) Polyinosinic-cytidylic acid complex (poly I: C) and viral infections in mice. Proc Soc Exp Biol Med 132:83–87

Lindsay HL, Trown PW, Brandt J, Forbes M (1969) Pyrogenicity of poly I·poly C in rabbits. Nature 223:717

Marquardt H (1973) Polyriboinosinic-polyribocytidylic acid prevents chemically-induced malignant transformation in vitro. Nature 246:228–229

Marquardt H (1981) Inhibition by polyriboinosinic-polyribocytidylic acid of malignant transformation in vitro induced by chemical carcinogens without affecting mutagenesis. Proc Am Assoc Cancer Res 22:109

Mathe G, Amiel L, Schwazenberg L, Schneider M, Hayat M, DeVassal F, Jasmin C, Rosenfeld C, Sakouhi M, Choay J (1970) Remission induction with poly IC in patients with acute lymphoblastic leukemia. Eur J Clin Biol Res 15:671–684

McIntyre OR, Rai K, Glidewell O, Holland JF (1977) Poly IC as adjunct to remission maintenance therapy in acute myelogenous leukemia. In: Terry WD, Windhorst D (eds) Immunotherapy of cancer. Present status of trials in man. Raven, New York

McNeill TA, Fleming WA, McCance DJ (1972) Interferon and haemopoietic colony inhibitor responses to poly I·poly C in rabbits and hamsters. Immunology 22:711–721

Merigan TC, Regelson W (1967) Interferon induction in man by a synthetic polyanion of defined composition. N Eng J Med 227:1283–1285

Minks MA, West DK, Benvin S, Baglioni C (1979) Structural requirements of double-stranded RNA for the activation of 2′,5′ oligo(A) polymerase and protein kinase of interferon-treated HeLa cells. J Biol Chem 254:10180–10183

Minks MA, West DK, Benvin S, Greene JJ, Ts'o POP, Baglioni C (1980) Activation of 2′,5′-oligo(A)polymerase and protein kinase of interferon-treated HeLa cells by 2′-O-methylated poly(inosinic acid)·poly(cytidylic acids). J Biol Chem 255:6403–6407

Morahan PS, Munson AE, Commerford SL, Hamilton LD (1972a) Antiviral activity and side effects of polyriboinosinic-cytidylic acid complexes as affected by molecular size. Proc Natl Acad Sci 69:842–846

Morahan PS, Regelson W, Munson AE (1972b) Pyran and polyribonucleotides: differences in biological activities. Antimicrob Agents Chemother 2:16–22

Nemes MM, Tytell AA, Lampson GP, Field AK, Hilleman MR (1969) Inducers of interferon and host resistance. VI. Antiviral efficacy of poly I: C in animal models. Proc Soc Exp Biol Med 132:776–783

O'Malley JA, Ho YK, Chakrabarti P, DiBerardino L, Chandra P, Orinda DAO, Byrd DM, Bardos TJ, Carter NA (1975) Antiviral activity of partially thiolated polynucleotides. Mol Pharmacol 11:61–69

O'Malley JA, Leong SS, Horoszewicz JS, Carter WA, Alderfer JL, Ts'o POP (1979) Polyinosinic acid-polycytidylic acid and its mismatched analogs: differential effects on human cell function. Mol Pharmacol 15:165–173

Philips FS, Fleisher M, Hamilton LC, Schwartz MK, Sternberg SS (1971) Polyinosinic-polycytidylic acid toxicity. In: Beers RF, Braun W (eds) Biological effects of polynucleotides. Springer, New York, pp 259–273

Phillips BM, Hartnagel RE, Kraus PJ, Tamayo RP, Fonseca EH, Kowalski RL (1971) Systemic toxicity of polyinosinic: polycytidylic acid in rodents and dogs. Toxicol Appl Pharmacol 18:220–230

Pitha PM, Marshall LW, Carter WA (1972) Interferon induction: rate of cellular attachment of poly I: C. J Gen Virol 15:89–92

Postic B, Sather GE (1970) Effect of poly I:C in mice injected with Japanese encephalitis virus. Ann NY Acad Sci 173:606–610

Purcell RH, London WT, Palmer AE, Kaplan PM, Gerin JL, Wagner J, Popper H, Lvovsky E, Wong DC, Levy HB (1976) Modification of chronic hepatitis-B virus infection in chimpanzees by administration of an interferon inducer. Lancet 2:757–761

Rhim JS, Heubner RJ (1971) Comparison of the antitumor effect of interferon and interferon inducers. Proc Soc Exp Biol Med 136:524–529

Rhim JS, Greenawalt C, Huebner RJ (1969) Synthetic double-stranded RNA: inhibitory effect on murine leukaemia and sarcoma viruses in cell cultures. Nature 222:1166–1168

Rice JM, Turner W, Chirigos MA, Rice NR (1970) Enhancement by poly·D-lysine of poly I: C-induced interferon production in mice. Appl Microbiol 19:867–869

Rice JM, Turner W, Chirigos MA, Spahn G (1971) Dose responsiveness and variation among inbred strains of mice in production of interferon after treatment with poly(I) -poly(C)[poly-D-lysine] complexes. Appl Microbiol 22:380–386

Richmond JY, Hamilton LD (1969) Foot-and-mouth disease virus inhibition induced in mice by synthetic double-stranded RNA. Proc Natl Acad Sci USA 64:81–87

Robinson RA, DeVita VT, Levy HB, Baron S, Hubbard SP, Levine AS (1976) A phase I–II trial of multiple dose polyriboinosinic-polyribocytidylic acid in patients with leukemia or solid tumors. J Natl Cancer Inst 57:599–602

Ruhl H, Vogt W, Bochert G, Schmidt S, Diamantstein T (1974) Stimulation of mouse lymphoid cells by polyanions in vitro. In: Lindahl-Kiessling K, Osoba D (eds) Lymphocyte recognition and effector substances. Academic, New York, pp 31–37

Salazar AM, Engel WK, Levy HB (1981) Poly ICLC in the treatment of postinfectious demyelinating encephalomyelitis. Arch Neurol 38:382–383

Schmidtke JR, Johnson AG (1971) Regulation of the immune system by synthetic polynucleotides: I. Characteristics of adjuvant action on antibody synthesis. J Immunol 106:1191–1200

Schultz RM, Papamatheakis JD, Stylos MA (1976) Augmentation of specific macrophage-mediated cytotoxicity: correlation with agents which enhance antitumor resistance. Cell Immunol 25:309–316

Schultz RM, Papamatheakis JD, Chirigos MS (1977a) Direct activation in vitro of mouse peritoneal macrophages by pyran copolymer (NSC 46015). Cell Immunol 29:403–409

Schultz RM, Papamatheakis JD, Chirigos MS (1977b) Interferon: an inducer of macrophage activation by polyanions. Science 197:674–676

Slamon DJ (1973) Protective effect of the double-stranded polyribonucleotide, polyinosinic-polycytidylic acid, against rat erythroblastosis induced by murine erythroblastosis virus. J Natl Cancer Inst 51:851–867

Slamon DJ (1975) Hemolytic anemia induced by murine, erythroblastosis virus-possible mechanisms of hemoylsis and effects of an interferon inducer. J Nat Cancer Inst 55:329–339

Steinberg AD, Baron S, Talal N (1969) The pathogenesis of autoimmunity in New Zealand mice. I. Induction of nucleic acid antibodies by polyinosinic·polycytidylic acid. Proc Natl Acad Sci USA 63:1102–1107

Stewart WE II (1979) The interferon system. Springer, Wien New York

Stewart WE II, DeClercq E (1974) Relationship of cytotoxicity and interferon inducing activity of polyriboinosinic-polyribocytidylic acid to the molecular weights of the homopolymers. J Gen Virol 23:83–89

Stewart WE II, DeClercq E, DeSomer P (1973) Specificity of interferon-induced enhancement of toxicity for double-stranded ribonucleic acids. J Gen Virol 18:237–246

Strayer DR, Carter WA, Brodsky I, Gillespie DH, Greene JJ, Ts'o POP (1981) Clinical studies with mismatched double-stranded RNA. Tex Rep Biol Med 42:663–671

Stringfellow DA (1973) Prostaglandin restoration of the interferon response of hyporeactive animals. Science 201:376–378

Stringfellow DA (1980) Interferon inducers: Theory and experimental application. In: Stringfellow DA (ed) Interferon and interferon inducers: clinical applications. Dekker, New York

Stringfellow DA, Weed SD (1980) Interferon induction by and toxicity of polyriboinosinic acid [Poly(rI)]·polyribocytidylic acid [Poly(rC)], mismatched analog Poly(rI)·Poly[r(C_{12} Uracil)$_n$], and Poly(rI)·Poly(rC)L-lysine complexed with carboxymethyl cellulose. Antimicrob Agents Chemother 17:988–992

Tomida M, Yamamoto Y, Hozumi M (1980) Inhibition of the leukemogenicity of myeloid leukemia cells in mice and in vivo induction of normal differentiation of the cells by poly(I)·poly(C). Gan 71:456–463

Ts'o POP, Alderfer JL, Levy J, Marshall LW, O'Malley JA, Horoszewicz JS, Carter WA (1976) An integrated and comparative study of the antiviral effects and other biological properties of the polyinosinic acid-polycytidylic acid and its mismatched analogues. Mol Pharmacol 12:299–312

Turner W, Chan SP, Chirigos MA (1970) Stimulation of humoral and cellular antibody formation in mice by poly Ir:Cr. Proc Soc Exp Biol Med 133:334–338

Vandeputte M, Datta SK, Billiau A, Desomer P (1970) Inhibition of polyoma-viurus oncogenesis in rats by polyriboinosinic-ribocytidylic acid. Eur J Cancer 6:323–327

Weinstein AJ, Gazdar AF, Sims HL, Levy HB (1971) Lack of correlation between interferon induction and antitumor effect of poly I·poly C. Nature 231:53–55

Worthington M, Baron S (1971) Late therapy with an interferon stimulator in an arbovirus encephalitis in mice. Proc Soc Exp Biol Med 136:323–327

Yaron M, Yaron I, Sinetana O, Eylan Herzberg M (1976) Hyaluronic acid produced by human synovial fibroblasts. Arthritis Rheum 19:1315–1320

Yaron M, Yaron I, Gurari-Rotman D (1977) Stimulation of prostaglandin E production in cultured human fibroblasts by poly(I)·poly(C) and human interferon. Nature 267:457–459

Yaron M, Yaron I, Wiletzki C, Zor U (1978) Interrelationship between stimulation of prostaglandin E and hyaluronate production by poly(I)·poly(C) and interferon in synovial fibroblast culture. Arthritis Rheum 21:694–698

Yaron M, Baratz M, Yaron I, Zor U (1979) Acute induction of joint inflammation in the rat by poly I·poly C. Inflammation 3:243–251

Young CW (1971) Interferon induction in cancer with some observations on the clinical effects of poly IC. Med Clin N Am 55:721–728

Zarling JM, Schlais J, Eskra L, Greene JJ, Ts'o POP, Carter WA (1980) Augmentation of human natural killer cell activity by polyinosinic acid-polycytidylic acid and its nontoxic mismatched analogues. J Immunol 124:1852–1857

CHAPTER 27

Monoclonal Antibodies to Interferons

D.C. BURKE and D.S. SECHER

A. Introduction: The Preparation and Use of Monoclonal Antibodies

I. Comparison of Monoclonal and Conventional Antibodies

The introduction of a technique for the production of monoclonal antibodies by hybrid myelomas (hybridomas) (KOHLER and MILSTEIN 1975) is leading to the widespread replacement of conventional antisera by monoclonal antibodies in many areas where antibodies are used. Conventional antisera generally contain a heterogeneous population of antibodies of different affinities and recognizing a variety of different antigenic determinants. The mixture of antibodies can vary not only from animal to animal, but even in successive bleeds from a single animal and this has led to difficulties in the standardization of antisera and of substances measured by antibodies. Monoclonal antibodies are chemically pure, recognize a single determinant with a unique affinity, and can be produced over a long period of time without any change of properties.

The possibility of producing large amounts of pure monoclonal antibodies allows the general use of antibodies as tools in purification. Antibodies from conventional antisera have had rather limited use in purification because the antisera are usually only available in very limited amounts and may contain antibodies of high affinity that bind the antigen so strongly that it can only be released from the antibody by conditions that destroy the antigen and/or the antibody. Finally the specificity of a conventional antiserum is dependent on the purity of the antigen used to immunize the animal and so it is difficult to obtain good antisera to antigens for which alternative methods of purification have not yet been developed. Highly specific monoclonal antibodies to minor components of a crude antigenic preparation can be isolated and, after coupling to a solid such as Sepharose, can be used as an affinity column to purify the corresponding antigen.

II. Production of Monoclonal Antibodies

The technique for the production of monoclonal antibodies has changed little since its introduction in 1975. A mouse or rat is immunized with a preparation containing the antigen to which antibodies are wanted. Usually test bleeds are taken and the level of serum antibodies determined as a measure of the progress of the immunization, but this may not always be necessary or even appropriate. Some 4 days before the fusion a solution of antigen is injected into the tail vein. The timing of this injection is quite critical; injection less than 3 or more than 5 days before the fusion results in a much lower yield of positive hybrids. Multiple injections between 3 and 5 days have also been advocated (STÄHLI et al. 1980) but a single injection is more common. For the fusion the spleen is removed asceptically from the immunized animal and a single-cell suspension prepared. The spleen cells (10^8) are mixed with $1–6 \times 10^7$ myeloma cells, pelleted by centrifugation and the cells fused by resuspending the pellet in the presence of polyethylene glycol (PEG). After fusion the cells are washed to remove the PEG and distributed into small culture wells (usually 50–200). These cultures are fed with a medium containing hypoxanthine, aminopterin and thymidine (HAT medium) that allows hybrid cells to grow, but not the unfused myeloma cells. About 2 weeks after the fusion, clones of hybrids should be visible in most if not all of the wells. The culture supernatants (spent medium) are tested for the presence of the desired antibody activity. Negative cultures are discarded and positive cultures purified by repeated cloning steps (either in soft agar or by dilution cloning). After the isolation of a pure clone of cells producing a single antibody, large amounts of the antibody can be produced either from spent culture medium or by injecting hybrid cells into mice (or rats if appropriate) where the cells may grow as subcutaneous or ascitic tumours producing much higher concentrations of antibody (2–20 mg/ml) in the serum or ascites fluid of the animal. Further details of the cell fusion protocol as used in the derivation of the NK 2 antibody described in Sect. C are given by SECHER and BURKE (1980) and MORSER et al. (1981).

B. Conventional Antibodies to Interferon

Early attempts to produce antibodies to interferons were unsuccessful (BURKE and ISAACS 1960; LINDENMANN 1960). In retrospect, as STEWART (1979) has pointed out, this was because of the extremely low antigenic mass being inoculated (no more than a few nanogram interferon) rather than because interferon was weakly or nonantigenic. However when sufficient interferon, with adjuvant, was used, then neutralizing antibody to mouse interferon was obtained (PAUCKER and CANTELL 1962), and the same group also showed that mouse, human and chick interferons were immunologically distinct from each other (PAUCKER 1965). When sufficient rabbit interferon (about 10^4 U/week for several months) was injected subcutaneously into guinea-pigs and rabbits, then guinea-pigs produced high titre neutralizing antibody to rabbit interferon, while rabbits developed no such antibody (LEVY-KOENIG et al. 1970a, b). Interferon was clearly antigenic, but not in the homologous species. It is interesting that rabbit cells in vitro and rabbits in vivo are sensitive to human interferon, yet human interferons are antigenic in rabbits (LEVY-KOENIG et al. 1970a; DUC-GOIRAN et al. 1971; MOGENSEN et al. 1975; BERG et al. 1975; HAVELL et al. 1975). The antigenic site (or sites) must thus be distinct from the site involved in cell recognition. Indeed PAUCKER et al. (1975) have reported that certain rabbit antisera to human interferon-α (leukocyte) were able to neutralize its activity for human cells, but not for rabbit cells.

Antibodies to human interferons have been prepared in rabbits, sheep and calves. For example, MOGENSEN et al. (1975) reported that by injecting a sheep with a total of about 3×10^8 U human leukocyte interferon, a neutralizing titre of about 10^6 was obtained. Despite the large amounts of human interferon that have been injected into human patients, there has been only one report of the production of antibodies to such interferon, in this case to interferon-β (fibroblast) (VALLBRACHT et al. 1981). Antisera to human interferon preparations have been used to distinguish the different types of interferon produced by a single cell type. It was found that antisera prepared against human leukocyte interferon were less effective against human fibroblast interferon, while antisera to human fibroblast interferon had no activity against human leukocyte interferon (BERG et al. 1975; HAVELL et al. 1975). When anti-human fibroblast interferon globulin was immobilized on a Sepharose column and human leukocyte interferon was passed through it, a small amount (about 1%) of the interferon was retained. This was neutralized by antibody to human fibroblast interferon, thus showing the presence of two antigenic species of human interferon – leukocyte (-α) and fibroblast (-β) – in the crude preparation. Different cells produce different relative amounts of these two when treated with viruses or double-stranded RNA, and some human cells produce a third antigenic type (-γ) when treated with mitogens or the appropriate antigen. Mouse cells also produce three species of interferon, mouse interferon-α showing some antigenic similarity to human interferon-α, while mouse and human interferon-β are antigenically distinct (KAWADE et al. 1980; STEWART and HAVELL 1980).

Since these antisera also precipitate the products obtained when mRNA preparations from interferon-producing mouse or human cells are incubated with a cell-free protein synthesis system (for a review see STEWART 1979), and since both mouse and human interferon-β are glycosylated, it is likely that the antigenic sites recognized by the antibodies do not involve the carbohydrate residues. Antisera, coupled to Sepharose, have also been used to purify both mouse and human interferons (see STEWART 1979). However the antibodies are polyclonal, and recognize a number of different antigenic sites, and since the antisera contain antibodies to the impurities present in the antigen, the product obtained by immunoprecipitation or immunochromatography will never be pure interferon, even though the antisera have been adsorbed with cell extracts, virus proteins and egg proteins (which contaminate the virus preparations) to make them more specific. The need for monoclonal antibodies was obvious.

C. NK2: A Monoclonal Antibody to Human Interferon-α

I. Isolation

When we first started the search for such an antibody in Spring 1977, highly purified human interferon was not available either for use as an antigen or for screening for the production of a monoclonal antibody. In the first screen (May–December 1977) mice were injected with relatively crude human interferon made by treatment of lymphoblastoid cells with Sendai virus, and screening was done by searching for neutralization of a small dose of interferon. This screen failed to produce a monoclonal antibody but identified a number of problems inherent in the screening procedure. This had to detect low antibody titres since it was known that cell culture supernatants typically had an antibody titre of about 0.1% of that in the mice used for fusion, in this case about 10^3. It was therefore necessary to be able to detect about 1 neutralizing unit and the screen was designed to be as sensitive as possible – using a small amount of interferon in a sensitive assay which gave a reproducible dose – response curve. The interferon dose was chosen so as to produce about 40% neutralization of the virus challenge and any partial neutralization was detected by movement up the dose–response curve. Such a sensitive assay produced a number of false positives and careful controls had to be used. In the event, the monoclonal antibody (NK2) that was isolated, altered virus growth in early screening by only about 3%, and if a less sensitive test had been used (e.g. the capacity to neutralize 10 U interferon), then NK2 would have been undetectable. The first screen was abandoned because of another artifact however; the isolation of clones that produced a substance that neutralized interferon, but did not release an immunoglobulin. The second, successful screen therefore incorporated a test to detect such secretion.

In this second screen (August 1978–January 1980, SECHER and BURKE 1980; MORSER et al. 1981) mice and rats were immunized with more highly purified interferon (specific activity between 0.72 and 2.4×10^7 U per milligram protein), a generous gift from Drs. K. FANTES and M. JOHNSTON, Wellcome Laboratories, Beckenham, Kent. The fusion was carried out with a mouse whose serum had a neutralizing titre of $10^{3.5}$, and the fused cells were plated out into 48 wells. Assay of the supernatant culture fluids showed that only one well (number 13) produced a slight, but reproducible neutralization of interferon (MORSER et al. 1981). When the cells from this well were cloned and the supernatant fluids tested for anti-interferon activity, a number of clones were positive but only one (clone 35) was active and also secreted immunoglobulin (SECHER and BURKE 1980). Recloning gave a series of subclones all of which produced immunoglobulin but whose anti-interferon activity appeared to vary considerably. The subclone (subclone 6) producing the most activity was designated NK2, grown in mice and the ascites fluid or the IgG fraction from the ascites fluid used for the subsequent experiments.

II. Properties

1. Characterization

The NK2 antibody was shown to be an IgG by growing NK2 cells in medium containing lysine ^{14}C for 24 h and analysing the culture supernatants by sodium dodecylsulphate polyacrylamide gel electrophoresis (SDS PAGE) (MORSER et al. 1981). Autoradiography of the dried polyacrylamide gel revealed a single chain (H) with the mobility of a γ-chain and a single light chain (L) with a mobility slightly greater than that of the light chain (K) of NSI, the myeloma line used for the fusion. SDS PAGE analysis of ^{125}I-labelled or unlabelled purified NK2 antibody confirmed that NK2 is an IgG. Ouchterlony analysis using commercial antisera suggested that the IgG belongs to the IgG1 subclass (J.M. JARVIS 1981, personal communication). In general, hybrids formed with NSI secrete two light chains: the specific antibody light chain and the NSI light chain. In this case the NSI light chain was presumably lost during the culturing and cloning of NK2. It may be that IgG molecules containing the NSI light chain H_2LK or H_2K_2) have a lower neutralization activity than those which have lost the NSI light chain and produce only H_2L_2

molecules, but since the (presumed) original HLK clone was not isolated it was not possible to derive HK clones to test this hypothesis.

2. Specificity

The antibody neutralized the antiviral effect of interferon because of the way in which it was selected. This was true whether a direct assay, as used in the initial screening, or an indirect assay, in which interferon was incubated with antibody followed by addition of normal mouse serum and sheep anti-mouse immunoglobulin, was used. However there was little neutralization of human interferon-β, even when using 500 µg/ml of immunoglobulin, nor any binding to interferon-β since passage of a partially purified preparation of interferon-β down a column of NK2 IgG bound to Sepharose led to negligible (0.6%) retention of interferon (MORSER et al. 1981). Thus although human interferons-α and -β show substantial homology (TANIGUCHI et al. 1980), the antigenic site recognized by NK2 is not present in interferon-β. The antibody also has no effect upon the activity of human interferon-γ (D.S. SECHER and K. CANTELL 1981, unpublished work). In view of these results, it was not surprising that the antibody did not bind a preparation of mouse interferon, which was a mixture of interferon-α and -β. It would be interesting to determine its effect on pure mouse interferon-α.

The antibody bound human interferon-α_2 synthesized in *Escherichia coli* (C. WEISSMANN and D.S. SECHER 1981, unpublished work). This is not surprising since interferon-α_2 is one of the main components of the lymphoblastoid interferon used as an antigen (ALLEN and FANTES 1980). It will be interesting to determine whether NK2 binds all the members of the human interferon-α family equally well.

III. Uses

1. Purification of Interferon

We have used NK2 to purify crude interferon prepared from leukocytes, from lymphoblastoid cells, or extracted from *E. coli* containing the gene coding for human interferon-α_2. For all these studies NK2 was grown in BALB/c × C3H mice as an ascitic tumour and the ascites fluid removed, depleted of cells and the IgG purified by ammonium sulphate precipitation and DEAE ion exchange chromatography. The purified IgG (2 mg per millilitre ascites fluid) was coupled to CNBr-activated Sepharose 4B and packed into a column for use as an immunoadsorbent. Crude interferon was passed through the column at neutral pH (6–8) and at a flow rate not exceeding 200 ml cm^{-2} h^{-1}. The column was then washed with phosphate-buffered saline containing ethylene glycol (to remove weakly attached proteins) until no more protein was eluted and then the interferon was eluted with 0.1 *M* citric acid. Columns of 0.5–50 ml NK2 Sepharose have been used to purify volumes of interferon up to 9.7 l (containing about 5×10^8 U) in a single passage through the column. Radiolabelled interferon has also been purified in this way (SECHER and BURKE 1980). The specific activity of interferon purified by NK2 Sepharose is around $0.5–2 \times 10^8$ U per milligram protein and yields ranging from 30% to well over 100% have been measured using biological (antiviral) assays. This variation is no doubt, partly a result of variability in the assay, but may also be due to the presence in different interferon preparations of variable amounts of interferons that do not bind or bind only weakly to the NK2 antibody. Using the immunoradiometric assay (IRMA – see Sect. C.III.2), consistantly high yields (80%–100%) were measured, but the assay only detects interferons that possess the NK2 antigenic site and any interferons that pass through the column because they lack the NK2 antigenic site would probably also be undetected in the assay. Purification factors of more than 5,000-fold have been measured in a single step starting from crude lymphoblastoid interferon (72,000 U/ml).

Interferon is ideally suited for purification by immunoadsorption chromatography since it is very stable at the low pH required for the dissociation of the interferon–antibody complex that forms on the column. The NK2 antibody also survives the acid wash and the columns may be used several times.

2. Immunoradiometric Assay

Radiolabelled interferon purified by monoclonal antibody immunoadsorption chromatography may be used in a classical radioimmunoassay (RIA) where an unknown concentration of interferon is measured by its ability to compete with the binding of radiolabelled interferon to an anti-interferon antibody. Where monoclonal antibodies are available the theoretical advantages of immunoradiometric assays (IRMA) can be realized. In these assays the antibody (and not the antigen) is radiolabelled and because the antibody may be added in excess the theoretical sensitivity is higher. In the past this advantage has not often been realized because of the difficulties in purifying a specific antibody from a conventional antisera but the ease of monoclonal antibodies is likely to lead to the widespread replacement of RIA by IRMA.

An IRMA for human leukocyte interferon using ^{125}I-labelled NK2 IgG has been described (SECHER 1981). In this assay a conventional sheep anti-interferon antibody is attached to the surface of a plastic bead (one 6.4 mm bead per assay) and incubated in the presence of interferon. The interferon binds to the antibody-coated bead and is detected after washing of the bead by the addition of ^{125}I-radiolabelled NK2. The radioactivity bound to the bead is measured and the interferon concentration in the sample deduced by reference to a standard curve. Interferon concentrations in the range 50–10,000 U/ml may be read directly from the standard curve. More concentrated samples are diluted by serial dilution and then assayed. Comparison of the titration curve with the standard curve allows calculation of the unknown concentration. Where the sensitivity limit is important (e.g. in serum interferon determination) the conditions of assay may be modified to increase sensitivity (WALKER et al. 1982). The IRMA offers several advantages over conventional (biological) assays for interferon. The antibody-coated beads and the radiolabelled antibody can both be stored for at least 1–2 months at 4 °C so assays may be carried out at short notice and completed within 24 h of beginning the assay. (Shorter incubation times or the simultaneous addition of interferon-containing sample and the labelled antibody may be used to reduce the assay time further if sensitivity of the assay is not critical.) The reproducibility of the assay is much better than with biological assays. Coefficients of variation below 10% have been measured for inter- and intra-assay variation. Serum samples may be assayed directly in the IRMA whereas for antiviral assays serum must be diluted at least 10 or 20 times because of the effect of substances other than interferon in serum that interfere with the assay. However biological assays will still be necessary to measure any interferons that do not possess the NK2 antigenic determinant and to confirm the biological activity of antigenically positive molecules.

3. Immunofluorescent Studies

Monoclonal antibodies are ideally suited to immunofluorescent studies and immunochemistry because of their high specificity and purity, which generally lead to a much lower background of nonspecific labelling. NK2 has been used in indirect immunofluorescence studies to confirm the observations obtained with a less pure sheep anti-interferon-α, that human natural killer cells synthesize interferon-α in response to contact with K 562 (erythroleukaemia) cells (E. SAKSELA 1981, personal communication). The same group has also shown that when human leukocytes are infected with Sendai virus in vitro it is only the monocytes and not, as previously reported, the B-lymphocytes that are labelled with NK2 IgG, suggesting that monocytes produce interferon-α in response to Sendai virus infection and B-lymphocytes do not produce any interferon-α (unless they produce one or more species lacking the NK2 antigenic site) (E. SAKSELA et al. 1983).

Indirect immunofluorescence with NK2 IgG has also been used to look for the binding of interferon-α to GM-258 fibroblasts (B. TYCKO and J. VILCEK 1981, personal communication). Even with a silicon video intensification camera, no binding of interferon could be seen after incubation of the cells with interferon at 5,000 U/ml for 1 h. Nonspecific labelling of the cells was not a problem even with NK2 IgG at 100 μg/ml. It seems that the number of molecules of interferon bound to the cells was below the detection limit of the assay system.

4. Applications of NK2-Purified Interferon

Leukocyte interferon purified by NK2 Sepharose affinity chromatography (NK2-IFN) has been used to investigate some aspects of the pharmacokinetics of interferon. SCOTT et al. (1981) have recently compared the reactions observed in volunteers injected with NK2-IFN or with partially purified IFN preparations of lower purity (PIF). Both preparations gave rise to similar changes in pulse, temperature, white blood cell counts and several subjective symptoms following intramuscular injection and in skin reactions following intradermal injection, suggesting that all these effects are consequence of the interferon-α types present in the NK2-IF and can no longer be ascribed to the presence of impurities in interferon preparations. It was also noted that indomethacin, a prostaglandin antagonist, eliminated the changes in pulse and body temperature, suggesting that these symptoms are mediated by prostaglandins. Whether these drugs also abolish any antiviral or antitumour properties of interferons remains to be determined.

Interferon purified by NK2 Sepharose has also been shown to induce changes in expression of the major human histocompatibility antigens (HL-A) on cells grown in vitro (BURRONE and MILSTEIN 1982) and to inhibit the growth of the lymphoblastoid Daudi cell line. Thus, a wide range of properties of interferon-α that have been tested have been found to be present in the NK2-positive population of molecules.

5. Use of NK2 as a Research Reagent

Monoclonal antibodies provide an ideal tool for distinguishing different antigens and different antigenic sites in a single molecule. They thus provide a way of specifically distinguishing one type of interferon from another, and since cells of the immune system often provide a mixture of interferons-α, -β, and -γ, NK2 provides a method of determining whether an interferon preparation contains interferon-α or not. This method has been used to show that the serum of patients suffering from systemic lupus erythematosus contains interferon-α (PREBLE et al. 1982), and that natural killer cells can produce interferon-α (see Sect. C.III.3).

D. Other Monoclonal Antibodies to Human Interferon-α

There have been two other reports of mouse monoclonal antibodies to human interferon-α. MONTAGNIER et al. (1980) immunized mice five times over 2.5 months with a total per mouse of 4×10^6 U interferon prepared from leukocytes (3×10^6 U/mg) and incorporated into liposomes. From 23 fusions a single hybridoma was selected for its ability to neutralize the effect of interferon in a cytopathic assay using vesicular stomatis virus. This hybridoma produced an IgG that neutralized leukocyte interferon, Namalwa interferon (partially) and interferon α_1-produced in *E. coli*, but, like NK2, not interferon-β.

STAEHELIN et al. (1981) used a different approach to the immunization of mice. They injected interferon preparations of much higher purity (10%–15%) and boosted with interferon further purified by SDS PAGE. The cultures produced in a single fusion were screened by a solid-phase binding assay in which interferon was attached to the plastic and the binding of antibodies from culture supernatants detected by the subsequent addition of ^{125}I-labelled anti-mouse immunoglobulin. A total of 13 specific hybridomas were isolated derived from at least 7 different B-cell clones. None of the hybrids nor even the serum of the immunized mouse neutralized crude leukocyte interferon although several of the monoclonals neutralized interferon fractions purified by high pressure liquid chromatography.

E. Monoclonal Antibodies to Human Interferon-β and -γ

HOCHKEPPEL et al. (1981) have recently reported the isolation of two stable hybrid cell lines that release antibody to human interferon-β. The mice were injected with purified interferon-β, followed by a final booster injection of interferon-β with the sugar moiety removed by enzyme degradation, 4 days before fusion. The hybrid cells were screened by using purified interferon-β in a binding assay to obtain a cell hybrid that secreted an antibody that neutralized interferon-β, but not interferon-α. The antibodies seemed to be directed against the protein part of interferon-β since removal of the sugar residues had no effect on the neutralizing titre. Use of antibody bound to a Sepharose column yielded purified interferon-β. Isolation of a hybrid cell secreting an antibody against interferon-β has also been reported by Y.H. TAN (1981, personal communication), which has been used to develop a radioimmunoassay. HOCHKEPPEL and DE LEY (1982) have also reported the isolation of a monoclonal antibody to human interferon-γ.

F. Monoclonal Antibodies to Mouse Interferon

The isolation of a hybrid cell producing a monoclonal antibody to mouse interferon-β has recently been reported (TRAPMAN et al. 1981) and, in addition, a rat cell producing a monoclonal antibody to both mouse interferon-α and -β (MANNELL et al. 1982).

References

Allen G, Fantes KH (1980) A family of structural genes for human lymphoblastoid (leukocyte-type) interferon. Nature 287:408–411

Berg K, Ogburn CA, Paucker K, Mogenson KE, Cantell K (1975) Affinity chromatography of human leukocyte and diploid cell interferons on sepharose-bound antibodies. J Immunol 114:640–644

Burke DC, Isaacs A (1960) Interferon: relation to heterologous interference and lack of antigenicity. Acta Virol 4:215–219

Burrone O, Milstein C (1982) The effect of interferon on the expression of human cell-surface antigens. Proc R Soc Lond [Biol] 299:133–135

Duc-Goiran P, Galliot B, Chany C (1971) Studies on virus-induced interferons produced by the human amniotic membrane and white blood cells. Arch Virol 34:232–243

Havell EA, Berman B, Ogburn CA, Berg K, Paucker K, Vilcek J (1975) Two antigenically distinct species of human interferon. Proc Nat Acad Sci USA 72:2185–2190

Hochkeppel HK, De Ley M (1982) Monoclonal antibody against human IFN-γ. Nature 296:258–259

Hochkeppel HK, Menge U, Collins J (1981) Monoclonal antibodies against human fibroblast interferon. Nature 291:500–501

Kawade Y, Yamamoto Y, Fujisawa J, Wanatabe Y (1980) Antigenic relationship between various interferon species. Ann N.Y. Acad Sci 350:422–427

Kohler G, Milstein C (1975) Continuous cultures of fused cells secreting antibody of predefined specificity. Nature 256:495–497

Levy-Koenig RE, Golgher RR, Paucker K (1970 a) Immunology of interferons. II. Heterospecific activities of human interferon and their neutralization by antibody. J Immunol 104:791–797

Levy-Koenig RE, Mundy MJ, Paucker K (1970 b) Immunology of interferons. I. Immune response to protective and nonprotective interferons. J Immunol 104:785–790

Lindenmann J (1960) Neuere Aspekte der Virus-Interferenz. Ergeb Microbiol Immunitaetsforsch 33:369–373

Mannell D, De Maeyer E, Kemeer R, Cacherd A, De Maeyer-Guignard J (1982) A rat monoclonal antibody against mouse α and β interferon of all molecular species. Nature 296:664–665

Montagnier L, Laurent AG, Gruest J (1980) Isolement d'un hybride cellulaire produisant un anticorps specifique de l'interferon leucocytaire humain. CR Acad Sci Paris 291:893–896

Mogensen KE, Pyhala L, Cantell K (1975) Raising antibodies to human leukocyte interferon. Acta Pathol Microbiol Scand 83:443–458

Morser J, Meager A, Burke DC, Secher DS (1981) Production and screening of cell hybrids producing a monoclonal antibody to human interferon-α. J Gen Virol 53:257–265

Paucker K (1965) The serological specificity of interferon. J Immunol 94:371–378

Paucker K, Cantell K (1962) Neutralization of interferon by specific antibody. Virology 18:145–147

Paucker K, Dalton BJ, Ogburn CA, Torma E (1975) Multiple active sites on human interferons. Proc Nat Acad Sci USA 72:4587–4591

Preble OT, Black RJ, Friedman RM, Klippel JH, Vilcek J (1982) Systemic lupus erthyematosus: presence in human serum of an unusual acid-labile leukocyte interferon. Science 216:429–431

Saksela E, Virtanen I, Hovi T, Secher DS, Kantell K (in press) Monocyte is the main producer of human leukocyte alpha interferons following Sendai Virus Induction. Progr Med Virol 30
Secher DS (1981) Immunoradiometric assay of human leukocyte interferon using monoclonal antibody. Nature 290:501–503
Secher DS, Burke DC (1980) A monoclonal antibody for largescale purification of human leukocyte interferon. Nature 285:446–450
Scott GM, Secher DS, Flowers D, Bate J, Cantell K, Tyrrell DAJ (1981) Toxicity of interferon. Br Med J 282:1345–1348
Staehelin T, Durrer B, Schmidt J, Takacs B, Stocker J, Miggiano V, Stahli C, Rubinstein M, Levy WP, Hershberg R, Pestka S (1981) Production of hybridomas secreting monoclonal antibodies to the human leukocyte interferons. Proc Nat Acad Sci USA 78:1848–1852
Stähli C, Staehelin T, Miggiano V, Schmidt J, Häring P (1980) High frequencies of antigen-specific hybridomas: dependence on immunisation parameters and prediction by spleen cell analysis. J Immunol Methods 32:297–304
Stewart WE II (1979) The interferon system. Springer, Wien, New York
Stewart WE II, Havell EA (1980) Characterization of a subspecies of mouse interferon cross-reactive on human cells and antigenically related to human leukocyte interferon. Virology 101:315–318
Taniguchi T, Mantei N, Schwarzstein M, Nagata S, Maramatsu M, Weissman C (1980) Human leukocyte and fibroblast interferon are structurally related. Nature 285:547–549
Trapman J, Bosveld IJ, Vonk WP, Heckman RCAP, De Jonge P, Van Vliet PW, Van Ewijk W (1981) A monoclonal antibody to murine interferon-β. In: De Maeyer E, Galasoo G, Schellekens HJ (eds) The biology of the interferon system. Elsevier, Amsterdam, pp 77–79
Vallbracht A, Treuner J, Flehmig B, Joester KE, Niethammer D (1981) Interferon-neutralizing antibodies in a patient treated with human fibroblast interferon. Nature 289:496–497
Walker JR, Nagington J, Scott GM, Secher DS (1982) An immunoradiometric assay of serum interferon using a monoclonal antibody. J Gen Virol 62:181–185

Subject Index

Handbook of Experimental Pharmacology

Continuation of "Handbuch der experimentellen Pharmakologie"

Editorial Board
G. V. R. Born, A. Farah,
H. Herken, A. D. Welch

Springer-Verlag
Berlin
Heidelberg
New York
Tokyo

Handbook of Experimental Pharmacology

Continuation of "Handbuch der experimentellen Pharmakologie"

Editorial Board
G.V.R. Born, A. Farah,
H. Herken, A.D. Welch

Springer-Verlag
Berlin
Heidelberg
New York
Tokyo

Volume 49
Ergot Alkaloids and Related Compounds

Volume 50: Part 1
Inflammation

Part 2
Anti-Inflammatory Drugs

Volume 51
Uric Acid

Volume 52
Snake Venoms

Volume 53
Pharmacology of Ganglionic Transmission

Volume 54: Part 1
Adrenergic Activators and Inhibitors I

Part 2
Adrenergic Activators and Inhibitors II

Volume 55
Psychotropic Agents

Part 1
Antipsychotics and Antidepressants I

Part 2
Anxiolytis, Gerontopsychopharmacological Agents and Psychomotor Stimulants

Part 3
Alcohol and Psychotomimetics, Psychotropic Effects of Central Acting Drugs

Volume 56, Part 1 + 2
Cardiac Glycosides

Volume 57
Tissue Growth Factors

Volume 58
Cyclic Nucleotides
Part 1: **Biochemistry**
Part 2: **Physiology and Pharmacology**

Volume 59
Mediators and Drugs in Gastrointestinal Motility
Part 1: **Morphological Basis and Neurophysiological Control**
Part 2: **Endogenis and Exogenous Agents**

Volume 60
Pyretics and Antipyretics

Volume 61
Chemotherapy of Viral Infections

Volume 62
Aminoglycosides

Volume 63
Allergic Reactions to Drugs

Volume 64
Inhibition of Folate Metabolism in Chemotherapy

Volume 65
Teratogenesis and Reproductive Toxicology

Volume 66
Part 1: **Glucagon I**
Part 2: **Glucagon II**

Volume 67
Part 1
Antibiotics Containing the Beta-Lactam Structure I

Part 2
Antibiotics Containing the Beta-Lactam Structure II